Overcoming Breast Cancer Therapy Resistance

Zodwa Dlamini
Editor

Overcoming Breast Cancer Therapy Resistance

From Mechanisms to Precision and AI-Powered Approaches

Springer

Editor
Zodwa Dlamini
SAMRC Precision Oncology Research Unit (PORU),
DSI/NRF SARChI Chair in Precision Oncology
and Cancer Prevention (POCP)
Pan African Cancer Research Institute (PACRI),
University of Pretoria
Pretoria, South Africa

ISBN 978-3-031-52859-0 ISBN 978-3-031-52860-6 (eBook)
https://doi.org/10.1007/978-3-031-52860-6

This Springer imprint is published by the registered company Springer Nature Switzerland AG
The registered company address is: Gewerbestrasse 11, 6330 Cham, Switzerland

Preface

Breast cancer is a pervasive and complex disease that affects millions of individuals worldwide. While significant progress has been made in the field of breast cancer treatment, one formidable challenge remains—drug resistance. The ability of breast cancer cells to develop resistance to therapies poses a significant hurdle in the quest for effective treatments. This book is dedicated to addressing this critical issue and delves into the multifaceted aspects of breast cancer drug resistance, shedding light on the mechanisms behind it and the innovative strategies being developed to overcome it.

The book is organized into four distinct parts, each contributing to a comprehensive understanding of the problem and potential solutions. The arrangement follows a logical flow, starting with an introduction to breast cancer and drug resistance, then delving into various types of drug resistance in breast cancer treatment, and finally exploring innovative strategies and future directions in overcoming drug resistance. Part I provides a foundational understanding of breast cancer and drug resistance. It explores the intricate molecular mechanisms that underlie drug resistance in breast cancer, setting the stage for the subsequent discussions. Part II takes a closer look at various types of drug resistance in breast cancer treatment. It examines the potential of targeted therapies, immunotherapy, endocrine therapy, and the challenges posed by chemoresistance. These chapters offer insights into both the promising approaches and the hurdles that need to be overcome in the battle against drug resistance. Part III explores innovative strategies and future directions to combat drug resistance. It dives into the role of alternative mRNA splicing, the influence of viral infections, the potential of natural products, and the transformative power of artificial intelligence. These cutting-edge approaches hold promise in revolutionizing breast cancer treatment. The final part of the book (IV) discusses future directions and advanced treatments that promise to contribute to overcoming drug resistance. It explores the impact of the microbiome, molecular profiling, and personalized medicine. It also highlights promising new strategies, including immunotherapy, gene therapy, epigenetic modulation, nanotechnology-based drug delivery systems, and combination therapies. Furthermore, it addresses disparities in breast cancer research and treatment, emphasizing the need for inclusivity in addressing these challenges.

Throughout the book, experts from diverse fields share their insights, research findings, and innovative approaches to tackle drug resistance in breast cancer. From the potential of natural products to the transformative impact of artificial intelligence, from the microbiome's role in treatment to the promise of personalized medicine, this book brings together a wealth of knowledge and ideas. The fight against drug resistance in breast cancer is ongoing, and it demands a multidisciplinary approach that considers all available avenues. The chapters within this book provide a glimpse into the cutting-edge research, the challenges faced, and the potential breakthroughs that lie ahead. We hope that this collection of insights and discoveries will serve as a valuable resource for researchers, clinicians, and anyone with an interest in the battle against breast cancer drug resistance. As we embark on this journey together, we remain committed to the relentless pursuit of solutions. The path may be complex, but it is illuminated by the collective expertise and determination of those dedicated to overcoming drug resistance in breast cancer. Together, we can pave the way for a brighter future in the battle against breast cancer treatment resistance.

Pretoria, South Africa Zodwa Dlamini

Contents

About the Editor

Zodwa Dlamini is Professor of Molecular Oncology and known for her unwavering commitment to advancing precision oncology. At the core of her career is her pivotal role as the Founding Director of the Pan African Cancer Research Institute (PACRI). Additionally, as the Director of the SAMRC Precision Oncology Research Unit (PORU) and a DSI/NRF SARChI Chair in Precision Oncology and Cancer Prevention (POCP), she is fully committed to advancing precision medicine in the battle against cancer. Beyond her institutional leadership, Professor Dlamini also serves as a distinguished member of the American Association for Cancer Research (AACR) Regional Advisory Committee on Sub-Saharan Africa. She additionally guides the AACR Pathology Resources in Africa Advisory Group, actively identifying strategies to address gaps in cancer pathology services across the African continent. Professor Dlamini extends her contributions to the African Organisation for Research and Training in Cancer (AORTIC), where she actively influences the organization's strategic direction and mission as a member of the Research Committee Scientific Advisory Board. Her dedication to advancing cancer research in Africa was honored with a Special Award from the Council and Executive of the African Society of Morphology and was then admitted as an "Honorary Fellow" of the West African College of Morphologists. Moreover, she is an Overseas Fellow of the Royal Society of Medicine (London), Professional Member of the New York Academy of Sciences (USA), and a member of the Academy of Science of South Africa, highlighting her contributions to the field of science. Through her multifaceted efforts, Professor Zodwa Dlamini remains steadfast in her commitment to shaping the ever-evolving landscape of cancer research, and her journey is driven by an unshakable belief that cancer can be conquered, paving the way for a healthier and more equitable world.

Part I
Understanding Breast Cancer and Drug Resistance

Introduction to Breast Cancer and Drug Resistance

Rodney Hull, Zukile Mbita, and Zodwa Dlamini

Abstract Breast cancer is the most prevalent cancer in women, worldwide. Thus, it has attained the number one spot as the most diagnosed cancer in most regions across the world. It is also the cancer with the highest mortality rates for women, worldwide. The soaring incidence, mortality, and recurrence rates can be partly attributed to late diagnosis and resistance to the current treatment strategies. These treatment regimens include chemotherapy, targeted therapy, immunotherapy, endocrine therapy, radiotherapy, and surgery. However, common mechanisms have evolved in cancers to counteract these treatments, resulting in cancer drug resistance. Resistance to treatment results in higher recurrence rates and increased mortality. These mechanisms can be targeted to reverse this resistance. Moreover, multiple treatments can be employed in order to bypass resistance. In addition to this, biomarkers for the development of resistance can be employed to detect the development of resistance at the early stages, allowing for treatments to be altered or supplemented with other drugs or treatments. There are also revolutionary treatments being developed to counteract resistance. These include the use of natural products to target novel pathways in cancer and be used to supplement other treatments. Nanomedicine and nanoparticles have been developed to assist in drug delivery. The more refined and precise delivery of drugs offered by nanotechnology can ensure efficient drug uptake and minimize efflux. Lastly, the development of personalized medicine, which is made possible using artificial intelligence and machine learning to analyze large omics databases, means that more precise customized treatments can be applied specifically to suit a single patient which may lower the chance of the development or resistance. Personalized medicine will allow the

R. Hull (✉) · Z. Dlamini
SAMRC Precision Oncology Research Unit (PORU), DSI/NRF SARChI Chair in Precision Oncology and Cancer Prevention (POCP), Pan African Cancer Research Institute (PACRI), University of Pretoria, Pretoria, South Africa
e-mail: rodney.hull@up.ac.za; zodwa.dlamini@up.ac.za

Z. Mbita
Department of Biochemistry, Microbiology and Biotechnology, School of Molecular and Life Sciences, University of Limpopo, Polokwane, South Africa
e-mail: Zukile.Mbita@ul.ac.za

Z. Dlamini (ed.), *Overcoming Breast Cancer Therapy Resistance*,
https://doi.org/10.1007/978-3-031-52860-6_1

detection of gene expression or pathway changes that will increase the chance of resistance development, which would allow for more appropriate therapies to be selected.

Keywords Low-to-middle income countries · Breast cancer subtypes · Resistance mechanisms · Novel targeted therapies · Novel immunotherapy · Personalized medicine · Targeted therapy

Introduction

Medical historians have traced the first mention of breast cancer to ancient Egypt where cases were documented. These historical writings also show that misunderstandings and misconceptions were rife in breast cancer. There are many reasons for the development of new treatments to replace existing ones. These reasons include the side effects of current treatments (Akram et al., 2017) and the development of resistance (Cleator et al., 2007). Drug resistance in breast cancer is a leading cause of mortality, forcing changes in treatments to try and ensure a long-term cure. As resistance develops, patients and oncologists are forced to change therapeutic strategies, which in turn could also result in the development of further resistance. Drug resistance also leads to disease recurrence. More accurate and timely diagnosis has resulted in an increase in breast cancer incidence by 0.5%, annually in the last four decades. These advances are not only the result of early detection but better public awareness. At the same time, modern treatment strategies have resulted in a dramatic decline in mortality (Giaquinto et al., 2022). Despite these advances, the ability to predict outcomes remains inconsistent. This situation is particularly true in younger and socially disadvantaged women, which suggests that there may be other factors involved.

Epidemiology and Classification of Breast Cancer

Worldwide, breast cancer is the leading cause of cancer-related deaths among women. As such, breast cancer is a major source of global concern. This concern is increased as both the incidence and mortality rates of breast cancer are on the rise (Bray et al., 2018; World Health Organisation, 2023). The incidence rate of breast cancer makes it the leading cancer in women, regardless of age. The disease is, however, more prevalent in women of a more advanced age; thus, age should be viewed as a risk factor increasing the chance of developing breast cancer. According to the WHO fact sheet on breast cancer, there were 2,300,000 new cases of breast cancer recorded in 2020 with 685,000 deaths attributed to it. In the last 5 years, the

WHO reported that 7.8 million women had been diagnosed with breast cancer (World Health Organisation, 2023). The prevalence of breast cancer has increased to such an extent that it has surpassed lung cancer as the most prevalent cancer (Sung et al., 2021). Statistics from the International Association of Cancer Registries (IACR) show that the highest prevalence of breast cancer is found in those countries that have a high human development index (HDI) or those considered to be High Income Countries (HIC). Consequently, this means that these countries are located in North America, Europe, and Oceania (Australia and New Zealand), and these continents have the highest incidence rates of breast cancer. However, these same continents and high-income countries with high HDIs have a comparatively low mortality rates compared to their high incidence rates. This is in stark contrast to Africa, which has the highest mortality rate of any continent (Fig. 1). This can be best described using the ratio of mortality to incidence. For North America and Europe this ratio is 0.16 and 0.2, respectively. While the ratio for Africa is 0.47. This means that nearly half of all diagnosed cases in Africa result in fatality compared to only a fifth of cases in Europe. One of the factors contributing to this is the frequency of the different subtypes of breast cancer found in the populations in these countries, with the more lethal and difficult-to-treat breast cancer subtypes being found more frequently in African populations.

There are five molecular subtypes of breast cancer (Table 1). This molecular classification is largely dependent on the presence of hormone receptors and other proteins specific to each type. The most common subtype is named luminal A or HR+/HER2− (ER-positive/HER2-negative). This subtype is defined by the presence of estrogen and progesterone receptors, while being negative for HER2 and low

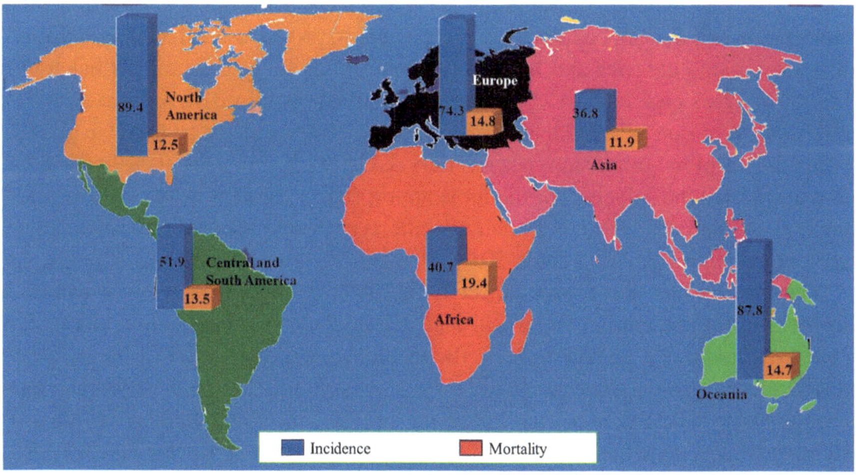

Fig. 1 Breast cancer incidence and mortality age-standardized rate by continent. North America and Oceania (Australia, New Zealand, Polynesia, and Micronesia) have the highest incidence rates. Asia and Africa have the lowest age-standardized rate (ASR) per 100,000 individuals. Despite this, Africa has higher mortality rates than North America, Oceania, and Europe. This implies that treatment outcomes in Africa are less favorable

Table 1 Breast cancer classification (Adapted from Eliyatkın et al. (2015))

Subtype	Estrogen receptor	HER2	Ki-67	Progesterone receptor	Growth	Prognosis
Luminal A	Positive	Negative	Low	Positive	Slow	Good
Luminal B	Positive	Negative	High or normal	Negative if KI-67 is normal	Fast	Worse
Luminal B like	Positive	Positive	Any level	Positive or negative	Fast	Worse
HER2 enriched	Negative	Positive	–	Negative	Faster	Bad but treatable
Triple-negative	Negative	Negative	–	Negative	Most aggressive	Worst

levels of proliferation promoting Ki-67 protein. These low levels of Ki-67 are one of the reasons for the luminal A cancers to progress slowly and have a better prognosis than most cancers. Luminal B breast cancers are also known as ER+/HER2+. These cancers are defined by the expression of the estrogen receptor but are HER2 negative. They can either express high levels of Ki-67 or lack the expression of progesterone receptors. Luminal B-like breast cancers are those that express both estrogen receptor and HER2 and both luminal B and luminal B-like are characterized by fast growth and have a worse prognosis than luminal A. The HER2-enriched breast cancer subtype expresses HER2 but niether the estrogen receptor nor the progesterone receptor. They grow faster than the previous three types and have a worse prognosis than the previous three types. However, this subtype is susceptible to treatment with therapies that target HER2. Finally, basal or triple-negative breast cancer (TNBC) does not express estrogen receptor, progesterone receptor, or HER2, It is the most aggressive and hardest to treat, and as such, generally, it has a poor prognosis. This type is more common in individuals with a BRCA1 mutation. It is also more common in individuals with African ancestry and can be found in younger women than in the other subtypes (Anders & Carey, 2009). This classification system allows for the selection of the most appropriate treatment as well as the development of therapies targeting each specific type based on the expression of the specific receptors (Sharma et al., 2010).

Despite the fact that breast cancer is the most commonly diagnosed cancer in women throughout the entire world and it is the second most common cause of cancer-related death among women, the incidence and death rates of breast cancer differ according to ethnicity. Studies on the variation between different ethnic groups show that the incidence rates for breast cancer are highest in those of European ancestry when it comes to HEER2+, in women of African ancestry with regard to TNBC and other breast cancer subtypes (Kong et al., 2020). The differences in the level of drug and xenobiotic metabolizing enzymes differ in different ethnicities, and this is only one of the factors that contribute to differences in drug resistance in different population groups. Other differences arise due to differences in socioeconomic status and lifestyle (Gerend & Pai, 2008; Harper et al., 2009; Echeverría et al., 2009).

Common Treatments and Resistance to these Therapies

Breast cancers are treated with a wide range of different therapeutic approaches (Table 2 and Fig. 2). These include surgery, chemotherapy, hormonal therapy, biological therapy, immunotherapy, and radiation therapy (Control et al., 2018). The choice of treatment depends on many factors. Some of these include the size and stage of cancer, the location of the tumor, histopathology, whether the tumor has already spread to the lymph nodes, the metastatic potential of the tumor, the age and health of the patient, the hormonal status of the patient and finally its molecular subtype (Cardoso et al., 2019). Endocrine therapy is used to treat breast cancers that express multiple hormone receptors on the surface of breast cancer cells, such as luminal A and B breast cancers. This is supplemented through the use of chemotherapy to supplement these treatments. HER 2-positive tumors (luminal B and HER2+) are most often treated with monoclonal antibodies (Tai et al., 2010; Harbeck et al., 2019; Waks & Winer, 2019). More recent treatment strategies that have been applied to breast cancer include immunotherapy, cyclin-dependent kinase inhibitors, tyrosine kinase inhibitors, microRNAs (miRNAs), use of repurposed drugs, nanomedicine, and electrochemotherapy (ECT).

It is estimated that the resistance of cancers to various drugs is responsible for up to 90% of cancer-related deaths (Łukasiewicz et al., 2021). Multidrug resistance (MDR) can reduce the effectiveness of chemotherapy which can lead to relapse or metastasis. Drug resistance can be classified as either innate or acquired resistance (Wang et al., 2019b). Intrinsic resistance that occurs before treatment, involving genetic mutations, pre-existing resistant sub-populations of cells, and increased activation of drug detoxifying enzyme pathways (Holohan et al., 2013). Acquired resistance, which results due to the exposure to the drug is the result of the activation of proto-oncogenes, altered epigenetic modifications, and mutations that lead to altered gene expression as well as changes in the tumor microenvironment (Holohan et al., 2013). Some of these resistance mechanisms include increased efflux of drugs, upregulated DNA repair, senescence escape, epigenetic modifications, tumor heterogeneity, TME, and epithelial-to-mesenchymal transition (EMT) (Holohan et al., 2013; Cosentino et al., 2021; He et al., 2021).

Cancers apart from TNBC can be targeted by targeting the hormone receptor, resulting in proliferation (Nilsson et al., 2001). For instance, activation of the estrogen receptor and the subsequent estrogen signaling pathway lead to the expression of genes such as *MYC* and *CCND1*, resulting in cell cycle progression (Prall et al., 1998) and increased growth factor, and transcription, leading to increased proliferation (Bocchinfuso & Korach, 1997). Endocrine therapies include selective ER modulators (SERMs), selective ER downregulators (SERDs), and aromatase inhibitors (AIs) (Aggelis & Johnston, 2019). These therapies are able to substantially reduce the recurrence rates of breast cancer as well as lowering the mortality rates (Lin & Winer, 2008). However, ER^+ metastatic breast cancer is known to develop resistance to endocrine therapy with the loss of ER expression only accounting for a small number of the cases where resistance develops (Shiino et al., 2016). The predominant

Table 2 Common drugs used to treat various types of breast cancer and the mechanisms underlying resistance to these drugs

Treatment	Drug resistance	Resistance mechanism	References
Aromatase inhibitors	Relapse after initial treatment	Exemestane (false aromatase enzyme substrate) alongside everolimus (an mTOR inhibitor)	(Carlini et al., 2007; Chin et al., 2007)
ER+			
Tamoxifen	Mutations in estrogen receptor	Fulvestrant-ER downregulatory	(Kang et al., 2005)
	CYP2D6 polymorphisms		(Li et al., 1997; Zakharchenko et al., 2011)
	cAMP/PKA 2 PI3K and MAPK pathways upregulated leading to transcription changes		
	PTEN mutations		(Razavi et al., 2018)
PI3K inhibitors	Increased toxicity	Everolimus (Afinitor) with the CDK4/6 inhibitor	(Hurvitz & Peddi, 2013)
Pictilisib and buparlisib	Increased toxicity		(Krop et al., 2016) (Dhakal et al., 2020)
ER+/PR+/HER2-			
ER downregulators	*PIK3CA* mutations	Piqray (PI3K inhibitor)	(Thorpe et al., 2015)
ER+/HER2			
CDK4/6 inhibitors	Increased toxicity	Combination of CDK4/6 inhibitors with FUL	(Turner et al., 2018; Killock, 2019)
HER2+			
Trastuzumab, pertuzumab, and 19H6-Hu	*PIK3CA* mutations	19H6-Hu (anti-HER2 antibody)	(Christianson et al., 1998)
	Truncated form of HER2 (P95HER2)	Pertuzumab is a monoclonal antibody that binds to the extracellular dimerization domain of HER2	(Warmerdam et al., 1991)
TNBC			
Chemotherapy by alkylating agents, antimetabolites, antitumor antibiotics, topoisomerase inhibitors, TKIs, and mitotic inhibitors	Epigenetic alterations	Epigenetic therapies	(Verweij et al., 1994)
	Enzyme system deactivation of drugs	Taxanes along with anthracyclines	(Miklavčič et al., 2014)
	TWIST overexpression due to NF-κB	Immunotherapy	(Loibl & Furlanetto, 2015)

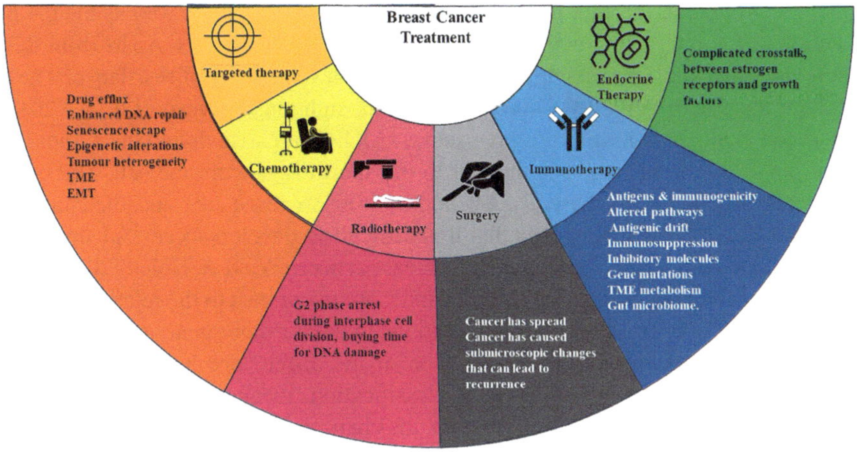

Fig. 2 Breast cancer treatment strategies and the mechanisms of resistance to these treatments. Breast cancers can be treated with multiple strategies (the middle circle), including targeted therapies, chemotherapy, radiation therapy, surgery, immunotherapy, and endocrine therapy. The outer circle shows the mechanisms developed by breast cancer cells to overcome these treatments

mechanism for the development of resistance is the ligand-independent ER reactivation (Miller et al., 2011). This can occur through multiple mechanisms which include gain-of-function mutations in ER, alterations in the interactions between ER and coactivators or corepressors, development of compensatory crosstalk between ER and growth factor receptors and finally, increased oncogenic signaling (Ma et al., 2015). For example, in 2018 Razavi and colleagues performed whole-exome sequencing on 1918 breast cancer patients to identify genetic alterations in various breast cancer types including those resistant to endocrine therapy. They identified mutations in ERBB2, which increased the activity of the protein and increased downstream signaling. They also identified loss-of-function mutations within the tumor suppressor gene Neurofibromin1 (NF1) (Razavi et al., 2018). These mutations were also commonly accompanied by alterations in MAPK genes and genes that regulate the transcription of Estrogen receptors (Razavi et al., 2018). Another approach is to prevent the recurrence of endocrine-resistant breast cancer, is to target dormant ER^+ breast cancer cells (Gawrzak et al., 2018; Zhang et al., 1997).

The Prevalence of Resistance in Breast Cancer

The development of chemoresistance has become a major problem in the control and management of breast cancer. Treatment resistance is exacerbated by relapses in the tumors that responded well to treatment in the early phases of the disease as well as resistance to multiple agents and strategies (Perez, 2009). The development of resistance can be caused by multiple changes at the molecular level, in the tumor microenvironment, through interaction with other cancer cells as well as the modification of the interaction between immune cells and cancer cells. Apart from this, there are other factors that can contribute to the development of resistance. These include the pH of cells, hypoxia and paracrine signaling (Mansoori et al., 2017; Nikolaou et al., 2018). Multidrug resistance (MDR) can arise due to the activity of multiple drug-resistance genes that act to transport drugs from the cell. The complex interplay between these factors contributing to resistance and the multiple mechanisms of resistance means that it is difficult to develop successful strategies to overcome resistance to treatments in breast cancer (Wind & Holen, 2011). The complexity and heterogeneity of breast cancer are in contrast to the relatively minor changes in gene expression, simple mutations in one or more genes (Organization, 2019). In addition to this the contribution of the differences between individual patients or tumors, regardless of their classification, means that patients respond differently to the same treatment. As such, the chances of a patient developing resistance cannot easily be predicted (Luque-Bolivar et al., 2020). The complexity and heterogeneity of breast cancer are in contrast to the relatively minor changes in gene expression, simple mutations are one or more genes (Organization, 2019).

Overcoming Resistance to Common Therapies

The primary strategy to counter the development of drug resistance has been to use a variety of drugs in different combinations. This strategy can be further complicated by multidrug resistant disease (Waks & Winer, 2019). Targeted therapy depends on the selection of a therapy based on the subtype of breast cancer and the stage at diagnosis (Kinnel et al., 2023). Targeted therapies have advanced in their specificity and effectiveness due to an increased understanding of the molecular changes that promote breast cancer development and progression. Potential molecular targets that have been investigated or used to overcome resistance include the Aryl hydrocarbon receptor (AhR), linked to increased drug efflux (Powell et al., 2013), nitric oxide synthase (NOS), linked to cisplatin resistance (Jin et al., 2015), Phosphoinositide 3 kinase (PI3K), involved in endocrine, HER-2, and cytotoxic therapy resistance (Paplomata & O'Regan, 2014), the Wnt/β-Catenin Pathway, which regulates cancer cell stemness (Zhong & Virshup, 2020) and Protein tyrosine kinase 6 (PTK6), which regulates anoikis resistance (Irie et al., 2010). Additional targets include those whose increased expression negates the effectiveness of drugs which act to inhibit them. These include epidermal growth factor receptor (EGFR (Ali & Wendt, 2017), Cyclin-Dependent Kinase 4/6 (CDK4/6) (Yang et al., 2017), Poly (ADP-Ribose) Polymerases (PARP) (O'Connor, 2015). Finally, human epidermal growth factor (HER-2) where antiHER2 therapy effectiveness is decreased due to decreased drug binding, lack of HER-2 downregulation, and alterations in apoptotic and cell cycle pathways (Zhang, 2021).

Studies have shown that immunotherapy can successfully be used to treat early-stage breast cancer patients with high levels of tumor-infiltrating lymphocytes

(TILs) even without accompanying chemotherapy treatment (Park et al., 2019). For non-responders, the improved understanding of tumor-immune interactions and the contribution of the TME, notably with the help of the latest technologies such as single-cell analyses and spatial transcriptomics, may provide new drug targets and strategies to overcome resistance (Aldea et al., 2021; Morad et al., 2021). For instance, single-cell transcriptome analysis was used to monitor HER2+ breast cancer patients undergoing a combination of CDK4/6 inhibitors. This analysis revealed an immunosuppressive population of immature myeloid cells that infiltrate resistant tumors. This study also showed that these cells can be targeted with cabozantinib, a tyrosine kinase inhibitor, used in combination with compounds that enhance immune checkpoint blockade (Wang et al., 2019a).

A 2018 global study estimated that 13% of cancers globally can be attributed to microbial infections, both bacterial and viral. The main causes of these infections were *H. pylori*, Human papilloma virus, Hepatitis B virus (HBV), and Hepatitis C virus (HCV) (de Martel et al., 2020). However, there are a vast number of microbes living within the human body. The microbiota is thought to play an important role in determining the severity and mortality of breast cancer. This is largely due to the generation of secondary metabolites with biological activity by these microbes, which can increase or decrease the risk of developing breast cancer, by changing energy intake and utilization or through the regulation of circulating steroid hormone levels. Breast tissue has a distinct microbial community which changes following the development of breast cancer (Parida & Sharma, 2019a, 2019b; Urbaniak et al., 2014; Smith et al., 2019). Additionally, this microbiota differs depending on the malignancy and type of breast cancer. The gut microbiota is known to play an important role in the development of breast cancer (Parida & Sharma, 2019a) and is expected to influence the effectiveness of endocrine therapy in the treatment of breast cancer due to the significant role played by the gut microbiota in estrogen metabolism (Brooks, 1984; Jerry, 2007; Truin et al., 2017). The gut microbiota achieves this by secreting the enzyme β-glucuronidase, which acts to deconjugate estrogens into their active forms (Parida & Sharma, 2019a).

Individual variations in the makeup of the gut microbiome depend on factors such as the individual's ethnicity, nutrition, BMI, use of antibiotics, and any current infections (Parida & Sharma, 2019a). Dysbiosis of the gut microbiota leads to a decline in the levels of circulating estrogens, a condition that is linked to many kinds of cancer (Helmink et al., 2019). Both the immune system and inflammatory response, both of which play a role in cancer development, can be regulated by the microbiota. The microbiota can also influence the effectiveness of immunotherapy such as checkpoint inhibitors (ICIs) and CTLA-4 (Li et al., 2019). The efficacy of many drugs that function to block immune-related molecules such as CTLA (Vétizou et al., 2015) or anti-PD-1 therapy (Gopalakrishnan et al., 2018; Sivan et al., 2015; Killock, 2018) are dependent on the presence of specific species of bacteria within the microbiome. The microbiome also regulates the response of tumors to radiation therapy (Shiao et al., 2021). The microbiota can also alter the metabolism of anticancer drugs. These include irinotecan, fluorouracil, and leucovorin (Bailly, 2019; Kang et al., 2015).

Chimeric antigen receptor cells are immune cells that have been modified to express molecules that are a combination of different cancer antigens, allowing them to recognize multiple cancer cells. These CAR-T or CAR-NK cells are a new immunotherapy that allows cancer cells to be specifically targeted using synthetic receptors that are specific to tumor cells expressed on their surface. There are promising breast cancer-specific targets for CAR cell therapy (Vitorino et al., 2021; Tóth et al., 2020; Szöőr et al., 2020).

Revolutionary Approaches to Reverse Resistance in Breast Cancer

Apart from adapting or improving existing therapies to overcome resistance, there are new revolutionary treatments that take advantage of new technologies such as the use of artificial intelligence to analyze large datasets. This would allow for the identification of new drug targets, active compounds, and biomarkers (Fig. 3). One exciting source of new drug targets are cancer promoting or specific protein isoforms or components of the alternative splicing machinery. Alternative splicing is the process where pre-mRNA is spliced to give rise to multiple mRNAs, which code for different protein isoforms. These isoforms may have completely different functions from each other, or they may share common functions (Abou Faycal et al., 2016). Alternative splicing is known to be dysregulated in cancers, including breast cancer. This can give rise to cancer promoting isoforms or isoforms which assist in promoting drug resistance. This includes isoforms of HER2, the estrogen receptor, caspase 9, and certain growth factor receptors (Gahete et al., 2022). Altered expression of spliceosome components and splicing regulators can also lead to a drastic change in the splicing pattern within a cancer cell that could promote drug resistance. These splicing factors may themselves be spliced to give rise to isoforms that promote the splicing of pro-oncogenic isoforms of other proteins (Gahete et al., 2022). As such, these splicing factors and proteasome components are viable targets to overcome drug resistance. Small molecule inhibitors of these spliceosome components and splicing regulators have been developed. In addition to this splice switching oligonucleotides have been developed that are complementary to splice sites or splice silencing sites on the target mRNA. By binding to these sites, they can stop the formation of pro-oncogenic or resistance promoting isoforms (Grollman, 1968; Havens & Hastings, 2016).

Precision medicine is the tailoring of treatments, detection, and monitoring of breast cancers based on individual variations, environment, genes, and lifestyles. Precision medicine offers great potential to improve the management of breast cancer (Collins & Varmus, 2015). The application of precision medicine has only become an option due to the development of new high throughput methods to study the "omics," such as genomics, transcriptomics, proteomics, epigenomics, metabolomics, and microbiomics (Naito & Urasaki, 2018). These omics technologies allow

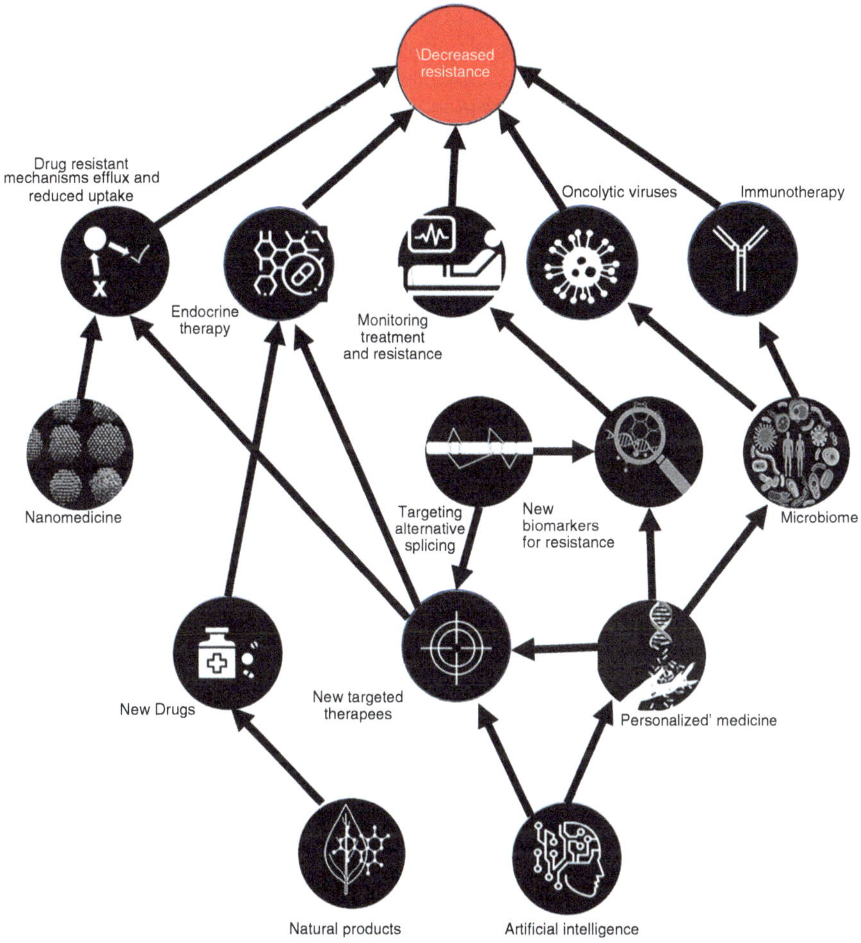

Fig. 3 Strategies for overcoming resistance to treatment in breast cancer. Artificial intelligence serves as the basis for the analysis of large amounts of omics data ranging from genomics to microbiomics. This data can be used to develop a personalized approach to medicine and will allow for the identification of biomarkers for the development of resistance. This in turn would allow for the modification of the treatment being used to overcome resistance. The microbiome analysis would allow for the identification of dysbiosis, which could result in suppression of the immune system or altered immune signaling. Rectifying this matter restores sensitivity to immunotherapy. Personalized medicine will also aid in the development of new targeted therapies. This will be aided by the identification of new processes to target, such as alternative splicing or a new source of potential drugs such as natural compounds

for the development of new biomarkers for improved prognosis and diagnosis. These predictive biomarkers would also help in the selection of the correct therapy and could be used to either predict the potential for resistance to develop or monitor treatment to detect the onset of treatment resistance (Lainetti et al., 2020).

Almost all current chemotherapy drugs originate from natural sources. These natural products are also the source of new drugs that are being developed. Research is centered on identifying highly active natural compounds, such as phytochemicals, that have anticancer activity and are suitable for modification to create synthetic compounds with improved pharmacokinetics. (Sharifi-Rad et al., 2019). One such compound is curcumin (Xiang et al., 2020) and has been modified to create curcumin analogs that effectively inhibit P-glycoprotein-mediated resistance in drug-resistant breast cancer (Gao et al., 2020). These synthetic analogs have reduced toxicity and increased solubility, making them far more appropriate and viable drugs (Liao et al., 2020). Other natural compounds that have been used as the basis for the design of synthetic derivatives include epigallocatechin and catechin. Both these compounds also inhibit P-glycoprotein (P-gp) activity preventing MDR as a result of drug efflux (Wong et al., 2021). Other natural products target drug resistance that results from apoptosis-resistance, metastatic processes, inflammation, necroptosis, autophagy, and proliferation.

Other advancements include the use of nanomedicine to improve drug delivery and targeting. Nanostructures can be used to overcome drug resistance by overcoming drug efflux, removal, and detoxification through this improved delivery or by shielding the drug (Lainetti et al., 2020). These nanoparticles can also be used to deliver drugs that are poorly soluble thereby improving drug uptake (Lainetti et al., 2020). Nanoparticles can also help to reduce side effects on normal tissue as the drug can be delivered specifically to the tumor cells (Cao et al., 2021).

Limitations to the Development in Implementation of Novel Strategies to Overcome Resistance in Breast Cancer

The limitations for the implementation of these new strategies to combat drug resistance in breast cancer are primarily due to limitations in current knowledge and technology combined with financial constraints. Other disadvantages involve ensuring the safety and efficacy of these new or modified treatments. An example of the limitations of current technology is the use of circulating tumor DNA (ctDNA) to identify genes that play a role in drug resistance and could be used as targets for the development of new drugs to counteract resistance. CtDNA could also serve as the source for the detection of biomarkers to monitor treatment and identify the development of resistance. However, in order for ctDNA to play a role in screening and the detection of resistance it must be able to detect a low burden of disease (Bettegowda et al., 2014). This may be a problem for current sequencing technologies, that cannot be overcome by increasing the intensity of sequencing or by using error correction techniques (Vasan et al., 2019).

Many of these new treatments and therapies are not guaranteed to be safe or have low toxicity. Many of the natural products isolated to serve as new drugs will need synthetic versions to be developed to overcome toxicity due to poor solubility or the compounds may have an innate cytotoxic effect that is not easily overcome or suitable for use as a treatment option. Drugs that inhibit components of the spliceosome may inhibit splicing to such a universal extent that they may disrupt proper cell function (Rymond, 2007).

Finally, when it comes to the cost of developing or putting these new therapies in place, and one of the most pressing issues is that the countries with increasing breast cancer burden and a disproportionately large mortality rate are the same countries that can ill afford the financial costs associated with implementing these new strategies. In addition, many of these new strategies involve the use of artificial intelligence to analyze data concerning genomics, transcriptomics, etc. However, these datasets are currently mostly generated in wealthier countries, and as such the genomic or transcriptomic patterns are characteristic of the population within these countries and not of those individuals in lower-income countries. This can only be rectified by ensuring that these individuals are more represented in any large datasets (Yamamoto et al., 2022).

Conclusion

This book aims to discuss the effect of the development of breast cancer on various therapies, the mechanism behind the development of this resistance, and the strategies being developed to overcome this resistance. The book is divided into four parts that follow a logical flow, starting with an introduction to breast cancer and drug resistance. Apart from this introductory chapter, this section also contains a chapter providing a detailed discussion of the mechanisms underlying drug resistance in breast cancer in order to shed light on how these complex and intricate molecular mechanisms hinder effective treatment. Part two of the book delves into various types of drug resistance in breast cancer treatment. The first chapter of this section will discuss the potential use of targeted therapies to overcome or counteract drug resistance and improve treatment outcomes in breast cancer. This will be followed by a chapter discussing the use of immunotherapy as a treatment for breast cancer and describing the mechanisms underlying the development of resistance to these treatments. In a similar manner, the following chapter will examine the use of endocrine therapy as a treatment for breast cancer and examine the mechanisms employed by breast cancers that contribute to the development of resistance to this therapeutic approach. The final chapter in part two will examine the mechanisms underlying chemoresistance in breast cancers.

Part three of the book will explore innovative strategies and future directions in overcoming drug resistance and will be initiated by a chapter discussing the contribution of alternative mRNA splicing to the development of drug resistance. It will then explore strategies based on correcting or changing these splicing events to restore treatment sensitivity. This will be followed by a chapter reviewing the relationship between viral infections and drug resistance in breast cancer, and how viral infections can contribute to the development of drug resistance.

The chapter will explore research into the development of effective strategies to overcome drug resistance by exploiting viral vulnerabilities for therapeutic intervention. The potential of natural products as a valuable resource in the battle against drug resistance will be explored in the following chapter. The chapter will describe the mechanisms by which this diverse range of bioactive compounds exert their anticancer effects. The final chapter in part three will discuss the potential of artificial intelligence to transform the way we approach overcoming drug resistance in breast cancer. It will discuss how the use of AI to analyze large sets of biological data collected from an individual in conjunction with machine learning can be used to develop personalized treatment and identify novel therapeutic targets.

The final part of the book discusses the future directions and advanced treatments that promise to contribute to overcoming drug resistance. The first chapter in this section will explore the application of research on the microbiome to the problem of drug resistance and reversing treatment outcomes in breast cancer. The chapter will delve into the relationship between the microbiome and breast cancer cells. It will then discuss the potential for microbiome-based interventions to reverse drug resistance. This will be followed by a chapter that focuses on the utilization of molecular profiling techniques and personalized medicine to manage drug resistance in breast cancer. This includes the use of biomarkers and the molecular alterations associated with drug resistance to develop personalized medicine strategies. The following two chapters will highlight promising new strategies to tackle drug resistance in breast cancer. The first of these will explore innovative therapeutic approaches such as immunotherapy, gene therapy, epigenetic modulation, nanotechnology-based drug delivery systems, and combination therapies that have the potential to overcome resistance to therapy in breast cancer. This will be followed by a chapter that will discuss the role played by effective drug delivery and how new advanced drug delivery systems can be used to overcome drug resistance in breast cancer. The final chapter in this section concerns not the development of a new technology or method to treat breast cancer, but rather addresses the disparities in breast cancer research and treatment regarding drug resistance. These include disparities in the ability to access healthcare, differences in the quality of care, and skewed representation in clinical trials leading to differential outcomes in breast cancer patients. It is imperative that these disparities must be addressed, and the chapter will discuss the various means this can be accomplished including inclusive research efforts, community engagement, and tailored interventions to overcome these disparities. This section of the book and the entire book will be closed off by a concluding chapter summarizing the book and discussing the way forward.

References

Abou Faycal, C., Gazzeri, S., & Eymin, B. (2016). RNA splicing, cell signaling, and response to therapies. *Current Opinion in Oncology, 28*, 58–64.

Aggelis, V., & Johnston, S. R. D. (2019). Advances in endocrine-based therapies for estrogen receptor-positive metastatic breast cancer. *Drugs, 79*, 1849–1866.

Akram, M., Iqbal, M., Daniyal, M., & Khan, A. U. (2017). Awareness and current knowledge of breast cancer. *Biological Research, 50*, 33.

Aldea, M., Andre, F., Marabelle, A., Dogan, S., Barlesi, F., & Soria, J.-C. (2021). Overcoming resistance to tumor-targeted and immune-targeted therapies. *Cancer Discovery, 11*, 874–899.

Ali, R., & Wendt, M. K. (2017). The paradoxical functions of EGFR during breast cancer progression. *Signal Transduction and Targeted Therapy, 2*, 16042.

Anders, C. K., & Carey, L. A. (2009). Biology, metastatic patterns, and treatment of patients with triple-negative breast cancer. *Clinical Breast Cancer, 9*(Suppl 2), S73–S81.

Bailly, C. (2019). Irinotecan: 25 years of cancer treatment. *Pharmacological Research, 148*, 104398.

Bettegowda, C., Sausen, M., Leary, R. J., Kinde, I., Wang, Y., Agrawal, N., Bartlett, B. R., Wang, H., Luber, B., Alani, R. M., Antonarakis, E. S., Azad, N. S., Bardelli, A., Brem, H., Cameron, J. L., Lee, C. C., Fecher, L. A., Gallia, G. L., GIBBS, P., Le, D., Giuntoli, R. L., Goggins, M., Hogarty, M. D., Holdhoff, M., Hong, S. M., Jiao, Y., Juhl, H. H., Kim, J. J., Siravegna, G., Laheru, D. A., Lauricella, C., Lim, M., Lipson, E. J., Marie, S. K., Netto, G. J., Oliner, K. S., Olivi, A., Olsson, L., Riggins, G. J., Sartore-Bianchi, A., Schmidt, K., Shih, L. M., Oba-Shinjo, S. M., Siena, S., Theodorescu, D., Tie, J., Harkins, T. T., Veronese, S., Wang, T. L., Weingart, J. D., Wolfgang, C. L., Wood, L. D., Xing, D., Hruban, R. H., Wu, J., Allen, P. J., Schmidt, C. M., Choti, M. A., Velculescu, V. E., Kinzler, K. W., Vogelstein, B., Papadopoulos, N., Diaz, L. A., & JR. (2014). Detection of circulating tumor DNA in early- and late-stage human malignancies. *Science Translational Medicine, 6*, 224ra24.

Bocchinfuso, W. P., & Korach, K. S. (1997). Mammary gland development and tumorigenesis in estrogen receptor knockout mice. *Journal of Mammary Gland Biology and Neoplasia, 2*, 323–334.

Bray, F., Ferlay, J., Soerjomataram, I., Siegel, R. L., Torre, L. A., & Jemal, A. (2018). Global cancer statistics 2018: GLOBOCAN estimates of incidence and mortality worldwide for 36 cancers in 185 countries. *CA: A Cancer Journal for Clinicians, 68*, 394–424.

Brooks, P. G. (1984). The relationship of estrogen and progesterone to breast disease. *The Journal of Reproductive Medicine, 29*, 530–538.

Cao, L., Zhu, Y., Wang, W., Wang, G., Zhang, S., & Cheng, H. (2021). Emerging nano-based strategies against drug resistance in tumor chemotherapy. *Frontiers in Bioengineering and Biotechnology, 9*, 798882.

Cardoso, F., Kyriakides, S., Ohno, S., Penault-Llorca, F., Poortmans, P., Rubio, I. T., Zackrisson, S., & Senkus, E. (2019). Early breast cancer: ESMO clinical practice guidelines for diagnosis, treatment, and follow-up†. *Annals of Oncology, 30*, 1194–1220.

Carlini, P., Michelotti, A., Ferretti, G., Ricci, S., Giannarelli, D., Pellegrini, M., Cresti, N., Di Cosimo, S., Bria, E., Papaldo, P., Fabi, A., Ruggeri, E. M., Milella, M., Alimonti, A., Salesi, N., & Cognetti, F. (2007). Clinical evaluation of the use of exemestane as further hormonal therapy after nonsteroidal aromatase inhibitors in postmenopausal metastatic breast cancer patients. *Cancer Investigation, 25*, 102–105.

Chin, Y. S., Beresford, M. J., Ravichandran, D., & Makris, A. (2007). Exemestane after non-steroidal aromatase inhibitors for post-menopausal women with advanced breast cancer. *Breast, 16*, 436–439.

Christianson, T. A., Doherty, J. K., Lin, Y. J., Ramsey, E. E., Holmes, R., Keenan, E. J., & Clinton, G. M. (1998). NH2-terminally truncated HER-2/neu protein: Relationship with shedding of the extracellular domain and with prognostic factors in breast cancer. *Cancer Research, 58*, 5123–5129.

Cleator, S., Heller, W., & Coombes, R. C. (2007). Triple-negative breast cancer: Therapeutic options. *The Lancet Oncology, 8*, 235–244.

Collins, F. S., & Varmus, H. (2015). A new initiative on precision medicine. *The New England Journal of Medicine, 372*, 793–795.

Control, C. F. D., Prevention, P. J. D. O. C., & Control. (2018). How is breast cancer treated.

Cosentino, G., Plantamura, I., Tagliabue, E., Iorio, M. V., & Cataldo, A. (2021). Breast cancer drug resistance: Overcoming the challenge by capitalizing on MicroRNA and tumor microenvironment interplay. *Cancers (Basel), 13*, 3691.

De Martel, C., Georges, D., Bray, F., Ferlay, J., & Clifford, G. M. (2020). Global burden of cancer attributable to infections in 2018: A worldwide incidence analysis. *The Lancet Global Health, 8*, e180–e190.

Dhakal, A., Antony Thomas, R., Levine, E. G., Brufsky, A., Takabe, K., Hanna, M. G., Attwood, K., Miller, A., Khoury, T., Early, A. P., Soniwala, S., O'connor, T., & Opyrchal, M. (2020). Outcome of everolimus-based therapy in hormone-receptor-positive metastatic breast cancer patients after progression on Palbociclib. *Breast Cancer (Auckl.), 14*, 1178223420944864.

Echeverría, S. E., Borrell, L. N., Brown, D., & Rhoads, G. (2009). A local area analysis of racial, ethnic, and neighborhood disparities in breast cancer staging. *Cancer Epidemiology, Biomarkers & Prevention, 18*, 3024–3029.

Eliyatkin, N., Yalçin, E., Zengel, B., Aktaş, S., & Vardar, E. (2015). Molecular classification of breast carcinoma: From traditional, old-fashioned way to A new age, and A new way. *Journal of Breast Health, 11*, 59–66.

Gahete, M. D., Herman-Sanchez, N., Fuentes-Fayos, A. C., Lopez-Canovas, J. L., & Luque, R. M. (2022). Dysregulation of splicing variants and spliceosome components in breast cancer. *Endocrine-Related Cancer, 29*, R123–r142.

Gao, L., Zhao, P., Li, Y., Yang, D., Hu, P., Li, L., Cheng, Y., & Yao, H. (2020). Reversal of P-glycoprotein-mediated multidrug resistance by novel curcumin analogues in paclitaxel-resistant human breast cancer cells. *Biochemistry and Cell Biology, 98*, 484–491.

Gawrzak, S., Rinaldi, L., Gregorio, S., Arenas, E. J., Salvador, F., Urosevic, J., Figueras-Puig, C., Rojo, F., Del Barco Barrantes, I., Cejalvo, J. M., Palafox, M., Guiu, M., Berenguer-Llergo, A., Symeonidi, A., Bellmunt, A., Kalafatovic, D., Arnal-Estapé, A., Fernández, E., Müllauer, B., Groeneveld, R., Slobodnyuk, K., Stephan-Otto Attolini, C., Saura, C., Arribas, J., Cortes, J., Rovira, A., Muñoz, M., Lluch, A., Serra, V., Albanell, J., Prat, A., Nebreda, A. R., Benitah, S. A., & Gomis, R. R. (2018). MSK1 regulates luminal cell differentiation and metastatic dormancy in ER(+) breast cancer. *Nature Cell Biology, 20*, 211–221.

Gerend, M. A., & Pai, M. (2008). Social determinants of black-white disparities in breast cancer mortality: A review. *Cancer Epidemiology, Biomarkers & Prevention, 17*, 2913–2923.

Giaquinto, A. N., Sung, H., Miller, K. D., Kramer, J. L., Newman, L. A., Minihan, A., Jemal, A., & Siegel, R. L. (2022). Breast cancer statistics, 2022. *CA: A Cancer Journal for Clinicians, 72*, 524–541.

Gopalakrishnan, V., Spencer, C. N., Nezi, L., Reuben, A., Andrews, M. C., Karpinets, T. V., Prieto, P. A., Vicente, D., Hoffman, K., Wei, S. C., Cogdill, A. P., Zhao, L., Hudgens, C. W., Hutchinson, D. S., Manzo, T., Petaccia De Macedo, M., Cotechini, T., Kumar, T., Chen, W. S., Reddy, S. M., Szczepaniak Sloane, R., Galloway-Pena, J., Jiang, H., Chen, P. L., Shpall, E. J., Rezvani, K., Alousi, A. M., Chemaly, R. F., Shelburne, S., Vence, L. M., Okhuysen, P. C., Jensen, V. B., Swennes, A. G., Mcallister, F., Marcelo Riquelme Sanchez, E., Zhang, Y., Le Chatelier, E., Zitvogel, L., Pons, N., Austin-Breneman, J. L., Haydu, L. E., Burton, E. M., Gardner, J. M., Sirmans, E., Hu, J., Lazar, A. J., Tsujikawa, T., Diab, A., Tawbi, H., Glitza, I. C., Hwu, W. J., Patel, S. P., Woodman, S. E., Amaria, R. N., Davies, M. A., Gershenwald, J. E., Hwu, P., Lee, J. E., Zhang, J., Coussens, L. M., Cooper, Z. A., Futreal, P. A., Daniel, C. R., Ajami, N. J., Petrosino, J. F., Tetzlaff, M. T., Sharma, P., Allison, J. P., Jenq, R. R., & Wargo, J. A. (2018). Gut microbiome modulates response to anti-PD-1 immunotherapy in melanoma patients. *Science, 359*, 97–103.

Grollman, A. P. (1968). Inhibitors of protein biosynthesis. V. Effects of emetine on protein and nucleic acid biosynthesis in HeLa cells. *The Journal of Biological Chemistry, 243*, 4089–4094.

Harbeck, N., Penault-Llorca, F., Cortes, J., Gnant, M., Houssami, N., Poortmans, P., Ruddy, K., Tsang, J., & Cardoso, F. (2019). Breast cancer. *Nature Reviews Disease Primers, 5*, 66.

Harper, S., Lynch, J., Meersman, S. C., Breen, N., Davis, W. W., & Reichman, M. C. (2009). Trends in area-socioeconomic and race-ethnic disparities in breast cancer incidence, stage at diagnosis, screening, mortality, and survival among women ages 50 years and over (1987–2005). *Cancer Epidemiology, Biomarkers & Prevention, 18*, 121–131.

Havens, M. A., & Hastings, M. L. (2016). Splice-switching antisense oligonucleotides as therapeutic drugs. *Nucleic Acids Research, 44*, 6549–6563.

He, J., Fortunati, E., Liu, D. X., & Li, Y. (2021). Pleiotropic roles of ABC transporters in breast cancer. *International Journal of Molecular Sciences, 22*, 3199.

Helmink, B. A., Khan, M. A. W., Hermann, A., Gopalakrishnan, V., & Wargo, J. A. (2019). The microbiome, cancer, and cancer therapy. *Nature Medicine, 25*, 377–388.

Holohan, C., Van Schaeybroeck, S., Longley, D. B., & Johnston, P. G. (2013). Cancer drug resistance: An evolving paradigm. *Nature Reviews Cancer, 13*, 714–726.

Hurvitz, S., & Peddi, P. (2013). Everolimus in postmenopausal hormone-receptor-positive advanced breast cancer. *Breast Diseases, 24*, 79–81.

Irie, H. Y., Shrestha, Y., Selfors, L. M., Frye, F., Iida, N., Wang, Z., Zou, L., Yao, J., Lu, Y., Epstein, C. B., Natesan, S., Richardson, A. L., Polyak, K., Mills, G. B., Hahn, W. C., & Brugge, J. S. (2010). PTK6 regulates IGF-1-induced anchorage-independent survival. *PLoS One, 5*, e11729.

Jerry, D. J. (2007). Roles for estrogen and progesterone in breast cancer prevention. *Breast Cancer Research, 9*, 102.

Jin, Z., Wang, W., Jiang, N., Zhang, L., Li, Y., Xu, X., Cai, S., Wei, L., Liu, X., Chen, G., Zhou, Y., Liu, C., Li, Z., Jin, F., & Chen, B. (2015). Clinical implications of iNOS levels in triple-negative breast cancer responding to neoadjuvant chemotherapy. *PLoS One, 10*, e0130286.

Kang, M. H., Wang, J., Makena, M. R., Lee, J. S., Paz, N., Hall, C. P., Song, M. M., Calderon, R. I., Cruz, R. E., Hindle, A., Ko, W., Fitzgerald, J. B., Drummond, D. C., Triche, T. J., & Reynolds, C. P. (2015). Activity of MM-398, nanoliposomal irinotecan (nal-IRI), in Ewing's family tumor xenografts is associated with high exposure of tumor to drug and high SLFN11 expression. *Clinical Cancer Research, 21*, 1139–1150.

Kang, S., Bader, A. G., & Vogt, P. K. (2005). Phosphatidylinositol 3-kinase mutations identified in human cancer are oncogenic. *Proceedings of the National Academy of Sciences of the United States of America, 102*, 802–807.

Killock, D. (2018). Immunotherapy: Gut bacteria modulate responses to PD-1 blockade. *Nature Reviews. Clinical Oncology, 15*, 6–7.

Killock, D. (2019). CDK4/6 inhibitors prolong OS. *Nature Reviews Clinical Oncology, 16*, 722.

Kinnel, B., Singh, S. K., Oprea-Ilies, G., & Singh, R. (2023). Targeted therapy and mechanisms of drug resistance in breast cancer. *Cancers (Basel), 15*, 1320.

Kong, X., Liu, Z., Cheng, R., Sun, L., Huang, S., Fang, Y., & Wang, J. (2020). Variation in breast cancer subtype incidence and distribution by race/ethnicity in the United States from 2010 to 2015. *JAMA Network Open, 3*, e2020303–e2020303.

Krop, I. E., Mayer, I. A., Ganju, V., Dickler, M., Johnston, S., Morales, S., Yardley, D. A., Melichar, B., Forero-Torres, A., Lee, S. C., De Boer, R., Petrakova, K., Vallentin, S., Perez, E. A., Piccart, M., Ellis, M., Winer, E., Gendreau, S., Derynck, M., Lackner, M., Levy, G., Qiu, J., He, J., & Schmid, P. (2016). Pictilisib for oestrogen receptor-positive, aromatase inhibitor-resistant, advanced or metastatic breast cancer (FERGI): A randomised, double-blind, placebo-controlled, phase 2 trial. *The Lancet Oncology, 17*, 811–821.

Lainetti, P. F., Leis-Filho, A. F., Laufer-Amorim, R., Battazza, A., & Fonseca-Alves, C. E. (2020). Mechanisms of resistance to chemotherapy in breast cancer and possible targets in drug delivery systems. *Pharmaceutics, 12*, 1193.

Li, J., Yen, C., Liaw, D., Podsypanina, K., Bose, S., Wang, S. I., Puc, J., Miliaresis, C., Rodgers, L., Mccombie, R., Bigner, S. H., Giovanella, B. C., Ittmann, M., Tycko, B., Hibshoosh, H., Wigler, M. H., & Parsons, R. (1997). PTEN, a putative protein tyrosine phosphatase gene mutated in human brain, breast, and prostate cancer. *Science, 275*, 1943–1947.

Li, W., Deng, Y., Chu, Q., & Zhang, P. (2019). Gut microbiome and cancer immunotherapy. *Cancer Letters, 447*, 41–47.

Liao, X., Bu, Y., & Jia, Q. (2020). Traditional Chinese medicine as supportive care for the management of liver cancer: Past, present, and future. *Genes Diseases, 7*, 370–379.

Lin, N. U., & Winer, E. P. (2008). Advances in adjuvant endocrine therapy for postmenopausal women. *Journal of Clinical Oncology, 26*, 798–805.

Loibl, S., & Furlanetto, J. J. C. B. C. R. (2015). Targeting the immune system in breast cancer: Hype or hope?: TILs and newer immune-based therapies being evaluated for HER2+ and TNBC. *Current Breast Cancer Reports, 7*, 203–209.

Łukasiewicz, S., Czeczelewski, M., Forma, A., Baj, J., Sitarz, R., & Stanisławek, A. (2021). Breast cancer-epidemiology, risk factors, classification, prognostic markers, and current treatment strategies-an updated review. *Cancers (Basel), 13*, 4287.

Luque-Bolivar, A., Pérez-Mora, E., Villegas, V. E., & Rondón-Lagos, M. (2020). Resistance and overcoming resistance in breast cancer. *Breast Cancer (Dove Med Press), 12*, 211–229.

Ma, C. X., Reinert, T., Chmielewska, I., & Ellis, M. J. (2015). Mechanisms of aromatase inhibitor resistance. *Nature Reviews Cancer, 15*, 261–275.

Mansoori, B., Mohammadi, A., Davudian, S., Shirjang, S., & Baradaran, B. (2017). The different mechanisms of cancer drug resistance: A brief review. *Advanced Pharmaceutical Bulletin, 7*, 339–348.

Miklavčič, D., Mali, B., Kos, B., Heller, R., & Serša, G. (2014). Electrochemotherapy: From the drawing board into medical practice. *Biomedical Engineering Online, 13*, 29.

Miller, T. W., Balko, J. M., Fox, E. M., Ghazoui, Z., Dunbier, A., Anderson, H., Dowsett, M., Jiang, A., Smith, R. A., Maira, S. M., Manning, H. C., González-Angulo, A. M., Mills, G. B., Higham, C., Chanthaphaychith, S., Kuba, M. G., Miller, W. R., Shyr, Y., & Arteaga, C. L. (2011). ERα-dependent E2F transcription can mediate resistance to estrogen deprivation in human breast cancer. *Cancer Discovery, 1*, 338–351.

Morad, G., Helmink, B. A., Sharma, P., & Wargo, J. A. (2021). Hallmarks of response, resistance, and toxicity to immune checkpoint blockade. *Cell, 184*, 5309–5337.

Naito, Y., & Urasaki, T. (2018). Precision medicine in breast cancer. *Chinese Clinical Oncology, 7*, 29.

Nikolaou, M., Pavlopoulou, A., Georgakilas, A. G., & Kyrodimos, E. (2018). The challenge of drug resistance in cancer treatment: A current overview. *Clinical & Experimental Metastasis, 35*, 309–318.

Nilsson, S., Mäkelä, S., Treuter, E., Tujague, M., Thomsen, J., Andersson, G., Enmark, E., Pettersson, K., Warner, M., & Gustafsson, J. A. (2001). Mechanisms of estrogen action. *Physiological Reviews, 81*, 1535–1565.

O'connor, M. J. (2015). Targeting the DNA damage response in cancer. *Molecular Cell, 60*, 547–560.

Organization, W. H. (2019). International agency for research on cancer.

Paplomata, E., & O'regan, R. (2014). The PI3K/AKT/mTOR pathway in breast cancer: Targets, trials and biomarkers. *Therapeutic Advances in Medical Oncology, 6*, 154–166.

Parida, S., & Sharma, D. (2019a). The microbiome-estrogen connection and breast cancer risk. *Cell, 8*, 1642.

Parida, S., & Sharma, D. (2019b). The power of small changes: Comprehensive analyses of microbial dysbiosis in breast cancer. *Biochimica Et Biophysica Acta. Reviews on Cancer, 1871*, 392–405.

Park, J. H., Jonas, S. F., Bataillon, G., Criscitiello, C., Salgado, R., Loi, S., Viale, G., Lee, H. J., Dieci, M. V., Kim, S. B., Vincent-Salomon, A., Curigliano, G., André, F., & Michiels, S. (2019). Prognostic value of tumor-infiltrating lymphocytes in patients with early-stage triple-negative breast cancers (TNBC) who did not receive adjuvant chemotherapy. *Annals of Oncology, 30*, 1941–1949.

Perez, E. A. (2009). Impact, mechanisms, and novel chemotherapy strategies for overcoming resistance to anthracyclines and taxanes in metastatic breast cancer. *Breast Cancer Research and Treatment, 114*, 195–201.

Powell, J. B., Goode, G. D., & Eltom, S. E. (2013). The aryl hydrocarbon receptor: A target for breast cancer therapy. *Journal of Cancer Therapy, 4*, 1177–1186.

Prall, O. W., Rogan, E. M., Musgrove, E. A., Watts, C. K., & Sutherland, R. L. (1998). C-Myc or cyclin D1 mimics estrogen effects on cyclin E-Cdk2 activation and cell cycle reentry. *Molecular and Cellular Biology, 18*, 4499–4508.

Razavi, P., Chang, M. T., Xu, G., Bandlamudi, C., Ross, D. S., Vasan, N., Cai, Y., Bielski, C. M., Donoghue, M. T. A., Jonsson, P., Penson, A., Shen, R., Pareja, F., Kundra, R., Middha, S., Cheng, M. L., Zehir, A., Kandoth, C., Patel, R., Huberman, K., Smyth, L. M., Jhaveri, K., Modi, S., Traina, T. A., Dang, C., Zhang, W., Weigelt, B., Li, B. T., Ladanyi, M., Hyman, D. M., Schultz, N., Robson, M. E., Hudis, C., Brogi, E., Viale, A., Norton, L., Dickler, M. N., Berger, M. F., Iacobuzio-Donahue, C. A., Chandarlapaty, S., Scaltriti, M., Reis-Filho, J. S., Solit, D. B., Taylor, B. S., & Baselga, J. (2018). The genomic landscape of endocrine-resistant advanced breast cancers. *Cancer Cell, 34*, 427–438.e6.

Rymond, B. (2007). Targeting the spliceosome. *Nature Chemical Biology, 3*, 533–535.

Sharifi-Rad, J., Ozleyen, A., Boyunegmez Tumer, T., Oluwaseun Adetunji, C., El Omari, N., Balahbib, A., Taheri, Y., Bouyahya, A., Martorell, M., Martins, N., & Cho, W. C. (2019). Natural products and synthetic analogs as a source of antitumor drugs. *Biomolecules, 9*, 679.

Sharma, G. N., Dave, R., Sanadya, J., Sharma, P., & Sharma, K. K. (2010). Various types and management of breast cancer: An overview. *Journal of Advanced Pharmaceutical Technology & Research, 1*, 109–126.

Shiao, S. L., Kershaw, K. M., Limon, J. J., You, S., Yoon, J., Ko, E. Y., Guarnerio, J., Potdar, A. A., Mcgovern, D. P. B., Bose, S., Dar, T. B., Noe, P., Lee, J., Kubota, Y., Maymi, V. I., Davis, M. J., Henson, R. M., Choi, R. Y., Yang, W., Tang, J., Gargus, M., Prince, A. D., Zumsteg, Z. S., & Underhill, D. M. (2021). Commensal bacteria and fungi differentially regulate tumor responses to radiation therapy. *Cancer Cell, 39*, 1202–1213.e6.

Shiino, S., Kinoshita, T., Yoshida, M., Jimbo, K., Asaga, S., Takayama, S., & Tsuda, H. (2016). Prognostic impact of discordance in hormone receptor status between primary and recurrent sites in patients with recurrent breast cancer. *Clinical Breast Cancer, 16*, e133–e140.

Sivan, A., Corrales, L., Hubert, N., Williams, J. B., Aquino-Michaels, K., Earley, Z. M., Benyamin, F. W., Lei, Y. M., Jabri, B., Alegre, M. L., Chang, E. B., & Gajewski, T. F. (2015). Commensal Bifidobacterium promotes antitumor immunity and facilitates anti-PD-L1 efficacy. *Science, 350*, 1084–1089.

Smith, A., Pierre, J. F., Makowski, L., Tolley, E., Lyn-Cook, B., Lu, L., Vidal, G., & Starlard-Davenport, A. (2019). Distinct microbial communities that differ by race, stage, or breast-tumor subtype in breast tissues of non-hispanic black and non-hispanic white women. *Scientific Reports, 9*, 11940.

Sung, H., Ferlay, J., Siegel, R. L., Laversanne, M., Soerjomataram, I., Jemal, A., & Bray, F. (2021). Global cancer statistics 2020: GLOBOCAN estimates of incidence and mortality worldwide for 36 cancers in 185 countries. *CA: A Cancer Journal for Clinicians, 71*, 209–249.

Szöőr, Á., Tóth, G., Zsebik, B., Szabó, V., Eshhar, Z., Abken, H., & Vereb, G. (2020). Trastuzumab derived HER2-specific CARs for the treatment of trastuzumab-resistant breast cancer: CAR T cells penetrate and eradicate tumors that are not accessible to antibodies. *Cancer Letters, 484*, 1–8.

Tai, W., Mahato, R., & Cheng, K. (2010). The role of HER2 in cancer therapy and targeted drug delivery. *Journal of Controlled Release, 146*, 264–275.

Thorpe, L. M., Yuzugullu, H., & Zhao, J. J. (2015). PI3K in cancer: Divergent roles of isoforms, modes of activation and therapeutic targeting. *Nature Reviews Cancer, 15*, 7–24.

Tóth, G., Szöllősi, J., Abken, H., Vereb, G., & Szöőr, Á. (2020). A small number of HER2 redirected CAR T cells significantly improves immune response of adoptively transferred mouse lymphocytes against human breast cancer xenografts. *International Journal of Molecular Sciences, 21*, 1039.

Truin, W., Roumen, R. M. H., Siesling, S., Van de Vijver, K. K., Tjan-Heijnen, V. C. G., & Voogd, A. C. (2017). Estrogen and progesterone receptor expression levels do not differ between lobular and ductal carcinoma in patients with hormone receptor-positive tumors. *Breast Cancer Research and Treatment, 164*, 133–138.

Turner, N. C., Slamon, D. J., Ro, J., Bondarenko, I., Im, S. A., Masuda, N., Colleoni, M., Demichele, A., Loi, S., Verma, S., Iwata, H., Harbeck, N., Loibl, S., André, F., Puyana Theall, K., Huang, X., Giorgetti, C., Huang Bartlett, C., & Cristofanilli, M. (2018). Overall survival

with Palbociclib and Fulvestrant in advanced breast cancer. *The New England Journal of Medicine, 379*, 1926–1936.
Urbaniak, C., Cummins, J., Brackstone, M., Macklaim, J. M., Gloor, G. B., Baban, C. K., Scott, L., O'hanlon, D. M., Burton, J. P., Francis, K. P., Tangney, M., & REID, G. (2014). Microbiota of human breast tissue. *Applied and Environmental Microbiology, 80*, 3007–3014.
Vasan, N., Baselga, J., & Hyman, D. M. (2019). A view on drug resistance in cancer. *Nature, 575*, 299–309.
Verweij, J., Clavel, M., & Chevalier, B. (1994). Paclitaxel (Taxol) and docetaxel (Taxotere): Not simply two of a kind. *Annals of Oncology, 5*, 495–505.
Vétizou, M., Pitt, J. M., Daillère, R., Lepage, P., Waldschmitt, N., Flament, C., Rusakiewicz, S., Routy, B., Roberti, M. P., Duong, C. P., Poirier-Colame, V., Roux, A., Becharef, S., Formenti, S., Golden, E., Cording, S., Eberl, G., Schlitzer, A., Ginhoux, F., Mani, S., Yamazaki, T., Jacquelot, N., Enot, D. P., Bérard, M., Nigou, J., Opolon, P., Eggermont, A., Woerther, P. L., Chachaty, E., Chaput, N., Robert, C., Mateus, C., Kroemer, G., Raoult, D., Boneca, I. G., Carbonnel, F., Chamaillard, M., & Zitvogel, L. (2015). Anticancer immunotherapy by CTLA-4 blockade relies on the gut microbiota. *Science, 350*, 1079–1084.
Vitorino, M., Baptista de Almeida, S., Alpuim Costa, D., Faria, A., Calhau, C., & Azambuja Braga, S. (2021). Human microbiota and immunotherapy in breast cancer - A review of recent developments. *Frontiers in Oncology, 11*, 815772.
Waks, A. G., & Winer, E. P. (2019). Breast cancer treatment. *Jama, 321*, 316.
Wang, Q., Guldner, I. H., Golomb, S. M., Sun, L., Harris, J. A., Lu, X., & Zhang, S. (2019a). Single-cell profiling guided combinatorial immunotherapy for fast-evolving CDK4/6 inhibitor-resistant HER2-positive breast cancer. *Nature Communications, 10*, 3817.
Wang, X., Zhang, H., & Chen, X. (2019b). Drug resistance and combating drug resistance in cancer. *Cancer Drug Resistance, 2*, 141–160.
Warmerdam, P. A., Van de Winkel, J. G., Vlug, A., Westerdaal, N. A., & Capel, P. J. (1991). A single amino acid in the second Ig-like domain of the human Fc gamma receptor II is critical for human IgG2 binding. *Journal of Immunology, 147*, 1338–1243.
Wind, N. S., & Holen, I. (2011). Multidrug resistance in breast cancer: From in vitro models to clinical studies. *International Journal of Breast Cancer, 2011*, 967419.
Wong, I. L. K., Wang, X. K., Liu, Z., Sun, W., Li, F. X., Wang, B. C., Li, P., Wan, S. B., & Chow, L. M. C. (2021). Synthesis and evaluation of stereoisomers of methylated catechin and epigallocatechin derivatives on modulating P-glycoprotein-mediated multidrug resistance in cancers. *European Journal of Medicinal Chemistry, 226*, 113795.
World Health Organisation. (2023). *Breast cancer* [online]. https://www.who.int/news-room/fact-sheets/detail/breast-cancer
Xiang, D. B., Zhang, K. Q., Zeng, Y. L., Yan, Q. Z., Shi, Z., Tuo, Q. H., Lin, L. M., Xia, B. H., Wu, P., & Liao, D. F. (2020). Curcumin: From a controversial "panacea" to effective antineoplastic products. *Medicine (Baltimore), 99*, e18467.
Yamamoto, Y., Kanayama, N., Nakayama, Y., & Matsushima, N. (2022). Current status, issues and future prospects of personalized medicine for each disease. *Journal of Personalized Medicine, 12*, 444.
Yang, C., Li, Z., Bhatt, T., Dickler, M., Giri, D., Scaltriti, M., Baselga, J., Rosen, N., & Chandarlapaty, S. (2017). Acquired CDK6 amplification promotes breast cancer resistance to CDK4/6 inhibitors and loss of ER signaling and dependence. *Oncogene, 36*, 2255–2264.
Zakharchenko, O., Greenwood, C., Lewandowska, A., Hellman, U., Alldridge, L., & Souchelnytskyi, S. (2011). Meta-data analysis as a strategy to evaluate individual and common features of proteomic changes in breast cancer. *Cancer Genomics Proteomics, 8*, 1–14.
Zhang, Q. X., Borg, A., Wolf, D. M., Oesterreich, S., & Fuqua, S. A. (1997). An estrogen receptor mutant with strong hormone-independent activity from a metastatic breast cancer. *Cancer Research, 57*, 1244–1249.

Zhang, Y. (2021). The root cause of drug resistance in HER2-positive breast cancer and the therapeutic approaches to overcoming the resistance. *Pharmacology & Therapeutics, 218*, 107677.
Zhong, Z., & Virshup, D. M. (2020). Wnt signaling and drug resistance in cancer. *Molecular Pharmacology, 97*, 72–89.

Mechanisms of Drug Resistance in Breast Cancer

McCabe Michelle, Dineo Disenyane, Benny Mosoane, Aristotelis Chatziioannou, Rodney Hull, and Zodwa Dlamini

Abstract The incidence of breast cancer has increased over the past decades making it the most common cancer in females worldwide. Multidrug resistance (MDR) has been one of the obstacles in decreasing death rates related to breast cancer. This chapter aims to explain the breast cancer subtypes, the underlying molecular mechanisms of development, and common treatment strategies and resistance associated with the various subtypes of breast cancer. This chapter will also shed light on the complexities that prevent effective treatment and identify potential viable drug targets to overcome related drug resistance.

Keywords Mechanisms · Drug resistance · Breast cancer · Trails · Pathways

---

M. Michelle (✉) · D. Disenyane
Department of Anatomical Pathology, Tshwane Academic Laboratory, National Health Laboratory Service, Faculty of Health Sciences, University of Pretoria, Pretoria, South Africa
e-mail: Michelle.Mccabe@nhls.ac.za; dineo.disenyane@nhls.ac.za

B. Mosoane
Department of Anatomical Pathology, National Health Laboratory Service (NHLS), University of Pretoria, Pretoria, South Africa
e-mail: Benny.Mosoane@nhls.ac.za

A. Chatziioannou
Centre of Systems Biology, Biomedical Research Foundation of the Academy of Athens, Athens, Greece
e-mail: achatzi@bioacademy.gr

R. Hull · Z. Dlamini
SAMRC Precision Oncology Research Unit (PORU), DSI/NRF SARChI Chair in Precision Oncology and Cancer Prevention (POCP), Pan African Cancer Research Institute (PACRI), University of Pretoria, Pretoria, South Africa
e-mail: rodney.hull@up.ac.za; zodwa.dlamini@up.ac.za

Z. Dlamini (ed.), *Overcoming Breast Cancer Therapy Resistance*,
https://doi.org/10.1007/978-3-031-52860-6_2

Introduction

Breast cancer (BC) is a highly heterogeneous disease and has been categorized into four main molecular subtypes, based on receptor expression profiles: i.e., (1) increased estrogen receptor (ER) expression (ER-positive [ER+]), (2) high progesterone receptor (PR) expression [PR+], (3) amplified human epidermal growth factor receptor expression [HER2+], and (4) no expression of any of the above receptors, triple-negative BC [TNBC] (The Cancer Genome Atlas, 2012; Orrantia-Borunda et al., 2022). The majority of invasive BC patients (~65–75%) have high ER expression, and the more common subtypes of ER+ BC are the luminal subtypes A and B (Weigelt et al., 2008; Nedeljkovi, 2019; Orrantia-Borunda et al., 2022).

Luminal A subtype represents approximately half of all BC patients and is characterized by concomitant increased ER and PR expressions. This subtype has increased PR levels and low protein Ki-67 levels, tends to have a slow growth rate, and a better prognosis (80% 5-year survival) with a longer time to relapse and treatment failure (Yersal & Barutca, 2014). Decreased PR levels and high Ki-67 levels are associated with the Luminal B subtype, having a poorer prognosis, progressive disease, and shorter time to relapse (The Cancer Genome Atlas, 2012; Nedeljkovi, 2019). Luminal B subtype has poorer outcomes with hormone-targeted (endocrine) therapy when compared to subtype A, however, resistance to this therapy remains a challenge for both subtypes (Yersal & Barutca, 2014; Pradubyat, 2023). The HER2+ subtype is also an aggressive form of BC and contributes to ~20–25% of patients, and shown to mainly benefit from HER2 targeted therapy (Herceptin) (Kreutzfeldt et al., 2020; Orrantia-Borunda et al., 2022). HER2 receptor overexpression triggers various signaling pathways, i.e., Ras/Raf/mitogen-activated protein kinase (MAPK), or PI3K/AKT (Phosphoinositide 3-kinases/ Protein kinase B), increasing cell growth, proliferation, and survival (Ruiz-Saenz et al., 2018; Mezynski et al., 2021). The TNBC subtype (~10–15%) is a highly diverse group and thus far portrays no distinct molecular signatures to assist with more targeted treatment strategies, therefore, limited to conventional chemotherapy and clinical trial drugs (Yin et al., 2020). Common aberrant gene expression profiles associated with TNBC include keratin 17, integrin-B4, MYC, cell cycle regulators CDK6, CCNE1, BRCA2, PTEN, MDM2, and TP53 (Zheng et al., 2023).

A study published by Lehmann et al. in 2011, categorized the TNBC group into seven subtypes based on genetic expression profile. These include the basal-like-1 (BL-1), basal-like-2 (BL2), immunomodulatory (IM), mesenchymal-like (ML), mesenchymal stem like (MSL), luminal androgen receptor, (LAR), and unstable (UNS) (Lehmann et al., 2011). More studies with larger cohorts are needed to further explore Lehmann's subtypes to comprehensively characterize and effectively treat TNBC according to specific molecular subtypes (Asleh et al., 2022). Another subtype known as the claudin-low BC subtype, has recently emerged as an additional independent group, described by a lack of genomic instability and mutations, low cell proliferation rates, and increased immune cells and stroma infiltration (Curtis et al., 2012; Sabatier et al., 2014). These breast tumors are reported to be mostly TNBC, ranging from 1.5% to 14% of BC tumors in various cohorts (Pereira et al., 2016) (Fig. 1).

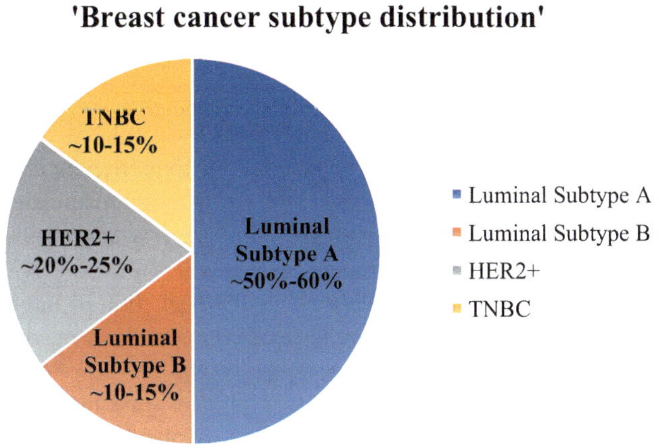

Fig. 1 Distribution of BC subtypes: Hormone receptor-positive (HR+) BC comprises Luminal subtype A (~50–60%) and Luminal subtype B (10–15%) of BC patients. HER2+ BC contributes to 20–25% of BC patients. The TNBC subtype is a highly diverse group with no unique underlying molecular alterations, contributing to ~10–15% of BC patients

Treatment

Standard of care for BC stages I, II, or III are routinely treated with surgery, followed by radiation and if necessary, systemic drug therapy, dependent on the subtype (hormone receptor-positive, HER2-positive, tumor grade, growth rate—Ki-67 index), overall patient health, and pre- or post-menopause status (Kroep & Wilma, 2020). Conventional chemotherapy for the treatment of BC includes anthracyclines, i.e., doxorubicin, epirubicin, taxanes—paclitaxel and docetaxel, Cyclophosphamide—Cytoxan, 5-fluorouracil (5-FU), and Platinum agents—cisplatin and carboplatin. Metastatic BC treatment includes chemotherapy using taxanes, anthracyclines, Ixabepilone, Eribulin, platinum agents, Capecitabine, and Gemcitabine (Andreopoulou & Sparano, 2013). Combination drug chemotherapy is often used to treat early BC, and advanced BC with single chemotherapy drugs (Fisusi & Akala, 2019; Kroep & Wilma, 2020). BC patients with overexpressed hormone receptors are treated with targeted hormone therapy (e.g., tamoxifen and aromatase inhibitor), whereas HER2+ BC will be treated with chemo and monoclonal antibody drugs trastuzumab, with or without pertuzumab (Montagna & Colleoni, 2019; Orrantia-Borunda et al., 2022). BC with a hormone receptor-positive subtype, HER2 negative status, and a BRCA mutation are treated with a PARP inhibitor, olaparib (Lynparza) to increase survival rates (Cortesi et al., 2021). Immunotherapy is another treatment option for BC that expresses the protein PD-L1, including metastatic BC (mBC) (Stage IV) and inflammatory breast cancer (IBC), where immunotherapy drug pembrolizumab is administered (Han et al., 2020; Kreutzfeldt et al., 2020). Treatment for recurrent BC is dependent on the cancer site it reoccurs in, and the initial therapy administered. Different treatment strategies are then provided to the patient, either hormone, targeted, immunotherapy, chemotherapy, or a combination of these after surgery and/or radiation.

Genetic and Molecular Mechanisms Contributing to Drug Resistance

Drug resistance accounts for approximately 90% of cancer-related deaths. Multidrug resistance (MDR) leads to relapse and metastasis due to inefficient chemotherapeutic drug targets. Resistance to drugs can be innate or acquired. Innate resistance is often seen in patients before the administration of therapy, and in the majority of cases due to mutations in key resistance-associated genes, the proliferation of existing insensitive cancer stem cell populations, or the activation of integral signaling pathways that protect the cell from external toxic compounds from entering the cell. Acquired resistance is mainly due to oncogene activation, genetic and epigenetic mutations leading to aberrant gene expression profiles, and tumor microenvironment (TME) alterations. Various mechanisms are involved in the development of drug resistance in BC, and more research is needed to highlight key molecular events and factors involved in overcoming resistance in BC cells. Molecular pathways thus far shown to be involved in the resistance of BC to current therapeutic strategies include the epidermal growth factor receptor (EGFR), RAS/RAF/MAPK, PI3K/Akt/mTOR, and Wnt/beta-catenin signaling pathways (Xu et al., 2020; Mezynski et al., 2021; Glaviano et al., 2023). Additional factors illustrated to contribute to treatment resistance include increased expression of drug efflux pumps (reduces the uptake of chemo into the cell), cancer stem cells (CSCs) (self-renewing cancer cells), genetic and epigenetic alterations of tumor suppressor genes (TP53), DNA repair genes (BRCA1/2), enhanced DNA and senescence escape and drug metabolism genes have also been shown to be associated with treatment resistance (Vaidya et al., 2022). Through the intricate and complex molecular mechanisms involved in cancer development, cancer cells develop various escaping methods to avoid cell death initiated by first-line treatments. This chapter focuses on the main molecular signaling pathways shown to be involved in BC development and resistance and highlights potential therapeutic approaches to overcome the challenge of drug resistance and improve BC patient outcomes.

Molecular Pathways

Hormone Receptor Pathway

Overactivated estrogen signaling correlates with the hormone receptor-positive (ER+) BC pathway, which accounts for approximately 75% of tumors. Anti-estrogen therapy (e.g., tamoxifen and raloxifene) is the standard of care for ER+ BC and has proven effective in preventing the development of BC in postmenopausal women with raised estrogen levels (Montagna & Colleoni, 2019; Ozyurt & Ozpolat, 2022). Resistance to this therapy however is a common problem, mainly due to factors such as estrogen receptor expression changes, ESR1 gene mutations, and increased PI3K signaling (Dustin et al., 2019; Ozyurt & Ozpolat, 2022). Estrogen receptor alpha (ERα), is a nuclear receptor that binds to estrogen (E2), and is involved in regulating the transcription of the genes involved in the cell cycle regulation, including Cyclin D1, MYC, BCL2 FOXM1, and CXCL12 (Harbeck et al., 2019). E2 binds to ERα, dimerizes, and becomes conformationally active, translocating to the nucleus to form a complex with activator protein 1 (AP1) and nuclear receptor corepressor (CoR) (Fig. 2). The activated receptor then binds to and regulates the transcription of many target genes involved in cell growth and differentiation (Frasor et al., 2003). Dysregulation of ERα expression therefore plays an

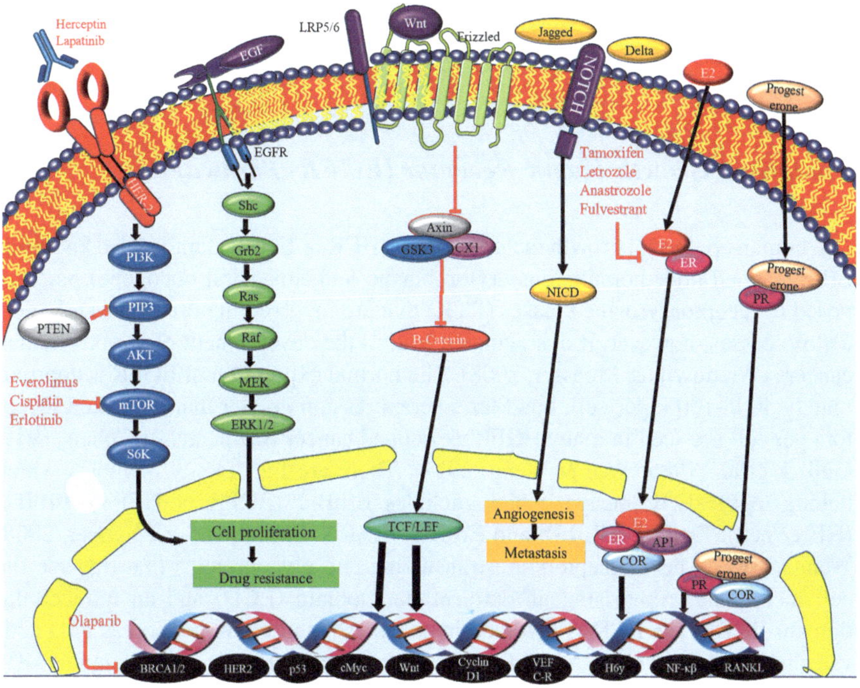

Fig. 2 Molecular mechanisms in the development of breast cancer and drug resistance. Many molecular pathways play a role in the development of BC as well as in innate and acquired resistance mechanisms to therapy. The EGFR/HER/ErbB family are receptor tyrosine kinases (RTK), and upon activation through EGFR-specific ligands, dimerize with other EGFR receptors (homodimerization) or family members (hetero-dimerization), resulting in activating conformational changes. EGFR recruits HER2, HER3, and HER4 in heterodimers, initiating intracellular TK activity, causing a cascade of intracellular mitotic signaling leading to multiple genes transcribed which are involved in cell proliferation, differentiation, cell cycle, apoptosis, cell survival, and migration. Activating EGFR (HER1/ErB1) can also stimulate alternative signaling pathways, i.e., PI3K/Akt/mTOR, RAS/RAF/MAPK, c-Jun N-terminal kinase (JNK), phospholipase C-gamma (PLCγ), and signal transducers and activators of transcription (STAT) pathway. ERα is activated by E2 and becomes conformationally active, translocates into the nucleus to form a complex with AP1 and CoR, and regulates many genes involved in the cell cycle, proliferation, and apoptosis. Cross-signaling between these pathways is common in drug-resistant mechanisms of BC

important role in the development of the majority of BC (luminal subtypes). The second estrogen receptor, ERβ, is homologous to ERα and can be stimulated by estrogen, but with a different affinity and a contradictory role of inhibiting proliferation and inducing cell dell (Mal et al., 2020). ERβ expression in some BC studies has even shown a more favorable prognosis linked to this subtype, however, contrary findings from other studies are also shown (Austin et al., 2018; Choi, 2022). More research is required to elucidate and understand the role of Erβ in BC.

Further development of new therapy strategies, including cyclin-dependent kinases, PI3K inhibitors, and selective estrogen receptor degraders (SERDs), is needed in ER+ BC patients and treatment resistance (Patel et al., 2023). Understanding the estrogen pathway and the physiological role of all the factors involved is critical for effective treatment innovative drug development and improvement of hormone receptor cancers.

Epidermal Growth Factor Receptor (EGFR) Pathway

The human epidermal growth factor receptor (HER or EGFR) family, also known as ErbB (named after homologous erythroblastic leukemia viral oncogene), is composed of receptor tyrosine kinases (RTK) that are involved in normal physiological cell processes, however, if dysregulated lead to the development of various human cancers (Wieduwilt & Moasser, 2008). The normal expression of EGFR is approximately 40 k–100 k per cell, however, overexpression greater than 1 million receptors per cell are seen in many EGFR associated cancer (Carpenter & Cohen, 1979; Gullick et al., 1986; Wee & Wang, 2017). There are four family members which belong to the ErB lineage, which includes ErbB-1 (EGFR or HER1), ErbB-2 (HER2/neu), ErbB-3 (HER3), and ErbB-4 (HER4) (Wieduwilt & Moasser, 2008; Wang, 2017). These receptors are transmembrane glycoproteins that traverse the cell membrane, comprising an extracellular domain (ECD) and an intracellular domain (ICD). The ECD is involved in specific ligand binding whereas ICD activates intracellular TK's. The EGFR extracellular domains consist of domains I-IV, with domain II particularly involved in homo- and hetero-dimerization formation with ErbB/HER RTK family members.

The intracellular domain (ICD), when phosphorylated or activated through ligand binding, regulates EGFR downstream signaling pathways. This occurs through the phosphorylation of 3 threonine/serine sites (Thr-654/Thr-669/Ser-671), and it has been shown when protein kinase C (PKC) phosphorylates Thr-654, it inhibits further kinase activity and EGFR-ligand binding (Aifa et al., 2006). EGFR-specific ligands include epidermal growth factor (EGF), heparin-binding EGF [HBEGF], transforming growth factor (TGF), epigen (EPG), epiregulin (EPR), amphiregulin (AR), and betacellulin (BTC) (Sanders et al., 2013). Upon binding, a conformational change of the receptor occurs, and EGFR can recruit HER2, HER3, and HER4 in heterodimers, initiating intracellular TK activity. This causes a cascade of intracellular mitotic signaling leading to the regulation of various genes involved in cell growth, proliferation, differentiation, cell cycle, apoptosis, cell survival, and migration. Activating EGFR (HER1/ErB1) also stimulates alternate signaling pathways, such as, i.e., the PI3K/Akt, Ras/Raf/MAPK, JNK, phospholipase C-gamma (PLCγ), and signal transducers and activators of transcription (STAT) pathway (Fig. 2) (Lemmon & Schlessinger, 2010; Appert-Collin et al., 2015). EGFR overexpression is linked to many cancers, including BC, non-small cell lung cancer, colon, ovarian, and head and neck cancer (Wang, 2017). In BC, EGFR overactivation is associated with larger tumor size, heterogeneous/complex phenotype, and poor clinical outcomes, more frequently seen in TNBC and inflammatory BC (IBC) (Ellis, 2004; Rakha et al., 2007). EGFR overexpression in BC is associated with metastasis, recurrence, and decreased survival. In one study, EGFR overexpression resulted in increased lung metastatic rates in BC compared to lower EGFR expression (Appert-Collin et al., 2015).

EGFR drug targets, i.e., tyrosine inhibitors (TKI) (e.g., lapatinib) and monoclonal antibodies (mAbs) (e.g., cetuximab, trastuzumab, and panitumumab) have been developed to target overexpressing EGFR tumors and shown to regain chemosensitivity in TNBC by reactivating apoptotic signaling networks (El Guerrab et al., 2016; Maennling et al., 2019). Downstream or parallel pathway signaling is another mechanism for the resistance to EGFR-directed therapies, including the activation of the PI3K/AKT pathway which stimulates cancer cell survival through activation of HER3 (Wieduwilt & Moasser, 2008). Additional factors such as EGFR sensitizing mutations (e.g., exon 19 deletion) and resistance mutations (T790M) to EGFR-TKIs, need to be taken into consideration and screened before initiating TKI or mAb treatment (Westover et al., 2018; Fu et al., 2022). Intrinsic and extrinsic resistance to EGFR-targeted therapies however remain a huge problem in effectively treating BC patients, and more research is required in the area of drug resistance in BC (Wheeler et al., 2008; Westover et al., 2018).

Cancer immunotherapy has become one of the most effective and promising treatment strategies in treatment-resistant BC, these include immune checkpoint blockade therapy, chimeric antigen receptor T cell (CAR-T), anti-cancer vaccines, and bispecific antibody (BsAb) antitumor immunotherapy (Khan et al., 2021; Gupta et al., 2022; Vafaei et al., 2022). BsAb therapy has become increasingly promising as it effectively targets immune effector cells and tumor cells and at the same time blocks two different oncogenic mediators (Han et al., 2017). More inhibitors targeting multiple kinases in the various signal transducing pathways are needed to overcome the challenge of drug resistance in the fight against BC and to overcome less toxic combination therapies.

Ras/Raf/MAPK Pathway

This pathway is activated by multiple growth factor (GF) ligands, hormones, stress signals, and mitogens binding to TK receptors, which play a pivotal part in cell proliferation, survival, and drug resistance in BC (McCubrey et al., 2007). Mutations in proto-oncogenes (e.g., Ras and B-Raf) or upstream EGFR, have been shown to cause aberrant constitutive signaling. The activation of Ras GTPase is the most important event in this pathway and is initiated by EGFR-ligand dimerization (Joneson & Bar-Sagi, 1997; Cargnello & Roux, 2011). This leads to tyrosine residue phosphorylation in the carboxyl terminus of the receptor, which recruits the growth factor binding protein 2 (Grb2) (Fig. 2). Grb2 consists of a SH2 domain flanked by two SH3 domains, and the N-terminal SH3 (nSH3) domain which binds the guanine nucleotide exchange factor, son of sevenless (SOS) (Li et al., 2001). SOS is then positioned adjacent to membrane-bound Ras, which activates the exchange of guanosine diphosphate (GDP) to guanosine-5′- triphosphate (GTP).

GTP-Ras subsequently activates Raf kinase, PI3K, and other signal transducing molecules. Activated Raf activates downstream MAPK enzyme kinase (MEK) and extracellular signal-regulated kinase (ERK), to phosphorylate and activate molecules involved in many cell processes, including proliferation and apoptosis (Santarpia et al., 2012). Raf has also been shown to play a role in doxorubicin and paclitaxel drug resistance in BC cells. Ras, Raf, MEK, and ERK1/2 downstream effector inhibitor molecules in combination therapies would perhaps prove clinically relevant, and inhibit the activation of survival signaling or enhance anti-proliferation processes. (McCubrey et al., 2007). Phosphorylated ERK1/2 could also serve as an effective biomarker to assist in predicting the success of ERK1/2 inhibitors. Emerging evidence suggests that these inhibitors could be useful in combination with apoptotic and cell cycle pathway inhibitors, such as Bcl-2 and heat shock protein (HSP) inhibitors (Chatterjee & Burns, 2017; Sugiura et al., 2021).

PI3K/Akt/mTOR Pathway

The PI3K/Akt/mTOR pathway also plays an important role in cell proliferation, survival, invasion, migration, apoptosis, and DNA repair (He et al., 2021). Its over-activation in cancer has also been linked to chemo- and targeted therapy resistance in BC (Dong et al., 2021). A negative regulator of PI3K includes the phosphatase and tensin homolog (PTEN), which dephosphorylates phosphatidylinositol (3,4,5)-tri-phosphate (PIP3) to PIP2, and downregulates AKT and other cell proliferation mediators (Fig. 2) (Liu et al., 2009). The activation of Akt phosphorylates PRAS40, in turn, activates the mammalian target of rapamycin complex 1 (mTORC1) and 40S ribosomal protein S6 kinase 1 (S6K1), which is involved in cell metabolism, anabolic growth, and protein synthesis (Saxton & Sabatini, 2017). Mutations in HER receptors, PI3K, Akt, as well as PTEN downregulation, have been correlated with an overactive PI3K/Akt/mTOR signaling pathway (Yuan & Cantley, 2008). Somatic variants in Phosphatidylinositol-4,5-bisphosphate 3-kinase catalytic subunit alpha (PIK3CA) occur in approximately 40% of ER+ and HER2- BC patients and the HER1–4 TK receptor signaling by various ligands also have been shown to lead to PI3K/AKT activation (Zardavas et al., 2014; Rasti et al., 2022). mTOR inhibitor, Rapamycin, and new mTOR inhibitors have been developed with better pharmacological and pharmacokinetic properties, and are available as potential inhibitors targeting this pathway (Lee et al., 2015). Oral mTOR inhibitor, everolimus, is administered to postmenopausal women with HR+ BC (Vilar et al., 2011).

The PI3K/Akt/mTOR pathway has also been associated with hormone therapy resistance, and Akt can independently trigger the ER pathway, without the need for estrogen. It is thought that mTOR inhibitors in combination with hormone therapy can overcome this treatment resistance (Alves & Ditzel, 2023). BOLERO-2 clinical trial assessed everolimus (EVE) plus exemestane (EXE) in postmenopausal women with advanced stage HR+ BC, who had disease progression or relapse aromatase inhibitor (AI) drugs. The results showed by adding EVE, significant improvement in progression-free survival in BC patients occurred (Piccart et al., 2014). Further research is required to discover new methods to completely inhibit mTOR catalytic activity and mTOR signaling and the metabolic network in cancer.

IL-6/JAK/STAT Pathway

Janus kinases (JAKs) and downstream signal transducers and activators of transcription (STAT) proteins are essential components of the interleukin-6 (IL-6)/JAK/STAT cytokine signaling, the pathway for tissue homeostasis, and also cancer development (Wehde et al., 2018). Activation of this pathway has been linked to EGFR overexpression in BC tumors (Rah et al., 2022). Metastatic BC (mBC) has also been shown to be regulated by uncontrolled inflammatory cells (chemokines, cytokines, and GFs) in the tumor microenvironment (TME) to promote tumor progression and escape immunity (Bates et al., 2018). Pro-inflammatory cytokines, such as IL-6 are secreted at increased levels in BC patients and mediate crosstalk between the TME and tumor cells. IL-6 modulates STAT3 target genes, which includes the cell cycle and apoptosis-regulating genes cyclin D1, Bcl-2, Bcl-xL, and VEGF (Fukada et al., 1996; Leslie et al., 2006). IL-6 signaling is facilitated through IL6 binding to a soluble form of IL-6Rα (sIL-6Rα), which recruits the transmembrane gp130, and activates downstream signaling which regulates certain immune responses (Mullberg et al., 1993; Riethmueller et al., 2016), These IL-6 induced inflammatory responses have also been linked to therapeutic resistance, angiogenesis, and poor clinical outcomes (DeMichele et al., 2009; Chalaris et al., 2011; Lo et al., 2011). Mutations in the *IL-6* promoter sequence have been linked with increased IL-6 levels and correlate with ER+ BC with poor prognoses (DeMichele et al., 2009). IL-6/JAK/STAT3 signaling is known to upregulate BC stem cells, leading to treatment resistance and metastasis. IL-6 is highly expressed in treatment-resistant BC cells, and chemoresistance mechanisms through upregulation of drug-resistant gene, MDR1 was demonstrated in BC cells (Conze et al., 2001). In addition, IL-6 inflammation has also been shown to activate resistance to trastuzumab in HER2+ BC cells (Korkaya et al., 2013). Based on these findings, IL-6/JAK/STAT3 is an actionable therapeutic target to sensitize tumor cells in therapy-resistant breast cancer.

WNT/β-Catenin Signaling Pathway

β-Catenin is a key factor in the canonical Wnt signaling pathway, which binds to E-cadherin for cell-cell adhesion in the cytoplasm (Xu et al., 2020). Wnt signaling remains in an off state when no extracellular Wnts are present. Cytoplasmic β-Catenin is degraded by the complex comprised mainly of adenomatous polyposis coli (APC), Axin, and glycogen synthase kinase 3β (GSK-3β) (Fig. 2). β-Catenin is first phosphorylated by GSK-3β at sites Thr41, Ser37, and Ser33, creating the recognition site for F-box protein β-TrCP ($SCF^{\beta\text{-}TrCP}$) ubiquitination and degradation. In the nucleus, histone deacetylases (HDACs) interact with TCF and LEF1, which form a complex to suppress Wnt target gene expression (Daniels & Weis, 2002). Wnt signaling is induced by Wnt ligands binding to the receptor Frizzleds (Fzds) and their coreceptors LRP5/6. Membrane E3 ligase ZNRF3 and RNF43 are important tumor suppressors by endorsing the degradation of Wnt receptors. Stem cell growth factor R-spondin proteins (RSPO1–4) are ZNRF3 and RNF43 opponents and induce auto-ubiquitination, removal of ZNRF3/RNF43 from the membrane, and Fzd ubiquitination. (Hao et al., 2012) GSK-3 and CK1 phosphorylates LRP6, which binds Axin, and Fzds binds Disheveled (Dvl), disassociating the destruction complex, promoting constitutive Wnt signaling (Davidson et al., 2005; Xu et al., 2020). Mutations in genes ZNRF3/RNF43 and recurrent translocations of RSPO2/RSPO3 are commonly seen in this pathway and have been seen in various cancers (Hao et al., 2016).

Invasive ductal carcinoma (IDC) and invasive lobular carcinoma (ILC) are the most common histological subtypes of BC, accounting for 70 ~ 75% and 10 ~ 14%, respectively (Harbeck et al., 2019). Most IDCs show membranous (~80%) and nuclear (~12%) β-Catenin expression, whereas ILCs lack membranous (~15%) and nuclear (0%) expression (Geyer et al., 2011). IDCs have been associated with a worse prognosis compared to ILCs, and convenes resistance to many cancer therapeutic strategies, through cancer stem cells, DNA repair mechanism, increased anti-apoptotic protein expressions (e.g., MYC), and MDR genes (Xu et al., 2020). Although Wnt pathogenic variants are not seen commonly in BC, approximately 50% of BC show increased levels of disheveled expression and stabilized β-catenin. A poor prognosis is seen in approximately 80% of BC and is associated with a lack of Frizzled-related protein 1 (FRP1) (Feng et al., 2018). Major mechanisms of drug resistance include epithelial-mesenchymal transition (EMT) and cancer stem cell (CSC) production (Zhong & Virshup, 2020). In BC, Wnt1 has been shown to upregulate Twist and promote the EMT-like phenotype SNAIL. (Takebe et al., 2011, Mani et al., 2008). Other Wnt targets, including ABCB1, CD44, CD24, and CD133, are also associated with CSC and resistance (Kahn & Kim, 2014; Martin-Orozco et al., 2019; Wang et al., 2020). In the TNBC subtype, increased β-catenin expression has been correlated with chemotherapy resistance (Merikhian et al., 2021).

Hedgehog Signaling Pathway

Hedgehog (Hh) signaling is involved in the cellular processes of organogenesis during fetal and postnatal development, including cellular proliferation, differentiation, and stem cell renewal in adult mammalian cells (Gupta et al., 2010). Stem cells have primary cilia (PC) which project from the cell's surface into the extracellular environment. PC is packed with a variety of receptors involved in Hh and Wnt signaling. Hh main role players include ligands, Sonic hedgehog (SHh), Indian Hedgehog (IHh) and Desert hedgehog (DHh), receptors Patched (PTCH) and Smoothened (SMO), suppressor of fused protein (SUFU), and glioma-associated oncogene (GLI) transcription factors (Skoda et al., 2018). In the absence of Hh ligand binding, the PTCH receptor remains localized at the base on the plasma membrane of the PC and suppresses the activity of receptor SMO, by transporting an SMO agonist molecule outside of the cell, preventing the activation of SMO located on the intracellular endosome membrane of PC (Fig. 3). In the event of Hh ligand binding to PTCH, the PTCH-Hh complex delocalizes and internalizes into the cell's cytoplasm where it becomes degraded by lysosomes. The SMO agonist now freely accumulates inside the cell and actives the SMO receptor, which transits to the plasma membrane where it signals downstream components to activate the GLI transcription factor, signaling the detachment of the SUFU–GLI structure, allowing its translocation into the nucleus, activating the transcription of Hh genes, i.e., *GLI* and *PTCH*.

Hh signaling has been shown to activate stemness and EMT of BC cells, through alternative mechanisms such as mutations in Hh target genes constitutive signaling (ligand-independent), autocrine signaling (Hh ligands produced by and responded to the same tumor cells), and paracrine signaling (Hh ligands produced by tumor cells to surrounding stroma cells, promoting growth and survival) (Scales & de Sauvage, 2009). Hh signaling has also been shown to be activated through crosstalk with alternative pathways, such as PI3K/AKT and Wnt signaling pathways, and these cancers reported to be linked to poor prognosis and endocrine treatment resistance in HR+ and TNBC (Bhateja et al., 2019). Clinical trials are currently evaluating the combination of targeted chemotherapy to frizzled receptors, including SMO inhibitors in treating treatment-resistant BC patients (Carballo et al., 2018; Landeros et al., 2023).

Notch Signaling Pathway

NOTCH signaling is a highly conserved pathway and comprised of a family of four notch receptors: NOTCH1–4 (Kumar et al., 2016). These are type-1 transmembrane proteins consisting of an ECD, binding (DLL1, 4, or Jagged 1, 2, Delta/Serrate/LAG-2 (DSL)) family ligands through juxtacrine signaling, and an intracellular transcriptional activation domain (TAD), allowing activation when in complex with

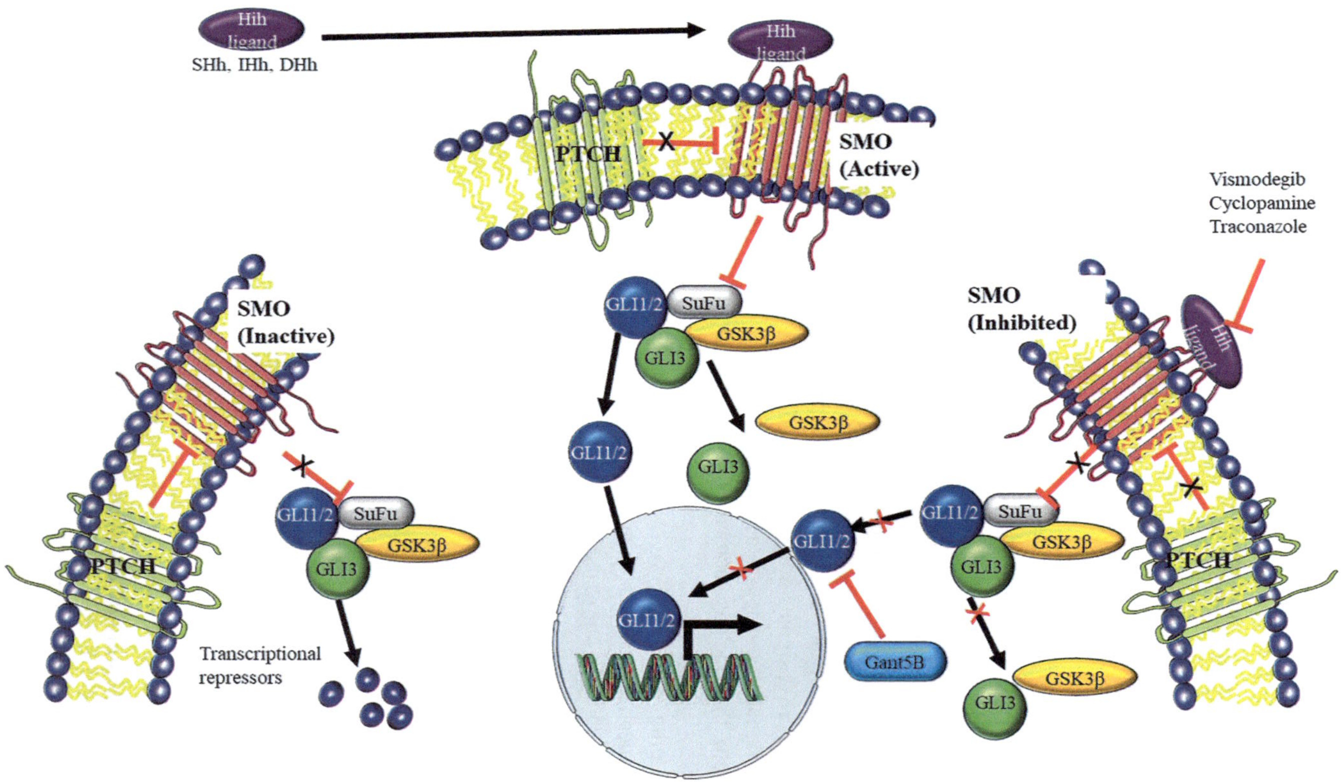

Fig. 3 Hedgehog signaling pathway. This image depicts the Hh signaling pathway in 3 states. (1) Off state: No Hh ligand binding, PTCH localizes in the membrane, suppresses, and prevents SMO activity. (2) On state: Hh ligand binds to PTCH, SMO becomes active and signals the Suppressor of fused (SUFU) to release glioma-associated oncogene homolog proteins (GLIs). GLI then translocates to the nucleus mediating the transcription of Hh target genes. (3) Drug target SMO inhibitor (e.g., vismodegib) inhibits SMO activity and prevents Hh target gene transcription

transcription factors (Fig. 2). Two mechanisms have been reported through which Notch signaling can be activated, (1) through adjacent ligand interaction or 2) Deltex activated endocytosis (Yamamoto et al., 2010). The precursor NOTCH receptor is transported to the endoplasmic reticulum (ER) where its ECD subunits are glycosylated for high-affinity binding to various ligands. It is then transported to the Golgi for S1 cleavage, producing a mature Notch heterodimer receptor protein which then moves to the plasma membrane on the cell surface (Zhou et al., 2022). Ligands that bind to this receptor are produced by a different cell and mediate metalloprotease (ADAM10) S2 proteolytic cleavage of NOTCH. NOTCH is then ready for S3 cleavage by gamma (γ)-secretase, and the NOTCH intracellular domain (NICD) is released into the cytoplasm where it translocates into the nucleus, forming important complexes with transcriptional activators, facilitating the many downstream NOTCH target gene expressions (Aster et al., 2017). Non-canonical signaling can also be mediated by Deltex, by causing non-ligand bound NOTCH receptors to be endocytosed into a gamma enzyme containing endosomes (ADAM), triggering S2 and S3 cleavage, and in turn triggering NOTCH signaling (Conner, 2016). NICD has also been shown to crosstalk with signaling pathways such as NF-κB, mTORC, TGF-β, AKT, and Wnt, to regulate target gene transcription (Xia et al., 2022). Targeting ECD glycosylation as well as posttranslational modifications of NICD (e.g., methylation, acetylation, and phosphorylation) is thought to be an effective strategy in drug development in inhibiting NOTCH signaling in BC, and further studies on the crosstalk of the Notch switchboard in multiple pathways is required to gain a deeper understanding to target this pathway (Antfolk et al., 2019).

Aryl Hydrocarbon Receptor

The Aryl Hydrocarbon Receptor (AhR) is a member of the basic helix-loop-helix/Per-Arnt-Sim (Bhlh/PAS) family and is involved in regulating different developmental processes, including the growth of the mammary gland. When AhR is unbound, it binds to two Hsp90 molecules in the cytosol, prostaglandin E synthase 3 (p23), and a molecule of hepatitis B virus X-associated protein 2 (XAP-2) (Stevens et al., 2009). When ligands bind to AhR, they become active. AhR mRNA in BC is overexpressed when compared to healthy tissues and therefore serves as a possible drug treatment target (Mohamed et al., 2019). AhR has also been shown to act as a tumor suppressor through the regulation of tumor suppressor-type miRNA (Paris et al., 2021). It has been shown that AhR inhibits cell proliferation through crosstalk with the ER and AhR inhibitor molecules prevent tumor invasion and metastasis in the TNBC subtype which is resistant to hormone treatment (Campbell et al., 2018).

Inducible Nitric Oxide Synthase

Inducible Nitric Oxide Synthase (iNOS) is an important facilitator of inflammation and generates nitric oxide (NO) from L-arginine. It is being implicated in numerous pathologies, including cancer, when overexpressed or dysregulated (Cinelli et al., 2020). There are three NOS isoforms, namely, neuronal NOS (nNOS), inducible NOS (iNOS), and endothelial NOS (eNOS) (Vanini et al., 2015). NOS converts into free radical nitric oxide (NO) when changing L-arginine to L-citrulline, and some studies illustrate a double role (oncogenic and tumor suppressive) in cancer. NO is concentration-dependent (Sheetal Korde Choudhari et al., 2013). Decreased NO levels in BC cells demonstrated ERK and hypoxia-induced factor one alpha (HIF-1α) activation caused tumor progression (Thomas et al., 2004). Increased concentrations of NO can lead to p53 activation, which leads to programmed cell death. NO has also been revealed to react with oxygen-free radicals and lead to peroxynitrite production, which subsequently can cause drug resistance (Bulut et al., 2005; Loibl et al., 2005; Glynn et al., 2010).

Preclinical and Clinical Trials in Breast Cancer

Drug repurposing is a process utilizing drugs already approved by the FDA, for new conditions that could potentially prove effective in resistance, stem cellness, and metastasis in cancer patients. Various drugs and interventions, i.e., antibiotics (Salinomycin), CAR-T cells, polymeric nanoparticles, immunotherapies, bispecific monoclonal antibodies targeting various cancer surface receptors, compounds targeting aldehyde dehydrogenase (ALDH1), SOX2 (SRY-box transcription factor 2), MYC, etc., which regulate pluripotency and cell stemness are currently being trialed. Table 1 illustrates current clinical trials with new drug and biological targets in treatment-resistant BC.

In one clinical trial (NTC01869192), the administration of docetaxel followed by capecitabine with anthracycline instead of fluorouracil (FU), showed significantly improved disease-free survival in TNBC patients, with no new severe side effects (Li et al., 2020). Capecitabine is a cancer drug that enzymatically converts to (FU) in tumor cells, where it inhibits DNA synthesis and tumor growth, through the RANK/RANKL protein expression pathway (Shao et al., 2022a). This drug in combination with standard-of-care chemotherapy shows promise as a novel therapeutic target.

In the management of HR+ BC, endocrine therapy in combination or standalone initially shows a pathological response, however, this effect decreases as resistance to treatment develops. Many studies have shown the interaction of estrogen with angiogenic pathways, which leads to treatment insensitivity. Clinical trial studies are, therefore, looking at antiangiogenesis and antiestrogenesis combination-type therapies.

Table 1 Clinical trial studies of therapeutic compounds directed against resistant, recurrent, and metastatic breast cancer

Clinical trial reference number (clinicaltrials.org)	Study title	Conditions	Drug/Biological/Intervention	Phase/Status	Reference
NCT01869192	Phase II trial for large ER- negative breast cancers.	Malignant breast neoplasm	Drugs: Epirubicin, cyclophosphamide, docetaxel, Capecitabine	Phase2 Completed	(Li et al., 2020)
NCT05075512	The efficacy and safety of Anlotinib combined with Fulvestrant in patients with advanced breast cancer.	Breast neoplasm	Drugs: Anlotinib, Fulvestrant	Phase2 Active	(Qian et al., 2022; Shao et al., 2022b)
NCT04504747	Real-time molecular analysis of breast cancer receiving neo-adjuvant chemotherapy.	Breast cancer	Molecular analysis of blood and tumor	Observational Recruiting	(Cui et al., 2021)
NCT02915445	EpCAM CAR-T for treatment of advanced solid tumors.	Breast cancer, recurrent	Biological: EpCAM CAR-T cells	Phase I Recruiting	(Cui et al., 2021)
NCT03065621	Neoadjuvant biomarker research study of Palbociclib combined with endocrine therapy in estrogen receptor positive/HER2 negative breast cancer (NeoRHEA).	Breast cancer	Drugs: Palbociclib, Capecit	Phase2 Completed	(Agostinetto et al., 2023)
NCT03323346	Phase II trial of disulfiram with copper in metastatic breast cancer.	Breast neoplasm female Metastatic breast cancer	Drug: Disulfiram	Phase 2, Recruiting	(Nasrollahzadeh et al., 2021; Deng et al., 2022)
NCT05452213	Comprehensive analysis of spatial, temporal and molecular patterns of Ribociclib efficacy and resistance in advanced breast cancer patients.	Breast neoplasm, Breast cancer, HER2-, ER+, PR+, Advanced breast cancer	Drug: Ribociclib	Phase 4, Recruiting	(Fasching et al., 2023)
NCT00002826	Drug resistance inhibition in treating women with recurrent or metastatic breast cancer.	Breast cancer	Drugs: Paclitaxel, Valspodar	Phase 2 completed	(Gadag et al., 2020)

(continued)

Table 1 (continued)

Clinical trial reference number (clinicaltrials.org)	Study title	Conditions	Drug/Biological/Intervention	Phase/Status	Reference
NCT03162627	Selumetinib and Olaparib in solid tumors.	Malignant breast neoplasm	Drugs: Selumetinib, Olaparib	Phase 1 Active	(Giudice et al., 2022)
NCT00238290	Trastuzumab and Letrozole in treating postmenopausal women with progressive advanced breast cancer.	Breast cancer	Drugs: Trastuzumab, Letrozole	Phase 2 completed	(Koeberle et al., 2011)
NCT00077363	Capecitabine and Tipifarnib in treating women with Taxane-resistant metastatic breast cancer.	Recurrent breast cancer Stage IV breast cancer	Drugs: Tipifarnib, Capecitabine	Phase 2 completed	(Li et al., 2012)
NCT04879888	Personalized vaccine for cancer immunotherapy.	Breast cancer female	Biological: Peptide pulsed dendritic cell	Phase 1 completed	(Fritah et al., 2022)
NCT01723774	PD 0332991 and Anastrozole for Stage 2 or 3 Estrogen receptor positive and HER2 negative breast cancer.	Breast neoplasms	Drugs: PD0332991, Anastrozole, Goserelin	Phase 2 Active	(Bagegni et al., 2017)
NCT01992952	Fulvestrant +/– Akt inhibition in advanced aromatase inhibitor resistant breast cancer.	ER+ breast cancer	Drugs: AZD5363, Fulvestrant	Phase 1 and Phase 2 Active	(Jones et al., 2020)
NCT00428896	A feasibility study with Iressa in resistant cytokeratin-positive tumor cells circulating in the blood of women with breast cancer.	Breast cancer	Drug: ZD1839	Phase 2 Complete	(Kalykaki et al., 2014; Gunzer et al., 2016)
NCT00694252	Lapatinib and Circulating Tumor Cells in Breast Cancer	Metastatic breast cancer	Drug: Lapatinib	Phase 2 Complete	(Agelaki et al., 2015)
NCT01953588	Fulvestrant and/or Anastrozole in treating postmenopausal patients with stage II-III breast cancer undergoing surgery.	ER+ breast cancer HER2-breast cancer Invasive ductal breast Cancer	Drugs: Fulvestrant, anastrozole	Phase 3 Active	(Ma et al., 2020)

Clinical trial reference number (clinicaltrials.org)	Study title	Conditions	Drug/Biological/Intervention	Phase/Status	Reference
NCT02444390	Molecular alterations associated with resistance to endocrine therapy and impacting treatment with mTOR inhibitor.	Procedure: Biopsy	The predictive value of p4EBP1 for an mTOR inhibitor	Phase N/A Complete	(Bachelot et al., 2019)
NCT00217399	Sorafenib and Anastrozole in treating postmenopausal women with metastatic breast cancer.	Recurrent breast cancer Stage IV breast cancer	Drugs: Sorafenib tosylate, anastrozole	Phases 1 and 2 Complete	(Moreno-Aspitia, 2010; Zhu & Zhou, 2015)
NCT02860000	Alisertib with or without Fulvestrant in treating patients with locally advanced or metastatic, endocrine-resistant breast cancer.	Estrogen receptor status HER2/Neu-, invasive, stage III, IIIa, IIIb, IIIc, IV	Drugs: Alisertib, Fulvestrant	Phase 2 Active	(Haddad et al., 2018, 2023)
NCT01231659	Safety and efficacy of RAD001 (Everolimus) in combination with Letrozole in the treatment of postmenopausal women with locally advanced or metastatic breast cancer.	Postmenopausal women Locally advanced metastatic breast cancer	Drugs: Everolimus, Letrozole	Phase 2 Complete	(Safra et al., 2018)
NCT02690480	Fulvestrant (F) + placebo vs F + Palbociclib first line for postmenopausal hormone receptor+ advanced breast cancer.	Breast neoplasms	Drugs: PD-0332991 (Palbociclib), Fulvestrant	Phase 2 Active	(Albanell et al., 2022)
NCT05455619	Evexomostat plus Alpelisib and Fulvestrant in women with the PIK3CA mutation with HR+/Her2- breast cancer.	HR+/HER2 Breast cancer Metastatic breast cancer	Drug: Evexomostat	Phase 2 Recruiting	(Cornelius et al., 2023)

(continued)

Table 1 (continued)

Clinical trial reference number (clinicaltrials.org)	Study title	Conditions	Drug/Biological/Intervention	Phase/Status	Reference
NCT02049957	Safety and efficacy study of Sapanisertib in combination with Exemestane or Fulvestrant in postmenopausal women with estrogen receptor positive/human epidermal growth factor receptor 2 negative (ER+/HER2-) metastatic breast cancer.	Breast cancer	Drugs: Sapanisertib, Fulvestrant, Exemestane	Phase 2 Complete	(Lim et al., 2021)
NCT01310231	A trial of standard chemotherapy with metformin (vs placebo) in women with metastatic breast cancer.	Metastatic breast cancer	Drugs: Metformin	Phase 2 Complete	(Pimentel et al., 2019)
NCT01670500	Cisplatin vs. doxorubicin/cyclophosphamide in BrCa.	Breast cancer	Drugs: Cisplatin, cyclophosphamide, doxorubicin	Phase 2 Active	(Tung et al., 2020)
NCT00031681	7-Hydroxystaurosporine and irinotecan hydrochloride in treating patients with metastatic or Unresectable solid tumors or triple-negative breast cancer (currently accruing only triple-negative breast cancer patients since 6/8/2007).	ER- breast Cancer	Drugs: 7-hydroxystaurosporine, irinotecan hydrochloride	Phase 2 Complete	(Fracasso et al., 2011)
NCT03829436	TPST-1120 as monotherapy and in combination with Nivolumab in subjects with advanced cancers.	Triple negative breast cancer	Drugs: Part 1 TPST-1120. Part 2 TPST-1120 + nivolumab. Part 3 TPST-1120	Phase 1 Complete	(Yarchoan et al., 2022)
NCT05700669	Study to assess safety and efficacy of AsiDNA in combination with Olaparib in participants with recurrent solid tumors.	Breast cancer	Drugs: AsiDNA, Olaparib	Phase 1 Recruiting	No results or preliminary data are available.

Clinical trial reference number (clinicaltrials.org)	Study title	Conditions	Drug/Biological/Intervention	Phase/Status	Reference
NCT04925284	Study of XB002 in subjects with solid tumors (JEWEL-101).	Triple-negative breast cancer Hormone receptor-positive breast Cancer	Drugs: XB002, Nivolumab, bevacizumab	Phase 1 Recruiting	(Johnson et al., 2022)
NCT02671097	Drug–drug interaction study using Rosuvastatin as a breast cancer-resistant protein (efflux transporter), organic anion-transporting polypeptide (OATP)1B1, and OATP1B3 (uptake transporters) probe substrate.	Healthy volunteers Pharmacokinetics Drug interaction	Drugs: Rosuvastatin, BAY1841788 (ODM-201)	Phase 1 Complete	(Zurth et al., 2022)
NCT00001383	A phase I study of Infusional paclitaxel with the P-glycoprotein antagonist PSC 833.	Breast cancer	Drugs: PSC 833, paclitaxel	Phase 1 Complete	(Nunes et al., 2021)
NCT02811497	A phase 1b trial of ATRC-101 in adults with advanced solid malignancies.	ER+ breast cancer HER2- breast cancer	Drugs: Azacitidine, Durvalumab	Phase 2 Complete	(Taylor et al., 2020)
NCT04244552	A phase 1b trial of ATRC-101 in adults with advanced solid malignancies.	Breast cancer	Biologicals: ATRC-10, Pembrolizumab Drug: Pegylated liposomal doxorubicin (PLD)	Phase 1 active	(Benjamin et al., 2020)

(continued)

Table 1 (continued)

Clinical trial reference number (clinicaltrials.org)	Study title	Conditions	Drug/Biological/Intervention	Phase/Status	Reference
NCT02009449	A phase 1 study of Pegilodecakin (LY3500518) in participants with advanced solid tumors.	Breast cancer	Drugs: Pegilodecakin, paclitaxel/ docetaxel, carboplatin/cisplatin, FOLFOX, gemcitabine/ nab-paclitaxel, Capecitabine, Pazopanib, Pembrolizumab, Paclitaxel, nivolumab, gemcitabine/carboplatin	Phase 1 active	(Naing et al., 2019)
NCT05585034	Phase 1, first-in-human, dose-finding, and expansion study to evaluate XmAb®808 in combination with Pembrolizumab in advanced solid tumors.	Triple-negative breast cancer	Biological: XmAb®808 Biological: Pembrolizumab	Phase 1, Recruiting	(Matossian et al., 2023)
NCT03454451	CPI-006 alone and in combination with Ciforadenant and with Pembrolizumab for patients with advanced cancers.	Triple-negative breast cancer	Drugs: CPI-006, CPI-006 + ciforadenant, CPI-006 + pembrolizumab	Phase 1, Active	(Luke et al., 2019)
NCT03517488	A study of XmAb®20,717 in subjects with selected advanced solid tumors.	Breast carcinoma	Biological: XmAb20717	Phase 1 Complete	(Shum et al., 2020)

Anlotinib is a new multitarget TKI drug, that inhibits various cytokine and growth factor receptors (GFR) such as vascular endothelial (VEGFR), fibroblast (FGFR), and platelet-derived growth factor receptors (PDGFR), and cytokine receptor c-kit (Shen et al., 2018). Early phase trials of anlotinib are effective with mono- and combination treatment regimens in advanced BC. A phase II study of anlotinib therefore aims to evaluate the efficacy and safety of anlotinib combined with hormone therapy (Qian et al., 2022; Shao et al., 2022b). Chimeric antigen receptor (CAR) T cell immunotherapy, utilizing a patient's immune cells to fight cancer cells, has been effective in the treatment of hematological cancers. Treating solid tumors, however, has proved to be more difficult, due to factors such as heterogeneity, TME, and EMT. More recently through research focused on tumor cell antigens, CARs have been modified to improve the specificity of solid tumor targeting. Epithelial cell adhesion molecule (EpCAM) is a cell surface protein that has been found overamplified in BC and linked with tumor growth, metastasis, and treatment resistance (Spizzo et al., 2003). Studies have shown inhibiting EpCAM has antitumor effects on BC cells, and the drug catumaxomab (EpCAM target) has been approved as a cancer therapeutic agent (Eyvazi et al., 2018). The fusion protein (EpCAM-CAR-T) targeting EpCAM on tumor cells, has also demonstrated improved tumor-inhibiting capability, inducing increased cytokine response and apoptotic cancer cell effects. (Zhou et al., 2019) An early phase I trial (NCT02915445) is currently being conducted in recurrent BC patients to study its effect on cancer cells (Cui et al., 2021).

Valspodar is a drug that inhibits P-glycoprotein and has been shown to increase the influx of mitoxantrone significantly and contributes greatly to efflux-mediated multidrug resistance (MDR) in cancer cells. Paclitaxel has also shown improved effectiveness in a clinical trial with MDR-BC patients pre-treated with valspodar (NCT00002826).

Ribociclib (CDK4/6 inhibitor) in combination with hormone therapy is a conventional first-line treatment regimen for advanced HR+ and HER2- BC, as it has consistently demonstrated significant overall survival (OS) compared to standalone hormone therapy. Intrinsic and extrinsic resistance to CDK4/6 inhibitors however is common, and predictive biomarkers in treatment response are also important factors in overcoming treatment resistance. An extensive study to identify and validate biomarkers pre-treatment and for the duration of the ribociclib clinical trial will also be conducted (NCT03065621).

Preclinical studies of selumetinib (MEK inhibitor) in combination with olaparib *(polyadenosine 5′-diphosphoribose polymerase (PARP) enzyme inhibitor)*, potentially show by targeting certain pathway targets (e.g., PI3K and MEK/ERK/MAPK) may improve PARP's effectiveness and maintain antitumor activity. The SOLAR clinical trial is an early phase trial combining these two drugs in solid tumors (including BC), to alter and reduce DNA damage repair, and the progression of mutant cells in these pathways (NCT03162627).

The biological Peptide pulsed Dendritic cell is used in the trial NCT04879888 to assess the response of neoantigen vaccines in BC patients, and the immunogenicity and safety of the vaccine.

Lapatinib is another drug that has shown effective in decreasing HER2−/+ circulating tumor cells (CTCs) in mBC patients, which suggests ongoing molecular alteration monitoring of CTCs during treatment with targeted agents could assist in early detection of pre-resistance to certain targets (NCT00694252).

RAF inhibitor, Sorafenib tosylate used in combination with aromatase inhibitors (AI) (anastrozole), may inhibit resistance before or after it occurs, by upregulation of cRAF and MAPK signaling, caused by CDK10 silencing (NCT00217399).

In another clinical trial (NCT01310231), metformin in combination with standard chemotherapy did not show any significant effect on the population regarding response, progression-free survival (PFS), or OS. The results demonstrated metformin administered in combination with standard chemotherapy in non-diabetic mBC patients was not effective.

An early phase (1b/2) open-label multicenter clinical trial will be conducted to assess the safety, tolerability, antitumor effect, pharmacokinetics, and dynamics of AsiDNA in combination with olaparib in recurrent BC patients (NCT05700669). Eligible patients are those whose tumors had advanced on receiving PARP therapy before. No preliminary data is available for this trial as yet.

Another clinical trial (NCT00238290) evaluates the combination of the drugs, trastuzumab, and letrozole, in suggesting that resistance to AI drugs such as letrazole and trastuzumab can be overcome in a fraction of BC patients by combining these two treatments. Preclinical data seems to show promise for a non-chemotherapy treatment strategy for a portion of HR+ and HER2+ BC patients.

Drugs, Tipifarnib, and Capecitabine most common severe toxicities experienced included neutropenia, nausea, vomiting, and neutropenia. Tipifarnib in combination with capecitabine did not prove more effective than capecitabine monotherapy in mBC patients treated before with anthracyclines or taxanes (NCT00077363).

The drug, ZD1839, based on preclinical data, demonstrates promise as a new BC treatment strategy in eliminating resistant cytokeratin-positive circulating tumor cells (occult tumor cells) (NCT00428896).

A phase I trial (NCT02009449) using several drugs in various combinations, including pegilodecakin (pegylated IL-10), paclitaxel, docetaxel, carboplatin, cisplatin, FOLFOX, capecitabine, zazopanib, pembrolizumab, nivolumab, and gemcitabine. In this study, pegilodecakin with anti-PD-1 monoclonal antibodies demonstrated a controllable safety and tolerability profile, and favorable antitumor effect, potentially providing an effective new treatment strategy for BC patients whose tumors have progressed when alternative cancer therapies.

Challenges and Limitations in Targeting Molecular Pathways

Although several therapeutic strategies have been developed to target stem cells, thus far no effective treatment exists, and greater efforts focusing on this area are needed to overcome the challenge of resistance in BC. The challenge with molecular mechanisms in cancer includes crosstalk and activation of alternative signaling pathways, increasing drug efflux pump regulation, a TME that comprises stromal cells, tumor-associated macrophages (TAMs) that protect cancer cells from the harmful effects of chemotherapy, and stiffness of the extracellular matrix in solid tumors are all challenging factors. Treatment strategies under investigation include using combination therapies that target multiple pathways and mechanisms, in the context of synthetic lethality, that inhibit important effector molecules in key cellular processes. Identifying biomarkers early in the course of treatment is also an essential issue to consider, in effective patient response prediction to targeted therapies.

Conclusion

The efficacy of targeted drugs to combat treatment resistance will include a combination type approach that includes stress-targeted drugs by targeting cellular stress responses and multiple signaling pathways, and comprehensive biomarker screening to direct appropriate targeted therapies. Further molecular characterization of the TNBC group, in addition to the alternative groups is required to gain deeper insights to improve molecular classification, identify key genes, develop more effective targeted treatment strategies, enhance and overcome the challenge of drug resistance with current treatment practices of hormone and anti-HER2 therapy in BC patients.

References

Agelaki, S., et al. (2015). Efficacy of lapatinib in therapy-resistant HER2-positive circulating tumor cells in metastatic breast cancer. *PLoS One, 10*(6), 1–16. https://doi.org/10.1371/journal.pone.0123683

Agostinetto, E., et al. (2023). Primary efficacy analyses of NeoRHEA, the neoadjuvant biomarker research study of palbociclib combined with endocrine therapy in estrogen receptor-positive/HER2 negative breast cancer. *Journal of Clinical Oncology, 41*(16_suppl), 522–522. https://doi.org/10.1200/jco.2023.41.16_suppl.522

Aifa, S., et al. (2006). Phosphorylation of Thr654 but not Thr669 within the juxtamembrane domain of the EGF receptor inhibits calmodulin binding. *Biochemical and Biophysical Research Communications, 347*(2), 381–387. https://doi.org/10.1016/j.bbrc.2006.05.200

Albanell, J., et al. (2022). Randomized phase II study of fulvestrant plus palbociclib or placebo in endocrine-sensitive, hormone receptor-positive/HER2–advanced breast cancer: GEICAM/2014–12 (FLIPPER). *European Journal of Cancer, 161*, 26–37. https://doi.org/10.1016/j.ejca.2021.11.010

Alves, C. L., & Ditzel, H. J. (2023). Drugging the PI3K/AKT/mTOR pathway in ER+ breast cancer. *International Journal of Molecular Sciences, 24*(5), 1–17. https://doi.org/10.3390/ijms24054522

Andreopoulou, E., & Sparano, J. (2013). Chemotherapy in patients with Anthracycline- and Taxane-pretreated metastatic breast cancer: An overview. *Current Breast Cancer Reports, 5*(1), 42–50. https://doi.org/10.1007/s12609-012-0097-1.Chemotherapy

Antfolk, D., et al. (2019). Decoding the PTM-switchboard of notch. *Biochimica et Biophysica Acta - Molecular Cell Research. Elsevier, 1866*(12), 118507. https://doi.org/10.1016/j.bbamcr.2019.07.002

Appert-Collin, A., et al. (2015). Role of ErbB receptors in cancer cell migration and invasion. *Frontiers in Pharmacology, 6*, 1–10. https://doi.org/10.3389/fphar.2015.00283

Asleh, K., Riaz, N., & Nielsen, T. O. (2022). Heterogeneity of triple negative breast cancer: Current advances in subtyping and treatment implications. *Journal of Experimental and Clinical Cancer Research. BioMed Central, 41*(1), 1–26. https://doi.org/10.1186/s13046-022-02476-1

Aster, J. C., Pear, W. S., & Blacklow, S. C. (2017). The varied roles of notch in cancer. *Annual Review of Pathology: Mechanisms of Disease, 12*, 245–275. https://doi.org/10.1146/annurev-pathol-052016-100127

Austin, D., et al. (2018). Estrogen receptor-beta is a potential target for triple negative breast cancer treatment. *Oncotarget, 9*(74), 33912–33930. https://doi.org/10.18632/oncotarget.26089

Bachelot, T. D., et al. (2019). mTORC1 activation assessed in metastatic sample to predict outcome in patients with metastatic breast cancer treated with everolimus-exemestan: Results from the SAFIRTOR study. *Journal of Clinical Oncology, 37*(15_suppl), 1024–1024. https://doi.org/10.1200/jco.2019.37.15_suppl.1024

Bagegni, N. A., et al. (2017). Phase II trial of neoadjuvant (neo) palbociclib (Palbo) plus anastrozole (ana) in endocrine resistant clinical stage 2/3 estrogen receptor positive and HER2 negative (ER+ HER2-) breast cancer (BC). *Journal of Clinical Oncology*, 35–38. https://doi.org/10.1200/JCO.2017.35.15

Bates, J. P., et al. (2018). Mechanisms of immune evasion in breast cancer. *BMC Cancer, 18*(556), 1–14. https://doi.org/10.1007/s00262-019-02443-4

Benjamin, J. E., et al. (2020). First-in-human phase Ib study of ATRC-101, an engineered version of a patient-derived antibody targeting a tumor-restricted ribonucleoprotein complex. *Journal of Clinical Oncology, 38*(15_suppl), TPS3168–TPS3168. https://doi.org/10.1200/jco.2020.38.15_suppl.tps3168

Bhateja, P., et al. (2019). The hedgehog signaling pathway: A viable target in breast cancer? *Cancers, 11*(8), 1126. https://doi.org/10.3390/cancers11081126

Bulut, A. S., et al. (2005). Significance of inducible nitric oxide synthase expression in benign and malignant breast epithelium: An immunohistochemical study of 151 cases. *Virchows Archiv, 447*(1), 24–30. https://doi.org/10.1007/s00428-005-1250-2

Campbell, P. S., et al. (2018). AhR ligand aminoflavone suppresses α6-integrin–Src–Akt signaling to attenuate tamoxifen resistance in breast cancer cells. *Journal of Cellular Physiology, 234*(1), 108–121. https://doi.org/10.1002/jcp.27013

Carballo, G. B., et al. (2018). 'A highlight on sonic hedgehog pathway', *cell communication and signaling. Cell Communication and Signaling, 16*(1), 1–15. https://doi.org/10.1186/s12964-018-0220-7

Cargnello, M., & Roux, P. P. (2011). Activation and function of the MAPKs and their substrates, the MAPK-activated protein kinases. *Microbiology and Molecular Biology Reviews, 75*(1), 50–83. https://doi.org/10.1128/mmbr.00031-10

Carpenter, G., & Cohen, S. (1979). Epidermal growth factor. *Annual review of biochemistry, 48*(1), 193–216.

Chalaris, A., et al. (2011). 'The soluble interleukin 6 receptor: Generation and role in inflammation and cancer. *European Journal of Cell Biology Elsevier GmbH, 90*(6–7), 484–494. https://doi.org/10.1016/j.ejcb.2010.10.007

Chatterjee, S., & Burns, T. F. (2017). Targeting heat shock proteins in cancer: A promising therapeutic approach. *International Journal of Molecular Sciences, 18*(9), 1978. https://doi.org/10.3390/ijms18091978

Choi, Y. (2022). Estrogen receptor β expression and its clinical implication in breast cancers: Favorable or unfavorable? *Journal of Breast Cancer, 25*(2), 75–93. https://doi.org/10.4048/jbc.2022.25.e9

Cinelli, M. A., et al. (2020). Inducible nitric oxide synthase: Regulation, structure, and inhibition. *Medicinal Research Reviews, 40*(1), 158–189. https://doi.org/10.1002/med.21599

Conner, S. D. (2016). *Regulation of notch signaling through intracellular transport, international review of cell and molecular biology*. Elsevier Inc. https://doi.org/10.1016/bs.ircmb.2015.12.002

Conze, D., Weiss, L., Regen, P. S., Bhushan, A., Weaver, D., Johnson, P., & Rincón, M. (2001). Autocrine production of interleukin 6 causes multidrug resistance in breast cancer cells. *Cancer Research, 61*(24), 8851–8858.

Cornelius, P., et al. (2023). The Amelia-1 study: A phase 1b/2 trial of evexomostat (SDX-7320) plus fulvestrant and alpelisib in patients with advanced breast cancer at risk for alpelisib-induced hyperglycemia. *Journal of Clinical Oncology, 41*(16_suppl), TPS1129–TPS1129. https://doi.org/10.1200/jco.2023.41.16_suppl.tps1129

Cortesi, L., Rugo, H. S., & Jackisch, C. (2021). An overview of PARP inhibitors for the treatment of breast cancer. *Targeted Oncology. Springer International Publishing, 16*(3), 255–282. https://doi.org/10.1007/s11523-021-00796-4

Cui, X., et al. (2021). CAR-T therapy: Prospects in targeting cancer stem cells. *Journal of Cellular and Molecular Medicine, 25*(21), 9891–9904. https://doi.org/10.1111/jcmm.16939

Curtis, C., et al. (2012). The genomic and transcriptomic architecture of 2,000 breast tumours reveals novel subgroups. *Nature, 486*(7403), 346–352. https://doi.org/10.1038/nature10983

Daniels, D. L., & Weis, W. I. (2002). ICAT inhibits β-catenin binding to tcf/lef-family transcription factors and the general coactivator p300 using independent structural modules. *Molecular Cell, 10*(3), 573–584. https://doi.org/10.1016/S1097-2765(02)00631-7

Davidson, G., et al. (2005). Casein kinase 1γ couples Wnt receptor activation to cytoplasmic signal transduction. *Nature, 438*(7069), 867–872. https://doi.org/10.1038/nature04170

DeMichele, A., et al. (2009). Host genetic variants in the interleukin-6 promoter predict poor outcome in patients with estrogen receptor-positive, node-positive breast cancer. *Cancer Research, 69*(10), 4184–4191. https://doi.org/10.1158/0008-5472.CAN-08-2989

Deng, X., et al. (2022). Editorial: Triple-negative breast cancer: Heterogeneity, tumor microenvironment and targeted therapy. *Frontiers in Oncology, 12*, 21–23. https://doi.org/10.3389/fonc.2022.1026566

Dong, C., et al. (2021). Activation of PI3K/AKT/mTOR pathway causes drug resistance in breast cancer. *Frontiers in Pharmacology, 12*, 1–16. https://doi.org/10.3389/fphar.2021.628690

Dustin, D., Gu, G., & Fuqua, S. A. W. (2019). ESR1 mutations in breast cancer. *Cancer, 125*, 3714–3728. https://doi.org/10.1002/cncr.32345

El Guerrab, A., et al. (2016). Anti-EGFR monoclonal antibodies and EGFR tyrosine kinase inhibitors as combination therapy for triple-negative breast cancer. *Oncotarget, 7*(45), 73618–73637. https://doi.org/10.18632/oncotarget.12037

Ellis, L. M. (2004). Epidermal growth factor receptor in tumor angiogenesis. *Hematology/Oncology Clinics of North America, 18*(5), 1007–1021. https://doi.org/10.1016/j.hoc.2004.06.002

Eyvazi, S., et al. (2018). Antibody based EpCAM targeted therapy of cancer, review and update. *Current Cancer Drug Targets, 18*(9), 857–868. https://doi.org/10.2174/1568009618666180102102311

Fasching, P. A., et al. (2023). CAPTOR-BC: Comprehensive analysis of spatial, temporal and molecular biomarkers predicting response and resistance to first-line treatment with ribociclib + ET in HR+, HER2- advanced breast cancer. *Journal of Clinical Oncology, 41*(16_suppl), TPS1124–TPS1124. https://doi.org/10.1200/jco.2023.41.16_suppl.tps1124

Feng, Y., et al. (2018). Breast cancer development and progression: Risk factors, cancer stem cells, signaling pathways, genomics, and molecular pathogenesis. *Genes and Diseases. Elsevier Ltd, 5*(2), 77–106. https://doi.org/10.1016/j.gendis.2018.05.001

Fisusi, F. A., & Akala, E. O. (2019). Drug combinations in breast cancer therapy. *Pharmaceutical Nanotechnology, 7*(1), 3–23. https://doi.org/10.2174/2211738507666190122111224

Fracasso, P. M., et al. (2011). A phase 1 study of UCN-01 in combination with irinotecan in patients with resistant solid tumor malignancies. *Cancer Chemotherapy and Pharmacology, 67*(6), 1225–1237. https://doi.org/10.1007/s00280-010-1410-1

Frasor, J., et al. (2003). Profiling of estrogen up- and down-regulated gene expression in human breast cancer cells: Insights into gene networks and pathways underlying estrogenic control of proliferation and cell phenotype. *Endocrinology, 144*(10), 4562–4574. https://doi.org/10.1210/en.2003-0567

Fritah, H., et al. (2022). The current clinical landscape of personalized cancer vaccines. *Cancer Treatment Reviews, 106*, 102383. https://doi.org/10.1016/j.ctrv.2022.102383

Fu, K., et al. (2022). Therapeutic strategies for EGFR-mutated non-small cell lung cancer patients with osimertinib resistance. *Journal of Hematology and Oncology. BioMed Central., 15*(1), 1–32. https://doi.org/10.1186/s13045-022-01391-4

Fukada, T., et al. (1996). Two signals are necessary for cell proliferation induced by a cytokine receptor gp130: Involvement of STAT3 in anti-apoptosis. *Immunity, 5*(5), 449–460. https://doi.org/10.1016/S1074-7613(00)80501-4

Gadag, S., et al. (2020). Combination therapy and nanoparticulate systems: Smart approaches for the effective treatment of breast cancer. *Pharmaceutics, 12*(6), 1–37. https://doi.org/10.3390/pharmaceutics12060524

Geyer, F. C., et al. (2011). B-catenin pathway activation in breast cancer is associated with triple-negative phenotype but not with CTNNB1 mutation. *Modern Pathology. United States & Canadian Academy of Pathology, 24*(2), 209–231. https://doi.org/10.1038/modpathol.2010.205

Giudice, E., et al. (2022). PARP inhibitors resistance: Mechanisms and perspectives. *Cancers, 14*(6), 1–15. https://doi.org/10.3390/cancers14061420

Glaviano, A., et al. (2023). PI3K / AKT/ mTOR signaling transduction pathway and targeted therapies in cancer. *Molecular Cancer. BioMed Central, 22*(1), 1–37. https://doi.org/10.1186/s12943-023-01827-6

Glynn, S. A., et al. (2010). Increased NOS2 predicts poor survival in estrogen receptor-negative breast cancer patients. *Journal of Clinical Investigation, 120*(11), 3843–3854. https://doi.org/10.1172/JCI42059

Gullick, W. J., et al. (1986). Expression of epidermal growth factor receptors on human cervical, ovarian, and vulval carcinomas. *Cancer Research, 46*(1), 2998607.

Gunzer, K., et al. (2016). A phase II study of afatinib, an irreversible ErbB family blocker, added to letrozole in patients with estrogen receptor-positive hormone-refractory metastatic breast cancer progressing on letrozole. *SpringerPlus. Springer International Publishing, 5*(1), 1–12. https://doi.org/10.1186/s40064-015-1601-7

Gupta, S., Takebe, N., & Lorusso, P. (2010). Review: Targeting the hedgehog pathway in cancer. *Therapeutic Advances in Medical Oncology, 2*(4), 237–250. https://doi.org/10.1177/1758834010366430

Gupta, S. L., et al. (2022). Immunotherapy: An alternative promising therapeutic approach against cancers. *Molecular Biology Reports Springer Netherlands, 49*(10), 9903–9913. https://doi.org/10.1007/s11033-022-07525-8

Haddad, T. C., et al. (2018). Phase i trial to evaluate the addition of alisertib to fulvestrant in women with endocrine-resistant, ER+ metastatic breast cancer. *Breast Cancer Research and Treatment Springer US, 168*(3), 639–647. https://doi.org/10.1007/s10549-017-4616-7

Haddad, T. C., et al. (2023). Evaluation of alisertib alone or combined with Fulvestrant in patients with endocrine-resistant advanced breast cancer. *JAMA Oncology, 9*(6), 815. https://doi.org/10.1001/jamaoncol.2022.7949

Han, X., et al. (2017). Recent advances of bispecific antibodies in solid tumors. *Journal of Hematology & Oncology, 10*(1), 1–16. https://doi.org/10.1186/s13045-017-0522-z

Han, Y., Liu, D., & Li, L. (2020). PD-1/PD-L1 pathway: Current research in cancer. *American Journal of Cancer Research, 10*(3), 727–742. http://www.ncbi.nlm.nih.gov/pubmed/32266087

Hao, H. X., Jiang, X., & Cong, F. (2016). Control of Wnt receptor turnover by R-spondin-ZNRF3/RNF43 signaling module and its dysregulation in cancer. *Cancers, 8*(6), 1–12. https://doi.org/10.3390/cancers8060054

Hao, H. X., et al. (2012). ZNRF3 promotes Wnt receptor turnover in an R-spondin-sensitive manner. *Nature. Nature Publishing Group, 485*(7397), 195–202. https://doi.org/10.1038/nature11019

Harbeck, N., et al. (2019). Breast cancer. *Nature Reviews Disease Primers, 5*(1), 66. https://doi.org/10.1038/s41572-019-0111-2

He, Y., et al. (2021). Targeting PI3K/Akt signal transduction for cancer therapy. *Signal Transduction and Targeted Therapy. Springer US, 6*(1), 425. https://doi.org/10.1038/s41392-021-00828-5

Johnson, M., et al. (2022). A first-in-human phase 1 study of the safety and pharmacokinetics of XB002 in patients with inoperable locally advanced or metastatic solid tumors. *Cancer Research, 82*(12_Supplement), CT254. https://doi.org/10.1158/1538-7445.am2022-ct254

Jones, R. H., et al. (2020). Fulvestrant plus capivasertib versus placebo after relapse or progression on an aromatase inhibitor in metastatic, oestrogen receptor-positive breast cancer (FAKTION): A multicentre, randomised, controlled, phase 2 trial. *The Lancet Oncology*. The Author(s). Published by Elsevier Ltd. This is an Open Access article under the CC BY 4.0 license, *21*(3), 345–357. https://doi.org/10.1016/S1470-2045(19)30817-4

Joneson, T., & Bar-Sagi, D. (1997). Ras effectors and their role in mitogenesis and oncogenesis. *Journal of Molecular Medicine, 75*(8), 587–593. https://doi.org/10.1007/s001090050143

Kahn, M., & Kim, Y. (2014). The role of the Wnt signaling pathway in cancer stem cells: Prospects for drug development. *Research and Reports in Biochemistry, 4*(1), 1–12. https://doi.org/10.2147/rrbc.s53823

Kalykaki, A., et al. (2014). Elimination of EGFR-expressing circulating tumor cells in patients with metastatic breast cancer treated with gefitinib. *Cancer Chemotherapy and Pharmacology, 73*(4), 685–693. https://doi.org/10.1007/s00280-014-2387-y

Khan, M., Maker, A. V., & Jain, S. (2021). The evolution of cancer immunotherapy. *Vaccine, 9*(6), 614. https://doi.org/10.3390/vaccines9060614

Koeberle, D., et al. (2011). Combination of trastuzumab and letrozole after resistance to sequential trastuzumab and aromatase inhibitor monotherapies in patients with estrogen receptor-positive, HER-2-positive advanced breast cancer: A proof-of-concept trial (SAKK 23/03). *Endocrine-Related Cancer, 18*(2), 257–264. https://doi.org/10.1530/ERC-10-0317

Korkaya, H., et al. (2013). Activation of an IL-6 Inflammatory Loop Mediates Trastuzumab Resistance in HER2 Overexpressing Breast Cancers by Expanding the Cancer Stem Cell Population Hasan. *Molecular Cell, 47*(4), 570–584. https://doi.org/10.1016/j.molcel.2012.06.014.Activation

Kreutzfeldt, J., et al. (2020). The trastuzumab era: Current and upcoming targeted HER2+ breast cancer therapies. *American Journal of Cancer Research, 10*(4), 1045–1067. http://www.ncbi.nlm.nih.gov/pubmed/32368385%0A, http://www.pubmedcentral.nih.gov/articlerender.fcgi?artid=PMC7191090

Kroep, Y. M. V. D. S. J. R., & Wilma, R. A. E. M. T. (2020). Chemotherapy resistance and stromal targets in breast cancer treatment: A review. *Molecular Biology Reports Springer Netherlands, 47*(10), 8169–8177. https://doi.org/10.1007/s11033-020-05853-1

Kumar, R., Juillerat-Jeanneret, L., & Golshayan, D. (2016). Notch antagonists: Potential modulators of cancer and inflammatory diseases. *Journal of Medicinal Chemistry, 59*(17), 7719–7737. https://doi.org/10.1021/acs.jmedchem.5b01516

Landeros, N., Castillo, I., & Pérez-Castro, R. (2023). Preclinical and clinical trials of new treatment strategies targeting cancer stem cells in subtypes of breast cancer. *Cell, 12*(5), 1–27. https://doi.org/10.3390/cells12050720

Lee, J. J. X., Loh, K., & Yap, Y. S. (2015). PI3K/Akt/mTOR inhibitors in breast cancer. *Cancer Biology and Medicine, 12*(4), 342–354. https://doi.org/10.7497/j.issn.2095-3941.2015.0089

Lehmann, B. D., et al. (2011). Identification of human triple-negative breast cancer subtypes and preclinical models for selection of targeted therapies. *Journal of Clinical Investigation, 121*(7), 2750–2767. https://doi.org/10.1172/JCI45014

Lemmon, M. A., & Schlessinger, J. (2010). Cell signaling by receptor tyrosine kinases. *Cell, 141*(7), 1117–1134. https://doi.org/10.1016/j.cell.2010.06.011

Leslie, K., et al. (2006). Cyclin D1 is transcriptionally regulated by and required for transformation by activated signal transducer and activator of transcription 3. *Cancer Research, 66*(5), 2544–2552. https://doi.org/10.1158/0008-5472.CAN-05-2203

Li, J., et al. (2020). Adjuvant capecitabine with docetaxel and cyclophosphamide plus epirubicin for triple-negative breast cancer (CBCSG010): An open-label, randomized, multicenter, phase III trial. *Journal of Clinical Oncology, 38*(16), 1774–1784. https://doi.org/10.1200/JCO.19.02474

Li, S., et al. (2001). Tyrosine phosphorylation of Grb2 by Bcr/Abl and epidermal growth factor receptor: A novel regulatory mechanism for tyrosine kinase signaling. *EMBO Journal, 20*(23), 6793–6804. https://doi.org/10.1093/emboj/20.23.6793

Li, T., et al. (2012). A phase II trial of capecitabine in combination with the farnesyltransferase inhibitor tipifarnib in patients with anthracycline-treated and taxane-resistant metastatic breast cancer: An eastern cooperative oncology group study (E1103). *Breast Cancer Research and Treatment, 134*(1), 345–352. https://doi.org/10.1007/s10549-012-2071-z

Lim, B., et al. (2021). Sapanisertib plus exemestane or fulvestrant in women with hormone receptor-positive/HER2-negative advanced or metastatic breast cancer. *Clinical Cancer Research, 27*(12), 3329–3338. https://doi.org/10.1158/1078-0432.CCR-20-4131

Liu, P., et al. (2009). Targeting the phosphoinositide 3-kinase (PI3K) pathway in cancer. *Nature Reviews. Drug Discovery, 8*(8), 627–644. https://doi.org/10.1038/nrd2926.Targeting

Lo, C. W., et al. (2011). IL-6 trans-signaling in formation and progression of malignant ascites in ovarian cancer. *Cancer Research, 71*(2), 424–434. https://doi.org/10.1158/0008-5472.CAN-10-1496

Loibl, S., et al. (2005). The role of early expression of inducible nitric oxide synthase in human breast cancer. *European Journal of Cancer, 41*(2), 265–271. https://doi.org/10.1016/j.ejca.2004.07.010

Luke, J. J., et al. (2019). Immunobiology, preliminary safety, and efficacy of CPI-006, an anti-CD73 antibody with immune modulating activity, in a phase 1 trial in advanced cancers. *Journal of Clinical Oncology, 37*(15_suppl), 2505–2505. https://doi.org/10.1200/jco.2019.37.15_suppl.2505

Ma, C., et al. (2020). Alternate: Neoadjuvant endocrine treatment (NET) approaches for clinical stage II or III estrogen receptor-positive HER2-negative breast cancer (ER+ HER2- BC) in postmenopausal (PM) women: Alliance A011106. *Journal of Clinical Oncology, 38*(15_suppl), 504–504. https://doi.org/10.1200/jco.2020.38.15_suppl.504

Maennling, A. E., et al. (2019). Molecular targeting therapy against egfr family in breast cancer: Progress and future potentials. *Cancers, 11*(12), 1826. https://doi.org/10.3390/cancers11121826

Mal, R., et al. (2020). Estrogen receptor Beta (ERβ): A ligand activated tumor suppressor. *Frontiers in Oncology, 10*, 1–14. https://doi.org/10.3389/fonc.2020.587386

Mani, S. A., et al. (2008). The epithelial-mesenchymal transition generates cells with properties of stem cells. *Cell, 133*(4), 704–715. https://doi.org/10.1016/j.cell.2008.03.027

Martin-Orozco, E., et al. (2019). WNT signaling in tumors: The way to evade drugs and immunity. *Frontiers in Immunology, 10*, 1–21. https://doi.org/10.3389/fimmu.2019.02854

Matossian, M., Chen, N., & Nanda, R. (2023). Exploiting therapeutic vulnerabilities in triple-negative breast cancer: Successes, challenges, and opportunities. *Current Breast Cancer Reports Springer US, 15*(3), 266–278. https://doi.org/10.1007/s12609-023-00492-4

McCubrey, J. A., et al. (2007). Roles of the Raf/MEK/ERK pathway in cell growth, malignant transformation and drug resistance. *Biochimica et Biophysica Acta-Molecular Cell Research, 1773*(8), 1263–1284. https://doi.org/10.1016/j.bbamcr.2006.10.001

Merikhian, P., Eisavand, M. R., & Farahmand, L. (2021). Triple-negative breast cancer: Understanding Wnt signaling in drug resistance. *Cancer Cell International. BioMed Central, 21*(1), 1–8. https://doi.org/10.1186/s12935-021-02107-3

Mezynski, M. J., et al. (2021). Targeting the PI3K and MAPK pathways to improve response to HER2-targeted therapies in HER2-positive gastric cancer. *Journal of Translational Medicine. BioMed Central, 19*(1), 1–16. https://doi.org/10.1186/s12967-021-02842-1

Mohamed, H. T., et al. (2019). Inflammatory breast cancer: Activation of the aryl hydrocarbon receptor and its target CYP1B1 correlates closely with Wnt5a/b-β-catenin signalling, the stem cell phenotype and disease progression. *Journal of Advanced Research Cairo University, 16*, 75–86. https://doi.org/10.1016/j.jare.2018.11.006

Montagna, E., & Colleoni, M. (2019). Hormonal treatment combined with targeted therapies in endocrine-responsive and HER2-positive metastatic breast cancer. *Therapeutic Advances in Medical Oncology, 11*, 1–10. https://doi.org/10.1177/1758835919894105

Moreno-Aspitia, A. (2010). Clinical overview of sorafenib in breast cancer. *Future Oncology, 6*(5), 655–663. https://doi.org/10.2217/fon.10.41

Mullberg, J., et al. (1993). The soluble interleukin-6 receptor is generated shedding*. *European Journal of Immunology, 23*, 473–480.

Naing, A., et al. (2019). Pegilodecakin combined with pembrolizumab or nivolumab for patients with advanced solid tumours (IVY): A multicentre, multicohort, open-label, phase 1b trial. *The Lancet Oncology. Elsevier Ltd, 20*(11), 1544–1555. https://doi.org/10.1016/S1470-2045(19)30514-5

Nasrollahzadeh, A., et al. (2021). Anti-proliferative activity of disulfiram through regulation of the AKT-FOXO axis: A proteomic study of molecular targets. *Biochimica et Biophysica Acta - Molecular Cell Research. Elsevier B.V., 1868*(10), 119087. https://doi.org/10.1016/j.bbamcr.2021.119087

Nedeljkovi, M. (2019). Mechanisms of chemotherapy resistance in triple-negative breast cancer—How we can rise to the challenge. *Cells, 8*(9), 957.

Nunes, M., et al. (2021). Generation of two paclitaxel-resistant high-grade serous carcinoma cell lines with increased expression of P-glycoprotein. *Frontiers in Oncology, 11*, 1–14. https://doi.org/10.3389/fonc.2021.752127

Orrantia-Borunda, E., Anchondo-Nuñez, P., & Acuña-Aguilar, L. (2022). Subtypes of breast cancer. In H. Mayrovitz (Ed.), *Breast cancer*. Exon Publications. https://doi.org/10.36255/exon-publications-breast-cancer-subtypes

Ozyurt, R., & Ozpolat, B. (2022). Molecular mechanisms of anti-estrogen therapy resistance and novel targeted therapies. *Cancers, 14*(21), 1–37. https://doi.org/10.3390/cancers14215206

Paris, A., et al. (2021). AhR and cancer: From gene profiling to targeted therapy. *International Journal of Molecular Sciences, 22*(2), 1–22. https://doi.org/10.3390/ijms22020752

Patel, R., et al. (2023). An emerging generation of endocrine therapies in breast cancer: A clinical perspective. *Npj Breast Cancer. Springer US, 9*(1), 1–12. https://doi.org/10.1038/s41523-023-00523-4

Pereira, B., et al. (2016). The somatic mutation profiles of 2,433 breast cancers refines their genomic and transcriptomic landscapes. *Nature Communications, 7*, 11479. https://doi.org/10.1038/ncomms11479

Piccart, M., et al. (2014). Everolimus plus exemestane for hormone receptor- positive, human epidermal growth factor receptor-2-negative advanced breast cancer: Overall survival results from BOLERO-2. *Annals of Oncology, 25*(12), 2357–2362. https://doi.org/10.1093/annonc/mdu456

Pimentel, I., et al. (2019). A phase II randomized clinical trial of the effect of metformin versus placebo on progression-free survival in women with metastatic breast cancer receiving standard chemotherapy. *Breast Elsevier Ltd, 48*, 17–23. https://doi.org/10.1016/j.breast.2019.08.003

Pradubyat, N. (2023). Molecular mechanisms of drug resistance in breast cancer and potential strategies for overcoming resistance: A literature review. *Oncología (Ecuador), 33*(1), 1–16. https://doi.org/10.33821/666

Qian, Y., et al. (2022). Efficacy and safety of anlotinib-based treatment in metastatic breast cancer patients. *Frontiers in Oncology, 12*, 1–8. https://doi.org/10.3389/fonc.2022.1042451

Rah, B., et al. (2022). JAK/STAT signaling: Molecular targets, therapeutic opportunities, and limitations of targeted inhibitions in solid malignancies. *Frontiers in Pharmacology, 13*, 1–19. https://doi.org/10.3389/fphar.2022.821344

Rakha, E. A., et al. (2007). Prognostic markers in triple-negative breast cancer. *Cancer, 109*(1), 25–32. https://doi.org/10.1002/cncr.22381

Rasti, A. R., et al. (2022). PIK3CA mutations drive therapeutic resistance in human epidermal growth factor receptor 2–positive breast cancer. *JCO Precision Oncology, 6*, 1–13. https://doi.org/10.1200/po.21.00370

Riethmueller, S., et al. (2016). Cleavage site localization differentially controls Interleukin-6 receptor proteolysis by ADAM10 and ADAM17. *Scientific Reports, 6*, 1–14. https://doi.org/10.1038/srep25550

Ruiz-Saenz, A., et al. (2018). HER2 amplification in tumors activates PI3K/Akt signaling independent of HER3. *Cancer Research, 78*(13), 3645–3658. https://doi.org/10.1158/0008-5472.CAN-18-0430

Sabatier, R., et al. (2014). Claudin-low breast cancers: Clinical, pathological, molecular and prognostic characterization. *Molecular Cancer, 13*(1), 1–14. https://doi.org/10.1186/1476-4598-13-228

Safra, T., et al. (2018). Everolimus plus letrozole for treatment of patients with HR + , HER2 – Advanced breast cancer progressing on endocrine therapy: An open-label, Phase II trial. *Clinical Breast Cancer. Elsevier Inc., 18*(2), e197–e203. https://doi.org/10.1016/j.clbc.2017.09.004

Sanders, J. M., et al. (2013). Molecular determinants of epidermal growth factor binding: A molecular dynamics study. *PLoS One, 8*(1), 8–10. https://doi.org/10.1371/journal.pone.0054136

Santarpia, L. L., Lippman, S., & El-Naggar, A. (2012). Targeting the mitogen-activated protein kinase RAS-RAF signaling pathway in cancer therapy. *Expert Opinion on Therapeutic Targets, 16*(1), 103–119. https://doi.org/10.1517/14728222.2011.645805.Targeting

Saxton, R. A., & Sabatini, D. M. (2017). mTOR signaling in growth, metabolism, and disease. *Cell, 169*(2), 361–371. https://doi.org/10.1016/j.cell.2017.03.035

Scales, S. J., & de Sauvage, F. J. (2009). Mechanisms of hedgehog pathway activation in cancer and implications for therapy. *Trends in Pharmacological Sciences, 30*(6), 303–312. https://doi.org/10.1016/j.tips.2009.03.007

Shao, M., et al. (2022a). Capecitabine inhibits epithelial-to-mesenchymal transition and proliferation of colorectal cancer cells by mediating the RANK/RANKL pathway. *Oncology Letters, 23*(3), 1–11. https://doi.org/10.3892/ol.2022.13216

Shao, Y., et al. (2022b). A real-world study of anlotinib as third-line or above therapy in patients with her-2 negative metastatic breast cancer. *Frontiers in Oncology, 12*, 1–11. https://doi.org/10.3389/fonc.2022.939343

Sheetal Korde, C., et al. (2013). Nitric oxide and cancer: A review. *World Journal of Surgical Oncology, 11*(118), 1–11. http://www.biomedcentral.com/content/pdf/1477-7819-11-118.pdf

Shen, G., et al. (2018). Anlotinib: A novel multi-targeting tyrosine kinase inhibitor in clinical development 11 medical and health sciences 1112 oncology and carcinogenesis. *Journal of Hematology & Oncology, 11*(1), 1–11.

Shum, E., et al. (2020). Preliminary clinical experience with XMAB20717, a PD-1 x CTLA-4 bispecific antibody, in patients with advanced solid tumors. *Journal for Immunotherapy of Cancer, 8*(3), A247–A248. https://doi.org/10.1136/jitc-2021-SITC2021.523

Skoda, A. M., et al. (2018). The role of the hedgehog signaling pathway in cancer: A comprehensive review. *Bosnian Journal of Basic Medical Sciences, 18*(1), 8–20. https://doi.org/10.17305/bjbms.2018.2756

Spizzo, G., et al. (2003). Correlation of COX-2 and ep-CAM overexpression in human invasive breast cancer and its impact on survival. *British Journal of Cancer, 88*(4), 574–578. https://doi.org/10.1038/sj.bjc.6600741

Stevens, E. A., Mezrich, J. D., & Bradfield, C. A. (2009). The aryl hydrocarbon receptor: A perspective on potential roles in the immune system. *Immunology, 127*(3), 299–311. https://doi.org/10.1111/j.1365-2567.2009.03054.x

Sugiura, R., Satoh, R., & Takasaki, T. (2021). Erk: A double-edged sword in cancer. Erk-dependent apoptosis as a potential therapeutic strategy for cancer. *Cell, 10*(10), 2509. https://doi.org/10.3390/cells10102509
Takebe, N., Warren, R. Q., & Ivy, S. P. (2011). Breast cancer growth and metastasis: Interplay between cancer stem cells, embryonic signaling pathways and epithelial-to-mesenchymal transition. *Breast Cancer Research, 13*(3), 1–11. https://doi.org/10.1186/bcr2876
Taylor, K., et al. (2020). An open-label, phase II multicohort study of an oral hypomethylating agent CC-486 and durvalumab in advanced solid tumors. *Journal for ImmunoTherapy of Cancer, 8*(2), e000883. https://doi.org/10.1136/jitc-2020-000883
The Cancer Genome Atlas. (2012). Comprehensive molecular portraits of human breast tumours. *Nature, 490*(7418), 1–10. https://doi.org/10.1038/nature11412
Thomas, D. D., et al. (2004). Signal-regulated kinase, and P53 are regulated by distinct threshold concentrations of nitric oxide. *Proceedings of the National Academy of Sciences of the United States of America, 101*(24), 8894–8899.
Tung, N., et al. (2020). TBCRC 031: Randomized phase II study of neoadjuvant cisplatin versus doxorubicin-cyclophosphamide in germline BRCA carriers with her2-negative breast cancer (the inform trial). *Journal of Clinical Oncology, 38*(14), 1539–1548. https://doi.org/10.1200/JCO.19.03292
Vafaei, S., et al. (2022). Combination therapy with immune checkpoint inhibitors (ICIs); a new frontier. *Cancer Cell International. BioMed Central, 22*(1), 1–27. https://doi.org/10.1186/s12935-021-02407-8
Vaidya, F. U., et al. (2022). Molecular and cellular paradigms of multidrug resistance in cancer. *Cancer Reports, 5*(12), 1–20. https://doi.org/10.1002/cnr2.1291
Vanini, F., Kashfi, K., & Nath, N. (2015). The dual role of iNOS in cancer. *Redox Biology. Elsevier, 6*, 334–343. https://doi.org/10.1016/j.redox.2015.08.009
Vilar, E., Perez-Garcia, J., & Tabernero, J. (2011). Pushing the envelope in the mTOR pathway: The second generation of inhibitors. *Molecular Cancer Therapeutics, 10*(3), 395–403. https://doi.org/10.1158/1535-7163.MCT-10-0905
Wang, H., et al. (2020). Role of CD133 in human embryonic stem cell proliferation and teratoma formation. *Stem Cell Research & Therapy, 11*(1), 1–14. https://doi.org/10.1186/s13287-020-01729-0
Wang, Z. (2017). ErbB receptors and cancer. *Methods in Molecular Biology, 1652*, 3–35. https://doi.org/10.1007/978-1-4939-7219-7_1
Wee, P., & Wang, Z. (2017). Epidermal growth factor receptor cell proliferation. *Cancers, 9*(52), 1–45. https://doi.org/10.3390/cancers9050052
Wehde, B. L., et al. (2018). Janus kinase 1 plays a critical role in mammary cancer progression. *Cell Reports, 25*(8), 2192–2207. https://doi.org/10.1016/j.celrep.2018.10.063.Janus
Weigelt, B., et al. (2008). Refinement of breast cancer classification by molecular characterization of histological special types. *Journal of Pathology, 216*, 141–150. https://doi.org/10.1002/path
Westover, D., et al. (2018). Mechanisms of acquired resistance to first-and second-generation EGFR tyrosine kinase inhibitors. *Annals of Oncology, 29*(Supplement 1), i10–i19. https://doi.org/10.1093/annonc/mdx703
Wheeler, D. L., et al. (2008). Mechanisms of acquired resistance to cetuximab: Role of HER (ErbB) family members. *Oncogene, 27*(28), 3944–3956. https://doi.org/10.1038/onc.2008.19
Wieduwilt, M. J., & Moasser, M. M. (2008). The epidermal growth factor receptor family: Biology driving targeted therapeutics. *Cellular and Molecular Life Sciences, 65*(10), 1566–1584. https://doi.org/10.1007/s00018-008-7440-8.The
Xia, R., et al. (2022). The role of hedgehog and notch signaling pathway in cancer. *Molecular Biomedicine. Springer Nature Singapore, 3*(1), 44. https://doi.org/10.1186/s43556-022-00099-8
Xu, X., et al. (2020). Wnt signaling in breast cancer: Biological mechanisms, challenges and opportunities. *Molecular Cancer, 19*(165), 1–35.

Yamamoto, S., Charng, W. L., & Bellen, H. J. (2010). Endocytosis and intracellular trafficking of notch and its ligands. *Current Topics in Developmental Biology, 92*(C), 165–200. https://doi.org/10.1016/S0070-2153(10)92005-X

Yarchoan, M., et al. (2022). A phase 1 study of TPST-1120 as a single agent and in combination with nivolumab in subjects with advanced solid tumors. *Journal of Clinical Oncology, 40*(16_suppl), 3107–3107. https://doi.org/10.1200/jco.2023.41.16_suppl.3107

Yersal, O., & Barutca, S. (2014). Biological subtypes of breast cancer: Prognostic and therapeutic implications. *World Journal of Clinical Oncology, 5*(3), 412–424. https://doi.org/10.5306/wjco.v5.i3.412

Yin, L., et al. (2020). Triple-negative breast cancer molecular subtyping and treatment progress. *Breast Cancer Research, 22*(1), 1–13. https://doi.org/10.1186/s13058-020-01296-5

Yuan, T. L., & Cantley, L. C. (2008). PI3K pathway alterations in cancer. *Oncogene, 27*(41), 5497–5510. https://doi.org/10.1038/onc.2008.245.PI3K

Zardavas, D., Phillips, W. A., & Loi, S. (2014). PIK3CA mutations in breast cancer: Reconciling findings from preclinical and clinical data. *Breast Cancer Research, 16*(1), 1–10. https://doi.org/10.1186/bcr3605

Zheng, Y., Li, S., & Tang, H. (2023). Molecular mechanisms of immunotherapy resistance in triple-negative breast cancer. *Frontiers in Immunology, 2*, 1–11. https://doi.org/10.3389/fimmu.2023.1153990

Zhong, Z., & Virshup, D. M. (2020). Wnt signaling and drug resistance in cancer. *Molecular Pharmacology, 97*(2), 72–89. https://doi.org/10.1124/MOL.119.117978

Zhou, B., et al. (2022). Notch signaling pathway: Architecture, disease, and therapeutics. *Signal Transduction and Targeted Therapy. Springer US, 7*(1), 1–33. https://doi.org/10.1038/s41392-022-00934-y

Zhou, Y., et al. (2019). Construction of chimeric antigen receptor-modified T cells targeting EpCAM and assessment of their anti-tumor effect on cancer cells. *Molecular Medicine Reports, 20*(3), 2355–2364. https://doi.org/10.3892/mmr.2019.10460

Zhu, X., & Zhou, W. (2015). The emerging regulation of VEGFR-2 in triple-negative breast cancer. *Frontiers in Endocrinology, 6*, 1–7. https://doi.org/10.3389/fendo.2015.00159

Zurth, C., et al. (2022). Clinical pharmacokinetics of the androgen receptor inhibitor Darolutamide in healthy subjects and patients with hepatic or renal impairment. *Clinical Pharmacokinetics. Springer International Publishing, 61*(4), 565–575. https://doi.org/10.1007/s40262-021-01078-y

Part II
Drug Resistance in Breast Cancer Treatment

Resistance to Targeted Therapy in Breast Cancer

Meshack Bida, Benny Mosoane, Zukile Mbita, Demetra Demetriou, Thabiso Victor Miya, Lloyd Mabonga, Talent Chipiti, and Zodwa Dlamini

Abstract The discoveries of breast cancer molecular subtypes and their deregulated pathways have given rise to the emergence of potential therapeutic targets and treatment options with excellent clinical outcomes. The HER2-amplified breast cancer remains the prototype in which the tyrosine kinase inhibitors are still being used clinically for molecular-targeted breast cancer treatment. Targeted therapy resistance in breast cancer (BC) can result from the proliferation of intrinsic and/or extrinsic instigators leading to relapse after a short remission. Intrinsic mechanisms (acquired before treatment) are a result of genetic mutations that result in a lack of target sensitivity in cancer cells. Extrinsic (acquired) resistance can result from; the emergence of the second proto-oncogene acting as the new driver gene, dysregulated expression of the drug targets as a result of new mutation, and alternations in tumor microenvironment (TME) post-treatment. To overcome the mutations and/or compensatory pathways that impart treatment resistance, often, combinational approaches to treatment are often required. Careful patient selection should be done before the start of targeted therapy to confirm the predictive response beforehand. Newer treatment agents are not without undesired side effects.

M. Bida (✉) · B. Mosoane
Department of Anatomical Pathology, National Health Laboratory Services (NHLS), University of Pretoria, Pretoria, South Africa
e-mail: meshack.bida@nhls.ac.za; Benny.Mosoane@nhls.ac.za

Z. Mbita
Department of Biochemistry, Microbiology and Biotechnology, School of Molecular and Life Sciences, University of Limpopo, Polokwane, South Africa
e-mail: Zukile.Mbita@ul.ac.za

D. Demetriou · T. V. Miya · L. Mabonga · T. Chipiti · Z. Dlamini
SAMRC Precision Oncology Research Unit (PORU), DSI/NRF SARChI Chair in Precision Oncology and Cancer Prevention (POCP), Pan African Cancer Research Institute (PACRI), University of Pretoria, Pretoria, South Africa
e-mail: dd.demetriou@up.ac.za; thabiso.miya@up.ac.za; Lloyd.Mabonga@up.ac.za; talent.chipiti@up.ac.za; zodwa.dlamini@up.ac.za

Z. Dlamini (ed.), *Overcoming Breast Cancer Therapy Resistance*,
https://doi.org/10.1007/978-3-031-52860-6_3

Keywords Molecular targets of therapy · Signaling pathways · Resistance to therapy · Tumor microenvironment · HER-2

Introduction

Breast cancer (BC) accounts for 24% of female cancers and is a leading contributor to female cancer-associated death globally (Bray et al., 2018). The origin of BC is multifactorial, and most studies point its foundation to hormones (estrogen and progesterone; endogenous or exogenous), diet (a high-calorie diet rich in animal fat and protein), reproductive factors (older age at first childbirth, lower parity and decreased duration of lactation), and genetics factors (Newcomb et al., 2011). BC presents clinically as an irregular mass, which may show overlying skin changes. Imaging reveals speculated mass with or without calcifications. On gross examination, BC appears irregular with stellate or nodular configuration and a gritty feel on cutting. The histologic appearance of cancer located in the milk duct shows duct carcinoma morphology while cancers from the lobules are termed lobular carcinoma. The spectrum of BC is, however, overly broad.

Several linear multistep pathways of BC pathogenesis have been described, largely based on hormone receptor status and morphology. For example, the estrogen receptor (ER) positive model acknowledges flat epithelial atypia, atypical ductal hyperplasia, and ER+ duct carcinoma in situ (DCIS) model as non-compelling forerunners of invasive BC whereas the ER-negative model recognizes ER-negative DCIS and micro glandular adenosis as precursors of ER-negative BC (Bombonati & Sgroi, 2011). Sporadic clonal evolution and cancer stem cell (CSC) models have been described at the cell of origin level model of BC. The molecular level model suggests that BC evolved along two divergent molecular pathways of progression, mainly related to hormone receptors. Classification of BC ER model hinges on the expression or lack of ER, progesterone receptor (PR) as well as human epidermal growth factor receptor 2 (HER2). The major subtypes are Luminal A which expresses ER and PR but not HER2; Luminal B expresses ER, PR, and HER2; HER2 enriched expresses HER2+ but not ER and PR; and triple-negative BC (TNBC) basal-like which does not express any of the three receptors. Histological staining has been used to classify BC into several subtypes as demonstrated in Fig. 1 (Kinnel et al., 2023).

Hormone-positive BC, Luminal A, and B are generally treated with endocrine therapy (ET), combined with chemotherapy. TNBCs are often aggressive and difficult to treat because they lack hormone receptors. Despite advanced technological breakthroughs in the treatment of BC, drug therapy resistance remains an obstacle. Drug therapy resistance accounts for nine out of ten cancer-related deaths (Łukasiewicz et al., 2021). This chapter will focus on the targeted therapies in drug-resistant BC and strategies to overcome drug-resistant BC.

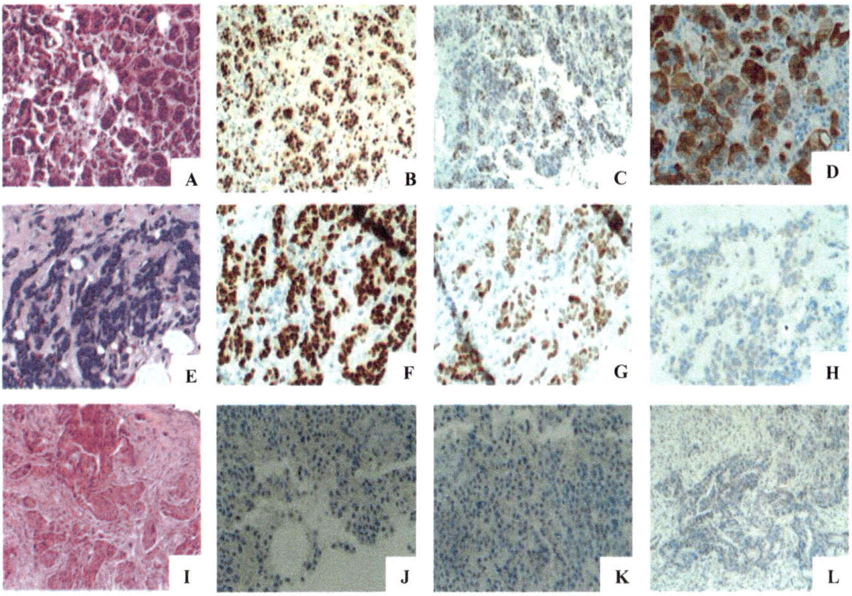

Fig. 1 Molecular types of breast cancer. A–D show Luminal B BC displaying micropapillary pattern, positive ER, PR, and HER-2 staining; E–H shows infiltrative duct carcinoma, which is positive ER and PR and negative HER-2; I–L shows a basal-like/triple negative infiltrative carcinoma, which is ER, PR, and HER-2 negative on immunohistochemistry

Drug-Resistant Breast Cancer

Mechanisms of drug resistance in BC can either be innate (intrinsic) or acquired, and Fig. 2 shows the mechanisms of BC drug resistance. Intrinsic mechanisms (acquired before treatment) are a result of genetic mutations that result in a lack of target sensitivity in cancer cells while acquired resistance is seen in the advanced stage of the disease. Acquired resistance in HER2-positive BC includes mechanisms such as losing the expression of the target that results from continual therapy, activating additional mechanisms that promote cell proliferation, and activating mutations downstream mutations from the target itself (Baselga et al., 2010). Other well-defined mechanisms of resistance in breast cancer include drug efflux, which results in decreased intracellular drug accumulation, which is via the ATP-binding cassette (ABC) transporter system (Kinnel et al., 2023). In various cancers, therapeutics damage the DNA of tumor cells; however, DNA damage response (DDR) in cancer can repair DNA lesions leading to drug resistance. With exposure to chemotherapy, cancer cells can become senescent (permeant cell proliferation arrest), only to acquire CSC-like properties to bolt tumor senescence and then resume progression (Milanovic et al., 2018).

At the epigenetic level, demethylation of the promoter regions of the oncogenes can cause acquired drug resistance due to increased gene expression. Epigenetic

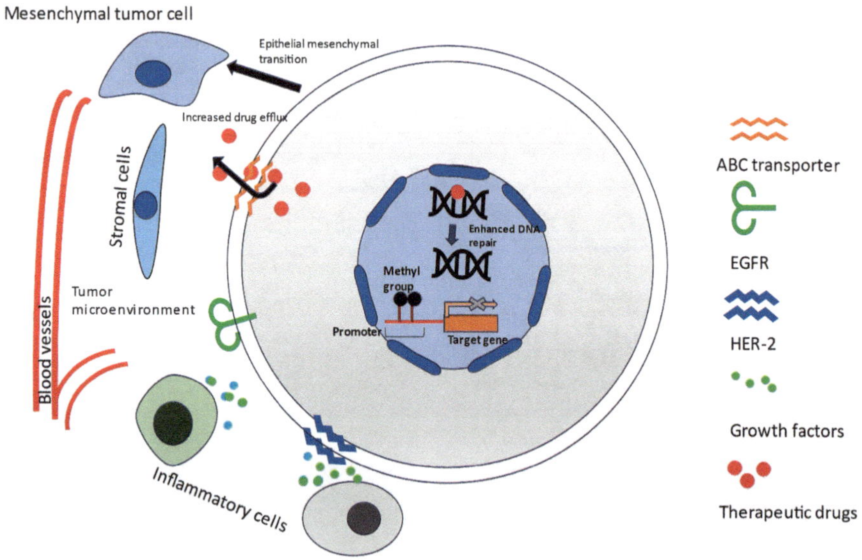

Fig. 2 Mechanisms of drug resistance in BC. These mechanisms include alteration from the epigenetic levels, DNA repair, cytoplasmic efflux transporter system, tumor microenvironment, and epithelial-mesenchymal transition

alteration has been associated with tamoxifen (TAM) resistance in BC due to decreased expression of ER (Zhu et al., 2016). There is a lot of work that is being done to understand the role players involved in TAM resistance in BC. Several types of non-protein coding RNAs, such as Long non-coding RNAs (LncRNAs) and microRNAs (miRNAs), are reported to contribute to this type of resistance. For example, Lnc-DC lncRNA was reported to induce TAM resistance by upregulating anti-apoptotic genes such as *Bcl2* and *Bcl-xL*. Additionally, microRNAs, small non-coding RNAs, which are epigenetic modulators that can affect gene expression via post-transcriptional modification, have been reported to play a role in treatment resistance. In BC, miRNA-27b, miRNA-134, and miRNA-21 were found to influence genes related to resistance, cell cycle, cell proliferation, and apoptosis (Zhu et al., 2016; Kinnel et al., 2023; Lu et al., 2015).

CSCs in BC play a major role in tumor heterogeneity, relapse, and metastasis. High expression of CSC biomarker, particularly CD133, and dysregulation of signaling pathways like the Notch, sonic hedgehog, Wnt/*B*-catenin, and JAK/STAT have been linked to drug resistance (Li et al., 2021; Zhao et al., 2016; Kapucuoğlu et al., 2015). Components of tumor microenvironment (TME); blood vessels, extracellular matrix, fibroblast, immune cells, and signaling molecules play a role in intrinsic and acquired treatment resistance (Wang et al., 2019). Hypoxic TME produces hypoxia-inducible factor (HIF-1α) that promotes epithelial-mesenchymal transition (EMT), an essential feature of TNBC (Nedeljković & Damjanović, 2019). During EMT cells lose E-cadherin function which leads to reduced cell-cell attachment and promotes metastasis.

Potential Targeted Therapies Directed At Various Molecular Pathways

Aryl Hydrocarbon Receptor

Studies show that repression of Aryl Hydrocarbon Receptor (AhR) can suppress mammary tumor development. Functional restoration of AhR repressor protein (AhRR) may have therapeutic benefits (Vogel et al., 2021; Yang et al., 2018). AhR is an intracytoplasmic protein belonging to the basic-helix-loop/Per-Arnt-Sim family, which is activated by ligands. When bound to the ligand, AhR translocates into the nucleus to form a heterodimer with AhR nuclear translocator protein (ARNT) that binds to DNA xenobiotic response elements (XRE) and coregulators that transcribes target genes (Lee et al., 2013). AhR crosstalk with the Wnt pathway has been described (Yang et al., 2018; Kinnel et al., 2023). AhR mRNA overexpression in BC makes it a viable treatment target. Conversely, loss of AhRR in BC has been correlated with decreased survival.

AhR has the potential to promote chemotherapy resistance in aggressive BC phenotypes through the Wnt5A/β-catenin signaling pathway (Yang et al., 2019). In BC cell lines, AhR confers apoptotic resistance (see Fig. 3) and serves as a mediator of metabolizing enzymes and transporters (Zhu & Cui, 2015). This transporting function contributes to the efflux of pharmaceutical compounds decreasing drug activity. Tamoxifen-resistant (TamR) MFC7 xenografts of BC subjected to ADM3100, an AhR antagonist, showed in vivo growth inhibition (Zhu & Cui, 2015). AhR has shown tumor suppressor effects via tumor suppressor miRNA and blocks proliferation via AhR crosstalk (Zhu & Cui, 2015; Yang et al., 2019; Campbell et al., 2018). Small molecules that act as AhR agonists such as dietary flavonoids and aminiflavone

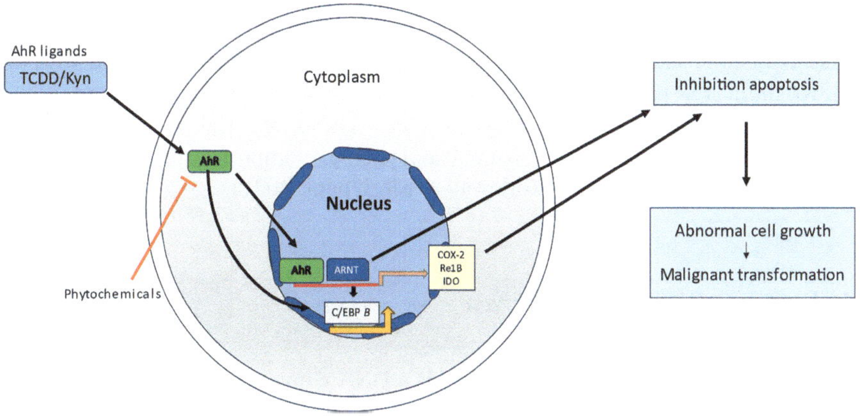

Fig. 3 The Aryl Hydrocarbon Receptor (AhR) located in the cytoplasm translocates to the nucleus, heterodimerizing with ARNT and binding to coregulators to affect transcription of target genes. This pathway allows the survival of cells by inhibition of apoptosis

(AF), can induce tumor suppressor-like qualities (Baker et al., 2020). AF inhibits expression of α-6-integrin which leads to the reduction of TamR cell viability (Campbell et al., 2018).

Inducible Nitrate Oxide Synthase

The inducible form of nitric oxide synthase (iNOS) has a calcium-dependent activity that enables it to produce nitric oxide (NO) in higher amounts (Vannini et al., 2015). In MFC-7 BC cells, low doses of NO of <300 nM lead to phosphorylation of ERK and HIF-1α which result in tumor progression (Thomas et al., 2004). NO >300 M was found to induce apoptosis phosphorylating P53 (Thomas et al., 2004). In some cancer cells, iNOS has been linked with cisplatin resistance with cisplatin sensitivity restored after attenuation of iNOS (Jin et al., 2015). iNOS expression attenuation in TNBC has shown a marked reduction in average tumor volume in patients treated with platinum-based chemotherapy in a study by Jin et al. (Jin et al., 2015).

PI3K/Akt/mTOR Pathway

One of the pathways that lead to cellular proliferation and tumorigenesis in BC is the phosphoinositide 3 kinase (PI3K)/Akt/mammalian target of the rapamycin pathway. PI3K catalytic subunit alpha (PI3KCA) mutations in exons 9 and 20 and the loss of phosphatase and TENsin homolog deleted on chromosome 10 (PTEN) are seen in the highest frequency in Luminal A BC cases (Paplomata & O'Regan, 2014; Chung et al., 2022). Combining inhibitors of mTOR like Everolimus and ET has shown the potential to overcome ET resistance in BC (Paplomata et al., 2013). Trastuzumab resistance in BC overexpressing HER-2 has been associated with the PI3K/Akt/mTOR pathway (Chung et al., 2022). Combination therapies have proven beneficial in overcoming treatment resistance. Holloway et al. demonstrated that Everolimus combined with trastuzumab and paclitaxel improves the overall survival rate in trastuzumab resistant (Holloway & Marignani, 2021).

Poly (ADP-Ribose) Polymerase

Poly (ADP-Ribose) Polymerase (PARP) is a DNA damage response (DDR) protein that detects and initiates an immediate cellular response to a single-stranded DNA breaks (SSB) by signaling the enzymatic machinery involved in the SSB repair. PARP detects an SSB, binds to the DNA, undergoes a structural alteration, and begins to synthesize a polymeric adenosine diphosphate ribose (PAR) chain, which acts as a signal for the other DNA-repairing effectors such as DNA polymerase beta (polβ), DNA ligase III (LigIII), and X-ray cross-complementing gene 1 (XRCC1) (London, 2015; Masson et al., 1998). The PAR chains are released from the DNA via Poly (ADP-ribose) glycohydrolase (PARG) after repairing the DNA (Isabelle et al., 2010). Figure 4 shows the effects of PARP in SSB.

Locally advanced and metastatic BC with germline or somatic mutation in BRCA1 or BRCA2 show deficiency in homologous recombination repair (HHR) of double-stranded DNA breaks (Desnoyers et al., 2022). The loss of HRR in BRCA mutant BC combined with PARP inhibitors (PARPi) results in the accumulation of DNA damage, cell cycle arrest, and apoptosis, a process called synthetic lethality (Desnoyers et al., 2022; Ashworth, 2008). PARPi prevents the release of PARP from the site of DNA damage, see Fig. 4 (Kyle et al., 2008). Examples of Food and Drug Administration (FDA) approved PARPi for locally and advanced and metastatic BC include olaparib and talazoparib (Cortesi et al., 2021). Drugs such as rucaparib, veliparib, and niraparib are still under clinical trials (Cortesi et al., 2021). Trapped PARPi can be removed from the chromatin by ubiquitin-regulated p97 ATP which suggests the role of p97 in PARPi resistance (Krastev et al., 2022). Resistance to orally administered PARPi develops over time in many patients (Li et al., 2020a). Several pathways can restore PARPi sensitivity when combined with agents that target particular pathways, see Table 1.

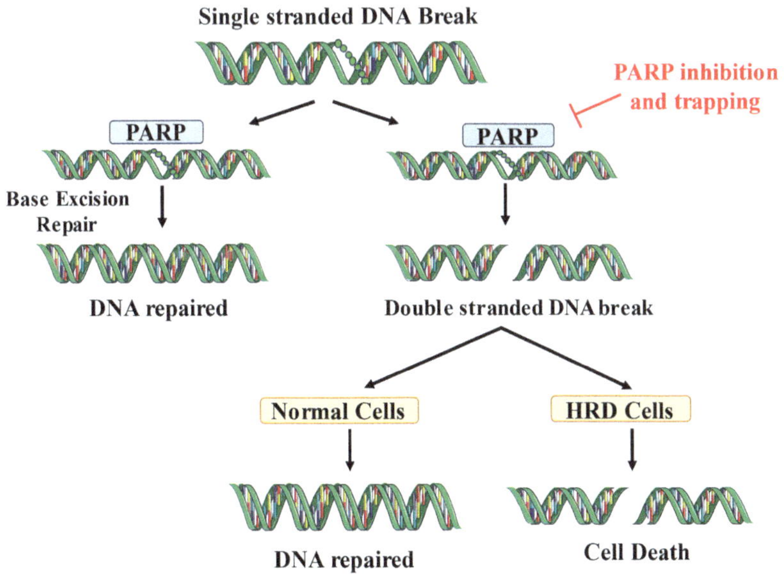

Fig. 4 The role of PARP in single-stranded DNA break (on the left) and the effect of PARP inhibition and PARP trapping in single-stranded DNA break (right). Entrapped PARP leads to double-stranded DNA breaks which require homologous recombination for cell survival to occur

Table 1 Target pathways that can restore PARPi sensitivity

Target pathway:	Active molecule	Therapeutic benefits of the combination PARPi	References
Kinases that control most DNA damage responses: Ataxia telangiectasia mutated and Rad3-related (ATR)	AZD6738 (ceralasertib)	Effective in treating cancers with BRCA1/2 mutations	(Janysek et al., 2021)
Cell cycle kinase inhibitors: WEE1 kinase that regulates G2/M checkpoint	AZD1775	Attunes olaparib sensitivity in TNBC	(Ha et al., 2020)
Transcription of oncogenes: Bromodomain containing 4 (BRD4)	BRD4 inhibitors	Cells become resensitized to PARPi by inducing homologous recombination deficiency	(Sun et al., 2018)

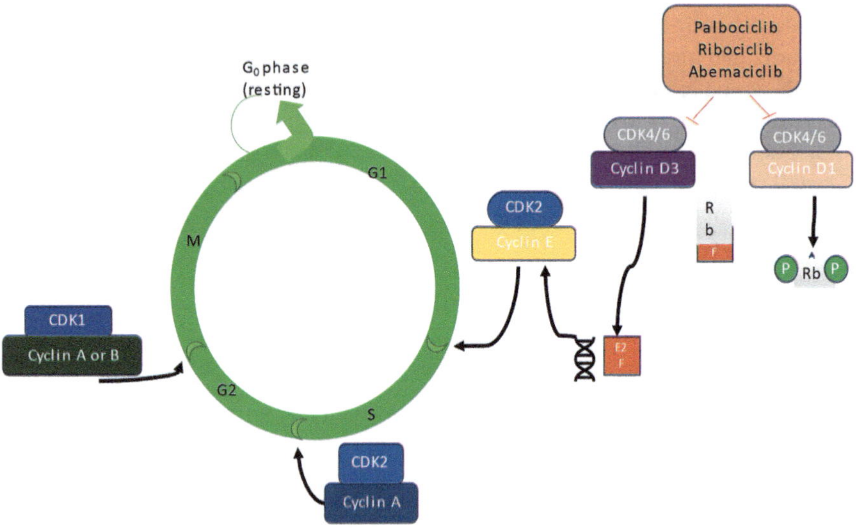

Fig. 5 Inhibition of cyclin-dependent kinase (CDK) 4/6 and how this affects cell cycle progression. CDK4/6 inhibitors prevent the phosphorylation of retinoblastoma protein (RB), and hypophosphorylated RB restrains the E2F transcription factor to prevent the transcriptional activities and result in arresting the cell cycle at the G1 phase

Cyclin-Dependent Kinase 4/6

The D cyclins (D1, D2, D3) and Cyclin-Dependent Kinase 4/6 (CDK4/6) initiate phosphorylation of substrates responsible for the progression of the cell cycle (Fig. 5). The substrates include retinoblastoma protein (pRB) and Cyclin D K inhibitors (CDKIs); p107 and p130 (Li et al., 2020b). Overexpression of cyclin D1 has been associated with BC recurrence and lack of response to TAM. There are

Table 2 Phase III trials of CDK5/6 in breast cancer

CDK5/6 inhibitor	Therapeutic results	References
Palbociclib	Combination with letrozole showed a median progression-free survival (PFS) of 24.8 months compared to PFS of 14.5 months in patients treated with letrozole and placebo.	(Finn et al., 2016)
Ribociclib	Combination with TAM showed longer overall survival than TAM alone.	(Lu et al., 2022)
Abemaciclib	Increase the efficacy of fulvestrant and letrozole.	(Lu et al., 2022)

promising therapeutic benefits of using CDK4/6 inhibitors in BC such as palbociclib, ribociclib, and abemaciclib (Li et al., 2020b, Nur Husna et al., 2018). These drugs are in phase III trials and Table 2 summarizes their therapeutic results.

Wnt/β-Catenin Pathway

In the Wnt signaling pathway, Wnt binds to Frizzled and LRP5/6 to activate phosphorylation of disheveled protein (Dvl). Dvl deactivates GSK-3B which inhibits degradation of B-catenin, a transcription factor that is often translocated into the nucleus (Pohl et al., 2017). This pathway regulates tissue stem cells in a non-pathologic setting (Zhong & Virshup, 2020). In cancer, it can stimulate the production of CSC and serve as a mechanism of treatment resistance (Zhong & Virshup, 2020). Several therapies that target nodes in this pathway are studied (Zhang & Wang, 2020), see Fig. 6.

In BC, Wnt mutations are not common (Feng et al., 2018). Expression of B-catenin has; however, been associated with chemoresistance in TNBC (Merikhian et al., 2021). B-catenin knock-off has shown improved re-sensitivity of cells to doxorubicin (DOX) and cisplatin (Xu et al., 2015). In BRCA-mutated TNBC cells, nuclear and cytoplasmic accumulation of B-catenin has been linked to the efflux of PARPi (Gangrade et al., 2018). Overexpression of Frizzled1 protein was found to be associated with multidrug resistance in BC cell subline MCF-7/ADM (Zhang et al., 2012).

Combination therapies that include targeting the Wnt/B-catenin pathway can combat certain types of drug resistance in BC. The agents inhibit nodes such as Wnt, Dvl, CBP, LRP5/6, and Porcupine (PORCN) (Zhang & Wang, 2020) (Fig. 6). PORCN is an O-acyltransferase that catalyzes palmitoylation of Wnt ligands and facilitates their secretion and biofunction (Yang et al., 2023). GNF-6231, a PORCN inhibitor showed inhibition of tumor activity in BC mouse models (Zhang & Wang, 2020). WNT974, another PORCN inhibitor shows BC stem cell proliferation when combined with buparlisib (PI3K inhibitor) (Solzak et al., 2017).

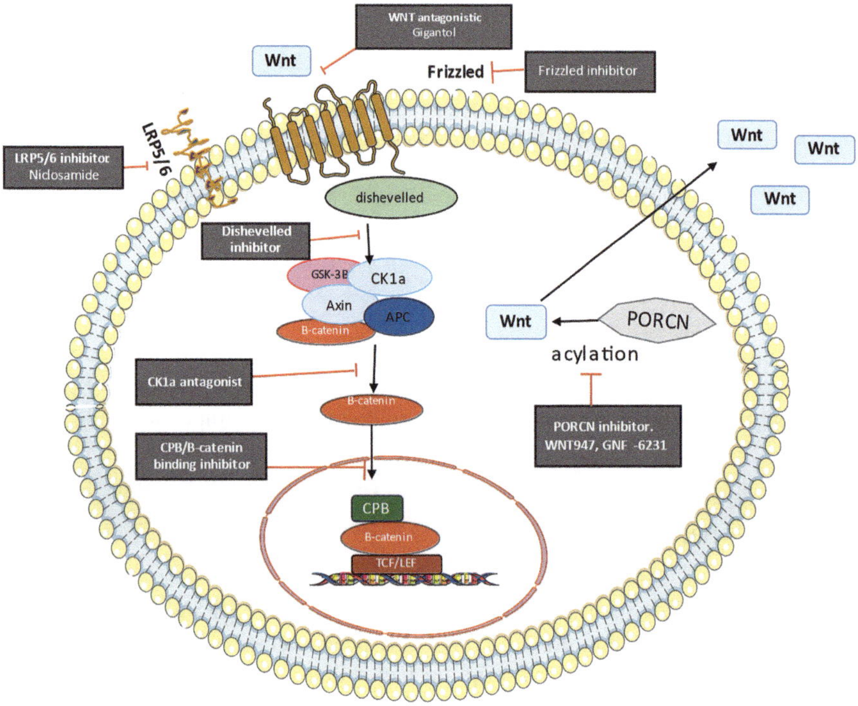

Fig. 6 Wnt signaling pathway and potential nodes of inhibition. Wnt binds to its receptors, Frizzled and LRP5/6 by recruiting disheveled (Dvl) that deactivates glycogen synthase kinase (GSK)-3*B* to prevent degradation of *B*-catenin. B-catenin then translocates into the nucleus to regulate the expression of genes. The figure demonstrates the nodes at which current therapies target this pathway

Epidermal Growth Factor Receptor

Epidermal Growth Factor Receptor (EGFR/HER1/ErbB1), a human epidermal growth factor receptor tyrosine kinase family member encompasses HER2/ErbB2, HER3/ErbB3, and HER4/ErbB4. When the ligand binds on the EGFR, several downstream pathways like Ras/MAPK, PI3K/Akt, STAT, PLCγ1/PKC, and Par6-atypical PKC become activated (Wieduwilt & Moasser, 2008) (Fig. 7). The results of the activated EGFR pathway are cell proliferation and survival. In BC, overexpression of EGFR is correlated with recurrence, metastasis, and lessened survival (Ali & Wendt, 2017). Unfortunately, EGFR inhibitors (depicted in Fig. 7) do not show any significant efficacy in BC (Ali & Wendt, 2017). Combining therapies that target more than one pathway may be efficacious in combating resistance of tyrosine kinase inhibitors in BC.

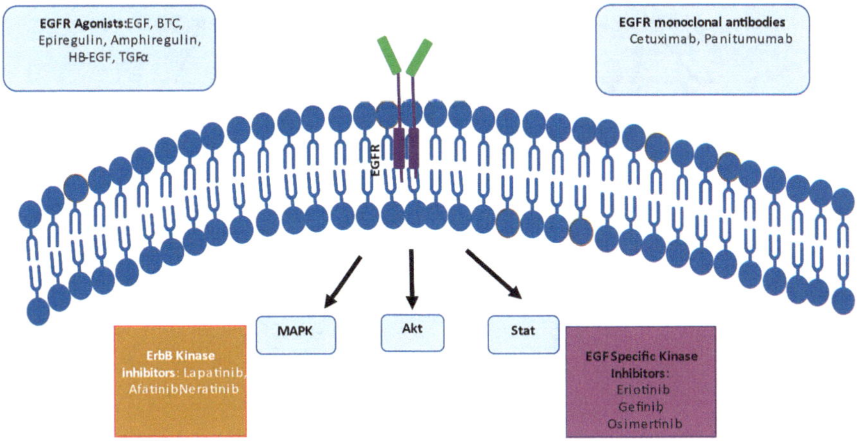

Fig. 7 Epidermal growth factor receptor (EGFR) pathway and drug inhibitors. Several antagonists of EGFR that include monoclonal antibodies have been developed to block ligand binding and several different kinases. All of the listed therapies are FDA-approved for various cancers except Neratinib

Human Epidermal Growth Factor Receptor-2 (HER-2)

The HER-2 oncogene, a member of the EGFR family is located on 17q12. HER-2 is one commonly overexpressed receptor in BC from this EGFR family. HER-2 in contrast to other members of the EGFR tyrosine kinase family, has no known ligand. HER-2 signaling pathway is activated by heterodimerization or homodimerization of EGFR or HER-3 to initiate the downstream signaling pathway EGFR, Fig. 8 (Hsu & Hung, 2016).

HER-2-positive BC cases account for 20% of BC cases and are characterized by complete, strong circumferential membranous staining in more than 10% of tumor cells on immunohistochemistry (Fig. 9). Equivocal cases can be confirmed on in situ hybridization test (whose interpretations are beyond the scope of this chapter). HER-2-positive BC cases are treated with HER-2 inhibitors that include trastuzumab, pertuzumab, neratinib, and lapatinib (Pernas & Tolaney, 2019).

HER-2-positive BCs can develop drug resistance due to reduced drug sensitivity, lack of HER-2 downregulation, dysregulated PI3K/Akt/mTOR pathway, dysregulated apoptosis and cell cycle, CDK4/6-cyclin D1 expression and immunodeficiency (Pernas & Tolaney, 2019; Zhang, 2021). Targeting of CDK4/6 inhibitor in BC has been found to re-sensitize tumors to anti-Her-2 therapy (Pernas & Tolaney, 2019). The combination of an mTOR inhibitor (Everolimus) with trastuzumab and paclitaxel has shown benefits in phase III trials (Hurvitz et al., 2015).

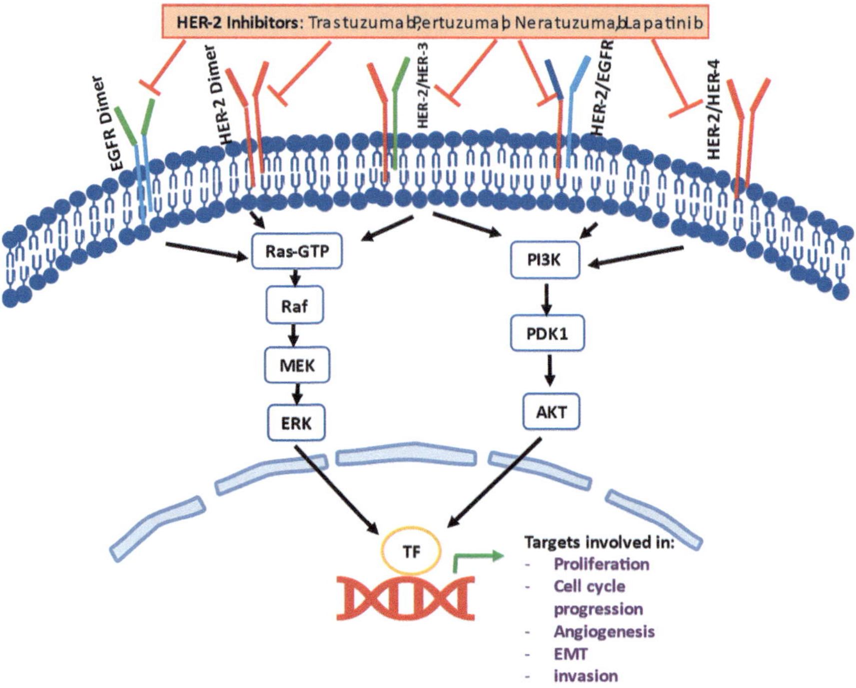

Fig. 8 Human epidermal growth factor receptor 2 (HER-2) in relation to other family members of Epidermal growth factor receptor (EGFR). Note the absence of ligand binding to the HER-2 receptor

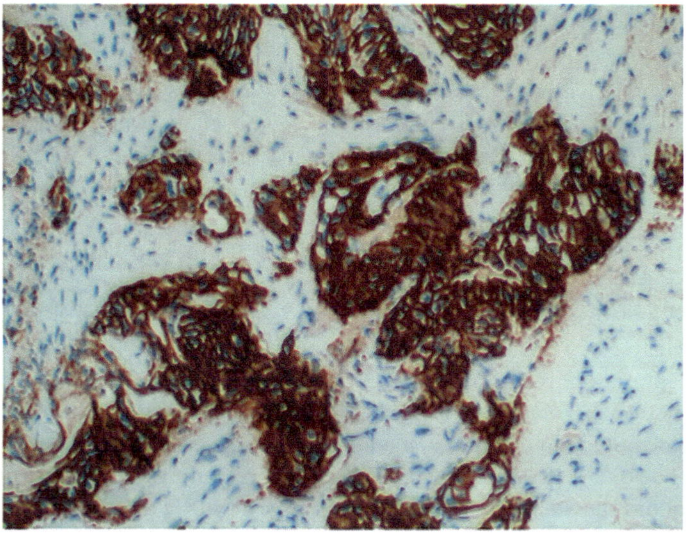

Fig. 9 Human epidermal growth factor receptor 2 (HER-2) immunohistochemistry expression with a score of 3+; intense complete circumferential membrane staining in > 10% of invasive tumor cells. An immunohistochemistry score of 3+ is required before the patient is put on anti-HER2 therapy (trastuzumab / Herceptin®)

The Vascular Endothelial Growth Factor

The main modulators in the emergence of tumor angiogenesis are represented by the vascular endothelial growth factor (VEGF) and its cell surface receptors. Bevacizumab, an anti-VEGF antibody is an anti-angiogenic agent used in therapy in cancer therapy. Bevacizumab is effectively used in combination with small molecule VEGF receptor kinase inhibitors (Masoud & Pagès, 2017). The VEGF ligand is a homodimeric structure stabilized by a disulfide knot and two symmetrically disposed intermolecular disulfide bridges with the monomers together. There are seven immunoglobulin-like structures on the extracellular domain of the three receptors of VEGF (Shibuya & Claesson-Welsh, 2006; Ferrara et al., 2003).

The members of the VEGF family bind to three different vascular endothelial growth factor receptors 1, 2, and 3(VEGFR1. VEGFR2, and VEGF3), all with different functions. VEGFR1 induces vascular differentiation and maintenance; VEGFR2 promotes vessel permeability and endothelial cell proliferation; and VEGFR3 activates the formation of lymphatic vessels. Neuropilin-1 and neuropilin-2 are VEGFR3 isoform-specific receptors that bind to the extracellular signaling protein, semaphorins which are involved in axonal growth. Binding of neuropilin-1 and neuropilin-2 to some VEGF1 isoforms become co-receptors which result in more VEGF binding to VEGFR2 (Bielenberg et al., 2006).

VEGF genes are upregulated within the hypoxia microenvironments, and they draw out a particular vascular phenotype. In human BC, the expression of VEGF serves as a prognostic factor, and it represents an important therapeutic target.

Several mechanisms are suggested in the unfolding of antiangiogenic therapy resistance in BC. One such mechanism relates to cancer cells producing different forms of alternative signals of angiogenesis which limit the efficacy of the drugs (Ayoub et al., 2022). The tumor vascularization escape can take place as induced by anti-angiogenesis treatment and hypoxia of TME (Loges et al., 2010).

Hormone Receptors as Targets of Therapy

BC cases that express hormone receptors such as estrogen receptor (ER) or progesterone receptor (PR) (or both) are sensitive to endocrine therapy. Estrogen and its receptors serve as important drivers in the progression of BC through the estrogen signaling pathway in patients with ER+ BC. Selective estrogen receptor modulators (SERM) are used to suppress the growth of tumor estrogen-dependent BC, particularly in ER-positive metastatic BC to recurrences (Chang et al., 2011). TAM was the prime approved drug. The aromatase inhibitors (letrozole, anastrozole, exemestane) are alternative therapies used to treat estrogen-dependent BC because they block the biosynthesis of androgens by inhibiting the aromatase enzyme thereby reducing estrogen levels in BC cells.

ET resistance is a great remonstrance within hormone expressing BC even though there is a proven efficacy of ER and PR targeted therapy, which also improves the quality of life. There are several pathways implicated in ET resistance. The HER tyrosine kinase receptor family (VEGF, FGF, and receptors for insulin/IGF1), AKT, proto-oncogene tyrosine-protein kinase Src, and stress-related kinases, play a key role in ET resistance particularly when their associated ligands are overexpressed or amplified. The link between the ER and growth factor receptor signaling with activation of the PI3K/Akt signaling pathway has been implicated in the development of ET resistance (Di Leo et al., 2015). Estrogen nuclear receptors and androgen receptors may be alternative stimulators of growth via post-translational modification which enables ER inhibition detour.

Simultaneous targeting of both EGFR and HER2 appears to be the most favorable approach in finding a way around ET resistance since the two pathways appear to be the key factors responsible for the ET resistance framework (Osborne & Schiff, 2011).

Pharmacologic Mechanisms of Target Therapy Agents

Molecular targeted therapy carries the advantage of the ability to effectively drug on the cell surface or cytoplasm of the cells of interest with a high level of specificity, with minimal toxicity in contrast to conventional chemotherapy. This implies that the agents are often administered in relatively low doses as compared to conventional chemotherapy. Most drug formulations are available as small molecules that can ensure successful delivery to the targeted cells. The relatively low molecular weight allows the agents to penetrate cells and target specific intracellular proteins (Ha et al., 2021). The targets include cell surface antigens, receptors, growth factors, and regulatory signaling transduction. The molecular targeted therapeutic agents fall into four main groups, namely, small molecules; monoclonal antibodies; gene therapy, and immunotherapeutic cancer vaccines (Lee et al., 2018).

Small Molecules

Small molecules are agents characterized by relatively low molecular weight of <900 Da. They can penetrate cells, to target specific proteins within the cells. Many of these compounds act by inactivating kinases and interrupting the signaling pathways which are dysregulated during carcinogenesis. Small molecules can be used to target proteasomes, cyclin-CDKs, and PARP. The small molecules as substances or drugs interfere with the functioning of certain molecules that participate in the proliferation and survival of tumor cells to block cancer growth (Bansal et al., 2023). BC cells may overexpress certain molecules that can start downstream signaling when activated, and result in the expression of genes that favor BC cell growth, proliferation, survival, migration, angiogenesis, and some key pathways of the cell cycle.

Monoclonal Antibodies

The Monoclonal Antibodies (mAbs) exhibit multifunctional roles such as directly attacking the actual cancer cells, assisting in delivering therapeutic drugs to targets, inhibiting cell growth, and also as immune checkpoint inhibitors (Fig. 10). Monoclonal antibodies have also been used to target specific cell surface receptors, such as Her2, especially in BC. Several side—effects have been detailed in the use of mAbs, which include breathing difficulties, skin rash, bleeding, headache, fever, muscle pain, trembling, fatigue, and nausea/vomiting. Nonetheless, mAbs have opened up newer opportunities due to their varied level of specificity which includes single antigen specificity, whereas bi- and/or trispecific mAbs cover more potential resistance in the course of treatment. The use of mAbs as immune checkpoint inhibitors seeks to explore the immune modulation of the immune effector cells in the tumor microenvironment to increase the efficacy of immune effector cells in cancer immune ablation (Behl et al., 2023).

The mAbs as drugs block specific targets on the cell surface of cancer cells by identifying cancer-specific antigens. The target might also be in the tumor microenvironment. The drugs have three main pertinent distinctive features: (1) tumor selectivity of mAbs that is target specific; (2) they can be restructured and attached with conjugators that are stable in circulation, but are split when delivered into a cell; and (3) humanized mAbs are not immunogenic and cause negligible systemic toxicity (Behl et al., 2023).

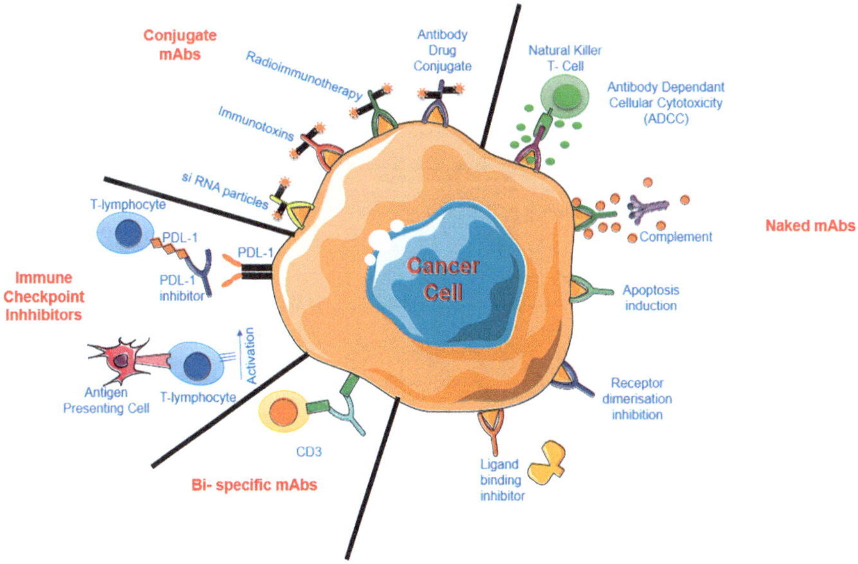

Fig. 10 Multiple levels of application of mononuclear antibodies (mAbs) in breast cancer treatment. This graphic demonstrates the breast cancer cell targets of immune check inhibitors, conjugate mAbs, naked mAbs, and bispecific mAbs

Immunotherapeutic Cancer Vaccines

Although breast cancer is characterized by limited immunogenicity, success in clinical trials of cancer immunotherapy looks promising to usher in a novel treatment of BC treatment in which the focal point of therapy becomes cancer vaccination. Vaccines target specific tumor-associated antigens (TAA) as well as tumor-specific antigens (TSA) (Fig. 11).

TAAs entail tumor differentiation antigens, tumor germline antigens, and overexpressed antigens. The tumor germline antigens, also called cancer-testis antigens (CTAs), are expressed in testicular, ovarian, and placental germ cells, with no expression in normal somatic cells (Ai et al., 2023). CTAs are expressed in numerous types of malignant tumor cells, BC included. The expression of CTAs has been reported in BC, such as New York Esophageal Squamous Cell Carcinoma-1 (NY-ESO1), melanoma-associated antigen 1 (MAGE-A1), and Kita-Kyushu Lung Cancer Antigen-1(KK-LC-1) (Bai & Yuan, 2022; Xiao et al., 2023). The detection of serum antibodies against CTAs has been dubbed as a practical biomarker to predict the clinical immunotherapeutic benefits (Yang et al., 2022).

Tumor differentiation antigens refer to the proteins that are present in neoplastic cells and premorbid cells of the tissue of origin for a particular tumor, for example, prostate-specific antigen (PSA), Melan-A/Mart-1, carcinoembryonic antigen (CEA), and glycoprotein P 100 (gp100). Overexpressed antigens are proteins that are expressed at some lower quantities in non-neoplastic cells and at higher quantities in neoplastic cells. Targeted antigens: HER2, human telomerase transcriptase

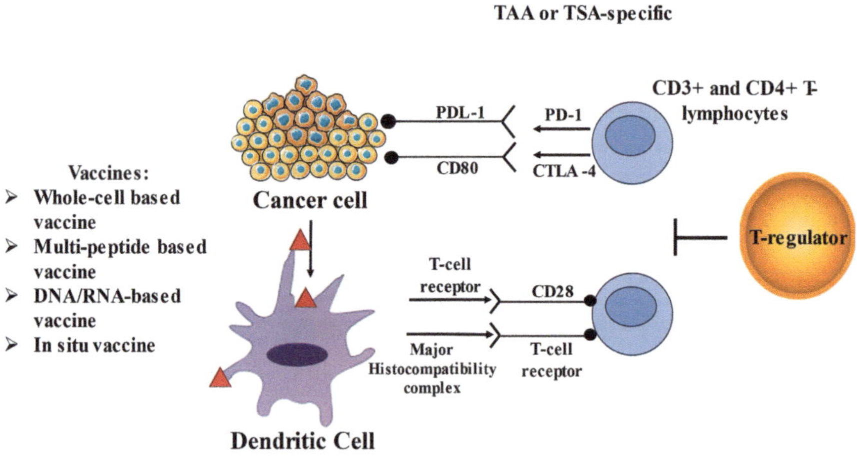

Fig. 11 The diagram represents the therapeutic BC vaccine platforms with the mechanisms of action. The vaccine platforms represented here are whole-cell based, multi-peptide, DNA/RNA-based, and in situ vaccination. Dendritic cells present the processed TAA or TSA to CD4+ and CD8+ T cells. The interaction of TAA/TSA generates specific effector T cells that lead to the killing of tumor cells. *Abbreviations*: CTLA-4, cytotoxic T lymphocyte-associated antigen 4; PD-1, programmed cell death protein 1; PDL-1, programmed death ligand 1; TAAs, tumor-associated antigens; TSAs, tumor-specific antigens

(hTERT), mucin 1(MUC-1), and survivin are frequently overexpressed in BC. The vaccines based on TAA must have sufficient immunogenicity to activate the poor-affinity TAA-reactive T cells that remain. T cells with strong TAA affinity are largely removed by central and peripheral immune tolerance mechanisms (Kondo et al., 2018).

TSAs expressed in neoplastic cells comprise oncoviral antigens and neoantigens (Feola et al., 2020). Neoantigens represent the genomic alterations products of point mutations, deletion mutations, or frameshift insertion. Other genomic alterations may include splice-site alterations resulting in exon skipping, the formation of chimeric fusion proteins, etc. Most cancers will acquire many genomic alterations during the tumorigenesis process and only a few neoantigens can elicit immunogenic response. TNBC is considered a likely fit candidate for immunotherapy and there are trials on neoantigens underway. The trials include the personalized synthetic long peptide (SLP) neoantigen vaccine administered with durvalumab and nab-paclitaxel (NCT03606967), the autologous dendritic cells (DCs) pulsed with tumor-specific neoantigen (NCT04105582), and neoantigen DNA vaccine administered with durvalumab (NCT03199040) which are enrolling TNBC patients (Karasaki et al., 2017). These vaccines elicit variable immune responses depending on the vaccine delivery platforms. Despite these promising ventures, only a few BC cases have been reported to benefit from neoantigen based (Zhang et al., 2022).

Gene Therapy

The study of the molecular basis of BC provides an opportunity for introducing gene therapy as an alternative treatment option. This strategy consists of transporting genetic material through a vector into target cells, which changes the genetic expression of the target genes. Since the technique involves targeting specific tumor cells normal cells are soared with less toxicity (Dastjerd et al., 2022).

Strategies to Overcome Resistance to Targeted Therapies

HER2+ BC can develop several resistance mechanisms to HER2 inhibitors limiting therapeutic options for the patients. There have been several approaches like antibody–drug conjugates (ADCs) developed, and some are in preclinical or clinical stages. These ADCs are either aimed at the HER2 receptor or downstream intracellular signaling (e.g., CDK4/6 inhibitors and PI3K/AKT/mTOR). The other approach commonly used is directed toward weakening the tumor through immunotherapy, blocking autophagy, or targeting genes within the HER2 amplicon). Furthermore, significant technical progress such as anti-HER2 immunotoxins and nanotherapies are emerging strategies to come around the challenge of resistance.

The main remonstrance that remains to be further elucidated is the appearance of therapeutic resistance mechanisms that are encountered shortly after the onset of therapy. These warrant compelling scrutiny and further investigation.

Limitations of Targeted Therapy in Breast Cancer

Most of the molecular targeted therapies are limited by the following: (1) Absence of potential molecules that are targeted due to lack of expression by tumor cells: Careful patient selection should be done before the start of targeted therapy to confirm the predictive response beforehand. (2) Mutational change of genes coding for the target proteins: Most tumors with a high mutational burden can modulate the tumor surface receptors and thus cause a misfit of the drug agent to the receptor site. (3) Resistance to treatment options already implemented: Cancers can use alternative pathways thus bypassing the targeted pathway in the course of treatment. Host factors that assist in immune-ablative therapy in the tumor microenvironment due to poor response of immune effector cells.

Conclusion

The use of targeted therapies has ushered in an era of personalized treatment in oncology practice. This is a rapidly evolving concept with several ongoing clinical trials (the pre-clinical phase) as well as the well-established modalities of cancer treatment (clinical phase). The complexity of pathways in tumorigenesis, tumor progression, and metastases however remains a challenge to monotherapeutic strategies and will most likely need multiple approaches to cancer treatment in breast cancer. The strategies for dealing with resistance to targeted therapies will also require further research.

References

Ai, H., Yang, H., Li, L., Ma, J., Liu, K., & Li, Z. (2023). Cancer/testis antigens: Promising immunotherapy targets for digestive tract cancers. *Frontiers in Immunology, 14*, 1190883.

Ali, R., & Wendt, M. K. (2017). The paradoxical functions of EGFR during breast cancer progression. *Signal Transduction and Targeted Therapy, 2*, 16042.

Ashworth, A. (2008). A synthetic lethal therapeutic approach: Poly(ADP) ribose polymerase inhibitors for the treatment of cancers deficient in DNA double-strand break repair. *Journal of Clinical Oncology, 26*, 3785–3790.

Ayoub, N. M., Jaradat, S. K., Al-Shami, K. M., & Alkhalifa, A. E. (2022). Targeting angiogenesis in breast cancer: Current evidence and future perspectives of novel anti-Angiogenic approaches. *Frontiers in Pharmacology, 13*, 838133.

Bai, R., & Yuan, C. (2022). Kita-Kyushu lung cancer Antigen-1 (KK-LC-1): A promising cancer testis antigen. *Aging and Disease, 13*, 1267–1277.

Baker, J. R., Sakoff, J. A., & Mccluskey, A. (2020). The aryl hydrocarbon receptor (AhR) is a breast cancer drug target. *Medicinal Research Reviews, 40*, 972–1001.

Bansal, I., Pandey, A. K., & Ruwali, M. (2023). Small-molecule inhibitors of kinases in breast cancer therapy: Recent advances, opportunities, and challenges. *Frontiers in Pharmacology, 14*, 1244597.

Baselga, J., Gelmon, K. A., Verma, S., Wardley, A., Conte, P., Miles, D., Bianchi, G., Cortes, J., Mcnally, V. A., Ross, G. A., Fumoleau, P., & Gianni, L. (2010). Phase II trial of pertuzumab and trastuzumab in patients with human epidermal growth factor receptor 2-positive metastatic breast cancer that progressed during prior trastuzumab therapy. *Journal of Clinical Oncology, 28*, 1138–1144.

Behl, A., Wani, Z. A., Das, N. N., Parmar, V. S., Len, C., Malhotra, S., & Chhillar, A. K. (2023). Monoclonal antibodies in breast cancer: A critical appraisal. *Critical Reviews in Oncology/Hematology, 183*, 103915.

Bielenberg, D. R., Pettaway, C. A., Takashima, S., & Klagsbrun, M. (2006). Neuropilins in neoplasms: Expression, regulation, and function. *Experimental Cell Research, 312*, 584–593.

Bombonati, A., & Sgroi, D. C. (2011). The molecular pathology of breast cancer progression. *The Journal of Pathology, 223*, 307–317.

Bray, F., Ferlay, J., Soerjomataram, I., Siegel, R. L., Torre, L. A., & Jemal, A. (2018). Global cancer statistics 2018: GLOBOCAN estimates of incidence and mortality worldwide for 36 cancers in 185 countries. *CA: A Cancer Journal for Clinicians, 68*, 394–424.

Campbell, P. S., Mavingire, N., Khan, S., Rowland, L. K., Wooten, J. V., Opoku-Agyeman, A., Guevara, A., Soto, U., Cavalli, F., Loaiza-Pérez, A. I., Nagaraj, G., Denham, L. J., Adeoye, O., Jenkins, B. D., Davis, M. B., Schiff, R., & Brantley, E. J. (2018). AhR ligand aminoflavone suppresses α6-integrin-Src-Akt signaling to attenuate tamoxifen resistance in breast cancer cells. *Journal of Cellular Physiology, 234*, 108–121.

Chang, B. Y., Kim, S. A., Malla, B., & Kim, S. Y. (2011). The effect of selective estrogen receptor modulators (SERMs) on the tamoxifen resistant breast cancer cells. *Toxicology Research, 27*, 85–93.

Chung, W. P., Huang, W. L., Lee, C. H., Hsu, H. P., Huang, W. L., Liu, Y. Y., & Su, W. C. (2022). PI3K inhibitors in trastuzumab-resistant HER2-positive breast cancer cells with PI3K pathway alterations. *American Journal of Cancer Research, 12*, 3067–3082.

Cortesi, L., Rugo, H. S., & Jackisch, C. (2021). An overview of PARP inhibitors for the treatment of breast cancer. *Targeted Oncology, 16*, 255–282.

Dastjerd, N. T., Valibeik, A., Rahimi Monfared, S., Goodarzi, G., Moradi Sarabi, M., Hajabdollahi, F., Maniati, M., Amri, J., & Samavarchi Tehrani, S. (2022). Gene therapy: A promising approach for breast cancer treatment. *Cell Biochemistry and Function, 40*, 28–48.

Desnoyers, A., Nadler, M., Wilson, B. E., Stajer, S., & Amir, E. (2022). Associations with response to poly(ADP-ribose) polymerase (PARP) inhibitors in patients with metastatic breast cancer. *npj Breast Cancer, 8*, 43.

Di Leo, A., Curigliano, G., Diéras, V., Malorni, L., Sotiriou, C., Swanton, C., Thompson, A., Tutt, A., & Piccart, M. (2015). New approaches for improving outcomes in breast cancer in Europe. *Breast, 24*, 321–330.

Feng, Y., Spezia, M., Huang, S., Yuan, C., Zeng, Z., Zhang, L., Ji, X., Liu, W., Huang, B., Luo, W., Liu, B., Lei, Y., Du, S., Vuppalapati, A., Luu, H. H., Haydon, R. C., He, T. C., & REN, G. (2018). Breast cancer development and progression: Risk factors, cancer stem cells, signaling pathways, genomics, and molecular pathogenesis. *Genes Diseases, 5*, 77–106.

Feola, S., Chiaro, J., Martins, B., & Cerullo, V. (2020). Uncovering the tumor antigen landscape: What to know about the discovery process. *Cancers (Basel), 12*(6), 1660.

Ferrara, N., Gerber, H. P., & Lecouter, J. (2003). The biology of VEGF and its receptors. *Nature Medicine, 9*, 669–676.

Finn, R. S., Martin, M., Rugo, H. S., Jones, S., Im, S. A., Gelmon, K., Harbeck, N., Lipatov, O. N., Walshe, J. M., Moulder, S., Gauthier, E., Lu, D. R., Randolph, S., Diéras, V., & Slamon,

D. J. (2016). Palbociclib and Letrozole in advanced breast cancer. *The New England Journal of Medicine, 375*, 1925–1936.

Gangrade, A., Pathak, V., Augelli-Szafran, C. E., Wei, H. X., Oliver, P., Suto, M., & Buchsbaum, D. J. (2018). Preferential inhibition of Wnt/β-catenin signaling by novel Benzimidazole compounds in triple-negative breast cancer. *International Journal of Molecular Sciences, 19*(5), 1524.

Ha, D. H., Min, A., Kim, S., Jang, H., Kim, S. H., Kim, H. J., Ryu, H. S., Ku, J. L., Lee, K. H., & Im, S. A. (2020). Antitumor effect of a WEE1 inhibitor and potentiation of olaparib sensitivity by DNA damage response modulation in triple-negative breast cancer. *Scientific Reports, 10*, 9930.

Ha, J., Park, H., Park, J., & Park, S. B. (2021). Recent advances in identifying protein targets in drug discovery. *Cell Chemical Biology, 28*, 394–423.

Holloway, R. W., & Marignani, P. A. (2021). Targeting mTOR and glycolysis in HER2-positive breast cancer. *Cancers (Basel), 13*, 2922.

Hsu, J. L., & Hung, M. C. (2016). The role of HER2, EGFR, and other receptor tyrosine kinases in breast cancer. *Cancer Metastasis Reviews, 35*, 575–588.

Hurvitz, S. A., Andre, F., Jiang, Z., Shao, Z., Mano, M. S., Neciosup, S. P., Tseng, L. M., Zhang, Q., Shen, K., Liu, D., Dreosti, L. M., Burris, H. A., Toi, M., Buyse, M. E., Cabaribere, D., Lindsay, M. A., Rao, S., Pacaud, L. B., Taran, T., & Slamon, D. (2015). Combination of everolimus with trastuzumab plus paclitaxel as first-line treatment for patients with HER2-positive advanced breast cancer (BOLERO-1): A phase 3, randomized, double-blind, multicentre trial. *The Lancet Oncology, 16*, 816–829.

Isabelle, M., Moreel, X., Gagné, J. P., Rouleau, M., Ethier, C., Gagné, P., Hendzel, M. J., & Poirier, G. G. (2010). Investigation of PARP-1, PARP-2, and PARG interactomes by affinity-purification mass spectrometry. *Proteome Science, 8*, 22.

Janysek, D. C., Kim, J., Duijf, P. H. G., & Dray, E. (2021). Clinical use and mechanisms of resistance for PARP inhibitors in homologous recombination-deficient cancers. *Translational Oncology, 14*, 101012.

Jin, Z., Wang, W., Jiang, N., Zhang, L., Li, Y., Xu, X., Cai, S., Wei, L., Liu, X., Chen, G., Zhou, Y., Liu, C., Li, Z., Jin, F., & Chen, B. (2015). Clinical implications of iNOS levels in triple-negative breast cancer responding to neoadjuvant chemotherapy. *PLoS One, 10*, e0130286.

Kapucuoğlu, N., Bozkurt, K. K., Başpinar, Ş., Koçer, M., Eroğlu, H. E., Akdeniz, R., & Akçil, M. (2015). The clinicopathological and prognostic significance of CD24, CD44, CD133, ALDH1 expressions in invasive ductal carcinoma of the breast: CD44/CD24 expression in breast cancer. *Pathology, Research and Practice, 211*, 740–747.

Karasaki, T., Nagayama, K., Kuwano, H., Nitadori, J. I., Sato, M., Anraku, M., Hosoi, A., Matsushita, H., Takazawa, M., Ohara, O., Nakajima, J., & Kakimi, K. (2017). Prediction and prioritization of neoantigens: Integration of RNA sequencing data with whole-exome sequencing. *Cancer Science, 108*, 170–177.

Kinnel, B., Singh, S. K., Oprea-Ilies, G., & Singh, R. (2023). Targeted therapy and mechanisms of drug resistance in breast cancer. *Cancers (Basel), 15*, 1320.

Kondo, Y., Fukuyama, T., Yamamura, R., Futawatari, N., Ichiki, Y., Tanaka, Y., Nishi, Y., Takahashi, Y., Yamazaki, H., Kobayashi, N., & Watanabe, M. (2018). Detection of KK-LC-1 protein, a cancer/testis antigen, in patients with breast cancer. *Anticancer Research, 38*, 5923–5928.

Krastev, D. B., Li, S., Sun, Y., Wicks, A. J., Hoslett, G., Weekes, D., Badder, L. M., Knight, E. G., Marlow, R., Pardo, M. C., Yu, L., Talele, T. T., Bartek, J., Choudhary, J. S., Pommier, Y., Pettitt, S. J., Tutt, A. N. J., Ramadan, K., & Lord, C. J. (2022). The ubiquitin-dependent ATPase p97 removes cytotoxic trapped PARP1 from chromatin. *Nature Cell Biology, 24*, 62–73.

Kyle, S., Thomas, H. D., Mitchell, J., & Curtin, N. J. (2008). Exploiting the Achilles heel of cancer: The therapeutic potential of poly(ADP-ribose) polymerase inhibitors in BRCA2-defective cancer. *The British Journal of Radiology, 81*(Special_issue_1), S6–S11.

Lee, H. H., Kim, W. T., Kim, D. H., Park, J. W., Kang, T. H., Chung, J. W., & Leem, S. H. (2013). Tristetraprolin suppresses AHRR expression through mRNA destabilization. *FEBS Letters, 587*, 1518–1523.

Lee, Y. T., Tan, Y. J., & Oon, C. E. (2018). Molecular targeted therapy: Treating cancer with specificity. *European Journal of Pharmacology, 834*, 188–196.

Li, H., Liu, Z. Y., Wu, N., Chen, Y. C., Cheng, Q., & Wang, J. (2020a). PARP inhibitor resistance: The underlying mechanisms and clinical implications. *Molecular Cancer, 19*, 107.

Li, Y., Wang, Z., Ajani, J. A., & Song, S. (2021). Drug resistance and cancer stem cells. *Cell Communication and Signaling: CCS, 19*, 19.

Li, Z., Zou, W., Zhang, J., Zhang, Y., Xu, Q., Li, S., & Chen, C. (2020b). Mechanisms of CDK4/6 inhibitor resistance in luminal breast cancer. *Frontiers in Pharmacology, 11*, 580251.

Loges, S., Schmidt, T., & Carmeliet, P. (2010). Mechanisms of resistance to anti-angiogenic therapy and development of third-generation anti-angiogenic drug candidates. *Genes & Cancer, 1*, 12–25.

London, R. E. (2015). The structural basis of XRCC1-mediated DNA repair. *DNA Repair (Amst), 30*, 90–103.

Lu, L., Ju, F., Zhao, H., & Ma, X. (2015). MicroRNA-134 modulates resistance to doxorubicin in human breast cancer cells by downregulating ABCC1. *Biotechnology Letters, 37*, 2387–2394.

Lu, Y. S., Im, S. A., Colleoni, M., Franke, F., Bardia, A., Cardoso, F., Harbeck, N., Hurvitz, S., Chow, L., Sohn, J., Lee, K. S., Campos-Gomez, S., Villanueva Vazquez, R., Jung, K. H., Babu, K. G., Wheatley-Price, P., De Laurentiis, M., Im, Y. H., Kuemmel, S., El-Saghir, N., O'Regan, R., Gasch, C., Solovieff, N., Wang, C., Wang, Y., Chakravartty, A., Ji, Y., & Tripathy, D. (2022). Updated overall survival of Ribociclib plus endocrine therapy versus endocrine therapy alone in pre- and perimenopausal patients with HR+/HER2- advanced breast cancer in MONALEESA-7: A phase III randomized clinical trial. *Clinical Cancer Research, 28*, 851–859.

Łukasiewicz, S., Czeczelewski, M., Forma, A., Baj, J., Sitarz, R., & Stanisławek, A. (2021). Breast cancer-epidemiology, risk factors, classification, prognostic markers, and current treatment strategies-An updated review. *Cancers (Basel), 13*, 4287.

Masoud, V., & Pagès, G. (2017). Targeted therapies in breast cancer: New challenges to fight against resistance. *World Journal of Clinical Oncology, 8*, 120–134.

Masson, M., Niedergang, C., Schreiber, V., Muller, S., Menissier-de Murcia, J., & de Murcia, G. (1998). XRCC1 is specifically associated with poly(ADP-ribose) polymerase and negatively regulates its activity following DNA damage. *Molecular and Cellular Biology, 18*, 3563–3571.

Merikhian, P., Eisavand, M. R., & Farahmand, L. (2021). Triple-negative breast cancer: Understanding Wnt signaling in drug resistance. *Cancer Cell International, 21*, 419.

Milanovic, M., Fan, D. N. Y., Belenki, D., Däbritz, J. H. M., Zhao, Z., Yu, Y., Dörr, J. R., Dimitrova, L., Lenze, D., Monteiro Barbosa, I. A., Mendoza-Parra, M. A., Kanashova, T., Metzner, M., Pardon, K., Reimann, M., Trumpp, A., Dörken, B., Zuber, J., Gronemeyer, H., Hummel, M., Dittmar, G., Lee, S., & Schmitt, C. A. (2018). Senescence-associated reprogramming promotes cancer stemness. *Nature, 553*, 96–100.

Nedeljković, M., & Damjanović, A. (2019). Mechanisms of chemotherapy resistance in triple-negative breast cancer-how we can rise to the challenge. *Cell, 8*, 957.

Newcomb, P. A., Trentham-Dietz, A., Hampton, J. M., Egan, K. M., Titus-Ernstoff, L., Warren Andersen, S., Greenberg, E. R., & Willett, W. C. (2011). Late age at first full term birth is strongly associated with lobular breast cancer. *Cancer, 117*, 1946–1956.

Nur Husna, S. M., Tan, H. T., Mohamud, R., Dyhl-Polk, A., & Wong, K. K. (2018). Inhibitors targeting CDK4/6, PARP and PI3K in breast cancer: A review. *Therapeutic Advances in Medical Oncology, 10*, 1758835918808509.

Osborne, C. K., & Schiff, R. (2011). Mechanisms of endocrine resistance in breast cancer. *Annual Review of Medicine, 62*, 233–247.

Paplomata, E., & O'Regan, R. (2014). The PI3K/AKT/mTOR pathway in breast cancer: Targets, trials and biomarkers. *Therapeutic Advances in Medical Oncology, 6*, 154–166.

Paplomata, E., Zelnak, A., & O'Regan, R. (2013). Everolimus: Side effect profile and management of toxicities in breast cancer. *Breast Cancer Research and Treatment, 140*, 453–462.

Pernas, S., & Tolaney, S. M. (2019). HER2-positive breast cancer: New therapeutic frontiers and overcoming resistance. *Therapeutic Advances in Medical Oncology, 11*, 1758835919833519.

Pohl, S. G., Brook, N., Agostino, M., Arfuso, F., Kumar, A. P., & Dharmarajan, A. (2017). Wnt signaling in triple-negative breast cancer. *Oncogene, 6*, e310.

Shibuya, M., & Claesson-Welsh, L. (2006). Signal transduction by VEGF receptors in regulation of angiogenesis and lymphangiogenesis. *Experimental Cell Research, 312*, 549–560.

Solzak, J. P., Atale, R. V., Hancock, B. A., Sinn, A. L., Pollok, K. E., Jones, D. R., & Radovich, M. (2017). Dual PI3K and Wnt pathway inhibition is a synergistic combination against triple negative breast cancer. *Npj Breast Cancer, 3*, 17.

Sun, C., Yin, J., Fang, Y., Chen, J., Jeong, K. J., Chen, X., Vellano, C. P., Ju, Z., Zhao, W., Zhang, D., Lu, Y., Meric-Bernstam, F., Yap, T. A., Hattersley, M., O'connor, M. J., Chen, H., Fawell, S., Lin, S. Y., Peng, G., & Mills, G. B. (2018). BRD4 inhibition is synthetic lethal with PARP inhibitors through the induction of homologous recombination deficiency. *Cancer Cell, 33*, 401–416.e8.

Thomas, D. D., Espey, M. G., Ridnour, L. A., Hofseth, L. J., Mancardi, D., Harris, C. C., & Wink, D. A. (2004). Hypoxic inducible factor 1alpha, extracellular signal-regulated kinase, and p53 are regulated by distinct threshold concentrations of nitric oxide. *Proceedings of the National Academy of Sciences of the United States of America, 101*, 8894–8899.

Vannini, F., Kashfi, K., & Nath, N. (2015). The dual role of iNOS in cancer. *Redox Biology, 6*, 334–343.

Vogel, C. F. A., Lazennec, G., Kado, S. Y., Dahlem, C., He, Y., Castaneda, A., Ishihara, Y., Vogeley, C., Rossi, A., Haarmann-Stemmann, T., Jugan, J., Mori, H., Borowsky, A. D., La Merrill, M. A., & Sweeney, C. (2021). Targeting the aryl hydrocarbon receptor signaling pathway in breast cancer development. *Frontiers in Immunology, 12*, 625346.

Wang, X., Zhang, H., & Chen, X. (2019). Drug resistance and combating drug resistance in cancer. *Cancer Drug Resistance, 2*, 141–160.

Wieduwilt, M. J., & Moasser, M. M. (2008). The epidermal growth factor receptor family: Biology driving targeted therapeutics. *Cellular and Molecular Life Sciences, 65*, 1566–1584.

Xiao, J., Huang, F., Li, L., Zhang, L., Xie, L., & Liu, B. (2023). Expression of four cancer-testis antigens in TNBC indicating potential universal immunotherapeutic targets. *Journal of Cancer Research and Clinical Oncology, 149*(16), 15003–15011.

Xu, J., Prosperi, J. R., Choudhury, N., Olopade, O. I., & Goss, K. H. (2015). β-Catenin is required for the tumorigenic behavior of triple-negative breast cancer cells. *PLoS One, 10*, e0117097.

Yang, P., Qiao, Y., Meng, M., & Zhou, Q. (2022). Cancer/testis antigens as biomarker and target for the diagnosis, prognosis, and therapy of lung cancer. *Frontiers in Oncology, 12*, 864159.

Yang, Q., Qin, T., An, T., Wu, H., Xu, G., Xiang, J., Lei, K., Zhang, S., Xia, J., Su, G., Wang, D., Xue, M., Kong, L., Zhang, W., Wu, S., & Li, Y. (2023). Novel PORCN inhibitor WHN-88 targets Wnt/β-catenin pathway and prevents the growth of Wnt-driven cancers. *European Journal of Pharmacology, 945*, 175628.

Yang, S. Y., Ahmed, S., Satheesh, S. V., & Matthews, J. (2018). Genome-wide mapping and analysis of aryl hydrocarbon receptor (AHR)- and aryl hydrocarbon receptor repressor (AHRR)-binding sites in human breast cancer cells. *Archives of Toxicology, 92*, 225–240.

Yang, T., Feng, Y. L., Chen, L., Vaziri, N. D., & Zhao, Y. Y. (2019). Dietary natural flavonoids treating cancer by targeting aryl hydrocarbon receptor. *Critical Reviews in Toxicology, 49*, 445–460.

Zhang, H., Zhang, X., Wu, X., Li, W., Su, P., Cheng, H., Xiang, L., Gao, P., & Zhou, G. (2012). Interference of frizzled 1 (FZD1) reverses multidrug resistance in breast cancer cells through the Wnt/β-catenin pathway. *Cancer Letters, 323*, 106–113.

Zhang, L., Zhou, X., Sha, H., Xie, L., & Liu, B. (2022). Recent Progress on therapeutic vaccines for breast cancer. *Frontiers in Oncology, 12*, 905832.

Zhang, Y. (2021). The root cause of drug resistance in HER2-positive breast cancer and the therapeutic approaches to overcoming the resistance. *Pharmacology & Therapeutics, 218*, 107677.

Zhang, Y., & Wang, X. (2020). Targeting the Wnt/β-catenin signaling pathway in cancer. *Journal of Hematology & Oncology, 13*, 165.

Zhao, H., Tang, H., Xiao, Q., He, M., Zhao, L., Fu, Y., Wu, H., Yu, Z., Jiang, Q., Yan, Y., Jin, F., & Wei, M. (2016). The hedgehog signaling pathway is associated with poor prognosis in breast cancer patients with the CD44+/CD24- phenotype. *Molecular Medicine Reports, 14*, 5261–5270.

Zhong, Z., & Virshup, D. M. (2020). Wnt signaling and drug resistance in cancer. *Molecular Pharmacology, 97*, 72–89.

Zhu, C., & Cui, L. (2015). The role of Ahr in anticancer drug resistance in breast cancer. *Journal of Bioanalysis & Biomedicine, 07*.

Zhu, J., Zou, Z., Nie, P., Kou, X., Wu, B., Wang, S., Song, Z., & He, J. (2016). Downregulation of microRNA-27b-3p enhances tamoxifen resistance in breast cancer by increasing NR5A2 and CREB1 expression. *Cell Death & Disease, 7*, e2454.

Resistance to Immunotherapy in Breast Cancer

Botle Precious Damane, Lorraine Tshegofatso Maebele, Malose Makgoka, Dikeledi Hendrika Mokone, Thanyani Victor Mulaudzi, Solomon Oladapo Rotimi, and Zodwa Dlamini

Abstract Breast cancer is the most common and second most deadly disease in women worldwide, with breast cancer screening resulting in a steady decline in mortality rate. However, early diagnosis of breast cancer for young black women has not improved the mortality rate due to aggressiveness, and the ability to grow faster resulting in potential metastasis and recurrence, especially in the triple-negative molecular subtype. This prompted the decision to first investigate the efficacy of immunotherapy, particularly immune checkpoint inhibitors (ICIs). However, ICIs are only successful in a small group of patients expressing programmed cell death ligand (PD-L1) and most patients develop toxicity and drug resistance. High levels of tumor-infiltrating T cells have been shown to be a favorable indicator of therapeutic response indicating that immunotherapy can be utilized to harness the power of the immune system to recognize and destroy cancer cells. This chapter will focus on the utilization of immunotherapy as a potential solution to overcome drug resistance in breast cancer. The chapter will explore various immunotherapeutic approaches, including ICIs, adoptive cell transfer, and bispecific antibody thera-

B. P. Damane (✉) · L. T. Maebele · M. Makgoka · T. V. Mulaudzi
Department of Surgery, Level 7, Bridge E, Steve Biko Academic Hospital, Faculty of Health Sciences, University of Pretoria, Pretoria, South Africa
e-mail: botle.damane@up.ac.za; lorraine.maebele@up.ac.za; malose.makgoka@up.ac.za; thanyani.mulaudzi@up.ac.za

D. H. Mokone
Department of Surgery, Dr George Mukhari Academic Hospital, Sefako Makgatho Health Sciences University, Pretoria, South Africa
e-mail: Dikeledi.Mokone@smu.ac.za

S. O. Rotimi
Department of Biochemistry, Covenant University, Ota, Nigeria
e-mail: ola.rotimi@covenantuniversity.edu.ng

Z. Dlamini
SAMRC Precision Oncology Research Unit (PORU), DSI/NRF SARChI Chair in Precision Oncology and Cancer Prevention (POCP), Pan African Cancer Research Institute (PACRI), University of Pretoria, Pretoria, South Africa
e-mail: zodwa.dlamini@up.ac.za

Z. Dlamini (ed.), *Overcoming Breast Cancer Therapy Resistance*,
https://doi.org/10.1007/978-3-031-52860-6_4

pies. These therapies aim to enhance the immune response against cancer cells and overcome mechanisms of drug resistance. By leveraging the body's natural defenses, immunotherapy holds promise in revolutionizing breast cancer treatment and improving patient outcomes.

Keywords Breast cancer · Immunotherapy · Drug resistance · Immune checkpoint inhibitors · Adoptive cell therapy

Introduction

The ability of the immune system to recognize and destroy precancerous cells is enabled by a process called immunosurveillance. This takes place during immunoselection where the immune system clears poorly immunogenic cancer cell variants. Immunosurveillance can also be avoided through immune subversion where cancer cells develop mechanisms to suppress immune responses (Zitvogel et al., 2006). Immunosurveillance was later described as cancer immunoediting divided into three stages. During the elimination phase, cancer cells are destroyed by the immune system. Should the immune system fail to get rid of cancer cell variants, the immune system becomes tolerant and allows cancer cells to survive within the equilibrium phase. Finally, cancer cells constantly mutate thus developing variants that can evade the immune system and continue to grow uncontrollably during the escape phase and become clinically detectable (Dunn et al., 2004a, 2004b). It is through this concept that scientists were able to discover that cancer cells express specific antigens that are useful for their identification. The challenge of mapping out the tumor antigen landscape is averted by advances in genome sequencing which allowed the discovery of diverse mutations as a result of genomic instability (Vesely & Schreiber, 2013).

An encounter with tumor antigens results in a pool of T cells that develop remembrance for these antigens. These T cells referred to as memory T cells can be harvested, multiplied, and engineered to specifically attack cancer cells. However, the architecture of the tumor microenvironment (TME) of solid cancers has made T cell engineering for solid tumors such as breast cancer (BC) a challenge (Ellis et al., 2021). Chimeric antigen receptor (CAR) T cells are autologous T cells genetically engineered to express chimeric receptors with a single-chain variable fragment with costimulatory molecules such as CD28, 4-1BB, and OX40 that bind to specific tumor antigens (Kudva & Modak, 2019; Toulouie et al., 2021). CAR T cells have a high affinity for target antigen and do not need activation by antigen-presenting cells indicating their potential in eliminating cancer cells (Toulouie et al., 2021). To leverage the benefits of CAR T cells and avert physical barriers posed by BC tumors. Wallstabe et al. 2019 generated microphysiological three-dimensional (3D) lung and breast cancer models that resemble architectural and phenotypical features of primary tumors. The study found that receptor tyrosine kinase-like orphan receptor 1-specific (ROR1-specific) CAR T cells can penetrate the core of the tumor and evoke anti-tumor activities. Tumor cells below and under the basement membrane were cleared out by ROR1 CAR T cells during migration to the core of the TME (Wallstabe et al., 2019).

Pembrolizumab was approved by the US Food and Drug Administration (FDA) in November 2020 for triple-negative breast cancer (TNBC) (Li et al., 2022). It is an anti-programmed death 1 (PD-1) monoclonal antibody administered to patients with metastatic TNBC (Schmid et al., 2020). Several other immunotherapy regimes have emerged as promising. These include other ICIs such as cytotoxic T-lymphocyte-associated antigen 4 (CTLA-4) blockades (Mina et al., 2019), adoptive T cell therapies such as the application of cytokine-induced killers (CIK) cells and cancer vaccines (Li et al., 2021b). However, it should be noted that immunotherapy is only successful in a certain group of patients. Furthermore, combination modalities have improved overall therapeutic response as opposed to single agent modalities; (Bayat Mokhtari et al., 2017; Boshuizen & Peeper, 2020) nevertheless, these therapies are still only successful in small group of patients (Boshuizen & Peeper, 2020). Moreover, cancer cells develop mechanisms to evade immunotherapies thus subjecting most patients to drug resistance (Bai et al., 2020). This chapter will, therefore, focus on the methods used to improve immunotherapy as a potential solution to overcome drug resistance in breast cancer. The chapter will also explore various immunotherapeutic approaches, including immune checkpoint inhibitors, adoptive cell transfer, and bispecific antibody therapies. These therapies aim to enhance the immune response against cancer cells and overcome mechanisms of drug resistance.

Classification of Immunotherapy Resistance to Breast Cancer Immunotherapies

There is a lack of consistency in terms of defining different types of resistance. Classification is mainly based on clinical outcomes (Vesely et al., 2022), namely: Primary resistance, acquired resistance, and adaptive resistance. Thus, primary resistance refers to the inability of cancers to respond to immunotherapeutic regimes. This is exacerbated by adaptive immune resistance which involves cancer cells manipulating the immune system to avoid clearance. Acquired resistance develops post-treatment whereby cancers respond to therapy but later relapse and progress (Sharma et al., 2017). Several factors are involved in resistance to immunotherapies, and these could be either intrinsic or extrinsic tumor factors. The intrinsic tumor factors could be due to the absence of neoantigens, defective antigen presentation machinery, genetic T cell exclusion, dysregulation of interferon signaling, or insensibility to T cells. The extrinsic factors could be due to an increase in immunosuppressive cells or inhibitory immune checkpoints (Sharma et al., 2017; Zhou et al., 2021).

Current Approaches in Breast Cancer Immunotherapeutic Interventions

Immune Checkpoint Inhibitors

Atezolizumab was the first immune checkpoint inhibitor to be approved by the FDA in March 2019 as immunotherapy for TNBC (Soare & Soare, 2019). This was followed by pembrolizumab for high-risk, early-stage TNBC in July 2021 (Bagegni et al., 2022). The efficacy of both immunotherapies has been substantially investigated both in terms of cost-effectiveness and efficaciousness by several studies (Isla et al., 2023; Zhang et al., 2018; West, 2018; Wu et al., 2018). In July 2021, the approval of atezolizumab was voluntarily withdrawn by the manufacturer (Valencia et al., 2022). Duan et al., 2020 also investigated the safety of anti-PD-1 and its ligand and found them to be favorably comparable in both survival outcomes and safety profile (Duan et al., 2020). The decision to focus on TNBC for clinical trials was based on the high immunogenic capacity of the disease including the expression of PD-L1 compared to other BCs. Several clinical trials reported an overall response rate (ORR) in TNBC patients with positive PD-L1 expression higher than other BCs (Howard et al., 2022) (Table 1). Additionally, metastatic breast cancer patients with positive PD-L1 expression showed significantly favorable response rate [odds ratio (OR) = 1.44, $p = 0.01$] and 1 year progression-free survival (PFS) (OR = 1.55, $p = 0.04$) compared to patients with a negative PD-L1 expression. Tumor-infiltrating lymphocytes (TILs) and increased frequency of infiltrated CD8+ T cells were shown to be the best predictors of ICI therapeutic responses (Zou et al., 2020).

The observation of TIL as a predictor of pathological complete response (pCR) to ICIs and favorable response in BC has revolutionized the understanding of how the immune system responds to this disease. This led to investigations of other immune checkpoints such as CTLA-4 (Wein et al., 2018). The expression of CTLA-4 in BC is associated with disease-free survival (DFS), overall survival (OS), and disease stage. CTLA-4 is expressed in both T and B-cells. Studies have shown an increased expression in regulatory T cells (Tregs) (Kern & Panis, 2021). Tregs constitutively express CTLA-4 as part of their mechanisms to suppress anti-cancer immunity (Sobhani et al., 2021). The levels of Tregs are highly increased in some patients with cancers (Saleh & Elkord, 2020).

Adoptive Cell Therapy

The ability of the immune system to distinguish cancer cells from normal cells and evoke processes to discriminately destroy these cells along with the ability to store memory of the first attack has encouraged the development of cancer immunotherapies to have a prolonged immunological effect with less toxicity (Beatty & Gladney,

Table 1 An update on clinical trials on the recently FDA approved, pembrolizumab for breast cancer immunotherapy

Clinical trial	Status	Trial number
Phase 2 study of imprime PGG and Pembrolizumab in patients with hormone receptor-positive or human epidermal receptor 2 negative [HR+/human epidermal growth factor receptor 2 (HER2)-] metastatic breast cancer (mBC)	Completed	NCT05159778
Neoadjuvant Pembrolizumab (Pbr)/nab-paclitaxel followed by Pbr/Epirubicin/ cyclophosphamide in TNBC	Completed	NCT03289819
Study to evaluate the efficacy and safety of Eribulin Mesylate in combination with Pembrolizumab in participants with metastatic triple-negative breast cancer (mTNBC)	Completed with results	NCT02513472
Study of Pembrolizumab (MK-3475) monotherapy for metastatic triple-negative breast cancer (MK-3475-086/ KEYNOTE-086)	Completed with results	NCT02447003
Effect of Pembrolizumab (Keytruda®) on biomarkers in early breast cancer.	Completed with results	NCT03197389
Ph II study of Pembrolizumab and Eribulin in patients with HR+/HER2- MBC previously treated with anthracyclines and Taxanes	Completed	NCT03222856
Niraparib in combination with Pembrolizumab in patients with triple-negative breast cancer or ovarian cancer	Completed with results	NCT02657889
Pilot study of paclitaxel plus Pembrolizumab in metastatic HER2-negative breast cancer	Completed with results	NCT03018080
Trial to evaluate efficacy and safety of Pembrolizumab and gemcitabine in HER2-negative ABC	Completed with results	NCT03025880
Study of single-dose cyclophosphamide +Pembrolizumab in patients with metastatic triple-negative breast cancer	Completed with results	NCT02768701
Phase 1b trial of Dinaciclib with Pembrolizumab for advanced breast cancer	Completed	NCT01676753
Study to assess the efficacy of Pembrolizumab plus radiotherapy in metastatic triple-negative breast cancer patients	Completed with results	NCT02730130

2015; Koury et al., 2018). Adoptive cell transfer (ACT) therapy utilizes immune cells modified ex vivo and infused into cancer patients to elicit an anti-tumor immune response with higher precision than surgery, chemo, or radiotherapy (Kiaei et al., 2023). The process of ACT involves, lympho-depletion which also assists with the elimination of immunosuppressive cells such as Tregs, cell administration followed by high doses of interleukin 2 (IL-2) (Koury et al., 2018; Rosenberg et al., 2008). ACT therapies include TIL, CAR T cells, engineered T cell receptor (TCR), and natural killer (NK) cells (Gautam et al., 2022). Their use in BC, therapeutic efficacy, and resistance will be discussed in more detail in the next sections.

Tumor-Infiltrating Lymphocytes (TILs) Therapy

Tumor-infiltrating lymphocytes (TILs) therapy is a form of adoptive therapy that involves the in vitro expansion of a patient's tumor-derived T lymphocytes followed by infusion into the patient (Koury et al., 2018) Fig. 1. When compared to primary tumors, TNBC tumors were shown to have significantly reduced infiltration lymphocytes. Increased TILs frequency is associated with improved survival (Park et al., 2019). Hence their consideration as surrogate biomarkers of T lymphocytes associated with anti-cancer immunity and ultimate use as predictive markers in early TNBCs. The heterogeneity of TILs and localization within the TME contribute to their functions against cancer cells with some favoring progression and others being anti-cancerous. Their identification as single cells limits their clinical value toward BC subtypes and thus must be further evaluated (Valenza et al., 2023).

Although clinical validity of the use of TILs as the surrogate marker was achieved by inter-pathologists-reproducibility studies, the analytical validity of TILs is yet to be determined due to the lack of a set golden standard. The International TILs Working Group has worked on standardizing methods to assess TILs in cancer tissues using hematoxylin and eosin (H&E). The ratio between lymphocytes and plasma cells infiltrating the stromal and the tumor is used as a measure of

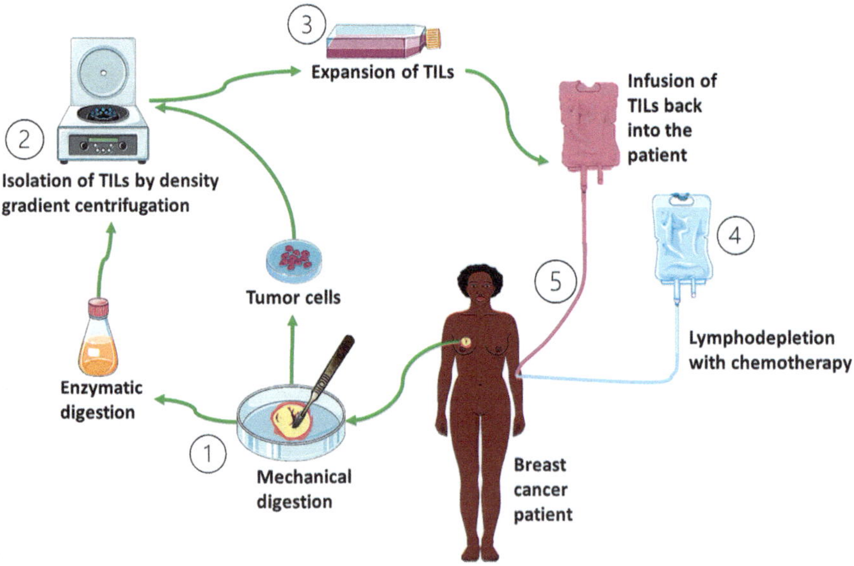

Fig. 1 Preparation of anti-tumor T cells for TILS therapy. (1) A patient's tumor is resected, and mechanical and enzymatic digestion of the tissue is performed to have a cell suspension. (2) Thereafter, the TILs are isolated from the cell suspension by density gradient centrifugation. (3) Isolated TILs will be expanded in the laboratory. (4) The patient will be treated with chemotherapy for the removal of lymphocytes from the patient's system before infusing (5) TILs back into the patient

assessment. A lymphocyte-predominant BC (LPBC) is then used as a description of BCs with >50% stromal lymphocytic infiltration (Salgado et al., 2015; El Bairi et al., 2021) and improves survival rate with every 10% increase in TILs (Stanton & Disis, 2016).

The HER2-BCs reduced the frequency of TILs, increased Tregs and PD-L1 expression, and therefore the worst prognosis compared to other BC subtypes which present with low, intermediate, or high infiltration of TILs. This feature is what presents TNBCs as the most responsive to ICI therapy. Therapeutic approaches that aim at increasing TILs might be beneficial to other BC subtypes to achieve better clinical outcomes. These could be in the form of other oncotherapeutic regimes such as chemoradiotherapy, targeted cytotoxic therapy, or vaccine therapy (Stanton & Disis, 2016). This is validated by a study done by Demaria et al. 2001 which indicated that neoadjuvant paclitaxel therapy resulted in histologically increased TILs as assessed by clinically complete response in 4 out of 6 BC patients who had low TILs before treatment (Demaria et al., 2001). However, the presence of immunosuppressive regulatory B-cells (Bregs) which induce activation of Tregs within TIL aggregates in the TME is a major challenge of therapeutic response in BCs. This group of cells is responsible for cancers acquiring immune tolerance and rendering cytotoxic TILs dysfunctional against cancer cells (Ishigami et al., 2019).

In personalized immunotherapy, a patient's tumor-infiltrating T cells are also depleted and infused back into the patient. Long-term exposure to cancer cells renders these T cells exhausted. Therefore, in personalized immunotherapy, only T cells that are still active toward the cancer cells are isolated and infused back into the patient. Interestingly, these neoantigens are unique to each patient. This treatment has shown a complete response in patients with metastatic BC, with one patient who was treated in 2018 remaining cancer free (Zacharakis et al., 2022; NIH, 2022). The approach also resolved therapeutic resistance posed by other TILs as previously indicated (Ishigami et al., 2019).

Chimeric Antigen Receptor (CAR) T Cell Therapy

The majority of CAR T cells are produced by the introduction of CARs into T cells via virus-derived vectors such as lenti/retroviruses or transposon-derived vectors such as the sleeping beauty (SB)/piggyBac (PB) transposon system as well as transient mRNA transfection (Dey et al., 2023; Lukjanov et al., 2021). CARs bind to a specific tumor antigen hence they can be engineered to target specific cancers. Although it has been challenging to apply CAR T cell therapy to solid cancers, recent advances have allowed the targeting of tumor-associated antigens such as mucin 1 (MUC1) (Jing et al., 2019), HER2, and Carcinoembryonic antigen (CEA) (Zhang et al., 2022). MUC1+ CAR T cells co-expressed with cytokine receptor linking the IL4 receptor exodomain with the IL7 receptor endodomain (4/7ICR) induced prolonged anti-cancer activity even in the suppressive TME (Bajgain et al., 2018). Recently FDA approved an investigational new drug application, MUC1*-CAR-1XX (huMNC2-CAR22; Minerva Biotechnologies) for CAR T cell targeting metastatic BC for clinical trials (Hunter, 2023). MUC1 is a transmembrane mucin overexpressed in several metastatic solid tumors and is considered a reliable diagnostic marker for metastatic progression (Horm & Schroeder, 2013).

In continual efforts to discover effective immunotherapy for BC, Price et al. 2018 found that HER2-CARs containing the 4-1BB costimulatory domain as opposed to CD28 have improved ability to induce anti-tumor activity while reducing T cells that display exhaustion in the brain metastatic BC. HER2-CAR T cells that were administered intraventricularly showed more efficiency indicating that the mode of delivery as well as CAR design have a significant role in the decision-making of multifocal BC brain metastases treatment (Priceman et al., 2018). In contrast to this study, complete remission was observed with the administration of even a small dose of HER2-CARs containing the CD28 costimulatory domain in HER2-positive JIMT-1 BC xenografts in severe combined immunodeficiency disease (SCID) mice (Tóth et al., 2020). The combination of HER2-CAR T cells with anti-PD1 antibody significantly increased the efficacy of therapy by inhibiting tumor growth and facilitating apoptosis (Li et al., 2020).

HER2-specific CAR T cells have also been shown to decipher drug resistance to chemotherapy. T cells expressing CARs containing the CD28 costimulatory domain derived from trastuzumab were generated and tested for cytotoxicity of HER2+ BC cell lines and xenografts resistant to the drug. A single dose of trastuzumab-derived HER2-specific CAR T cells is specific and can penetrate the TME and efficiently eradicate BC tumors (Szöőr et al., 2020). Although CARs can successfully eradicate cancer cells, mechanisms of cancer cells to develop intrinsic resistance to HER2-specific CAR T cells are eminent. Cancer cells induce interferon-gamma (IFN-γ) signaling dysregulation in HER2-specific CAR T cells. A protein encoded by a gene that is specifically regulated by IFN-γ signaling, interferon regulatory factor 1 (IRF1) was impaired in resistant HER2-specific CAR T cells. Furthermore, knocking out the Interferon Gamma Receptor 1 (IFNGR1) gene, JAK1 or STAT1 using CRISPR–Cas9 technology, or downregulating its expression with shRNAs from parental BT474 cells resulted in dysregulation of IFN-γ signaling leading to HER2-CAR T cells. The same results were observed in coculture assays with HER2-T cell bispecific antibodies (TCBs) (Arenas et al., 2021).

Engineered T Cell Receptor Therapy

T Cell Receptor (TCR) therapies conquer the limitations of CAR T cell therapy which only focuses on targeting surface antigen by providing a wider range of antigens and overcoming challenges posed by the immunosuppressive TME and its heterogeneous nature. Antigens that can be targeted for TCR-T cell therapy can recognize epitopes from both surface and intracellular proteins presented by the major histocompatibility complex (MHC) although limited to the human leukocyte antigen (HLA) allele presenting the epitope. This increases sensitivity thus allowing improved tumor cell detection and destruction (Baulu et al., 2023). The most abundant CD8 + T cells expressed TCRs are composed of an alpha (α-) and a beta (β) -chain with a small subset (1–10%) consisting of gamma (γ) and delta (δ)-chains (Tsimberidou et al., 2021). The gamma delta (γδ) T cells are the most studied subgroup connecting innate and adaptive immunity. These cells can either be pro- or anti-tumorous (Li et al., 2021a; Schönefeldt et al., 2021; Kabelitz et al., 2020). One of the best features of γδ T cells is their ability to evoke immunity without the need for TCR–MHC interaction. This is complemented by the ability to detect tumors without specific surveillance of tumor-associated antigens (TAAs) but through NK cell receptors (Zlatareva & Wu, 2023).

TNBCs are abundant in cancer stem cells which promote metastasis and drug resistance. γδ T cells isolated from healthy individuals effectively recognized and eliminated primary TNBC cancer stem cells. An activating receptor, natural killer group 2D (NKG2D) acts as the mediator of anti-cancer activity of γδ T cells and was upregulated during their expansion. Orthotopical transplants of breast cancer stem cells into the mammary gland of non-obese diabetic (NOD) SCID mice were treated with γδ T cells and no significant increase in overall survival of mice was observed, as reported by Raute et al., 2022. This led the authors to investigate if cancer stem cells were still sensitive to treatment and found that γδ T cells had lost the capacity to destroy the tumor cells. However, secretion molecules that assist in γδ T cell-killing capacity remained intact. However, further studies indicated that they could still migrate to cancers. Ultimately, the authors found the expression of mammary stem cell proteins was significantly reduced in xenograft-derived tumor cells indicating that BC cancer stem cells developed resistance by restructuring their signature while maintaining the patient's molecular tumor subtype (Raute et al., 2022).

Natural Killer Cell Therapy

The involvement of NK cells in anti-cancer mechanisms also holds promise for their use in cellular immunotherapy. NK cells evoke anti-cancer immune responses without the need for MHC engagement, thus their genetic modifications can heighten their functionality and ability to overcome cancer-escaping mechanisms (Chu et al., 2022). Their most powerful resources for modulating cancer mechanisms are through the induction of cytokine responses. The presence of active IL-2 and IL-15 can enhance the survival and cytotoxicity of NK cells (Fig. 2). Immune checkpoint inhibitors such as anti-PD-1, anti-PD-L1, or CTLA-4 can block the interaction between the co-inhibitory receptors and ligands interaction between NK cells and tumor cells preventing inhibitory effects on the NK cell as a result enhancing its activity (Fig. 2). NK cells express CD16 enabling their interaction with Fc regions of antibodies linked to tumor antigens to initiate antibody-dependent cellular cytotoxicity (ADCC) (Wang et al., 2022) (Maskalenko et al., 2022) or immunomodulation through bi- or tri-specific antibody activities (Fig. 2) (Maskalenko et al., 2022) (Kiaei et al., 2023).

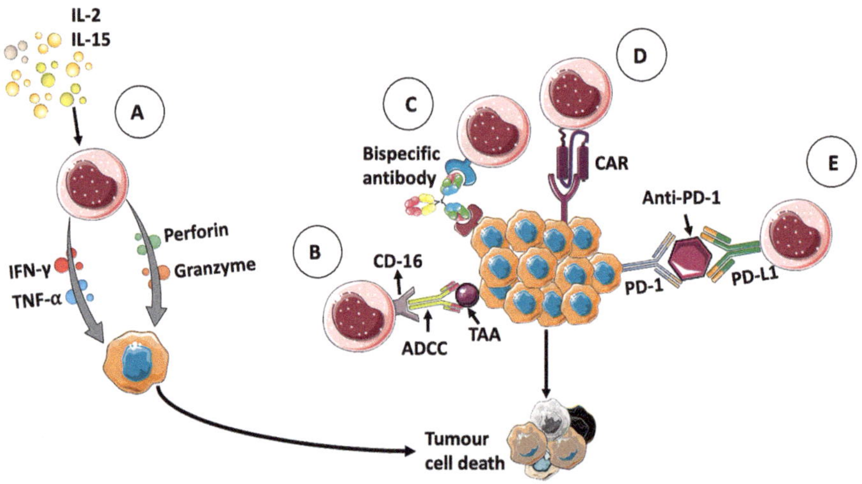

Fig. 2 Methods of enhancing NK therapy. (**a**) Demonstrates the use of cytokines such as IL-2 and IL-15 to enhance NK cell survival and cytotoxicity. (**b**) The ADCC is generated by the monoclonal antibody linking CD16 of the NK cell to TAA expressed on the tumor cell surface. (**c**) Using bispecific antibodies to redirect NK cells to tumor cells through interacting with NK's CD16 and tumor cell's antigen. (**d**) NK cells can be engineered ex vivo to express CAR molecules specific to tumor antigens not expressed on MHC class I molecules. (**e**) Immune checkpoint inhibitors bind to and block the interaction between immune checkpoint molecules with NK cell co-inhibitory molecules. These methods enhance interaction between NK cells and tumor cells, and consequently augmenting NK cell cytotoxicity eradicating tumor cells

Immunomodulation by a bispecific antibody with a tribody structure consisting of two HER2-specific single-chain variable fragments (scFv) linked to fragment antigen binding for interacting with CD16 expressed on NK cells and γδ T Cell in solid cancers was evaluated. Study findings indicated that the bispecific antibody enhanced NK cell-mediated cytolysis in HER2-expressing breast, pancreatic ductal adenocarcinoma (PDAC), and ovarian tumor cells (Oberg et al., 2018). Chimeric antigen receptor-engineered NK cell therapy employs the use of NK cells obtainable from multiple sources including cell lines, PBMCs, cord blood, and induced pluripotent stem cells with an enhanced cytotoxic function through the incorporation of CAR receptor (Wang et al., 2022). An epidermal growth factor receptor (EGFR)-specific CAR-NK cells containing an anti-EGFR single-chain variable fragment (scFv) region capable of recognizing an EGFR receptor on TNBC cells exhibited their potential use as therapeutic strategies for treating TNBC patients. These cells were shown to kill TNBC cells overexpressing EGFR in vitro and in vivo consequently inhibiting TNBC progression (Liu et al., 2020). Expanded NK cells from healthy controls and BC patients were equally efficient at lysing BC cell lines indicating that autologous treatment of NK cells derived from the same patient can be useful as immunotherapy (Shenouda et al., 2017).

Bispecific Antibody Therapy

Bispecific antibodies (BsAbs) are a heterogeneous family of antibodies with recognition of two specific antigens or epitopes on the same target triggering two different immunological responses (Fig. 3) (Labrijn et al., 2019). The use of BsAbs in cancer immunotherapy relies on the recruitment of T cells and activation of memory T cells (Labrijn et al., 2019; Kamakura et al., 2021). Upon recognition of cancer cells within the TME, a crosslink between cancer cells and T cells is initiated allowing specific recognition of tumor cells without the need for MHC engagement (Offner et al., 2006).

Because memory T cells are already present with the TME, crosslinking with tumor cells by tumor-accumulated BsAbs stimulates T cell activation. This results in the expansion of activated T cells and secretion of cytotoxic and proinflammatory cytokines which promotes contact-independent cell killing and the Fas ligand/Fas-mediated apoptosis, respectively. Circulating T cells are recruited to the TME by proinflammatory cytokines and other intrinsic signaling molecules such as the CXCR3. Tumor cells /BsAbs immune synapses are generated and activated T cells initiate perforin and granzyme mechanisms for the destruction of cancer cells.

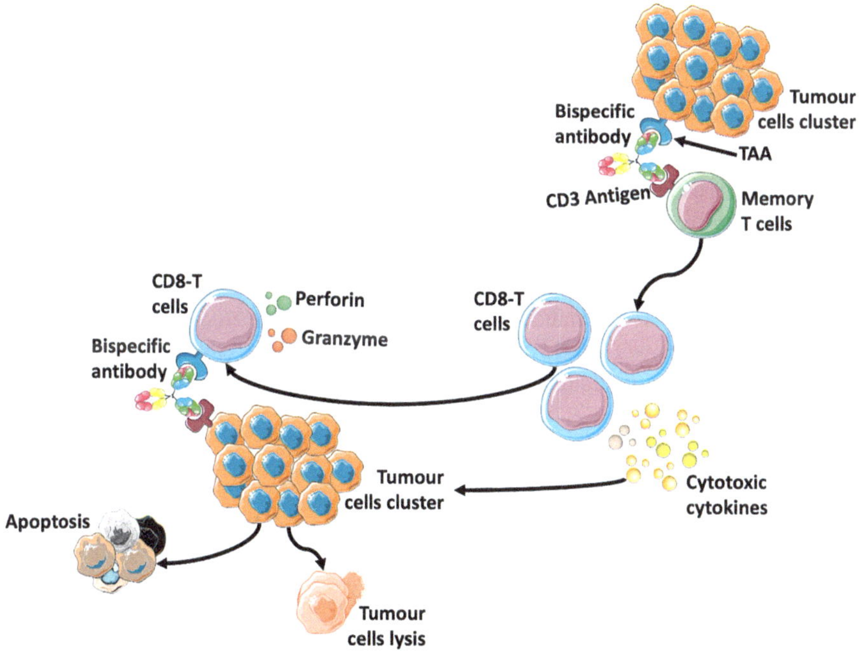

Fig. 3 Bispecific antibodies. Bispecific antibodies have specificity for both CD3 expressed on memory T cells and TAA which activates memory T cells, as a result inducing cytotoxic T cell proliferation. Thereafter, cytotoxic T cells will initiate cell-dependent cytotoxicity or cell-independent cytotoxicity through the secretion of cytokines resulting in tumor cell apoptosis or cytolysis

Adjacent tumor cells will also be destroyed by continuous cross-linking with tumor cells (Fig. 3). However, although promising, none of the BsAbs have been approved for cancer immunotherapy thus far due to therapeutic efficacy complicated by the complexity of the TME (Kamakura et al., 2021).

To investigate the potential therapeutic efficacy of BsAbs in BC, Liu et al. 2021 developed a novel BsAb referred to as F7AK3 fused with a single-chain variable fragment (ScFv) of anti-CD3 with human anti-trophoblast cell surface antigen 2 (TROP2), its Fc part. The innovation was encouraged by the approval of an anti-TROP2 antibody–drug conjugate, Sacituzumab govitecan, which was approved by the FDA for metastatic TNBC in 2020. An increased binding affinity was observed between F7AK3 with TROP2 protein. The half maximal effective concentration (EC_{50}) value of the MCF7 cell line in response to F7AK3 treatment was significantly increased compared to another BC cell line. This correlated well with the expression levels of TROP2. The antibodies were also shown to specifically target cancer cells within the TME (Liu et al., 2021).

Another novel BsAb that is clinically [ClinicalTrials.gov (NCT02892123)] being tested on patients with locally advanced or metastatic HER2-expressing or HER2-amplified cancers is zanidatamab (ZW25) for safety, tolerability, and effectiveness. Zanidatamab targets two non-overlapping domains of HER2. Patients had favorable tolerance to the antibodies administered at different dosages. The final recommended dose was 20 mg/kg every 2 weeks; however, BC was excluded. Though there was no mortality reported, six grade 3 treatment-related adverse events were seen in 4 of 132 patients with diarrhea being the most reported followed by infusion reactions. The efficaciousness was therefore verified only in biliary tract cancer and colorectal cancer (Meric-Bernstam et al., 2022).

Intrinsic resistance to HER2-T cell bispecific antibodies (HER2-TCBs) therapy was tested by treating mice with PBMC: BT474 cocultures with HER2-TCB. Six months later, the BT-R cells had a tenfold increased IC50 compared to parental cells. Silencing IFNGR1 resulted in resistance in 3D cultures and in vivo. BT-R cells also developed resistance to trastuzumab-based second-generation HER2-TCBs in both settings. JAK2 was downregulated as a potential consequence of IFN-γ signaling dysregulation while pSTAT1 levels decreased with IFN-γ therapy (Labrijn et al., 2019).

Combinations of Cancer Immunotherapy in Breast Cancer

Several combination therapies are now used as first-line for multiple cancers. These mainly involve chemotherapy and ICIs (Lu et al., 2022). The pembrolizumab and chemotherapy combination therapy was approved by the FDA on the 13th of November 2020 for PD-L1 positive metastatic TNBC patients (Li et al., 2022). It was shown in a phase 3 clinical trial that early TNBC patients who received adjuvant chemotherapy and pembrolizumab combination therapy exhibited a significantly higher pCR compared to patients who received placebo and neoadjuvant chemotherapy (Schmid et al., 2020). Other clinical trials conducted to assess the effectiveness of Pembrolizumab with other therapies are indicated in Table 1.

The ALICE trial was one of the first investigations of the safety and efficacy of the combination of atezolizumab with anthracyclines used for the treatment of mTNBC. Patients treated with this combination therapy had significantly improved progression-free survival (PFS) compared to patients administered with the placebo-chemotherapy combination. Improved therapeutic outcome was also observed in patients with PD-L1-negative tumors (Røssevold et al., 2022). However, it should be noted that on September 08, 2020, the FDA raised concerns regarding the efficacy and potential safety of atezolizumab and paclitaxel in mTNBCs (FDA, 2020).

This warrants the need to further investigate combination therapies that have potential efficacy for BCs more for the hard-to-treat TNBC. Thus, a study has looked at identifying biomarkers for CAR T cell therapies that can be used in combination with antibody–drug conjugates to improve efficacy and safety for BC therapy. Data was collected from The Cancer Genome Atlas to assess BC subtypes with the 200 most upregulated gene expression. Of the previously identified potential specific tumor-associated antigen genes, TACSD2 (protein TROP-2), SLC39A6 (protein LIV-1), ERBB2 (protein HER2), and ERBB3 (protein HER3), the current study identified fibroblast growth factor receptor-4 (FGFR4), carcinoembryonic antigen-related cell adhesion molecule 6 (CEACAM6), GDNF family receptor alpha 1 (GFRA1), integrin beta-6 (ITGB6) and ectonucleotide pyrophosphatase/phosphodiesterase 1 (ENPP1) which could be used for the development of novel CAR T cells therapy in combination with antibody–drug conjugates in BC (Schettini et al., 2021).

Overcoming Immune Resistance and Enhancing Responses

PEGylation of nanoparticles prevents them from being stuck within the reticuloendothelial system thus keeping them longer in circulation (Cheng et al., 2019). Seeing that PEGylated liposomal doxorubicin (DOX), Lipo-Dox® was approved for metastatic BC (Aloss & Hamar, 2023), the approach was used to develop HER2+ methoxy-polyethylene glycol (mPEG) to improve the efficacy of PEGylated liposomal doxorubicin (PLD) therapy in BC (Cheng et al., 2019). Nanoparticles improve the efficacy of DOX by ensuring its delivery and accumulation in the TME. However, the most prominent adverse event seen with DOX is cardiotoxicity (Aloss & Hamar, 2023) followed by vomiting and alopecia (O'Brien et al., 2004). PLD therapy showed over 200- and 28-fold increased cytotoxicity to HER2 + MCF7 cells and drug-resistant MDA-MB-361 cells, respectively (Cheng et al., 2019). To overcome efflux pump (EP) mediated drug resistance, BsAbs with specificity for extracellular domains of EPs and tumor-associated antigens (TAA) were developed. Antibodies had a high binding affinity and their efficacy to destroy cancer cells remained the same as monotherapy and in addition with other cancer therapies. Less off-tumor toxicity was shown thus indicating that they provide promising novel targeted therapies for patients with drug-resistant cancers (Arathoon et al., 2021).

Conventional DCs (cDCs) present antigens to T cells and modulate their function. Upon activation, T cells proliferate and survive. There are two subtypes of CDCs, namely, cDC1 and cDC2. Each has its transcription factors but among others, cDC1 depends on BATF3 for proliferation (Böttcher & Reis e Sousa, 2018). These Batf3-dependent cDC1s were used to induce anti-tumor T cell immunity in orthotopic tumor mouse models with anti-PD-L1 resistant tumors. Immunohistochemical analysis of tumor samples showed decreased CD8+ T cells with an abundance of CD163+ tumor-associated macrophages (TAMs) in AT-3, B16, and 4 T1 tumors compared to MC38 tumors in response to anti-PD-L1 therapy indicating that the latter models do not respond well to therapy. These models were then treated with a combinatorial therapeutic regimen referred to as in situ immunomodulation (ISIM) which comprised intratumoral sequential administration of Flt3L, radiotherapy, and TLR3/CD40 agonists. Migration and increased infiltration of CD103+ DCs were observed in TME, lymph nodes, and circulation. Moreover, lymph nodes had high infiltration of TAA-loaded cDC1s facilitated by TLR3/CD40 stimulation compared to control lymph nodes of mice treated with PBS. An increase in ISIM-induced CD8+ T cell infiltration results in upregulation of the expression of PD-1 on CD8+ TILs and a concurrent increase in susceptibility to anti-PD-L1 therapy due to ISIM-induced tumor-specific CD8+ T cell infiltrations. Taken together, these results have provided evidence of the ability of cDCs to overcome mechanisms of intratumoral T cell exclusion and increase their sensitivity to immune checkpoint therapy (Oba et al., 2020).

Resistance to BC immunotherapy is conferred by low tumor mutation burden which generates fewer TAAs and thus reduced antigen presentation capacity. To develop methods to overcome resistance in BC, Wu et al. engineered smart nanovesicles from autologous DC-derived small extracellular vesicles (sEVs) for active and personalized immunotherapeutic treatment in BC. These sEVs expressed surface membrane-bound IL2. A combination of lipopolysaccharides (LPS) and stimulator of interferon genes (STING) agonist-induced the expression of costimulatory molecules on the surface of the nanovesicle needed to produce an enhanced version of such active immunotherapy (ep13nsEV). This IL2-ep13nsEV smart nanovesicle could target lymphocytes, prime T cells induce active anti-cancer immunity in patient-derived xenografts, and improve therapeutic response to ICIs (Wu et al., 2023).

Challenges and Limitations

The initial attempt to treat patients with a high concentration of CAR T cells resulted in a patient experiencing a lot of distress within a few minutes after administration before going into a coma. This patient ultimately died 5 days later with organs, mostly the lungs infiltrated with CAR T cells resulting in the discovery that the cause of death was the expression of HER2 in pulmonary epithelial cells (Johnson & June, 2017). CAR T cell exhaustion may occur as they enter solid tumors. Moreover, CAR T cells target tumor-associated antigens which may lead to mistargeting (Zhao & Cao, 2019).

Alpha-beta T cell (αβT cell) immune systems cannot be transferred between individuals unless all of the HLA molecules are precisely matched. Transferring γδ T cells between individuals may be less restricted and allow the use of γδ T cells from normal volunteers who would serve as "universal donors" (Tsimberidou et al., 2021). The αβTCR cells are restricted to tumor antigens presented on MHC molecules and this reduces their targets as many tumor antigens are not presented on MHC molecules (Fuentes-Antrás et al., 2020). The process of generating quality engineered TCR and CAR T cells is costly and overly complex as it involves highly regulated good manufacturing processes (GMP). Other challenges include the limitation of the T cell persistence through costimulatory molecule paucity, immune suppressive TME, and the tumor's capacity to generate immune escape mechanisms varying among tumor types and patients (Shafer et al., 2022).

There are thorny problems associated with CAR-NK cells despite their impressive therapeutic potential hampering their approval. CAR-NK cell function may be suppressed by the presence of transforming growth factor beta (TGF-β), Indoleamine 2,3-dioxygenase (IDO), IL-10, PD-1, and prostaglandin E2 (PGE2) secreted by tumor cells. Furthermore, NK cells are difficult to transport and store since they are sensitive to cryopreservation. Thawing reduces their survival rate as well as cytotoxic ability (Wang et al., 2022). Lastly, transfused NK cell proliferation in patients is restricted by Tregs and myeloid-derived suppressor cells (MDSCs) (Kiaei et al., 2023).

Conclusion and Future Perspectives

Immunotherapy is a recent advance in oncology that has revolutionized breast cancer treatment and improved the survival of patients with advanced disease. Mono- or combination therapies have exhibited positive patient clinical outcomes. However, the development of severe immune-related adverse events (irAEs), low response rate, resistance, manufacturing, transportation, and storage poses a challenge in their clinical applications. This calls for the development of novel immunotherapy strategies or exploring ways of improving these therapies to be effective and feasible in clinical application. This should include a better characterization of BC TME as many therapies are challenged by its heterogeneity. Moreover, predictive markers indicating therapy response or resistance in early stage and metastatic stages for all breast cancer subtypes should also be explored. It is quite impressive that the number of clinical trials exploring various immunotherapeutic strategies is increasing across all BC subtypes, however, more population groups should be studied such as patients from lower socioeconomic population groups, for example, black patients as they present with aggressive disease, recurrence, and high mortality rates.

Exploring ways of reducing costs and improving the production, transportation, and storage of adoptive cell therapies can improve their feasibility in clinical applications.

References

Aloss, K., & Hamar, P. (2023). Recent preclinical and clinical Progress in liposomal doxorubicin. *Pharmaceutics, 15*, 893.

Arathoon, R., Briante, R., O'connor, A., Tan, C., Klein, P., Morgan, J., Ponath, P., Presta, L., Zhai, Q., Mohanty, S., & Zhang, P. (2021). 282 bispecific antibodies (BsAbs) targeting ABCB1/PgP and CD47 provide a multi-modal, tumor-specific approach to combat drug resistant cancers. *Journal for ImmunoTherapy of Cancer, 9*, A306–A306.

Arenas, E. J., Martínez-Sabadell, A., Rius Ruiz, I., Román Alonso, M., Escorihuela, M., Luque, A., Fajardo, C. A., Gros, A., Klein, C., & Arribas, J. (2021). Acquired cancer cell resistance to T cell bispecific antibodies and CAR T targeting HER2 through JAK2 down-modulation. *Nature Communications, 12*, 1237.

Bagegni, N. A., Davis, A. A., Clifton, K. K., & Ademuyiwa, F. O. (2022). Targeted treatment for high-risk early-stage triple-negative breast cancer: Spotlight on Pembrolizumab. *Breast Cancer (Dove Med Press), 14*, 113–123.

Bai, R., Chen, N., Li, L., Du, N., Bai, L., Lv, Z., Tian, H., & Cui, J. (2020). Mechanisms of cancer resistance to immunotherapy. *Frontiers in Oncology, 10*, 1290.

Bajgain, P., Tawinwung, S., D'elia, L., Sukumaran, S., Watanabe, N., Hoyos, V., Lulla, P., Brenner, M. K., Leen, A. M., & Vera, J. F. (2018). CAR T cell therapy for breast cancer: Harnessing the tumor milieu to drive T cell activation. *Journal for ImmunoTherapy of Cancer, 6*, 34.

Baulu, E., Gardet, C., Chuvin, N., & Depil, S. (2023). TCR-engineered T cell therapy in solid tumors: State of the art and perspectives. *Science Advances, 9*, eadf3700.

Bayat Mokhtari, R., Homayouni, T. S., Baluch, N., Morgatskaya, E., Kumar, S., Das, B., & Yeger, H. (2017). Combination therapy in combating cancer. *Oncotarget, 8*, 38022–38043.

Beatty, G. L., & Gladney, W. L. (2015). Immune escape mechanisms as a guide for cancer immunotherapy. *Clinical Cancer Research, 21*, 687–692.

Boshuizen, J., & Peeper, D. S. (2020). Rational cancer treatment combinations: An urgent clinical need. *Molecular Cell, 78*, 1002–1018.

Böttcher, J. P., Reis, E., & Sousa, C. (2018). The role of type 1 conventional dendritic cells in cancer immunity. *Trends Cancer, 4*, 784–792.

Cheng, Y.-A., Chen, I. J., Su, Y.-C., Cheng, K.-W., Lu, Y.-C., Lin, W.-W., Hsieh, Y.-C., Kao, C.-H., Chen, F.-M., Roffler, S. R., & Cheng, T.-L. (2019). Enhanced drug internalization and therapeutic efficacy of PEGylated nanoparticles by one-step formulation with anti-mPEG bispecific antibody in intrinsic drug-resistant breast cancer. *Biomaterials Science, 7*, 3404–3417.

Chu, J., Gao, F., Yan, M., Zhao, S., Yan, Z., Shi, B., & Liu, Y. (2022). Natural killer cells: A promising immunotherapy for cancer. *Journal of Translational Medicine, 20*, 240.

Demaria, S., Volm, M. D., Shapiro, R. L., Yee, H. T., Oratz, R., Formenti, S. C., Muggia, F., & Symmans, W. F. (2001). Development of tumor-infiltrating lymphocytes in breast cancer after neoadjuvant paclitaxel Chemotherapy. *Clinical Cancer Research, 7*, 3025–3030.

Dey, A., Ghosh, S., Jha, S., Hazra, S., Srivastava, N., Chakraborty, U., & Roy, A. G. (2023). Recent advancement in breast cancer treatment using CAR T cell therapy:- A review. *Advances in Cancer Biology - Metastasis, 7*, 100090.

Duan, J., Cui, L., Zhao, X., Bai, H., Cai, S., Wang, G., Zhao, Z., Zhao, J., Chen, S., Song, J., Qi, C., Wang, Q., Huang, M., Zhang, Y., Huang, D., Bai, Y., Sun, F., Lee, J. J., Wang, Z., & Wang, J. (2020). Use of immunotherapy with programmed cell death 1 vs programmed cell death ligand 1 inhibitors in patients with cancer: A systematic review and meta-analysis. *JAMA Oncology, 6*, 375–384.

Dunn, G. P., Old, L. J., & Schreiber, R. D. (2004a). The immunobiology of cancer immunosurveillance and immunoediting. *Immunity, 21*, 137–148.

Dunn, G. P., Old, L. J., & Schreiber, R. D. (2004b). The three Es of cancer immunoediting. *Annual Review of Immunology, 22*, 329–360.

El Bairi, K., Haynes, H. R., Blackley, E., Fineberg, S., Shear, J., Turner, S., De Freitas, J. R., Sur, D., Amendola, L. C., Gharib, M., Kallala, A., Arun, I., Azmoudeh-Ardalan, F., Fujimoto, L., Sua, L. F., Liu, S.-W., Lien, H.-C., Kirtani, P., Balancin, M., El Attar, H., Guleria, P., Yang, W., Shash, E., Chen, I. C., Bautista, V., Do Prado Moura, J. F., Rapoport, B. L., Castaneda, C., Spengler, E., Acosta-Haab, G., Frahm, I., Sanchez, J., Castillo, M., Bouchmaa, N., Md Zin, R. R., Shui, R., Onyuma, T., Yang, W., Husain, Z., Willard-Gallo, K., Coosemans, A., Perez, E. A., Provenzano, E., Ericsson, P. G., Richardet, E., Mehrotra, R., Sarancone, S., Ehinger, A., Rimm, D. L., Bartlett, J. M. S., Viale, G., Denkert, C., Hida, A. I., Sotiriou, C., Loibl, S., Hewitt, S. M., Badve, S., Symmans, W. F., Kim, R. S., Pruneri, G., Goel, S., Francis, P. A., Inurrigarro, G., Yamaguchi, R., Garcia-Rivello, H., Horlings, H., Afqir, S., Salgado, R., Adams, S., Kok, M., Dieci, M. V., Michiels, S., Demaria, S., Loi, S., El Bairi, K., Haynes, H. R., Blackley, E., Fineberg, S., Shear, J., Turner, S., De Freitas, J. R., Sur, D., Amendola, L. C., Gharib, M., Kallala, A., Arun, I., Azmoudeh-Ardalan, F., Fujimoto, L., Sua, L. F., Liu, S.-W., Lien, H.-C., Kirtani, P., Balancin, M., El Attar, H., Guleria, P., Yang, W., Shash, E., Chen, I. C., Bautista, V., Do Prado Moura, J. F., et al. (2021). The tale of TILs in breast cancer: A report from the international immuno-oncology biomarker working group. *Npj Breast Cancer, 7*, 150.

Ellis, G. I., Sheppard, N. C., & Riley, J. L. (2021). Genetic engineering of T cells for immunotherapy. *Nature Reviews Genetics, 22*, 427–447.

FDA. (2020). *FDA issues alert about efficacy and potential safety concerns with atezolizumab in combination with paclitaxel for treatment of breast cancer* [Online]. U.S.A. Food & Drug Administration. Retrieved August 08, 2023, from https://www.fda.gov/drugs/resources-information-approved-drugs/fda-issues-alert-about-efficacy-and-potential-safety-concerns-atezolizumab-combination-paclitaxel

Fuentes-Antrás, J., Guevara-Hoyer, K., Baliu-Piqué, M., García-Sáenz, J., Pérez-Segura, P., Pandiella, A., & Ocaña, A. (2020). Adoptive cell therapy in breast cancer: A current perspective of next-generation medicine. *Frontiers in Oncology, 10*, 605633.

Gautam, N., Elleson, K. M., Ramamoorthi, G., & Czerniecki, B. J. (2022). Current state of cell therapies for breast cancer. *Cancer Journal, 28*, 301–309.

Horm, T. M., & Schroeder, J. A. (2013). MUC1 and metastatic cancer: Expression, function and therapeutic targeting. *Cell Adhesion & Migration, 7*, 187–198.

Howard, F. M., Pearson, A. T., & Nanda, R. (2022). Clinical trials of immunotherapy in triple-negative breast cancer. *Breast Cancer Research and Treatment, 195*, 1–15.

Hunter, E. (2023). *FDA approved IND for CAR T cell that target metastases-causing breast cancer tumor* [Online]. Pharmacy Times. Retrieved July 28, 2023, from https://www.pharmacytimes.com/view/fda-approved-ind-for-car-t-cell-that-target-metastases-causing-breast-cancer-tumor

Ishigami, E., Sakakibara, M., Sakakibara, J., Masuda, T., Fujimoto, H., Hayama, S., Nagashima, T., Sangai, T., Nakagawa, A., Nakatani, Y., & Otsuka, M. (2019). Coexistence of regulatory B cells and regulatory T cells in tumor-infiltrating lymphocyte aggregates is a prognostic factor in patients with breast cancer. *Breast Cancer, 26*, 180–189.

Isla, D., Lopez-Brea, M., Espinosa, M., Arrabal, N., Pérez-Parente, D., Carcedo, D., & Bernabé-Caro, R. (2023). Cost-effectiveness of atezolizumab versus pembrolizumab as first-line treatment in PD-L1-positive advanced non-small-cell lung cancer in Spain. *Cost Effectiveness and Resource Allocation, 21*, 6.

Jing, X., Liang, H., Hao, C., Yang, X., & Cui, X. (2019). Overexpression of MUC1 predicts poor prognosis in patients with breast cancer. *Oncology Reports, 41*, 801–810.

Johnson, L. A., & June, C. H. (2017). Driving gene-engineered T cell immunotherapy of cancer. *Cell Research, 27*, 38–58.

Kabelitz, D., Serrano, R., Kouakanou, L., Peters, C., & Kalyan, S. (2020). Cancer immunotherapy with γδ T cells: Many paths ahead of us. *Cellular & Molecular Immunology, 17*, 925–939.

Kamakura, D., Asano, R., & Yasunaga, M. (2021). T cell bispecific antibodies: An antibody-based delivery system for inducing antitumor immunity. *Pharmaceuticals (Basel), 14*, 1172.

Kern, R., & Panis, C. (2021). CTLA-4 expression and its clinical significance in breast cancer. *Archivum Immunologiae et Therapiae Experimentalis, 69*, 16.

Kiaei, S. Z. F., Nouralishahi, A., Ghasemirad, M., Barkhordar, M., Ghaffari, S., Kheradjoo, H., Saleh, M., Mohammadzadehsaliani, S., & Molaeipour, Z. (2023). Advances in natural killer cell therapies for breast cancer. *Immunology and Cell Biology, 101*, 705–726.

Koury, J., Lucero, M., Cato, C., Chang, L., Geiger, J., Henry, D., Hernandez, J., Hung, F., Kaur, P., Teskey, G., & Tran, A. (2018). Immunotherapies: Exploiting the immune system for cancer treatment. *Journal of Immunology Research, 2018*, 9585614.

Kudva, A., & Modak, S. (2019). Chapter 9 - Immunotherapy for neuroblastoma. In S. K. Ray (Ed.), *Neuroblastoma*. Academic Press.

Labrijn, A. F., Janmaat, M. L., Reichert, J. M., & Parren, P. W. H. I. (2019). Bispecific antibodies: A mechanistic review of the pipeline. *Nature Reviews Drug Discovery, 18*, 585–608.

Li, P., Yang, L., Li, T., Bin, S., Sun, B., Huang, Y., Yang, K., Shan, D., Gu, H., & Li, H. (2020). The third generation anti-HER2 chimeric antigen receptor mouse T cells alone or together with anti-PD1 antibody inhibits the growth of mouse breast tumor cells expressing HER2 in vitro and in immune competent mice. *Frontiers in Oncology, 10*, 1143.

Li, Y., Li, G., Zhang, J., Wu, X., & Chen, X. (2021a). The dual roles of human γδ T cells: Anti-tumor or tumor-promoting. *Frontiers in Immunology, 11*, 619954.

Li, Y., Miao, W., He, D., Wang, S., Lou, J., Jiang, Y., & Wang, S. (2021b). Recent progress on immunotherapy for breast cancer: Tumor microenvironment, nanotechnology and more. *Frontiers in Bioengineering and Biotechnology, 9*, 680315.

Li, Y., Zhang, H., Merkher, Y., Chen, L., Liu, N., Leonov, S., & Chen, Y. (2022). Recent advances in therapeutic strategies for triple-negative breast cancer. *Journal of Hematology & Oncology, 15*, 121.

Liu, H., Bai, L., Huang, L., Ning, N., Li, L., Li, Y., Dong, X., Du, Q., Xia, M., Chen, Y., Zhao, L., Li, Y., Meng, Q., Wang, J., Duan, Y., Ming, J., Yuan, A. Q., & Yang, X.-P. (2021). Bispecific antibody targeting TROP2xCD3 suppresses tumor growth of triple negative breast cancer. *Journal for ImmunoTherapy of Cancer, 9*, e003468.

Liu, Y., Zhou, Y., Huang, K. H., Fang, X., Li, Y., Wang, F., An, L., Chen, Q., Zhang, Y., Shi, A., Yu, S., & Zhang, J. (2020). Targeting epidermal growth factor-overexpressing triple-negative breast cancer by natural killer cells expressing a specific chimeric antigen receptor. *Cell Proliferation, 53*, e12858.

Lu, L., Zhan, M., Li, X. Y., Zhang, H., Dauphars, D. J., Jiang, J., Yin, H., Li, S. Y., Luo, S., Li, Y., & He, Y. W. (2022). Clinically approved combination immunotherapy: Current status, limitations, and future perspective. *Current Research in Immunology, 3*, 118–127.

Lukjanov, V., Koutná, I., & Šimara, P. (2021). CAR T-cell production using nonviral approaches. *Journal of Immunology Research, 2021*, 6644685.

Maskalenko, N. A., Zhigarev, D., & Campbell, K. S. (2022). Harnessing natural killer cells for cancer immunotherapy: Dispatching the first responders. *Nature Reviews Drug Discovery, 21*, 559–577.

Meric-Bernstam, F., Beeram, M., Hamilton, E., Oh, D. Y., Hanna, D. L., Kang, Y. K., Elimova, E., Chaves, J., Goodwin, R., Lee, J., Nabell, L., Rha, S. Y., Mayordomo, J., El-Khoueiry, A., Pant, S., Raghav, K., Kim, J. W., Patnaik, A., Gray, T., Davies, R., Ozog, M. A., Woolery, J., & Lee, K. W. (2022). Zanidatamab, a novel bispecific antibody, for the treatment of locally advanced or metastatic HER2-expressing or HER2-amplified cancers: A phase 1, dose-escalation and expansion study. *The Lancet Oncology, 23*, 1558–1570.

Mina, L. A., Lim, S., Bahadur, S. W., & Firoz, A. T. (2019). Immunotherapy for the treatment of breast cancer: Emerging new data. *Breast Cancer (Dove Med Press), 11*, 321–328.

NIH. (2022). *NIH study advances personalized immunotherapy for metastatic breast cancer* [Online]. Turning Discovery into Health: National Institutes of Health. Retrieved August 03, 2023, from https://www.nih.gov/news-events/news-releases/nih-study-advances-personalized-immunotherapy-metastatic-breast-cancer

O'brien, M. E. R., Wigler, N., Inbar, M., Rosso, R., Grischke, E., Santoro, A., Catane, R., Kieback, D. G., Tomczak, P., Ackland, S. P., Orlandi, F., Mellars, L., Alland, L., & Tendler, C. (2004). Reduced cardiotoxicity and comparable efficacy in a phase III trial of pegylated liposomal doxorubicin HCl (CAELYX™/Doxil®) versus conventional doxorubicin for first-line treatment of metastatic breast cancer. *Annals of Oncology, 15*, 440–449.

Oba, T., Long, M. D., Keler, T., Marsh, H. C., Minderman, H., Abrams, S. I., Liu, S., & Ito, F. (2020). Overcoming primary and acquired resistance to anti-PD-L1 therapy by induction and activation of tumor-residing cDC1s. *Nature Communications, 11*, 5415.

Oberg, H. H., Kellner, C., Gonnermann, D., Sebens, S., Bauerschlag, D., Gramatzki, M., Kabelitz, D., Peipp, M., & Wesch, D. (2018). Tribody [(HER2)(2)xCD16] is more effective than Trastuzumab in enhancing γδ T cell and natural killer cell cytotoxicity against HER2-expressing cancer cells. *Frontiers in Immunology, 9*, 814.

Offner, S., Hofmeister, R., Romaniuk, A., Kufer, P., & Baeuerle, P. A. (2006). Induction of regular cytolytic T cell synapses by bispecific single-chain antibody constructs on MHC class I-negative tumor cells. *Molecular Immunology, 43*, 763–771.

Park, J. H., Jonas, S. F., Bataillon, G., Criscitiello, C., Salgado, R., Loi, S., Viale, G., Lee, H. J., Dieci, M. V., Kim, S. B., Vincent-Salomon, A., Curigliano, G., André, F., & Michiels, S. (2019). Prognostic value of tumor-infiltrating lymphocytes in patients with early-stage triple-negative breast cancers (TNBC) who did not receive adjuvant chemotherapy. *Annals of Oncology, 30*, 1941–1949.

Priceman, S. J., Tilakawardane, D., Jeang, B., Aguilar, B., Murad, J. P., Park, A. K., Chang, W. C., Ostberg, J. R., Neman, J., Jandial, R., Portnow, J., Forman, S. J., & Brown, C. E. (2018). Regional delivery of chimeric antigen receptor-engineered T cells effectively targets HER2(+) breast cancer metastasis to the brain. *Clinical Cancer Research, 24*, 95–105.

Raute, K., Strietz, J., Andrieux, G., Thomas, O. S., Kistner, K. M., Zintchenko, M., Aichele, P., Zhou, H., Weber, W., Boerries, M., Swamy, M., Maurer, J., & Minguet, S. (2022). Breast cancer stem cell-derived tumors escape from γδ T cell immunosurveillance <em>in vivo</em> by modulating γδ T cell ligands. *bioRxiv. Cancer Immunology Research, 11*(6), 810–829. 2022.04.04.486931.

Rosenberg, S. A., Restifo, N. P., Yang, J. C., Morgan, R. A., & Dudley, M. E. (2008). Adoptive cell transfer: A clinical path to effective cancer immunotherapy. *Nature Reviews Cancer, 8*, 299–308.

Røssevold, A. H., Andresen, N. K., Bjerre, C. A., Gilje, B., Jakobsen, E. H., Raj, S. X., Falk, R. S., Russnes, H. G., Jahr, T., Mathiesen, R. R., Lømo, J., Garred, Ø., Chauhan, S. K., Lereim, R. R., Dunn, C., Naume, B., & Kyte, J. A. (2022). Atezolizumab plus anthracycline-based chemotherapy in metastatic triple-negative breast cancer: The randomized, double-blind phase 2b ALICE trial. *Nature Medicine, 28*, 2573–2583.

Saleh, R., & Elkord, E. (2020). FoxP3+ T regulatory cells in cancer: Prognostic biomarkers and therapeutic targets. *Cancer Letters, 490*, 174–185.

Salgado, R., Denkert, C., Demaria, S., Sirtaine, N., Klauschen, F., Pruneri, G., Wienert, S., Van Den Eynden, G., Baehner, F. L., Penault-Llorca, F., Perez, E. A., Thompson, E. A., Symmans, W. F., Richardson, A. L., Brock, J., Criscitiello, C., Bailey, H., Ignatiadis, M., Floris, G., Sparano, J., Kos, Z., Nielsen, T., Rimm, D. L., Allison, K. H., Reis-Filho, J. S., Loibl, S., Sotiriou, C., Viale, G., Badve, S., Adams, S., Willard-Gallo, K., & Loi, S. (2015). The evaluation of tumor-infiltrating lymphocytes (TILs) in breast cancer: Recommendations by an international TILs working group 2014. *Annals of Oncology, 26*, 259–271.

Schettini, F., Barbao, P., Brasó-Maristany, F., Galván, P., Martínez, D., Paré, L., de Placido, S., Prat, A., & Guedan, S. (2021). Identification of cell surface targets for CAR-T cell therapies and antibody-drug conjugates in breast cancer. *ESMO Open, 6*, 100102.

Schmid, P., Cortes, J., Pusztai, L., Mcarthur, H., Kümmel, S., Bergh, J., Denkert, C., Park, Y. H., Hui, R., Harbeck, N., Takahashi, M., Foukakis, T., Fasching, P. A., Cardoso, F., Untch, M., Jia, L., Karantza, V., Zhao, J., Aktan, G., Dent, R., & O'shaughnessy, J. (2020). Pembrolizumab for early triple-negative breast cancer. *New England Journal of Medicine, 382*, 810–821.

Schönefeldt, S., Wais, T., Herling, M., Mustjoki, S., Bekiaris, V., Moriggl, R., & Neubauer, H. A. (2021). The diverse roles of γδ T cells in cancer: From rapid immunity to aggressive lymphoma. *Cancers (Basel), 13*, 6212.

Shafer, P., Kelly, L. M., & Hoyos, V. (2022). Cancer therapy with TCR-engineered T cells: Current strategies, challenges, and prospects. *Frontiers in Immunology, 13*, 835762.

Sharma, P., Hu-Lieskovan, S., Wargo, J. A., & Ribas, A. (2017). Primary, adaptive, and acquired resistance to cancer immunotherapy. *Cell, 168*, 707–723.

Shenouda, M. M., Gillgrass, A., Nham, T., Hogg, R., Lee, A. J., Chew, M. V., Shafaei, M., Aarts, C., Lee, D. A., Hassell, J., Bane, A., Dhesy-Thind, S., & Ashkar, A. A. (2017). Ex vivo expanded natural killer cells from breast cancer patients and healthy donors are highly cytotoxic against breast cancer cell lines and patient-derived tumours. *Breast Cancer Research, 19*, 76.

Soare, G. R., & Soare, C. A. (2019). Immunotherapy for breast cancer: First FDA approved regimen. *Discoveries (Craiova), 7*, e91.

Sobhani, N., Tardiel-Cyril, D. R., Davtyan, A., Generali, D., Roudi, R., & Li, Y. (2021). CTLA-4 in regulatory T cells for cancer immunotherapy. *Cancers, 13*, 1440.

Stanton, S. E., & Disis, M. L. (2016). Clinical significance of tumor-infiltrating lymphocytes in breast cancer. *Journal for Immunotherapy of Cancer, 4*, 59.

Szöőr, Á., Tóth, G., Zsebik, B., Szabó, V., Eshhar, Z., Abken, H., & Vereb, G. (2020). Trastuzumab derived HER2-specific CARs for the treatment of trastuzumab-resistant breast cancer: CAR T cells penetrate and eradicate tumors that are not accessible to antibodies. *Cancer Letters, 484*, 1–8.

Tóth, G., Szöllősi, J., Abken, H., Vereb, G., & Szöőr, Á. (2020). A small number of HER2 redirected CAR T cells significantly improves immune response of adoptively transferred mouse lymphocytes against human breast cancer xenografts. *International Journal of Molecular Sciences, 21*, 1039.

Toulouie, S., Johanning, G., & Shi, Y. (2021). Chimeric antigen receptor T-cell immunotherapy in breast cancer: Development and challenges. *Journal of Cancer, 12*, 1212–1219.

Tsimberidou, A.-M., Van Morris, K., Vo, H. H., Eck, S., Lin, Y.-F., Rivas, J. M., & Andersson, B. S. (2021). T-cell receptor-based therapy: An innovative therapeutic approach for solid tumors. *Journal of Hematology & Oncology, 14*, 102.

Valencia, G. A., Rioja, P., Morante, Z., Ruiz, R., Fuentes, H., Castaneda, C. A., Vidaurre, T., Neciosup, S., & Gomez, H. L. (2022). Immunotherapy in triple-negative breast cancer: A literature review and new advances. *World Journal of Clinical Oncology, 13*, 219–236.

Valenza, C., Taurelli Salimbeni, B., Santoro, C., Trapani, D., Antonarelli, G., & Curigliano, G. (2023). Tumor infiltrating lymphocytes across breast cancer subtypes: Current issues for biomarker assessment. *Cancers (Basel), 15*, 767.

Vesely, M. D., & Schreiber, R. D. (2013). Cancer immunoediting: Antigens, mechanisms, and implications to cancer immunotherapy. *Annals of the New York Academy of Sciences, 1284*, 1–5.

Vesely, M. D., Zhang, T., & Chen, L. (2022). Resistance mechanisms to anti-PD cancer immunotherapy. *Annual Review of Immunology, 40*, 45–74.

Wallstabe, L., Göttlich, C., Nelke, L. C., Kühnemundt, J., Schwarz, T., Nerreter, T., Einsele, H., Walles, H., Dandekar, G., Nietzer, S. L., & Hudecek, M. (2019). ROR1-CAR T cells are effective against lung and breast cancer in advanced microphysiologic 3D tumor models. *JCI insight, 4*, e126345.

Wang, X., Yang, X., Yuan, X., Wang, W., & Wang, Y. (2022). Chimeric antigen receptor-engineered NK cells: New weapons of cancer immunotherapy with great potential. *Experimental Hematology & Oncology, 11*, 85.

Wein, L., Luen, S. J., Savas, P., Salgado, R., & Loi, S. (2018). Checkpoint blockade in the treatment of breast cancer: Current status and future directions. *British Journal of Cancer, 119*, 4–11.

West, H. J. (2018). *Choosing between Atezolizumab and Pembrolizumab in lung cancer* [Online]. Targeted Oncology: MJH Life Science. Retrieved July 24, 2023, from https://www.targetedonc.com/view/choosing-between-atezolizumab-and-pembrolizumab-in-lung-cancer

Wu, K., Lyu, F., Wu, S.-Y., Sharma, S., Deshpande, R. P., Tyagi, A., Zhao, D., Xing, F., Singh, R., & Watabe, K. (2023). Engineering an active immunotherapy for personalized cancer treatment and prevention of recurrence. *Science Advances, 9*, eade0625.

Wu, Y., Lin, L., Shen, Y., & Wu, H. (2018). Comparison between PD-1/PD-L1 inhibitors (nivolumab, pembrolizumab, and atezolizumab) in pretreated NSCLC patients: Evidence from a Bayesian network model. *International Journal of Cancer, 143*, 3038–3040.

Zacharakis, N., Huq, L. M., Seitter, S. J., Kim, S. P., Gartner, J. J., Sindiri, S., Hill, V. K., Li, Y. F., Paria, B. C., Ray, S., Gasmi, B., Lee, C.-C., Prickett, T. D., Parkhurst, M. R., Robbins, P. F., Langhan, M. M., Shelton, T. E., Parikh, A. Y., Levi, S. T., Hernandez, J. M., Hoang, C. D., Sherry, R. M., Yang, J. C., Feldman, S. A., Goff, S. L., & Rosenberg, S. A. (2022). Breast cancers are immunogenic: Immunologic analyses and a phase II pilot clinical trial using mutation-reactive autologous lymphocytes. *Journal of Clinical Oncology, 40*, 1741–1754.

Zhang, C., Durer, S., Thandra, K. C., & Kasi, A. (2022). *Chimeric antigen receptor T-cell therapy* [Online]. National Library of Medicine, National Canter for Biotechnology Information: StatPearls Publishing. Retrieved July 28, 2023, from https://www.ncbi.nlm.nih.gov/books/NBK537294/

Zhang, Y., Zhou, H., & Zhang, L. (2018). Which is the optimal immunotherapy for advanced squamous non-small-cell lung cancer in combination with chemotherapy: Anti-PD-1 or anti-PD-L1? *Journal for Immunotherapy of Cancer, 6*, 135.

Zhao, L., & Cao, Y. J. (2019). Engineered T cell therapy for cancer in the clinic. *Frontiers in Immunology, 10*, 2250.

Zhou, B., Gao, Y., Zhang, P., & Chu, Q. (2021). Acquired resistance to immune checkpoint blockades: The underlying mechanisms and potential strategies. *Frontiers in Immunology, 12*, 693609.

Zitvogel, L., Tesniere, A., & Kroemer, G. (2006). Cancer despite immunosurveillance: immunoselection and immunosubversion. *Nature Reviews Immunology, 6*, 715–727.

Zlatareva, I., & Wu, Y. (2023). Local γδ T cells: Translating promise to practice in cancer immunotherapy. *British Journal of Cancer, 129*, 393–405.

Zou, Y., Zou, X., Zheng, S., Tang, H., Zhang, L., Liu, P., & Xie, X. (2020). Efficacy and predictive factors of immune checkpoint inhibitors in metastatic breast cancer: A systematic review and meta-analysis. *Therapeutic Advances in Medical Oncology, 12*, 1758835920940928.

Resistance to Endocrine Therapy in Breast Cancer

Demetra Demetriou, Richard Khanyile, Zukile Mbita, and Zodwa Dlamini

Abstract The foremost cause of female deaths is due to breast cancer. The most frequent type of breast cancer is hormone-dependent breast cancer, being either progesterone- or estrogen receptor-positive and in certain cases, both. Breast cancer treatments include radiation, surgery, endocrine therapy, targeted therapy, immunotherapy, or chemotherapy. A regular treatment for patients with estrogen receptor-positive tumors is endocrine treatment. Various compounds can directly target estrogen receptors or can suppress estrogen production. The introduction of gene therapy, targeted treatment, or biological drugs can reduce mortality rates and enhance the patients' quality of life. Endocrine therapy resistance is on the rise leading to a major burden for treatment and poor survival for patients. Novel endocrine therapy and combinational therapy are solutions to overcome endocrine therapy resistance and to increase patient survival rates.

Keywords Endocrine therapy · Resistance · Breast cancer · Hormone receptor · Estrogen · Progesterone · HER2 · BRCA · Combinational therapy · Overcoming resistance

---

D. Demetriou (✉) · Z. Dlamini
SAMRC Precision Oncology Research Unit (PORU), DSI/NRF SARChI Chair in Precision Oncology and Cancer Prevention (POCP), Pan African Cancer Research Institute (PACRI), University of Pretoria, Pretoria, South Africa
e-mail: dd.demetriou@up.ac.za; zodwa.dlamini@up.ac.za

R. Khanyile
SAMRC Precision Oncology Research Unit (PORU), DSI/NRF SARChI Chair in Precision Oncology and Cancer Prevention (POCP), Pan African Cancer Research Institute (PACRI), University of Pretoria, Hatfield, South Africa

Department of Medical Oncology, Faculty of Health Sciences, Steve Biko Academic Hospital, University of Pretoria, Hatfield, South Africa
e-mail: richard.khanyile@up.ac.za

Z. Mbita
Department of Biochemistry, Microbiology and Biotechnology, School of Molecular and Life Sciences, University of Limpopo, Polokwane, South Africa
e-mail: Zukile.Mbita@ul.ac.za

Z. Dlamini (ed.), *Overcoming Breast Cancer Therapy Resistance*,
https://doi.org/10.1007/978-3-031-52860-6_5

Introduction to Endocrine Therapy

Breast cancer (BC) is a global burden and the need for early diagnosis is pivotal. Treatments of BC contain radiation, surgery, endocrine therapy, targeted therapy, immunotherapy, or chemotherapy (Fig. 5.1). Endocrine therapy is a common treatment for BC, especially for hormone receptor-positive BC. Breast cancer cells that have been removed are tested for progesterone or estrogen receptors. Receptors are protein structures on or in a cell that can bind to certain molecules in the blood such as hormones. Cancer growth can be stimulated if progesterone or estrogen binds to the receptors. ER-positive (ER+) cancers are BC that have estrogen receptors. PR-positive (PR+) cancers are BC that have progesterone receptors. Breast cancer cells (BCC) may present either one, a single or both of these receptors. BC is classified into hormone receptor positive (HR+) if they possess these receptors or hormone receptor negative (HR-) if they do not possess these receptors. BC that has low levels of the human epidermal growth factor receptor 2 (HER2) protein and not one of the receptors is known to be triple-negative breast cancer (TNBC). Triple-positive breast cancers (TPBC) are ER+, PR+, and have high levels of HER2 protein. By preventing the attachment of the hormones to the receptor with example drugs, the growth and spreading of the cancer is decreased.

The clinician can be assisted in the decision-making process by knowing the hormone receptor status (HRS). If the cancer is ER+ and/or PR+, hormone therapy drugs can be used to stop estrogen attachment or lower estrogen levels. This treatment is beneficial for HR+ cancers but will not work for cancers that are HR-.

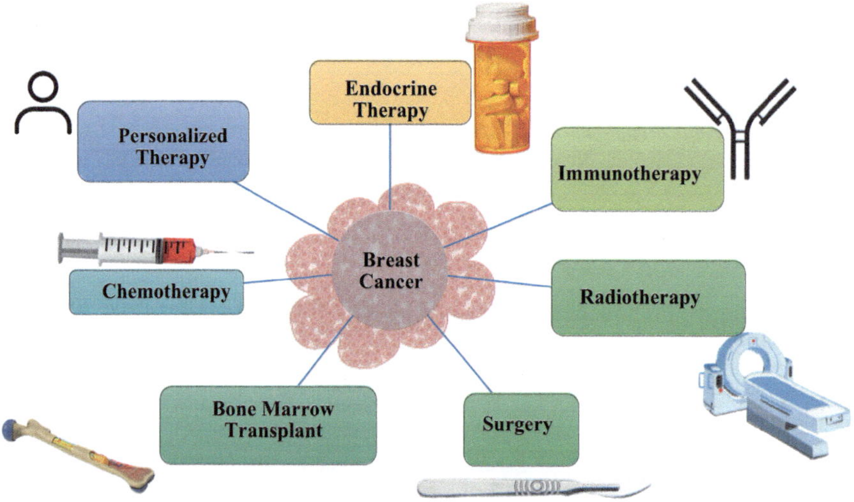

Fig. 5.1 *Various breast cancer treatments. Treatments include radiation, surgery, immunotherapy, endocrine therapy, or chemotherapy*. Endocrine therapy is the preferred choice

Hormone Receptor Testing

BC can be tested for estrogen and progesterone receptors through immunohistochemistry (IHC) or gene expression profiles (Goldhirsch et al., 2011; Gerratana et al., 2015). Intracellular proteins in tissues and various cell surfaces are characterized by IHC. Markers can be used to confirm tissue origins, characterize various tumor subtypes, distinguish primary versus metastatic tumors, and provide additional information that can be used for diagnosis, prognosis, decision-making for treatment, or treatment evaluation (Zaha, 2014). The assessment of the hormone receptors can guide therapy decisions. Hormone receptor testing (HRT) can ensure that patients who will benefit from endocrine therapy will receive treatment and those who will not benefit from the therapy, will not be susceptible to unwanted side effects. Previously, dextran-coated charcoal/ligand binding assay (DCC/LBA) was the common method used for HRT. Alternative assays, for example, enzyme immunoassay (EIA) and enzyme-linked immunosorbent assay (ELISA) became available and more commonly used (Nofech-Mozes et al., 2012). In the late 1980s—early 1990s, formalin-fixed paraffin-embedded (FFPE) IHC samples replaced the DCC assay due to its advantages such as the use of FFPE samples that prolonged tissue storage, smaller amounts of tissue required, staining and histology correlation, and storage of the samples for future testing (Nofech-Mozes et al., 2012).

Today, IHC is the most frequently preferred method to assess hormone receptor status (HRS). IHC must be performed reliably and accurately across laboratories. Based on the HRS results, the tumor is HR+ if 1% of the cells tested have progesterone and/or estrogen receptors. Otherwise, it will be HR-. HR+ cancers tend to grow more slowly than HR- cancers. Patients with HR+ cancers have an improved prognosis, but reoccurrence is still a huge burden. HR- cancers grow faster and often reoccur in the first few years after treatment. HR- cancers are more common in menopausal women. Women who have a mutation in the breast cancer 1 (BRCA1) gene, younger women (<40 years) and black women commonly have TNBC. TNBCs grow and spread fast and hormone therapy will not benefit them as they are HR-cancers. Drugs that target HER2 are also not very helpful as they have low levels of HER2. Chemotherapy can, however, still be useful. TPBC can be treated with drug—or hormone therapy that targets HER2.

ER+ BC is the most common breast cancer subtype (Hanker et al., 2020). Estrogen has an important role in the development and growth of female reproductive and mammary phenotypes (Nilsson et al., 2001). Through genomic regulation, such as the transcription of genes that support survival, and non-genomic regulation, such as the activation of cellular signaling, estrogen-induced activation of ERα and ERβ nuclear receptors supports the proliferation and survival of tumor breast tissue and normal breast tissue.

Endocrine Therapy

For decades, endocrine therapies have been used for BC treatment. Endocrine therapy is preferred as its toxicity is less than other treatments and can be used for metastatic breast cancer (MBC), pre-operatively (neoadjuvant) or post-operatively (adjuvant) (Palmieri et al., 2014; Shioi et al., 2014). The first systemic treatment for HR+ BC and the oldest endocrine treatment is ovarian suppression; however, it has been replaced by ovarian irradiation (Beatson, 1896; Paterson and Russell, 1959). It is important to know how normal transcription works to understand how endocrine therapy can play a role. Various tissues such as breasts, ovaries, adipose tissues, and adrenal glands produce androgens. Aromatase is used to change androgens into estrogens. When estrogen binds to the ER, the ER dimerizes and moves to the nucleus, where it binds coactivators (CoA) and triggers transcription (Fig. 5.2a). Endocrine therapy treatments include aromatase inhibitors (AI), Selective estrogen receptor modulators (SERMs) and Selective estrogen receptor downregulators (SERDs) (Siris et al., 1999; Aggelis and Johnston, 2019). In post-menopausal patients, AIs lower estrogen levels by preventing the transition of androgens to estrogens (Fig. 5.2b). SERMs are generally utilized in premenopausal individuals and compete with estrogen for binding to the receptor (Fig. 5.2c). SERDs can promote ER protein degradation, block ER transcriptional activity or impair ER mobility (Fig. 5.2d; Wittmann et al., 2007; Wardell et al., 2011; Guan et al., 2019).

Aromatase and Aromatase Inhibitors

The aromatase enzyme comes from the cytochrome P450 family and results from the Cytochrome P450 Family 19 Subfamily A Member 1 (CYP19A1) gene located on chromosome 15 (Chen et al., 1988; Thompson and Siiteri, 1974). Aromatase is also known as estrogen synthase or estrogen synthetase, and it is responsible for the crucial step in the synthesis of estrogen by catalyzing the rate-limiting and last step, the aromatization of androgens to estrogens, through three oxidation reactions of the androstenedione A ring (Chumsri et al, 2011). The first two reactions are common steps of the P450 cytochrome proteins but the third reaction is unique (Akhtar et al., 2011). BC tissues have shown increased aromatase expression which led to elevated levels of estrogens when compared to non-cancerous tissues and is a molecule of interest for this reason (Harada, 1997).

Richard Santen and colleagues used aminoglutethimide, an anti-epileptic drug, as a treatment for breast cancer and demonstrated its effectiveness in breast cancer treatment in the late 1970s (Santen et al., 2009). Aminoglutethimide inhibited the aromatase enzyme which resulted in the lower estrogens levels, however, aminoglutethimide also inhibited Cytochrome P450, family 11 (CYP11) which required cortisol replacement and was thus not commonly used (McDonnell, 1999; Fisher et al., 1994). From there on, various drugs and options have been tested to inhibit aromatase. Current AIs are organized into two subtypes, namely non-steroidal and steroidal AIs. Table 5.1 displays a few examples of non-steroidal and steroidal aromatase inhibitors.

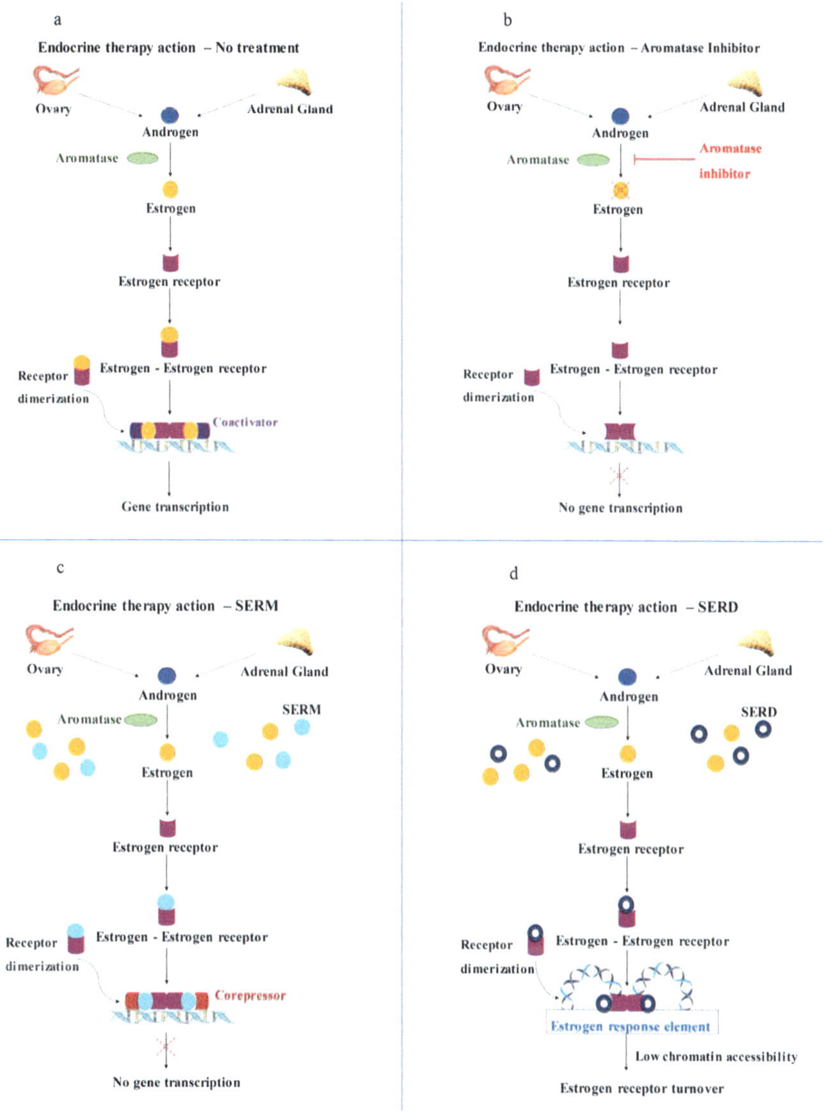

Fig. 5.2 *Simple illustration of normal estrogen receptor gene transcription and endocrine therapy action via Aromatase inhibitors, Selective estrogen receptor modulators (SERMs), and Selective estrogen receptor downregulators (SERDs) on breast cancer.* (**a**) Breasts, ovaries, adipose tissues, and adrenal glands produce androgens. Aromatase is used to change androgens into estrogens. Upon estrogen binding, the ER dimerizes and translocate to the nucleus, where ER dimers bind coactivators (CoA). Transcription begins. (**b**) AI blocks estrogen production through the inhibition of the aromatization of androgens to estrogens. Since no estrogens are produced, there is no binding to the receptors and no transcription. (**c**) SERMs compete with estrogen to prevent it from attaching to the ER. Although SERM-bound ER dimers interact with chromatin at estrogen response elements (ERE), the corepressors (CoR) are linked to prevent transcription. (**d**) SERD-ER complex cannot establish an open chromatin conformation which leads to activated transcription of the gene resulting in ER turnover and SERD-ER degradation

Table 5.1 Non-steroidal and steroidal aromatase inhibitors

Non-steroidal aromatase inhibitors	Steroidal aromatase inhibitors
Letrozole—Femara®	Exemestane—Aromasin®
Aminoglutethimide	Formestane
Anastrozole—Arimidex®	
Rogletimide	
Fadrozole	
Vorozole	

As a result of binding-site saturation brought on by non-steroidal aromatase inhibitors' non-covalent attachment to the heme moiety of the aromatase enzyme, androgen binding is prevented (McDonnell, 1999; Chen et al., 1988). Through competitive inhibition of androgens, these inhibitors are reversible. Steroidal aromatase inhibitors are irreversible inhibitors that bind to the aromatase substrate-binding site and are converted to a reactive intermediate substrate. Due to the enzyme's inherent ability to inactivate itself, these inhibitors are also referred to as "suicide inhibitors" (Santen et al., 2009, Brodie et al., 1981). Other steroid biosyntheses will not be influenced by selective aromatase inhibition due to the specificity of the aromatase enzyme. However, there is a lot that is still unknown and future investigation is required.

Although patients' resistance to AIs in the adjuvant setting and in cases of metastatic breast cancer sometimes limits their effectiveness, AIs are nevertheless widely regarded as effective treatments. Regardless of the sequence, there is no proof of cross-resistance between steroidal and non-steroidal AIs (Miller et al., 2008, Thürlimann et al., 1997, Carlini et al., 2001).

Selective Estrogen Receptor Modulators

SERMs are synthetic non-steroidal anti-estrogen compounds that influence target sites in the body by competing with estrogen and modulate ER activity by changing the cofactors that it associates with (Nilsson and Koehler, 2005). SERMs can be categorized based on chemical structure namely tetrahydronaphthalenes, triphenylethylene, phenylindoles, and benzothiophenes. Table 5.2 shows each category and examples of each.

Tamoxifen was the first SERM and is known to have antagonistic or antiproliferative effects in breast tissue and agonistic on the heart, uterus, and bone (Jordan, 2008). As a derivative of triphenylethylene, Tamoxifen was first approved in the United Kingdom in 1973, followed by approval from the Food and Drug Administration (FDA) in the United States of America in 1977 to be used as a treatment for advanced BC. Tamoxifen was approved for the risk reduction of BC in pre- and post-menopausal women and high-risk women (Park and Jordan, 2002) and is used to this day as an anti-cancer treatment. Tamoxifen has also shown

Table 5.2 SERMs categories and examples

Category	Examples
Tetrahydronaphthalenes	Lasofoxifene
Triphenylethylenes	Tamoxifen or "tamoxifen-like" compounds
Phenylindoles	Bazedoxifene and pipindoxifene
Benzothiophenes	Raloxifene and arzoxifene

beneficial estrogen-like effects on selective estrogen target organs (Kristensen et al., 1994; Park and Jordan, 2002; Love et al., 1992). Raloxifene hydrochloride is another example of a non-steroidal benzothiophene that binds to ER and blocks the estrogen-induced DNA transcription in the endometrium and breast; however, it is not as strong as tamoxifen due to its short half-life and poor bioavailability (Snyder et al., 2000; Gottardis and Jordan, 1987). Raloxifene has been shown to lower low-density lipoproteins (LDL) and improve bone mineral density without the stimulation of the endometrium which opens the idea to use raloxifene as an osteoporosis prevention and treatment (Delmas et al., 1997).

Selective Estrogen Receptor Downregulators

SERDs are now considered an essential treatment for BC due to endocrine resistance with the use of SERMs and AI. SERDs have changed the direction of anticancer research and are a rising field of interest as they are capable of blocking and reducing ER signaling in drug-resistant cases. SERDs have been studied to find alternative solutions with no agonist activity with improved antagonist potency when compared to tamoxifen (Johnston, 2005). SERDs can attach and cause the degradation of ER which will prevent dimerization and stop the ER signaling pathway (Xiong et al., 2016). Unlike SERMs, SERDs are "pure anti-estrogens" as they do not have any estrogenic effects (Wang et al., 2018). SERDs lead to a decrease in ER levels and an increase in ER turnover (Kieser et al., 2010) resulting in silenced gene expression of estrogen-regulated genes, inactivation of ER AF-1 and AF-2 signaling pathways and disturbance of nuclear localization. An example of an FDA approved SERDs is Fulvestrant. Fulvestrant is a steroidal anti-estrogen that competes with estrogen for ER binding. It is referred to be a first-generation SERD and was used to treat post-menopausal women who had received previous endocrine therapy and had metastatic ER+ breast cancer (Nathan and Schmid, 2017). It caused denaturation, a structural alteration that accelerated the breakdown of estrogen receptors (Wardell et al., 2020). Other compounds are also being developed as potential SERDs (Table 5.3).

Various steroidal and non-steroidal compounds have the potential to be effective SERDs. Non-steroidal moieties such as benzothiophene, Indole, 6,7-dihydro-5-benzo (7) annulene, Indazole, oxabicycloheptane, chromenes, and cinnamic acid showed increased SERDs activity (Bhatia et al., 2023).

Table 5.3 Various SERDs in clinical trials

SERD:	Trial phase	Reference
Rintodestrant G1T48	I	Dees et al. (2019)
AZD9496	I	Weir et al. (2016)
LSZ102	I	Tria et al. (2018)
Brilanestrant GDC0810	II	Cheung et al. (2019)
Fulvestrant-3 boronic acid ZB71	II	Guo et al. (2018)
Camizestrant AZD9833	III	Gangl et al. (2020)
Giredestrant GDC-9545	III	Hernando et al. (2021)
Amcenestrant SAR439859	III	Campone et al. (2020)

Endocrine Therapy Resistance

Although the mortality rate and recurrence of BC have been reduced with endocrine therapy (Nayar et al., 2019), acquired and de novo resistance is a major challenge. Up to 20% of tumors might develop metastatic illness and recur (Pan et al., 2017). Mechanisms of endocrine resistance include epigenetic-, somatic-, or tumor micro-environmental changes. In ER+ metastatic breast cancer (MBC), endocrine resistance also exists. In 10% of endocrine-resistant breast tumors, the ER expression is lost (Shiino et al., 2016) and is typically fueled by ER reactivation that is not ligand dependent. The resistance can be caused by changes in the coactivator/corepressor–ER interaction, compensatory cross-talking between oncogenic signaling pathways, growth factor receptors, and ER or ER gain-of-function mutations (Ma et al., 2015). Activation of ER by cross-talking leads to tumor endocrine therapy resistance. (Nardone et al., 2015). A common endocrine resistance mechanism is due to genomic changes in components in various pathways. Various approaches have been investigated to discover new mechanisms of resistance and how to overcome it. These approaches include molecular profiling of biopsies and correlation studies of the molecular alterations with anti-proliferative response (Giltnane et al., 2017, Guerrero-Zotano et al., 2018, Dunbier et al., 2013), identification of resistant genes through high-throughput functional genetic screens (Nagarajan et al., 2020; Xu et al., 2020; Miller et al., 2011; Xiao et al., 2018; Fox et al., 2011) and next generation sequencing (NGS) of patients with acquired drug resistance (Razavi et al., 2018; O'Leary et al., 2018).

Epigenic Changes

Epigenetics is the study of the mechanisms and compounds that can maintain several states of gene activity within the setting of the same DNA sequence (Cavalli and Heard, 2019). Covalent changes in DNA, histone proteins, and chromatin encode epigenetic information through their structure and function (Szczepanek et al., 2023). The mechanisms of epigenetics include cell development, cell maintenance, cell differentiation, genomic stability, and gene transcription regulation (Kim et al., 2023). Genetic or genomic information is not changed by epigenetic modifications. The three main categories of epigenetics include DNA methylation, noncoding RNAs (ncRNAs), and histone modifications (Kim et al., 2023). Epigenetic changes contribute to the heterogeneity of cancer and aberrant epigenetic regulation is highly associated with breast cancer development. Tumor suppressor genes are silenced as a result of epigenetic alterations or epimutations, and this can stimulate the growth of tumors by activating oncogenes (Szczepanek et al., 2023). For instance, BRCA1 can change epigenetics through physical interactions and/or transcriptional regulation, which are often referred to as epigenetic modifiers. Epimutations can work alone or in conjunction with others. BRCA1 can also directly ubiquitylates histones. BRCA1/2-associated hereditary BC is characterized by DNA methylation changes. In BRCA1/2 mutational genes, cancer cells are unable to correctly repair DNA damage which leads to tumor development and proliferation. The expression of genes involved in cell signaling, proliferation, DNA repair mechanisms, and differentiation is impacted by alterations in DNA methylation, which promotes the growth of tumors (Sharma et al., 2010).

Somatic Changes

Somatic changes are changes to DNA and are not passed on to the next generation. These changes randomly. Cancer genetic research has focused on the characterization of the driver somatic mutations and investigates the linkage of driver mutations to clinical phenotypes that can be used to provide insights into treatments and treatment responses (Mathioudaki et al., 2020). The most frequent somatic events include the mutations in the tumor protein P53 (TP53), Cadherin-1 (CDH1), MYC, phosphatidylinositol-4,5-bisphosphate 3-kinase, catalytic (PIK3CA), mitogen-activated protein kinase 7 (MAP2K7), GATA Binding Protein 3 (GATA3), and AKT serine/threonine kinase 1 (AKT1); duplications in the epidermal growth factor receptor 2 (ERBB2) and deletions in the phosphatase and tensin homolog (PTEN) or mitogen-activated protein kinase 4 (MAP2K4). The correlation between mutation rates and the subtype of BC tumors can vary depending on sample numbers and study designs (Ademuyiwa et al., 2017; Pereira et al., 2016; Nik-Zainal et al., 2016; Ellis et al., 2012). The somatic landscapes of cancer have not yet been compared across all nations and ethnic groups. When compared to sporadic breast cancers, patients with germline mutations in the BRCA1/2 gene exhibit greater genetic abnormalities (Ingvarsson, 1999). An aggressive and particular pathway of chromosomal damage in BC patients may be indicated by an increase in somatic alterations during tumor growth (Ingvarsson, 1999). Most somatic mutations are frameshift mutations that cause a premature stop codon and result in the decreased production of functional BRCA proteins (Rebbeck et al., 2018).

Approximately 30% of the processes that amplify the PI3K/AKT/mTOR signaling pathway, which is mostly associated with BC, are caused by somatic mutations in PIK3CA (Shimoi et al., 2018). As important prognostic indicators, PIK3CA mutations are frequent in ER-positive/HER2 tumors (Elwy et al., 2017; Berger et al., 2013). Exons 9 and 20 are where the majority of PIK3CA somatic mutations are found (Zhang et al., 2013). In BC, somatic TP53 mutations are also common (Zhang et al., 2018). Next generation sequencing (NGS) was used to build a genomic model of BC, and genome-wide association studies (GWAS) found several loci related to BC (Easton et al., 2007; Chen et al., 2013; Cai et al., 2014). Whole genome amplification (WGA) was also used to identify novel partner and localizer of BRCA2 (PALB2), BRCA1 and BRCA2 mutations in breast and ovarian cancer (Kraus et al., 2017).

Tumor Microenvironment

Endocrine resistance can be caused by the tumor microenvironment. These components include exosomes, hypoxia, immune cells, cancer-associated fibroblasts (CAFs), inflammatory responses, and extracellular matrix (ECM). CAFs have an important role in tumor progression via proliferation growth factors, ECM remodeling and cytokine secretion (Houthuijzen and Jonkers, 2018). Epithelial-to-mesenchymal transition (EMT) in ER+ cancers can be promoted by CAFs (Soon et al., 2013) and CAF can secrete growth factors or cytokines that can lead to that contribute to drug resistance (Brechbuhl et al., 2017). Brechbuhl et al. (2017) found that CD146-negative reduces tamoxifen sensitivity leading to poor outcomes, reduces ER expression, and activates receptor tyrosine kinases (RTKs) in Michigan Cancer Foundation-7 (MCF7) cells (Brechbuhl et al., 2017). Extracellular vesicles (EVs) have the ability to transport proteins, DNA, and RNA across cells, which can accelerate the development of cancer (Desrochers et al., 2016). ECM components can influence the response to anti-estrogen therapy. For instance, in the mouse model of ER+ breast cancer, enhanced displacement of collagen I increased ECM stiffness or density and encouraged tamoxifen resistance (Jallow et al., 2019).

Anti-estrogen treatment induces the transforming growth factor beta (TGFβ) cytokine in breast cancer cells which leads to immunosuppression and anti-estrogen resistance (Joffroy et al., 2010). Research has demonstrated that the tumor microenvironment communicates with the ER directly and mediates ligand-independent ER activation (Dunbier et al., 2013; Stender et al., 2017).

Overcoming Endocrine Therapy Resistance

Inhibition of Downstream Signaling Pathways

According to studies, endocrine resistance can be overcome by upregulating signaling pathways such PI3K/AKT/mTOR and MAPK as well as tyrosine kinase receptor (TKR) expression and activity. In the absence of estradiol, ER phosphorylation and activation are induced when TKRs are activated via mutations or amplification of intracellular signal transduction pathways (Hanker et al., 2020; Rani et al., 2019;

Giuliano et al., 2011; Hartkopf et al., 2020). The MAPK and PI3K pathways downstream of growth factor receptors (GFRs) coordinate and cross-talk to drive cancer cell survival and proliferation. Various feedback loops have been investigated where the inhibition of one pathway leads to activation of the other (Turke et al., 2012; Carracedo et al., 2008). AKT is one of the downstream targets of PI3K that promotes anti-apoptotic responses and cellular proliferation (Datta et al., 1999). By inhibiting this target, the apoptotic response improves and proliferation decreases. It has been demonstrated that inhibiting mTOR, another downstream target of the PI3K pathway, lowers endocrine resistance. Everolimus and exemestane have been proven to extend progression-free survival (PFS) in advanced ER+/HER2-BC following progression on non-steroidal AIs (Baselga et al., 2012; Hortobagyi et al., 2016). Abelson (ABL) tyrosine kinases is a Src-like non-receptor protein kinase that acts downstream of the platelet-derived growth factor (PDGFR) that regulates apoptosis, cell proliferation, stress responses, cell migration, and adhesion (Dibb et al., 2004; Yuan et al., 1996; Brasher and Van Etten, 2000). Inhibition of ABL can lead to effective cancer treatment (Schindler et al., 2000).

Novel Endocrine Therapies

Existing clinical treatments have been able to limit the progression of BC and metastasis, but multidrug resistance, immunosuppression, and abnormal metabolism remain a huge burden for BC treatment. The "Warburg effect" may be reversed by adenosine 5′-monophosphate (AMP)-activated protein kinase (AMPK), which has the ability to control metabolic reprogramming. An essential regulator of eukaryotic cells' energy homeostasis and metabolism, AMPK is a highly conserved serine/threonine kinase (Hardie et al., 2012). AMPK participates in a variety of biological processes, including lipid synthesis, glucose metabolism, protein synthesis, immunological responses, cell cycle regulation, and other biological processes. The activation of AMPK phosphorylation has been shown to have many anti-response multidrug resistance (MDR), triggering apoptosis, kicking off autophagy, limiting proliferation, stimulating immunological response, and suppressing metastasis, according to a number of studies (Mihaylova and Shaw, 2011; Tan et al., 2019; Haikala et al., 2019; Faubert et al., 2013). However, some studies demonstrated that activation of AMPK and abnormal expression in cancer cells can play a key role in promoting cancer cell survival, metastasis, and proliferation under stress conditions (Jeon et al., 2012; Liu et al., 2016, 2020). As a result, other molecules, such as tamoxifen, can be employed in conjunction with AMPK to control the progression of cancer by AMPK's and its downstream targets' activity (Yan et al., 2020).

The cancer cell membrane and cytoplasm both contain the protein known as programmed death ligand 1 (PD-L1). PD L1 can be monitored by T cells that can regulate cancer cell escape (Wu et al., 2019). Suppressing PD-L1 is regarded as a powerful cancer therapy. PD-L1 is phosphorylated at the Ser195 location by AMPK, which causes PD-L1 to be glycosylated and degraded, demonstrating its therapeutic potential for cancer (Cha et al., 2018). Additionally, AMPK activation can enhance the effects of PD-1 inhibition by increasing PGC-1 expression (Chamoto et al., 2017). Agents that can restore the functioning of apoptotic pathways are a viable alternative for advanced drug-resistant malignancies since dysregulation of apoptosis is a prevalent resistance mechanism in breast cancer. The process of planned cell death known as apoptosis is crucial for healthy immunological response, cell growth, and regular cell turnover (Green, 2022). Apoptosis is tightly controlled and essential for removing damaged cells and preserving the health of the organism. The identification and study of apoptosis-inducing targets may be a potential strategy against resistant BC since therapy resistance avoids apoptosis.

Epigenetic changes are reversible and can be restored to their normal state through epigenetic therapy making epigenetic research a promising field of interest. Epigenetic therapy is a therapeutic approach that focuses on chemical modifications that affect gene activity in cancer cells. For BC, epigenetic therapy aims to restore normal tumor suppressor gene expression which inhibits cancer cell growth (Szczepanek et al., 2023). RNA inhibitors, DNA methyltransferase inhibitors (DNMTi), and histone deacetylase inhibitors (HDACi) are three types of epigenetic therapy for breast cancer that are frequently used (Sharma et al., 2010; Ascoët and De Waard, 2020). Epigenetic therapy has also advanced to include various inhibitors and miRNAs (Shukla et al., 2019). Small molecule inhibitors targeting HDACis and DNA hypomethylating compounds have been shown to re-sensitize agents to endocrine therapy (Oronsky et al., 2014; Zucchetti et al., 2019). This shows the potential that novel epigenetic approaches can overcome endocrine therapy resistance.

HDACi can inhibit the activity of enzymes that remove acetyl groups from histones leading to the activation of tumor suppressor genes and chromatin changes. DNMT inhibitors can inhibit the enzyme activity that adds methyl groups to DNA resulting in the blockage in the expression of the tumor suppressor gene. Inhibitors of epigenetic enzymes are known as "epi-drugs" and new potential epi-drugs are being studied (Dawson et al., 2012; Stefansson and Esteller, 2013; Plass et al., 2013; You and Jones, 2012; Berdasco and Esteller, 2010). MicroRNAs (miRNAs) are a key interest as they are involved in various pathways and might be a novel approach to overcome endocrine therapy resistance (Zamarbide Losada et al., 2023). MiRNAs are an important regulator of gene expression and influence tumorigenesis and can regulate drug resistance, metastasis, and tumor progression (Adams et al., 2014). MiRNAs can be used for gene therapy by introducing the miRNAs into cancer cells that express a low level of a particular miRNA and can be used for therapeutic or diagnostic purposes (Gorur et al., 2021; Valcourt and Day, 2020; Qattan, 2020). Examples of miRNA with potential therapeutic value include the following:

- MiR-34a can induce apoptosis and inhibit the proliferation of BCC (Xia et al., 2018; Wu et al., 2014; Mohammady et al., 2019).
- MiR-155 is involved in the proliferation and inflammatory processes of BCC and is a potential and novel therapeutic target (Zaleska et al., 2017; Zhang et al., 2020, 2022; Abtin et al., 2018; Shang et al., 2022).

- MiR-200 is involved in the invasion and metastasis of BC via epithelial-mesenchymal transition (EMT) regulation. Increased miR-200 expression can reduce the ability of cancer cells to invade and migrate (Fkih M'hamed et al., 2017; Yoo et al., 2015; Khalighfard et al., 2018).

Many more miRNAs are being investigated for their potential use as therapeutic agents and to overcome endocrine therapy resistance. RNA inhibitors can block mRNA transcription and translation which affects the regulation of gene expression and is used as replacement therapy (Szczepanek et al., 2022).

Combinatorial Approaches to Enhance Endocrine Therapy Response

Combinational approaches align with the saying that two heads are better than one. Treatments are often combined to increase the effects and/or the mechanism of therapy. Combinational therapy represents a promising treatment strategy for improved systemic control of the disease. Polychemotherapy is better tolerated by patients and due to its multidirectional activity, which includes immunomodulatory, antiangiogenic, and anti-proliferative activity may provide superior clinical benefits for cancer (Wysocki et al., 2022; Cazzaniga et al., 2019, 2021). Given the biological similarities between metronomic chemotherapy and CDK4/6i, the combination of endocrine therapy with anti-proliferative drugs such as CDK4/6i has the potential to be a treatment, particularly in low- and middle-income countries. However, the combination of endocrine therapy and chemotherapy is still controversial (André et al., 2013). Blocking both HER2 and ER mutations simultaneously has demonstrated synergistic anti-cancer efficacy both in vivo and in vitro (Croessmann et al., 2019, Nayar et al., 2019) and the combinational therapy of neratinib and fulvestrant has shown promising activity in metastatic ER+/HER2-mutated BC (Smyth et al., 2020).

HDACi treatment for ER+ cells resulted in an increase in the effectiveness of anti-proliferative endocrine therapy. The restoration of endocrine sensitivity has also shown encouraging effects when HDACis and tamoxifen are combined (Munster et al., 2011). HDACi therapy combined with azacytidine—resulted in ER re-expression and effective resistance to anti-estrogen therapy (Buocikova et al., 2020). Tamoxifen-resistant cell proliferation can be inhibited by the bromodomain and extra-terminal motif (BET) inhibitor, JQ1, in combination with SERDs (Yellapu et al., 2022). Additionally, miRNAs can be utilized in conjunction with additional anti-cancer medications to improve treatment outcomes and lessen side effects (Xue et al., 2016, Gong et al., 2022, Lindholm et al., 2019, Dwivedi et al., 2022). The MONALEESA-1 trial compared biological response to neoadjuvant letrozole alone and combined with ribociclib. The results reported greater Ki67 reduction in the combinational therapy (Curigliano et al., 2016). Complete cell cycle arrest was observed in the NeoPalAna research, which evaluated neoadjuvant treatment using a combination of anastrozole and palbociclib (Ma et al., 2017). In comparison to letrozole alone, the combined therapy of neoadjuvant letrozole and palbociclib boosted the Ki67 decrease, according to the phase II PALLET trial (Johnston et al., 2019). There are many other trials currently testing combinational therapeutic approaches for example the ongoing DxCARTES trial NCT03819010 and the ongoing phase III trial NCT03969121 (Cussac et al., 2019).

Challenges and Limitations of Endocrine Therapy

There are still many unknown factors regarding endocrine resistance. Further investigation is required to fully understand what causes the resistance and how it can be overcome. BC is a very complex cancer and hence shows the need for adequate and accurate treatment. BC is highly heterogeneous and can be multidrug resistant which can cause recurrence and metastasis (Mansoori et al., 2017). Cross influences of various treatments can have a negative alternative effect and can lead to poor outcomes. Drugs or treatments' lack of selectivity and high toxicity is another challenge. Musculoskeletal pain and menopausal symptoms are common problems for patients receiving adjuvant endocrine therapy that influences the quality of life of the patient and must be closely monitored (Choo et al., 2019). Clinical adverse effects linked to PI3K/AKT/mTOR include diarrhea, rashes, hyperglycemia, stomatitis, and pneumonitis and have led to a high percentage of treatment patient discontinuation (Sirico et al., 2023). Novel mutations in various genes and pathways make it difficult to study potential drugs. The PI3K/AKT/mTOR pathway frequently mutates and promotes treatment resistance which makes targeting this pathway difficult. The identification of mutational drivers remains a major challenge (Cerma et al., 2023). Treatment affordability or lack of resources is another barrier to overcoming endocrine therapy resistance. Potential treatments might only be available in developed countries and may be too expensive (André et al., 2013). Another challenge also includes the effective delivery of miRNA to the cancer cells. MiRNA must be effectively delivered to influence the target cell (Shinde et al., 2023).

Conclusion

By understanding the underlying mechanisms of endocrine therapy resistance and implementing innovative strategies, researchers aim to improve treatment outcomes and provide new avenues for patients with HR+ breast cancer. The ability to treat clinically metastatic ER+ breast cancer is hampered by resistance to endocrine therapy, even though early-stage ER+ breast tumors are responsive to these treatments. Improved adjuvant approaches to lessen metastatic recurrence may be addressed by new and existing targeted therapeutics for ER+ breast cancer. Inhibiting PI3K,

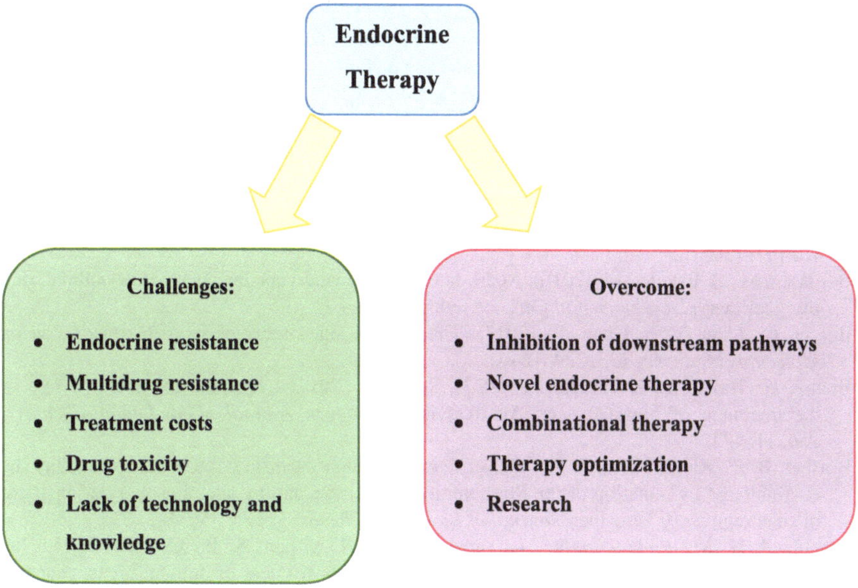

Fig. 5.3 *Challenges and overcoming endocrine therapy resistance*. Endocrine resistance has various challenges, but this can be overcome to improve the treatment of breast cancer

CDK4/6, and mTOR have been found to increase the effectiveness of endocrine therapy, and new medications that target additional elements of important pathways, such as the PI3K/AKT/mTOR pathway, are now being researched. Combinational therapy can also contribute to more effective BC treatment. As the molecular mechanisms of endocrine resistance are diverse, optimal sequencing, and combination strategies must be investigated and developed that can be used to overcome endocrine therapy resistance (Fig. 5.3).

References

Abtin, M., Alivand, M. R., Khaniani, M. S., Bastami, M., Zaeifizadeh, M., & Derakhshan, S. M. (2018). Simultaneous downregulation of Mir-21 and Mir-155 through oleuropein for breast cancer prevention and therapy. *Journal of Cellular Biochemistry, 119*, 7151–7165.

Adams, B. D., Kasinski, A. L., & Slack, F. J. (2014). Aberrant regulation and function of Micrornas in cancer. *Current Biology, 24*, R762–R776.

Ademuyiwa, F. O., Tao, Y., Luo, J., Weilbaecher, K., & Ma, C. X. (2017). Differences in the mutational landscape of triple-negative breast cancer in African Americans and Caucasians. *Breast Cancer Research and Treatment, 161*, 491–499.

Aggelis, V., & Johnston, S. R. D. (2019). Advances in endocrine-based therapies for Estrogen receptor-positive metastatic breast cancer. *Drugs, 79*, 1849–1866.

Akhtar, M., Wright, J. N., & Lee-Robichaud, P. (2011). A review of mechanistic studies on aromatase (Cyp19) and 17α-Hydroxylase-17, 20-lyase (Cyp17). *The Journal of Steroid Biochemistry and Molecular Biology, 125*, 2–12.

André, N., Banavali, S., Snihur, Y., & Pasquier, E. (2013). Has the time come for Metronomics in Low-income and middle-income countries? *The Lancet Oncology, 14*, E239–E248.

Ascoët, S., & De Waard, M. (2020). Diagnostic and therapeutic value of aptamers in envenomation cases. *International Journal of Molecular Sciences, 21*, 3565.

Baselga, J., Campone, M., Piccart, M., Burris, H. A., 3rd, Rugo, H. S., Sahmoud, T., et al. (2012). Everolimus in postmenopausal hormone-receptor-positive advanced breast cancer. *The New England Journal of Medicine, 366*, 520–529.

Beatson, G. T. (1896). On the treatment of inoperable cases of carcinoma of the mamma: Suggestions for a new method of treatment, with illustrative cases. *Trans Med Chir Soc Edinb, 15*, 153–179.

Berdasco, M., & Esteller, M. (2010). Aberrant epigenetic landscape in cancer: How cellular identity goes awry. *Developmental Cell, 19*, 698–711.

Berger, C., Qian, Y., & Chen, X. (2013). The P53-Estrogen receptor loop in cancer. *Current Molecular Medicine, 13*, 1229–1240.

Bhatia, N., Hazra, S., & Thareja, S. (2023). Selective Estrogen receptor degraders (Serds) for the treatment of breast cancer: An overview. *European Journal of Medicinal Chemistry, 256*, 115422.

Brasher, B. B., & Van Etten, R. A. (2000). C-Abl has high intrinsic tyrosine kinase activity that is stimulated by mutation of the Src homology 3 domain and by autophosphorylation at two distinct regulatory Tyrosines. *Journal of Biological Chemistry, 275*, 35631–35637.

Brechbuhl, H. M., Finlay-Schultz, J., Yamamoto, T. M., Gillen, A. E., Cittelly, D. M., Tan, A.-C., et al. (2017). Fibroblast subtypes regulate responsiveness of luminal breast cancer to Estrogenfibroblasts regulate Estrogen response in er+ breast cancer. *Clinical Cancer Research, 23*, 1710–1721.

Brodie, A. M. H., Garrett, W. M., Hendrickson, J. R., Tsai-Morris, C.-H., Marcotte, P. A., & Robinson, C. H. (1981). Inactivation of aromatase in vitro by 4-Hydroxy-4-Androstene-3, 17-Dione and 4-Acetoxy-4-Androstene-3, 17-Dione and sustained effects in vivo. *Steroids, 38*, 693–702.

Buocikova, V., Rios-Mondragon, I., Pilalis, E., Chatziioannou, A., Miklikova, S., Mego, M., et al. (2020). Epigenetics in breast cancer therapy—New strategies and future nanomedicine perspectives. *Cancers, 12*, 3622.

Cai, Q., Zhang, B., Sung, H., Low, S.-K., Kweon, S.-S., Lu, W., et al. (2014). Genome-wide association analysis in east Asians identifies breast cancer susceptibility loci at 1q32. 1, 5q14. 3 and 15q26. 1. *Nature Genetics, 46*, 886–890.

Campone, M., Bardia, A., Ulaner, G. A., Chandarlapaty, S., Gosselin, A., Doroumian, S., et al. (2020). Abstract P5-11-02: Dose-escalation study of Sar439859, an Oral selective Estrogen receptor degrader, in postmenopausal women with Estrogen receptor-positive and human epidermal growth factor receptor 2-negative metastatic breast cancer. *Cancer Research, 80*, P5–P11.

Carlini, P., Frassoldati, A., De Marco, S., Casali, A., Ruggeri, E. M., Nardi, M., et al. (2001). Formestane, a steroidal aromatase inhibitor after failure of non-steroidal aromatase inhibitors (anastrozole and letrozole): Is a clinical benefit still achievable? *Annals of Oncology, 12*, 1539–1543.

Carracedo, A., Ma, L., Teruya-Feldstein, J., Rojo, F., Salmena, L., Alimonti, A., et al. (2008). Inhibition of Mtorc1 leads to Mapk pathway activation through a Pi3k-dependent feedback loop in human cancer. *The Journal of Clinical Investigation, 118*, 3065–3074.

Cavalli, G., & Heard, E. (2019). Advances in epigenetics link genetics to the environment and disease. *Nature, 571*, 489–499.

Cazzaniga, M. E., Munzone, E., Bocci, G., Afonso, N., Gomez, P., Langkjer, S., et al. (2019). Pan-European expert meeting on the use of metronomic chemotherapy in advanced breast cancer patients: The Penelope project. *Advances in Therapy, 36*, 381–406.

Cazzaniga, M. E., Cordani, N., Capici, S., Cogliati, V., Riva, F., & Cerrito, M. G. (2021). Metronomic chemotherapy. *Cancers, 13*, 2236.

Cerma, K., Piacentini, F., Moscetti, L., Barbolini, M., Canino, F., Tornincasa, A., et al. (2023). Targeting Pi3k/Akt/Mtor pathway in breast cancer: From biology to clinical challenges. *Biomedicines [Online], 11*, 109.

Cha, J.-H., Yang, W.-H., Xia, W., Wei, Y., Chan, L.-C., Lim, S.-O., et al. (2018). Metformin promotes antitumor immunity via endoplasmic-reticulum-associated degradation of pd-L1. *Molecular Cell, 71*, 606–620.

Chamoto, K., Chowdhury, P. S., Kumar, A., Sonomura, K., Matsuda, F., Fagarasan, S., et al. (2017). Mitochondrial activation chemicals synergize with surface receptor pd-1 blockade for T cell-dependent antitumor activity. *Proceedings of the National Academy of Sciences, 114*, E761–E770.

Chen, S., Besman, M. J., Sparkes, R. S., Zollman, S., Klisak, I., Mohandas, T., et al. (1988). Human aromatase: Cdna cloning, southern blot analysis, and assignment of the gene to chromosome 15. *DNA, 7*, 27–38.

Chen, F., Chen, G. K., Stram, D. O., Millikan, R. C., Ambrosone, C. B., John, E. M., et al. (2013). A genome-wide association study of breast cancer in women of African ancestry. *Human Genetics, 132*, 39–48.

Cheung, K. W. K., Yoshida, K., Cheeti, S., Chen, B., Morley, R., Chan, I. T., et al. (2019). Gdc-0810 pharmacokinetics and transporter-mediated drug interaction evaluation with an endogenous biomarker in the first-in-human, dose escalation study. *Drug Metabolism and Disposition, 47*, 966–973.

Choo, S. B., Saifulbahri, A., Zullkifli, S. N., Fadzil, M. L., Redzuan, A. M., Abdullah, N., et al. (2019). Adjuvant endocrine therapy side-effects among postmenopausal breast cancer patients in Malaysia. *Climacteric, 22*, 175–181.

Chumsri, S., Howes, T., Bao, T., Sabnis, G., & Brodie, A. (2011). Aromatase, aromatase inhibitors, and breast cancer. *The Journal of Steroid Biochemistry and Molecular Biology, 125*, 13–22.

Croessmann, S., Formisano, L., Kinch, L. N., Gonzalez-Ericsson, P. I., Sudhan, D. R., Nagy, R. J., et al. (2019). Combined blockade of activating Erbb2 mutations and er results in synthetic lethality of er+/Her2 mutant breast cancer. *Clinical Cancer Research, 25*, 277–289.

Curigliano, G., Pardo, P. G., Meric-Bernstam, F., Conte, P., Lolkema, M. P., Beck, J. T., et al. (2016). Ribociclib plus letrozole in early breast cancer: A presurgical, window-of-opportunity study. *The Breast, 28*, 191–198.

Cussac, A. L., Pérez-García, J., Guerrero, Á., Bermejo, B., Gil, M., Carañana, V., et al. (2019). Abstract Ct219: Neoadjuvant letrozole and palbociclib in stage ii-Iiib hr [+]/Her2 [−] breast cancer with oncotype dx recurrence score®(Rs) 18-25 or 26-100. Analysis of Rs changes at surgery (Dxcartes trial). *Cancer Research, 79*, Ct219–Ct219.

Datta, S. R., Brunet, A., & Greenberg, M. E. (1999). Cellular survival: A play in three Akts. *Genes & Development, 13*, 2905–2927.

Dawson, M. A., Kouzarides, T., & Huntly, B. J. P. (2012). Targeting epigenetic readers in cancer. *New England Journal of Medicine, 367*, 647–657.

Dees, E. C., Aftimos, P. G., Van Oordt, H., De Vries, E. G. E., Neven, P., Pegram, M. D., et al. (2019). Dose-escalation study of G1t48, an Oral selective Estrogen receptor degrader (Serd), in postmenopausal women with er+/Her2-locally advanced or metastatic breast cancer (Abc). *Annals of Oncology, 30*, V121–V122.

Delmas, P. D., Bjarnason, N. H., Mitlak, B. H., Ravoux, A.-C., Shah, A. S., Huster, W. J., et al. (1997). Effects of raloxifene on bone mineral density, serum cholesterol concentrations, and uterine endometrium in postmenopausal women. *New England Journal of Medicine, 337*, 1641–1647.

Desrochers, L. M., Antonyak, M. A., & Cerione, R. A. (2016). Extracellular vesicles: Satellites of information transfer in cancer and stem cell biology. *Developmental Cell, 37*, 301–309.

Dibb, N. J., Dilworth, S. M., & Mol, C. D. (2004). Switching on kinases: Oncogenic activation of Braf and the Pdgfr family. *Nature Reviews Cancer, 4*, 718–727.

Dunbier, A. K., Ghazoui, Z., Anderson, H., Salter, J., Nerurkar, A., Osin, P., et al. (2013). Molecular profiling of aromatase inhibitor–treated postmenopausal breast tumors identifies immune-

related correlates of resistancegenomic profiling predicts response to aromatase inhibitor treatment. *Clinical Cancer Research, 19*, 2775–2786.
Dwivedi, S., Pareek, P., Vishnoi, J. R., Sharma, P., & Misra, S. (2022). Downregulation of Mirna-21 and cancer stem cells after chemotherapy results in better outcome in breast cancer patients. *World Journal Of Stem Cells, 14*, 310.
Easton, D. F., Pooley, K. A., Dunning, A. M., Pharoah, P. D. P., Thompson, D., Ballinger, D. G., et al. (2007). Genome-wide association study identifies novel breast cancer susceptibility loci. *Nature, 447*, 1087–1093.
Ellis, M. J., Ding, L., Shen, D., Luo, J., Suman, V. J., Wallis, J. W., et al. (2012). Whole-genome analysis informs breast cancer response to aromatase inhibition. *Nature, 486*, 353–360.
Elwy, F., Helwa, R., El Leithy, A. A., Assem, M. M., & Hassan, N. H. A. (2017). Pik3ca mutations in Her2-positive breast cancer patients; frequency and clinicopathological perspective in Egyptian patients. *Asian Pacific Journal Of Cancer Prevention: Apjcp, 18*, 57.
Faubert, B., Boily, G., Izreig, S., Griss, T., Samborska, B., Dong, Z., et al. (2013). Ampk is a negative regulator of the Warburg effect and suppresses tumor growth in vivo. *Cell Metabolism, 17*, 113–124.
Fisher, B., Costantino, J. P., Redmond, C. K., Fisher, E. R., Wickerham, D. L., Cronin, W. M., et al. (1994). Endometrial cancer in tamoxifen-treated breast cancer patients: Findings from the National Surgical Adjuvant Breast and Bowel Project (Nsabp) B-14. *Jnci: Journal Of The National Cancer Institute, 86*, 527–537.
Fkih M'hamed, I., Privat, M., Trimeche, M., Penault-Llorca, F., Bignon, Y.-J., & Kenani, A. (2017). Mir-10b, Mir-26a, Mir-146a and Mir-153 expression in triple negative vs non triple negative breast cancer: Potential biomarkers. *Pathology & Oncology Research, 23*, 815–827.
Fox, E. M., Miller, T. W., Balko, J. M., Kuba, M. G., Sánchez, V., Smith, R. A., et al. (2011). A Kinome-wide screen identifies the insulin/Igf-I receptor pathway as a mechanism of escape from hormone dependence in breast Cancerinsulin/Igf-I receptors and Antiestrogen resistance. *Cancer Research, 71*, 6773–6784.
Gangl, E. T., Markandu, R., Sharma, P., Sykes, A., Pop-Damkov, P., Gutierrez, P. M., et al. (2020). Preclinical pharmacokinetic and metabolic characterization of the next generation Oral Serd Azd9833. *Cancer Research, 80*, 1042–1042.
Gerratana, L., Fanotto, V., Bonotto, M., Bolzonello, S., Minisini, A. M., Fasola, G., et al. (2015). Pattern of metastasis and outcome in patients with breast cancer. *Clinical & Experimental Metastasis, 32*, 125–133.
Giltnane, J. M., Hutchinson, K. E., Stricker, T. P., Formisano, L., Young, C. D., Estrada, M. V., et al. (2017). Genomic profiling of er+ breast cancers after short-term Estrogen suppression reveals alterations associated with endocrine resistance. *Science Translational Medicine, 9*, Eaai7993.
Giuliano, M., Schifp, R., Osborne, C. K., & Trivedi, M. V. (2011). Biological mechanisms and clinical implications of endocrine resistance in breast cancer. *Breast, 20*(Suppl 3), S42–S49.
Goldhirsch, A., Wood, W. C., Coates, A. S., Gelber, R. D., Thürlimann, B., & Senn, H. J. (2011). Strategies for subtypes—Dealing with the diversity of breast cancer: Highlights of the St Gallen international expert consensus on the primary therapy of early breast cancer 2011. *Annals of Oncology, 22*, 1736–1747.
Gong, C., Cheng, Z., Yang, Y., Shen, J., Zhu, Y., Ling, L., et al. (2022). A 10-Mirna risk score-based prediction model for pathological complete response to neoadjuvant chemotherapy in hormone receptor-positive breast cancer. *Science China Life Sciences, 65*, 2205–2217.
Gorur, A., Bayraktar, R., Ivan, C., Mokhlis, H. A., Bayraktar, E., Kahraman, N., et al. (2021). Ncrna therapy with Mirna-22-3p suppresses the growth of triple-negative breast cancer. *Molecular Therapy-Nucleic Acids, 23*, 930–943.
Gottardis, M. M., & Jordan, V. C. (1987). Antitumor actions of Keoxifene and tamoxifen in the N-Nitrosomethylurea-induced rat mammary carcinoma model. *Cancer Research, 47*, 4020–4024.
Green, D. R. (2022). The mitochondrial pathway of apoptosis part I: The Bcl-2 protein family. *Cold Spring Harbor Perspectives in Biology, 14*, A041046.

Guan, J., Zhou, W., Hafner, M., Blake, R. A., Chalouni, C., Chen, I. P., et al. (2019). Therapeutic ligands antagonize Estrogen receptor function by impairing its mobility. *Cell, 178*, 949–963.

Guerrero-Zotano, A. L., Stricker, T. P., Formisano, L., Hutchinson, K. E., Stover, D. G., Lee, K.-M., et al. (2018). Er+ breast cancers resistant to prolonged neoadjuvant letrozole exhibit an E2f4 transcriptional program sensitive to Cdk4/6 Inhibitorse2f4 activity mediates resistance to Antiestrogen therapy. *Clinical Cancer Research, 24*, 2517–2529.

Guo, S., Zhang, C., Bratton, M., Mottamal, M., Liu, J., Ma, P., et al. (2018). Zb716, a steroidal selective Estrogen receptor degrader (Serd), is orally efficacious in blocking tumor growth in mouse xenograft models. *Oncotarget, 9*, 6924.

Haikala, H. M., Anttila, J. M., Marques, E., Raatikainen, T., Ilander, M., Hakanen, H., et al. (2019). Pharmacological reactivation of Myc-dependent apoptosis induces susceptibility to anti-pd-1 immunotherapy. *Nature Communications, 10*, 620.

Hanker, A. B., Sudhan, D. R., & Arteaga, C. L. (2020). Overcoming endocrine resistance in breast cancer. *Cancer Cell, 37*, 496–513.

Harada, N. (1997). Aberrant expression of aromatase in breast cancer tissues. *The Journal of Steroid Biochemistry and Molecular Biology, 61*, 175–184.

Hardie, D. G., Ross, F. A., & Hawley, S. A. (2012). Ampk: A nutrient and energy sensor that maintains energy homeostasis. *Nature Reviews Molecular Cell Biology, 13*, 251–262.

Hartkopf, A. D., Grischke, E. M., & Brucker, S. Y. (2020). Endocrine-resistant breast cancer: Mechanisms and treatment. *Breast Care (Basel), 15*, 347–354.

Hernando, C., Ortega-Morillo, B., Tapia, M., Moragón, S., Martínez, M. T., Eroles, P., et al. (2021). Oral selective Estrogen receptor degraders (Serds) as a novel breast cancer therapy: Present and future from a clinical perspective. *International Journal of Molecular Sciences, 22*, 7812.

Hortobagyi, G. N., Chen, D., Piccart, M., Rugo, H. S., Burris, H. A., 3rd, Pritchard, K. I., et al. (2016). Correlative analysis of genetic alterations and Everolimus benefit in hormone receptor-positive, human epidermal growth factor receptor 2-negative advanced breast cancer: Results from Bolero-2. *Journal of Clinical Oncology, 34*, 419–426.

Houthuijzen, J. M., & Jonkers, J. (2018). Cancer-associated fibroblasts as key regulators of the breast cancer tumor microenvironment. *Cancer and Metastasis Reviews, 37*, 577–597.

Ingvarsson, S. (1999). Molecular genetics of breast cancer progression. *Seminars in Cancer Biology, 9*, 277–288.

Jallow, F., O'leary, K. A., Rugowski, D. E., Guerrero, J. F., Ponik, S. M., & Schuler, L. A. (2019). Dynamic interactions between the extracellular matrix and Estrogen activity in progression of er+ breast cancer. *Oncogene, 38*, 6913–6925.

Jeon, S.-M., Chandel, N. S., & Hay, N. (2012). Ampk regulates Nadph homeostasis to promote tumour cell survival during energy stress. *Nature, 485*, 661–665.

Joffroy, C. M., Buck, M. B., Stope, M. B., Popp, S. L., Pfizenmaier, K., & Knabbe, C. (2010). Antiestrogens Induce Transforming Growth Factor B–Mediated Immunosuppression In Breast Cancer antiestrogens Induce Immunosuppression In Breast Cancer. *Cancer Research, 70*, 1314–1322.

Johnston, S. R. D. (2005). Selective oestrogen receptor modulators and Downregulators for breast cancer—Have they lost their way. *Breast Cancer Research, 7*, 119–130.

Johnston, S., Puhalla, S., Wheatley, D., Ring, A., Barry, P., Holcombe, C., et al. 2019. Randomized phase ii study evaluating palbociclib in addition to letrozole as neoadjuvant therapy in Estrogen receptor-positive early breast cancer: Pallet trial.

Jordan, V. C. (2008). Tamoxifen: Catalyst for the change to targeted therapy. *European Journal of Cancer, 44*, 30–38.

Khalighfard, S., Alizadeh, A. M., Irani, S., & Omranipour, R. (2018). Plasma Mir-21, Mir-155, Mir-10b, and let-7a as the potential biomarkers for the monitoring of breast cancer patients. *Scientific Reports, 8*, 17981.

Kieser, K. J., Kim, D. W., Carlson, K. E., Katzenellenbogen, B. S., & Katzenellenbogen, J. A. (2010). Characterization of the pharmacophore properties of novel selective Estrogen receptor Downregulators (Serds). *Journal of Medicinal Chemistry, 53*, 3320–3329.

Kim, A., Mo, K., Kwon, H., Choe, S., Park, M., Kwak, W., et al. (2023). Epigenetic regulation in breast cancer: Insights on Epidrugs. *Epigenomes, 7*, 6.
Kraus, C., Hoyer, J., Vasileiou, G., Wunderle, M., Lux, M. P., Fasching, P. A., et al. (2017). Gene panel sequencing in familial breast/ovarian cancer patients identifies multiple novel mutations also in genes others than Brca1/2. *International Journal of Cancer, 140*, 95–102.
Kristensen, B., Ejlertsen, B., Dalgaard, P., Larsen, L., Holmegaard, S. N., Transbøl, I., et al. (1994). Tamoxifen and bone metabolism in postmenopausal Low-risk breast cancer patients: A randomized study. *Journal of Clinical Oncology, 12*, 992–997.
Lindholm, E. M., Ragle Aure, M., Haugen, M. H., Kleivi Sahlberg, K., Kristensen, V. N., Nebdal, D., et al. (2019). Mirna expression changes during the course of neoadjuvant bevacizumab and chemotherapy treatment in breast cancer. *Molecular Oncology, 13*, 2278–2296.
Liu, P., Ye, F., Xie, X., Li, X., Tang, H., Li, S., et al. (2016). Mir-101-3p is a key regulator of tumor metabolism in triple negative breast cancer targeting Ampk. *Oncotarget, 7*, 35188–35198.
Liu, Q. Q., Huo, H. Y., Ao, S., Liu, T., Yang, L., Fei, Z. Y., et al. (2020). Tgf-B1-induced epithelial-mesenchymal transition increases fatty acid oxidation and Oxphos activity via the P-Ampk pathway in breast cancer cells. *Oncology Reports, 44*, 1206–1215.
Love, R. R., Mazess, R. B., Barden, H. S., Epstein, S., Newcomb, P. A., Jordan, V. C., et al. (1992). Effects of tamoxifen on bone mineral density in postmenopausal women with breast cancer. *New England Journal of Medicine, 326*, 852–856.
Ma, C. X., Reinert, T., Chmielewska, I., & Ellis, M. J. (2015). Mechanisms of aromatase inhibitor resistance. *Nature Reviews Cancer, 15*, 261–275.
Ma, C. X., Gao, F., Luo, J., Northfelt, D. W., Goetz, M., Forero, A., et al. (2017). Neopalana: Neoadjuvant palbociclib, a cyclin-dependent kinase 4/6 inhibitor, and anastrozole for clinical stage 2 or 3 Estrogen receptor–positive breast Cancerneoadjuvant Palbo and anastrozole for er+ breast cancer. *Clinical Cancer Research, 23*, 4055–4065.
Mansoori, B., Mohammadi, A., Davudian, S., Shirjang, S., & Baradaran, B. (2017). The different mechanisms of cancer drug resistance: A brief review. *Advanced Pharmaceutical Bulletin, 7*, 339.
Mathioudaki, A., Ljungström, V., Melin, M., Arendt, M. L., Nordin, J., Karlsson, Å., et al. (2020). Targeted sequencing reveals the somatic mutation landscape in a Swedish breast cancer cohort. *Scientific Reports, 10*, 19304.
Mcdonnell, D. P. (1999). The molecular pharmacology of Serms. *Trends In Endocrinology & Metabolism, 10*, 301–311.
Mihaylova, M. M., & Shaw, R. J. (2011). The Ampk signalling pathway coordinates cell growth, autophagy and metabolism. *Nature Cell Biology, 13*, 1016–1023.
Miller, W. R., Bartlett, J., Brodie, A. M. H., Brueggemeier, R. W., Di Salle, E., Lønning, P. E., et al. (2008). Aromatase inhibitors: Are there differences between steroidal and nonsteroidal aromatase inhibitors and do they matter? *The Oncologist, 13*, 829–837.
Miller, T. W., Balko, J. M., Fox, E. M., Ghazoui, Z., Dunbier, A., Anderson, H., et al. (2011). Erα-dependent E2f transcription can mediate resistance to Estrogen deprivation in human breast Cancererα drives resistance to Estrogen deprivation therapy. *Cancer Discovery, 1*, 338–351.
Mohammady, M., Ghetmiri, S. I., Baharizade, M., Morowvat, M. H., & Torabi, S. (2019). Expanding the biotherapeutics realm via Mir-34a:"potent clever little" agent in breast cancer therapy. *Current Pharmaceutical Biotechnology, 20*, 665–673.
Munster, P. N., Thurn, K. T., Thomas, S., Raha, P., Lacevic, M., Miller, A., Melisko, M., Ismail-Khan, R., Rugo, H., Moasser, M., & Minton, S. E. (2011). A phase II study of the histone deacetylase inhibitor vorinostat combined with tamoxifen for the treatment of patients with hormone therapy-resistant breast cancer. *British journal of cancer, 104*(12), 1828–1835.
Nagarajan, S., Rao, S. V., Sutton, J., Cheeseman, D., Dunn, S., Papachristou, E. K., et al. (2020). Arid1a influences Hdac1/Brd4 activity, intrinsic proliferative capacity and breast cancer treatment response. *Nature Genetics, 52*, 187–197.
Nardone, A., De Angelis, C., Trivedi, M. V., Osborne, C. K., & Schiff, R. (2015). The changing role of Er in endocrine resistance. *The Breast, 24*, S60–S66.

Nathan, M. R., & Schmid, P. (2017). A review of Fulvestrant in breast cancer. *Oncology and Therapy, 5*, 17–29.

Nayar, U., Cohen, O., Kapstad, C., Cuoco, M. S., Waks, A. G., Wander, S. A., et al. (2019). Acquired Her2 mutations in Er(+) metastatic breast cancer confer resistance to Estrogen receptor-directed therapies. *Nature Genetics, 51*, 207–216.

Nik-Zainal, S., Davies, H., Staaf, J., Ramakrishna, M., Glodzik, D., Zou, X., et al. (2016). Landscape of somatic mutations in 560 breast cancer whole-genome sequences. *Nature, 534*, 47–54.

Nilsson, S., & Koehler, K. F. (2005). Oestrogen receptors and selective oestrogen receptor modulators: Molecular and cellular pharmacology. *Basic & Clinical Pharmacology & Toxicology, 96*, 15–25.

Nilsson, S., Makela, S., Treuter, E., Tujague, M., Thomsen, J., Andersson, G. R., et al. (2001). Mechanisms of Estrogen action. *Physiological Reviews, 81*, 1535–1565.

Nofech-Mozes, S., Vella, E. T., Dhesy-Thind, S., Hagerty, K. L., Mangu, P. B., Temin, S., et al. (2012). Systematic review on hormone receptor testing in breast cancer. *Applied Immunohistochemistry & Molecular Morphology, 20*, 214–263.

O'leary, B., Cutts, R. J., Liu, Y., Hrebien, S., Huang, X., Fenwick, K., et al. (2018). The genetic landscape and clonal evolution of breast cancer resistance to palbociclib plus Fulvestrant in the Paloma-3 Trialgenetic landscape of palbociclib-resistant breast cancer. *Cancer Discovery, 8*, 1390–1403.

Oronsky, B., Oronsky, N., Knox, S., Fanger, G., & Scicinski, J. (2014). Episensitization: Therapeutic tumor Resensitization by epigenetic agents: A review and reassessment. *Anti-Cancer Agents In Medicinal Chemistry (Formerly Current Medicinal Chemistry-Anti-Cancer Agents), 14*, 1121–1127.

Palmieri, C., Patten, D. K., Januszewski, A., Zucchini, G., & Howell, S. J. (2014). Breast cancer: Current and future endocrine therapies. *Molecular and Cellular Endocrinology, 382*, 695–723.

Pan, H., Gray, R., Braybrooke, J., Davies, C., Taylor, C., Mcgale, P., et al. (2017). 20-year risks of breast-cancer recurrence after stopping endocrine therapy at 5 years. *New England Journal of Medicine, 377*, 1836–1846.

Park, W.-C., & Jordan, V. C. (2002). Selective estrogen receptor modulators (Serms) and their roles in breast cancer prevention. *Trends in Molecular Medicine, 8*, 82–88.

Paterson, R., & Russell, M. H. (1959). Clinical trials in malignant disease: Part ii—Breast cancer: Value of irradiation of the ovaries. *Journal of the Faculty of Radiologists, 10*, 130–133.

Pereira, B., Chin, S.-F., Rueda, O. M., Vollan, H.-K. M., Provenzano, E., Bardwell, H. A., et al. (2016). The somatic mutation profiles of 2,433 breast cancers refine their genomic and transcriptomic landscapes. *Nature Communications, 7*, 11479.

Plass, C., Pfister, S. M., Lindroth, A. M., Bogatyrova, O., Claus, R., & Lichter, P. (2013). Mutations in regulators of the epigenome and their connections to global chromatin patterns in cancer. *Nature Reviews Genetics, 14*, 765–780.

Qattan, A. (2020). Novel Mirna targets and therapies in the triple-negative breast cancer microenvironment: An emerging Hope for a challenging disease. *International Journal of Molecular Sciences, 21*, 8905.

Rani, A., Stebbing, J., Giamas, G., & Murphy, J. (2019). Endocrine resistance in hormone receptor positive breast cancer-from mechanism to therapy. *Front Endocrinol (Lausanne), 10*, 245.

Razavi, P., Chang, M. T., Xu, G., Bandlamudi, C., Ross, D. S., Vasan, N., et al. (2018). The genomic landscape of endocrine-resistant advanced breast cancers. *Cancer Cell, 34*, 427–438.

Rebbeck, T. R., Friebel, T. M., Friedman, E., Hamann, U., Huo, D., Kwong, A., et al. (2018). Mutational Spectrum in a worldwide study of 29,700 families with Brca1 or Brca2 mutations. *Human Mutation, 39*, 593–620.

Santen, R. J., Brodie, H., Simpson, E. R., Siiteri, P. K., & Brodie, A. (2009). History of aromatase: Saga of an important biological mediator and therapeutic target. *Endocrine Reviews, 30*, 343–375.

Schindler, T., Bornmann, W., Pellicena, P., Miller, W. T., Clarkson, B., & Kuriyan, J. (2000). Structural mechanism for Sti-571 inhibition of Abelson tyrosine kinase. *Science, 289*, 1938–1942.

Shang, M., Wu, Y., Wang, Y., Cai, Y., Jin, J., & Yang, Z. (2022). Dual antisense oligonucleotide targeting Mir-21/Mir-155 synergize photodynamic therapy to treat triple-negative breast cancer and inhibit metastasis. *Biomedicine & Pharmacotherapy, 146*, 112564.

Sharma, S., Kelly, T. K., & Jones, P. A. (2010). Epigenetics in cancer. *Carcinogenesis, 31*, 27–36.

Shiino, S., Kinoshita, T., Yoshida, M., Jimbo, K., Asaga, S., Takayama, S., et al. (2016). Prognostic impact of discordance in hormone receptor status between primary and recurrent sites in patients with recurrent breast cancer. *Clinical Breast Cancer, 16*, E133–E140.

Shimoi, T., Hamada, A., Yamagishi, M., Hirai, M., Yoshida, M., Nishikawa, T., et al. (2018). Pik 3 ca mutation profiling in patients with breast cancer, using a highly sensitive detection system. *Cancer Science, 109*, 2558–2566.

Shinde, S. S., Ahmed, S., Malik, J. A., Hani, U., Khanam, A., Ashraf Bhat, F., et al. (2023). Therapeutic delivery of tumor suppressor Mirnas for breast cancer treatment. *Biology, 12*, 467.

Shioi, Y., Kashiwaba, M., Inaba, T., Komatsu, H., Sugai, T., & Wakabayashi, G. (2014). Long-term complete remission of metastatic breast cancer, induced by a steroidal aromatase inhibitor after failure of a non-steroidal aromatase inhibitor. *The American Journal of Case Reports, 15*, 85.

Shukla, S., Penta, D., Mondal, P., & Meeran, S. M. (2019). Epigenetics of breast cancer: Clinical status of epi-drugs and phytochemicals. In A. Ahmad (Ed.), *Breast cancer metastasis and drug resistance: Challenges and Progress*. Springer International Publishing.

Sirico, M., D'angelo, A., Gianni, C., Casadei, C., Merloni, F., & De Giorgi, U. (2023). Current state and future challenges for Pi3k inhibitors in cancer therapy. *Cancers, 15*, 703.

Siris, E. S., Schussheim, D. H., & Muchmore, D. B. (1999). Chapter 42 - Selective Estrogen Receptor Modulators. In C. J. Rosen, J. Glowacki, & J. P. Bilezikian (Eds.), *The aging skeleton*. Academic Press.

Smyth, L. M., Piha-Paul, S. A., Won, H. H., Schram, A. M., Saura, C., Loi, S., et al. (2020). Efficacy and determinants of response to her kinase inhibition in Her2-mutant metastatic breast cancer. *Cancer Discovery, 10*, 198–213.

Snyder, K. R., Sparano, N., & Malinowski, J. M. (2000). Raloxifene hydrochloride. *American Journal of Health-System Pharmacy, 57*, 1669–1675.

Soon, P. S., Kim, E., Pon, C. K., Gill, A. J., Moore, K., Spillane, A. J., et al. (2013). Breast cancer-associated fibroblasts induce epithelial-to-mesenchymal transition in breast cancer cells. *Endocrine-Related Cancer, 20*, 1–12.

Stefansson, O. A., & Esteller, M. (2013). Epigenetic modifications in breast cancer and their role in personalized medicine. *The American Journal of Pathology, 183*, 1052–1063.

Stender, J. D., Nwachukwu, J. C., Kastrati, I., Kim, Y., Strid, T., Yakir, M., et al. (2017). Structural and molecular mechanisms of cytokine-mediated endocrine resistance in human breast cancer cells. *Molecular Cell, 65*, 1122–1135.

Szczepanek, J., Skorupa, M., & Tretyn, A. (2022). Microrna as a potential therapeutic molecule in cancer. *Cell, 11*, 1008.

Szczepanek, J., Skorupa, M., Jarkiewicz-Tretyn, J., Cybulski, C., & Tretyn, A. (2023). Harnessing epigenetics for breast cancer therapy: The role of Dna methylation, histone modifications, and Microrna. *International Journal of Molecular Sciences, 24*, 7235.

Tan, W., Zhong, Z., Carney, R. P., Men, Y., Li, J., Pan, T., & Wang, Y. (2019). *Deciphering the metabolic role of Ampk in cancer multi-drug resistance* (pp. 56–71). Elsevier.

Thompson, E. A., & Siiteri, P. K. (1974). Utilization of oxygen and reduced nicotinamide adenine dinucleotide phosphate by human placental microsomes during aromatization of androstenedione. *Journal of Biological Chemistry, 249*, 5364–5372.

Thürlimann, B., Paridaens, R., Serin, D., Bonneterre, J., Roche, H., Murray, R., et al. (1997). Third-line hormonal treatment with exemestane in postmenopausal patients with advanced breast cancer progressing on aminoglutethimide: A phase ii multicentre multinational study. *European Journal of Cancer, 33*, 1767–1773.

Tria, G. S., Abrams, T., Baird, J., Burks, H. E., Firestone, B., & Gaither, L. A. (2018). Discovery of Lsz102, a potent, orally bioavailable selective Estrogen receptor degrader (Serd) for the treatment of Estrogen receptor positive breast cancer. *Journal of Medicinal Chemistry, 61*, 2837–2864.

Turke, A. B., Song, Y., Costa, C., Cook, R., Arteaga, C. L., Asara, J. M., et al. (2012). Mek inhibition leads to Pi3k/Akt activation by relieving a negative feedback on Erbb receptors. *Cancer Research, 72*, 3228–3237.

Valcourt, D. M., & Day, E. S. (2020). Dual regulation of Mir-34a and notch Signaling in triple-negative breast cancer by antibody/Mirna nanocarriers. *Molecular Therapy-Nucleic Acids, 21*, 290–298.

Wang, L., Guillen, V. S., Sharma, N., Flessa, K., Min, J., Carlson, K. E., et al. (2018). New class of selective Estrogen receptor degraders (Serds): Expanding the toolbox of Protac degrons. *ACS Medicinal Chemistry Letters, 9*, 803–808.

Wardell, S. E., Marks, J. R., & Mcdonnell, D. P. (2011). The turnover of Estrogen receptor A by the selective Estrogen receptor degrader (Serd) Fulvestrant is a saturable process that is not required for antagonist efficacy. *Biochemical Pharmacology, 82*, 122–130.

Wardell, S. E., Yllanes, A. P., Chao, C. A., Bae, Y., Andreano, K. J., Desautels, T. K., et al. (2020). Pharmacokinetic and pharmacodynamic analysis of Fulvestrant in preclinical models of breast cancer to assess the importance of its Estrogen receptor-A degrader activity in antitumor efficacy. *Breast Cancer Research and Treatment, 179*, 67–77.

Weir, H. M., Bradbury, R. H., Lawson, M., Rabow, A. A., Buttar, D., Callis, R. J., et al. (2016). Azd9496: An oral estrogen receptor inhibitor that blocks the growth of er-positive and Esr1-mutant breast Tumors in preclinical modelspharmacology of Serd inhibitor in breast cancer models. *Cancer Research, 76*, 3307–3318.

Wittmann, B. M., Sherk, A., & Mcdonnell, D. P. (2007). Definition of functionally important mechanistic differences among selective estrogen receptor Down-regulators. *Cancer Research, 67*, 9549–9560.

Wu, M.-Y., Fu, J., Xiao, X., Wu, J., & Wu, R.-C. (2014). Mir-34a regulates therapy resistance by targeting Hdac1 and Hdac7 in breast cancer. *Cancer Letters, 354*, 311–319.

Wu, Y., Chen, W., Xu, Z. P., & Gu, W. (2019). Pd-L1 distribution and perspective for cancer immunotherapy—Blockade, knockdown, or inhibition. *Frontiers in Immunology, 10*, 2022.

Wysocki, P. J., Lubas, M. T., & Wysocka, M. L. (2022). Metronomic chemotherapy in prostate cancer. *Journal of Clinical Medicine, 11*, 2853.

Xia, Y., Deng, X., Cao, M., Liu, S., Zhang, X., Xiao, X., et al. (2018). Nanodiamond-based layer-by-layer nanohybrids mediate targeted delivery of Mir-34a for triple negative breast cancer therapy. *RSC Advances, 8*, 13789–13797.

Xiao, T., Li, W., Wang, X., Xu, H., Yang, J., Wu, Q., et al. (2018). Estrogen-regulated feedback loop limits the efficacy of Estrogen receptor–targeted breast cancer therapy. *Proceedings of the National Academy of Sciences, 115*, 7869–7878.

Xiong, R., Zhao, J., Gutgesell, L., Tonetti, D., & Thatcher, G. (2016). Novel selective estrogen receptor downregulators developed using endocrine-independent breast cancer cell lines. *Cancer Research, 76*, 3902–3902.

Xu, G., Chhangawala, S., Cocco, E., Razavi, P., Cai, Y., et al. (2020). Arid1a determines luminal identity and therapeutic response in Estrogen-receptor-positive breast cancer. *Nature Genetics, 52*, 198–207.

Xue, J., Chi, Y., Chen, Y., Huang, S., Ye, X., Niu, J., et al. (2016). Mirna-621 sensitizes breast cancer to chemotherapy by suppressing Fbxo11 and enhancing P53 activity. *Oncogene, 35*, 448–458.

Yan, J.-B., Lai, C.-C., Jhu, J.-W., Gongol, B., Marin, T. L., Lin, S.-C., et al. (2020). Insulin and metformin control cell proliferation by regulating Tdg-mediated Dna demethylation in liver and breast cancer cells. *Molecular Therapy-Oncolytics, 18*, 282–294.

Yellapu, N. K., Ly, T., Sardiu, M. E., Pei, D., Welch, D. R., Thompson, J. A., et al. (2022). Synergistic anti-proliferative activity of Jq1 and Gsk2801 in triple-negative breast cancer. *BMC Cancer, 22*, 627.

Yoo, B., Kavishwar, A., Ross, A., Wang, P., Tabassum, D. P., Polyak, K., et al. (2015). Combining Mir-10b–targeted Nanotherapy with Low-dose doxorubicin elicits durable regressions of metastatic breast Cancerregression of metastatic cancer using Mirna Nanotherapy. *Cancer Research, 75*, 4407–4415.

You, J. S., & Jones, P. A. (2012). Cancer genetics and epigenetics: Two sides of the same coin? *Cancer Cell, 22*, 9–20.

Yuan, Z.-M., Huang, Y., Whang, Y., Sawyers, C., Weichselbaum, R., Kharbanda, S., et al. (1996). Role for C-Abl tyrosine kinase in growth arrest response to Dna damage. *Nature, 382*, 272–274.

Zaha, D. C. (2014). Significance of immunohistochemistry in breast cancer. *World Journal of Clinical Oncology, 5*, 382–392.

Zaleska, K., Przybyła, A., Kulcenty, K., Wichtowski, M., Mackiewicz, A., & Suchorska, W. (2017). Wound fluids affect Mir-21, Mir-155 and Mir-221 expression in breast cancer cell lines, and this effect is partially abrogated by intraoperative radiation therapy treatment. *Oncology Letters, 14*, 4029–4036.

Zamarbide Losada, J. N., Sulpice, E., Combe, S., Almeida, G. S., Leach, D. A., Choo, J., et al. (2023). Apoptosis-modulatory Mir-361-3p as a novel treatment target in endocrine-responsive and endocrine-resistant breast cancer. *The Journal of Endocrinology, 256*, e220229.

Zhang, L., Shi, L., Zhao, X., Wang, Y., & Yue, W. (2013). Pik3ca gene mutation associated with poor prognosis of lung adenocarcinoma. *Oncotargets and Therapy, 6*, 497–502.

Zhang, Y., Xiong, S., Liu, B., Pant, V., Celii, F., Chau, G., et al. (2018). Somatic Trp53 mutations differentially drive breast cancer and evolution of metastases. *Nature Communications, 9*, 3953.

Zhang, Z., Zhang, L., Yu, G., Sun, Z., Wang, T., Tian, X., et al. (2020). Exosomal Mir-1246 and Mir-155 as predictive and prognostic biomarkers for trastuzumab-based therapy resistance in Her2-positive breast cancer. *Cancer Chemotherapy and Pharmacology, 86*, 761–772.

Zhang, Q., Huang, Y., Yang, R., Mu, J., Zhou, Z., & Sun, M. (2022). Poly-antioxidants for enhanced anti-Mir-155 delivery and synergistic therapy of metastatic breast cancer. *Biomaterials Science, 10*, 3637–3646.

Zucchetti, B., Shimada, A. K., Katz, A., & Curigliano, G. (2019). The role of histone deacetylase inhibitors in metastatic breast cancer. *The Breast, 43*, 130–134.

Resistance to Chemotherapy in Breast Cancer

Richard Khanyile, Thabiso Victor Miya, Nare Sekoba, Emad Rakha, and Zodwa Dlamini

Abstract Breast cancer (BC) is the most frequently diagnosed cancer in women and the leading cause of death for women worldwide. Conventional clinical treatment of BC entails surgery, radiation therapy, hormone therapy, chemotherapy (CT), and targeted therapies. CT plays a critical role in cancer treatment and is linked with improved prognosis in BC patients. However, tumors can become resistant to CT which results in recurrence, treatment failure, and mortality. The underlying mechanisms of chemoresistance in BC are not fully elucidated. This is due to the heterogeneous nature of this disease and the wide spectrum of CT regimens used. Furthermore, current treatment strategies to overcome chemoresistance showed limited success. Therefore, novel and efficacious strategies are urgently needed to overcome chemoresistance in BC. This review sheds light on various mechanisms underlying chemoresistance in BC, including genetic factors, cancer

R. Khanyile (✉)
SAMRC Precision Oncology Research Unit (PORU), SARChI Chair in Precision Oncology and Cancer Prevention (POCP), Pan African Cancer Research Institute (PACRI), University of Pretoria, Pretoria, South Africa

Department of Medical Oncology, Faculty of Health Sciences, Steve Biko Academic Hospital, University of Pretoria, Hatfield, South Africa
e-mail: richard.khanyile@up.ac.za

T. V. Miya · Z. Dlamini
SAMRC Precision Oncology Research Unit (PORU), DSI/NRF SARChI Chair in Precision Oncology and Cancer Prevention (POCP), Pan African Cancer Research Institute (PACRI), University of Pretoria, Pretoria, South Africa
e-mail: thabiso.miya@up.ac.za; Zodwa.Dlamini@up.ac.za

N. Sekoba
Department of Natural Sciences, Faculty of Health Sciences, University of Fort Hare, East London, South Africa
e-mail: NSekoba@ufh.ac.za

E. Rakha
School of Medicine, University of Nottingham and Department of Cellular Pathology, Nottingham University Hospitals NHS Trust City Hospital Campus, Nottingham, UK
e-mail: emad.rakha@nottingham.ac.uk

Z. Dlamini (ed.), *Overcoming Breast Cancer Therapy Resistance*,
https://doi.org/10.1007/978-3-031-52860-6_6

stem cells, and drug efflux. Novel strategies that can be used to combat chemoresistance in BC are also discussed. Novel drug delivery methods, gene therapy, and combining CT with other therapeutic strategies like immunotherapy are some of them. We highlight that further understanding the mechanisms involved in BC chemoresistance can help to develop novel and efficacious treatment strategies and ameliorate current strategies to overcome chemoresistance.

Keywords Breast cancer · Chemotherapy resistance · Genetic factors · Cancer stem cells · Novel drug delivery systems · Gene therapy · Immunotherapy

Introduction

Overview of Breast Cancer and Its Prevalence

Breast cancer (BC) is the most common cancer worldwide. Around 2.3 million patients were diagnosed with BC in 2020, and 685,000 BC-related deaths among women (29.7%) were noted globally in the same year. High mortality rates of BC are the result of distant metastasis (DM) involving vital organs such as the lungs, brain, liver, bone, and other organs (Shah et al., 2018). Less than 10% of BC is present in metastatic disease at first presentation while DM is the end stage of progression of all types of BC that are not controlled by local and systemic treatments. Involvement of the draining lymph nodes is present in 30%–40% of operable breast cancer. Invasive ductal carcinoma (70–75%) and invasive lobular (12–15%) are the most prevalent histological subtypes of BC. The histological classification and clinical pathologies parameters (tumor size, histological grade, and vascular invasion) are amongst several factors that are used to categorize patients with BC to determine prognosis and suggest the most suitable course of treatment (Giuliano et al., 2017; Cardoso et al., 2019). A molecular technique called gene expression profiling is utilized to categorize BC into distinct intrinsic subtypes. BC is routinely categorized based on the expression of crucial genes such as the human epidermal growth factor (HER2), progesterone receptors (PR), and estrogen receptors (ER). These molecular subtypes as well as the level of Ki67 labeling index are associated with different degrees of chemosensitivity and can be used as predictors of CT response (Ruddy & Ganz, 2019; Harbeck et al., 2019). The BC molecular subtypes include triple-negative (ER, PR, and HER2 negative and typically has high Ki67 index), luminal A-like (ER+ and PR+ HER2- and has low Ki67 index), luminal B-like (ER+ and HER2- with PR- and/or high Ki67 index), luminal B-like HER2+ (ER+, PR+/− Ki67 index high/low and HER2+), and HER2+ (HER2+, ER-, PR-) (Ruddy & Ganz, 2019; Harbeck et al., 2019; Fragomeni et al., 2018). In contrast to luminal B (20–30%), the most prevalent molecular subtype, Luminal A (30–40%), has a good prognosis and a low recurrence. The prognosis is worse for luminal B tumors, which are more frequently of a higher histological grade and have a higher rate of proliferation (Johnson et al., 2021). An increased incidence of local or regional recurrences and a poor prognosis are associated with the HER2 subtype (12–20%)

(Fragomeni et al., 2018; Blows et al., 2010). The most aggressive subtype, but least common, triple-negative subtypes (10–15%), is associated with and is linked with higher recurrence rates, poor prognosis, distant metastases, and shorter disease-free intervals and survival time. Currently, surgery, radiation, hormone therapy, and targeted therapy are treatment options for BC. Nevertheless, for patients with high-risk BC, such as the triple-negative and HER2+ subtypes, CT is still the go-to treatment (Society, 2022). CT is amongst the treatment strategies for BC which has led to a decrease in BC-related mortality rates and has also ameliorated the prognosis of this disease (Fig. 6.1). However, the onset of BC is sporadic because of mutated genes that advance progression and also promote CT resistance (chemoresistance) (Pavitra et al., 2023).

Chemoresistance is defined as the cancer cells' insensitivity to treatment, leading to BC chemotherapy failure (Ji et al., 2019). Drug resistance is categorized into intrinsic resistance and acquired resistance, according to drug responsiveness (Nikolaou et al., 2018). The drug resistance spectrum can also be divided into two categories: original primary drug resistance and multidrug resistance (MDR). The four main mediators of intrinsic resistance are drug breakdown, altered expression and/or function of the drug target, altered drug transport across the cellular membrane, altered drug interaction efficiency with the drug's molecular target, and altered drug transport (Sherlach & Roepe, 2014; Mansoori et al., 2017). Nuclear receptors or membrane transporters that are ATP-dependent can promote intrinsic cellular resistance (Synold et al., 2001). Conversely, acquired resistance is determined by environmental or genetic factors that mediate the development of drug-resistant cancer cell clones or cause mutation in the enzymes associated with pertinent metabolic pathways (Gottesman, 2002; Mansoori et al., 2017).

The outcomes of numerous attempts to overcome BC's chemoresistance to currently available chemotherapeutic agents are still unsatisfactory (Ji et al., 2019).

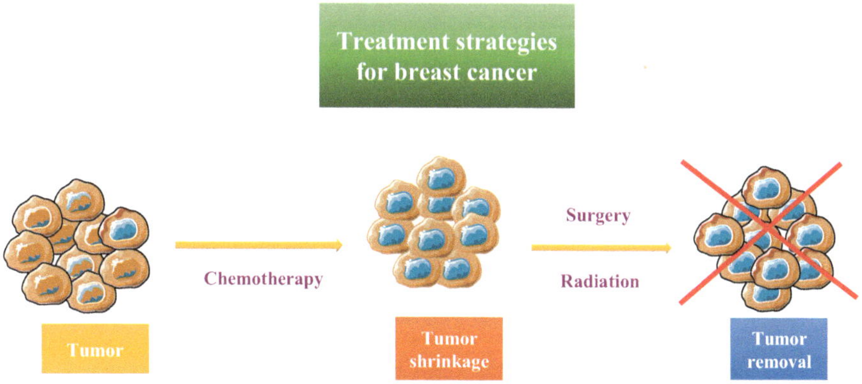

Fig. 6.1 *A schematic diagram of neoadjuvant therapy of breast cancer showing the impacts of chemotherapy in treating cancer that is followed by surgical removal of tumor bed or residual tumor with or without.* Tumors are initially exposed to chemotherapy; however, some tumors can survive (chemoresistance) resulting in a lack of response in the neoadjuvant setting or tumor recurrence in the adjuvant setting

Therefore, further understanding of the underlying mechanisms of chemoresistance in BC is critically important as it will assist in creating novel and effective therapeutic strategies. In return, this will help to combat chemoresistance and improve clinical outcomes in BC patients. This chapter will summarize factors leading to chemoresistance, mechanisms of resistance to CT agents, challenges in combating chemoresistance in BC treatment, strategies to combat chemoresistance in BC treatment, identification of predictive biomarkers, advances in CT drug development, and lastly, strategies to sensitize resistant BC tumors to CT.

Mechanisms of Chemotherapy Resistance in Breast Cancer

Some of the mechanisms involved in chemoresistance in BC include the modulation of immune, macrophage, and other immune and inflammatory cells linked to cancer, the heterogeneity of cancer cells, and interactions between cancer cells and the tumor microenvironment in addition to the wide range of CT regimens with various monochemotherapy and polychemotherapy. Furthermore, chemoresistance is linked to other intrinsic factors such as pH, paracrine signaling, hypoxia, and the tumor microenvironment as well as the existence of other cancer cell clones within the tumors (Nikolaou et al., 2018; Mansoori et al., 2017). The mechanisms underlying CT resistance in BC include epithelial-mesenchymal transitions (EMT), cancer stem cells, transport proteins, cell membrane drug absorption, transport, efflux, alterations of specific cancer-associated genes (oncogenes and tumor-suppressor genes), and alterations in DNA damage repair (Fig. 6.2) (Nikolaou et al., 2018; Ji et al., 2019).

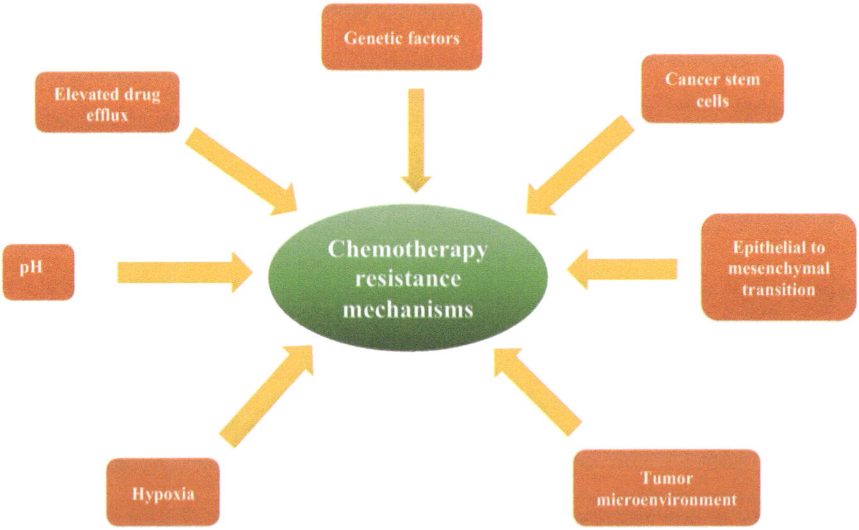

Fig. 6.2 *A schematic diagram showing several mechanisms of chemoresistance in breast cancer.* These include genetic factors, cancer stem cells, elevated drug efflux, etc

Genetic Factors Influencing Chemoresistance in Breast Cancer

Multidrug Resistance Gene (*MDR1*)

The multidrug resistance gene (*MDR1*) plays a crucial role in the chemoresistance of BC (Gao et al., 2013b). The ATP-binding cassette (ABC)-containing drug efflux transporter P-glycoprotein (Pg-p), which is encoded by *MDR1*, is crucial for controlling intracellular drug concentrations that affect a cell's sensitivity to chemotherapeutic treatments. Elevated levels of MDRP1/P-gp in breast cancer are associated with chemoresistance through which intracellular drug contents reduce to sublethal levels (Kuo, 2007). MDR1 encodes an anti-apoptotic gene, p53, which contributes to chemotherapy resistance by resisting chemotherapy-mediated apoptosis (Li et al., 2017b). Another protein encoded by MRD1 which is linked to chemoresistance is GST-π (Gao et al., 2013a). Increased activity of GST-π results in reduced efficacy of anti-cancer drugs and promotes their efflux in cells (Ściskalska & Milnerowicz, 2020).

Twist-Related Protein 1 Gene (*TWIST1*)

Twist-related protein 1 gene (*TWIST1*) encodes for a transcription factor (TF) called Twist 1. Twist 1 controls EMT, a process by which cells acquire mesenchymal characteristics (vimentin and N-cadherin) while losing epithelial characteristics (E-cadherin) (Fig. 6.3) (Kang & Massagué, 2004). Upregulation of Twist 1 promotes invasion and metastasis of BC cells through recognizing and attaching to E-box sequence on the promoter regions of E-cadherin, resulting in repression of E-cadherin transcription, thus promoting an invasive, migratory BC tumor which facilitates chemoresistance (Lo et al., 2007). Furthermore, research has shown that NF-κB elevates *TWIST1* expression, to promote chemoresistance (Pham et al., 2007). *TWIST1* overexpression has also been associated with hormone resistance in BC tumors via downregulation of ER-α activity (Vesuna et al., 2012).

Epigenetic Factors Influencing Chemoresistance

One of the first-line treatments for ER-positive BC is endocrine therapy (ET), as it is expressed in 2/3 of patients (Magnani et al., 2012). ET was successfully utilized in luminal BC patients where it elevated overall survival (OS) (Fontes-Sousa et al., 2019). However, cancer can develop resistance to ET and in some cases, patients can undergo tumor recurrence (Fontes-Sousa et al., 2019). Notably, epigenetic machinery is involved in the mechanisms that induce ET resistance. For example, ESR1-promoter hypermethylation in ER-positive cell lines has been linked with ER downregulation and ET resistance (Stone et al., 2015; Achinger-Kawecka et al., 2020). Additionally, progesterone receptor (PR) expression may be directly

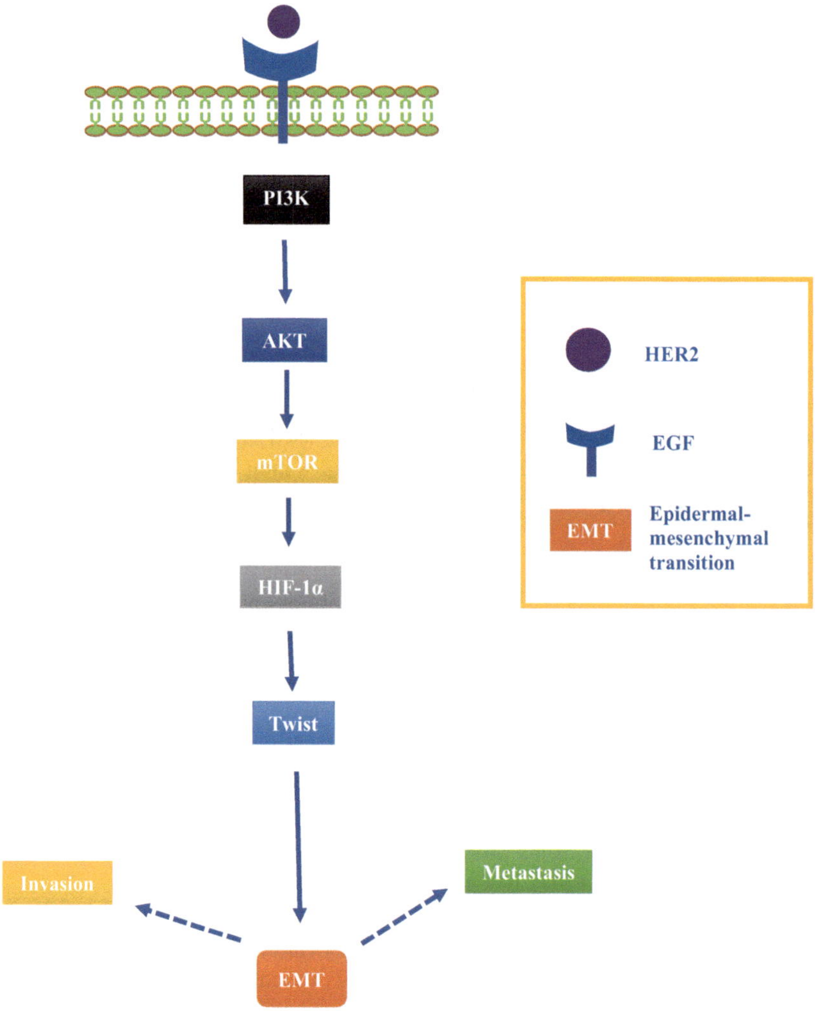

Fig. 6.3 *A schematic diagram showing the PI3K pathway and the involvement of Twist in EMT activation which results in invasion and metastasis of BC tumor*. HER2 human epidermal growth factor receptor 2, PI3K phosphatidylinositol 3-kinase, EGFR epidermal growth factor receptor, mTOR mammalian target of rapamycin, Akt Ser/Thr kinase, HIF-1α hypoxia-inducible factor-1α, EMT mesenchymal transition

impacted by transcriptional ER regulation. Notably, ER-positive sections of the tumor also express PR (Lustberg & Ramaswamy, 2009). The first exon of the PR gene contains a CpG island, and approximately 40% of PR-negative BC cases are linked with hypermethylation of the PR-promoter (Lapidus et al., 1996). The activation of PR expression in a hormone cell-free BC cell results in a decrease in the expression of ESR1, which is associated with hypermethylation of the ESR1 promoter, according to a study using BC cell line models (Verde et al., 2018). These results imply that methylation may regulate PR and ER in human BC cell lines and that methylation may facilitate gene-cross regulation. Therefore, novel therapeutic interventions aimed at epigenetic modifications might be linked with hormone-negative BC patients (Lainetti et al., 2020).

Fibroblast growth factor receptor 1 (FGFR1) has been associated with BC cell proliferation, development, migration, and survival (Drago et al., 2019). Additionally, it is known that FGFR1 is a prognostic factor that lowers patient survival in hormone receptor (HR)-positive tumors and induces estrogen resistance. The amplification of *FGFR1* is associated with resistance to inhibitors of PI3K, CDL4/6, and ER thus, rendering resistance to various drug therapies (Drago et al., 2019). In triple-negative cancers, higher *FGFR1* expression has also been linked to worse OS and prognosis, and it is a crucial gene for tumor cell survival. A second fibroblast growth factor, FGF2, has been associated with the chemoresistance of triple-negative breast cancer (TNBC) patients. The overexpression of FGF-2 assists in radiotherapy resistance and metastasis induction (Li et al., 2015). Additionally, FGF-2 overexpression also assists in the modulation of cell cycle and cell survival. Furthermore, it was shown that subpopulations of chemoresistant cells overexpressed FGF2, which decreased prognosis and also triggered metastases (Li et al., 2015). Furthermore, the cell death and sensitivity to CT of chemically resistant cells increased when these cells were treated and downregulated (Hu et al., 2016). *Mitogen-activated protein kinase 8* (*MAPK8*) also called *c-Jun N-terminal kinase 1* (*JNK1*) has been linked with cancer cell survival through regulation of autophagy via B-cell lymphoma-2 (BCL-2) phosphorylation (Wu et al., 2019). Furthermore, *JNK1* has been linked to chemoresistance in cancer cells. The expression of *JNK1* sensitizes P-glycoprotein overexpression, resulting in resistance to doxorubicin which is a chemotherapeutic drug used to treat various cancers including BC, Kaposi's sarcoma, and bladder cancer, among others. Lastly, blockage of MAPK or JNK pathway has been reported to decrease breast cancer resistance protein (ABCG2) transporter expression and also results in tumor cell autophagy (Wu et al., 2019; Xiang et al., 2020).

MicroRNAs

MicroRNAs (miRNAs) have been reported to be involved in the modulation of the sensitivity of BC cells to CT. Notably, miR-326 and miR-451 were shown to mediate the downregulation of the expression of *MRP1* and *MDR1* genes, respectively. This downregulation led to the upregulation of the sensitivity of MCF-7 cells to doxorubicin (Kovalchuk et al., 2008; Liang et al., 2010). On the other hand, some miRNAs can induce BC cells to proliferate without estrogen and also develop resistance toward ET via downregulation of ER-α expression (Levin, 2014). For example, miR-873, Let-7b/Let-7i (Muluhngwi & Klinge, 2015), miR-221/222, and miR-342-3p (He et al., 2013) induced resistance to tamoxifen via p27Kip1 and ER-α inhibition. Furthermore, miRNA also modulates ER-α posttranslational modification to elevate ET resistance (Muluhngwi & Klinge, 2015). miRNA-129-5p can inhibit ATP-binding cassette subfamily B member 1 (ABCB1) from being involved in MDR reversal (Luan et al., 2016). miR-200c has been reported to restore the chemosensitivity of cancer cells toward paclitaxel through *ZEB1*, *ZEB2*, and *TUBB3* gene suppression (Cochrane et al., 2009). MiR-125b has been shown to render chemoresistance to paclitaxel by suppressing Bcl-2 antagonist killer 1 (Bak1) (Zhou et al., 2010). Lastly, miR-218 targets *BRCA1*, thereby regulating cisplatin chemosensitivity in BC (He et al., 2015).

Cancer Stem Cells and Their Contribution to Treatment Resistance

Studies have demonstrated that a population of cells with stem cell characteristics induces BC carcinogenesis. This population of oncogenic cells is called cancer stem cells (CSCs). Besides facilitating tumor formation and progression, CSCs also enable tumor progression, metastasis, and acquisition of the chemoresistant phenotype (Fig. 6.4; Yang et al., 2017; Dittmer, 2018). Previous studies have demonstrated that the ATP-binding cassette (ABC) transporters ABCC, ABCG, ABCB, and Pg-p are all overexpressed in BC CSCs (Ji et al., 2019; Palomeras et al., 2018). These transporters can assist BC CSCs in pumping out CT agents and also elevate crucial processes that are involved in tumor progression such as cell migration, invasion, and EMT (Das et al., 2019; Nassar et al., 2020). Furthermore, overexpression of ALDH1, ABCG2, CD10, CD24, CD133, CD44, GPR77, and EpCAM which are BC CSC surface biomarkers, are key inducers of chemoresistance in BC CSC (Ji et al., 2019). GPR77 and CD10 cell-surface markers were reported to promote the formation of tumors and chemoresistance through the provision of a BC CSC

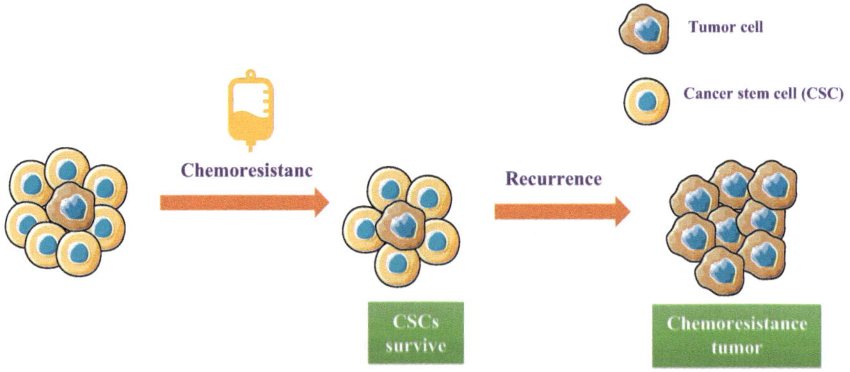

Fig. 6.4 *A schematic diagram of CSCs and their role in resistance to CT.* Besides enabling tumorigenesis, CSCs also induce tumor metastasis and chemoresistance. Moreover, CSCs that survive chemotherapy attain chemoresistance thereby enhancing crucial processes involved in carcinogenesis. *CSCs* Cancer stem cells, *CT* Chemotherapy. (Created in BioRender.com)

survival niche (Su et al., 2018). Furthermore, a high ratio of CD44/CD24 and ALDH1+ was reported to be unaltered during metastasis (Li et al., 2017a). These findings provide evidence that these BC CSC biomarkers have the potential to monitor cancer progression, metastasis, and therapeutics, and can be used in clinical therapeutics (Cao et al., 2021).

Epithelial to Mesenchymal Transition (EMT)

Polarized epithelial cells are transformed into mesenchymal cells by a process known as EMT. These cells have elevated migration, extracellular matrix component production, and metastasis capabilities (Kalluri & Weinberg, 2009). EMT involves the induction of numerous signaling and transcription factors (Kokudo et al., 2008). BC CSCs bearing various phenotypes such as CD44+/CD24−/low have been reported to show EMT attributes (Mani et al., 2008). According to Liu and colleagues, BC CSCs with the CD44+/CD24/low phenotype isolated primary human breast cells showed enhanced expression of the EMT markers zinc finger E-box binding homeobox 1 (ZEB1), matrix metalloproteinase 1, and vimentin (Liu et al., 2014). The notch pathway is recognized as the regulator of EMT in BC. Induction of the notch pathway results in the phosphatidylinositol 3-kinase/protein kinase B pathway expression. This pathway is central to cell growth and proliferation, and it does this by mediating NF-κB transcriptional activity (Li et al., 2016). Additionally, through influencing downstream effectors such as VEGF, MMP-9, survivin, and cyclin D1, NF-B induces EMT (Cohen et al., 2010; Li et al., 2014). The ability of epithelial cells to metastasize when exposed to NF-κB inhibitors is reduced, highlighting the significance of NF-B in EMT (Huber et al., 2004).

Tumor cells often release cytokines that are central to EMT regulation. Epithelial cell irradiation results in the synthesis of interleukin-6 which induces JAK/STAT pathway activation. In return, different downstream effectors such as Notch2, Jagged1, and DLL4 become expressed resulting in EMT induction (Kim et al., 2016). Tumor necrosis factor-α (TNFα), one of the inflammatory cytokines, mediates tumor metastasis and induces EMT in BC cells by activating Twist1 expression (Li et al., 2012). Transforming growth factor-β (TGF β) is commonly linked with the initiation of EMT in BC.

Hypoxia induces the expression of HEY1 and HES1 effectors through Notch20 activation to reduce E-cadherin expression and induce EMT (Chen et al., 2010). Moreover, hypoxia also has an effect on cadherin expression to induce EMT through cyclooxygenase-2 expression (Bocca et al., 2014). miRNAs also play a crucial role in the modulation of EMT in BC. Downregulation of miRNA-190a in BC tissues has been reported to promote metastasis and EMT (Yu et al., 2018). Notably, the upregulation of miRNA-27a was reported to promote EMT in BC cells by affecting the WD repeat domain containing 7 and F-box expression (Gao et al., 2019).

Tumor Microenvironment and Chemoresistance

The tumor microenvironment (TME) comprises numerous proteins, including growth factors, cytokines, the extracellular matrix, and several cells with varying genotypes and phenotypes, corroborating the heterogeneity of the tumor. The TME is also composed of an extensive number of blood vessels that feed the tumor with nutrition and oxygen. Studies have shown that TME plays a role in the response of tumors to CT (Nikolaou et al., 2018; Mansoori et al., 2017; Ji et al., 2019). As tumors proliferate, vast usage of energy and nutrients is evident and the alteration of the TME such as hypoxia and acidity accompanies tumor proliferation (Yeldag et al., 2018). Insufficient oxygen is linked with chemoresistance activation genes which result in the proliferation of cells that are resistant to hypoxia (Nikolaou et al., 2018). Therefore, hypoxia affects the efficacy of CT drugs. Similarly, reduced TME pH results in tumor resistance, cell proliferation, metastasis, and reduced efficacy of antitumor drugs. The acidic environment impairs the transportation of antitumor drugs. However, in an alkaline TME, the cytotoxicity of antitumor drugs increases (Nikolaou et al., 2018). Thus, hypoxia renders the TME more acidic, thereby inducing cell resistance to CT drugs (Nedeljković & Damjanović, 2019).

Tumor Hypoxia

Hypoxia serves as the major barrier in cancer treatment and occurs in proliferating tumors. As breast tumors grow, they tend to develop hypoxia, which triggers metabolic adaptation by increasing tumor glycolysis resulting in an aggressive tumor. Studies have shown that hypoxia can render chemotherapeutic drugs ineffective through the increase of metabolic enzyme expression (Shannon et al., 2003). Tsuruo and colleagues reported that hypoxia-induced chemoresistance in cancer cells by decreasing topoisomerase II (Topo II) expression (Tsuruo et al., 2003). Moreover, hypoxia-induced upregulation of MRP expression is another mechanism of chemoresistance. Studies have also shown that chemoresistant cancer cells can restore chemotherapy sensitivity by mediating glycolysis pathway inhibition in anoxic environment (Xu et al., 2005). A heterodimer called hypoxia-inducible factor-1 (HIF-1) is present in both humans and mammals in hypoxic environments. HIF-1 comprises two subunits, namely HIF-1α and HIF-1β. HIF-1α is particularly vulnerable to oxygen concentration and is susceptible to degradation in hyperoxic environments. As such, HIF-1α is the one that determines HIF-1 activity. P-gp is encoded by the *MDR1* gene which is a type of hypoxia-responsive gene. Moreover, HIF-1 can modulate P-gp expression through binding to hypoxia response elements (HRE) found on MDR1 (KM, 2002). Studies have reported that HIF-1/HIF-2 can bind with HRE on the promoter of breast cancer resistance protein (BCRP) and induce its overexpression (Vannini et al., 2008; Martin et al., 2008).

Tumor Tissue pH

The modification of pH contributes to tumor cell proliferation, metastasis, as well as chemoresistance. This occurs through elevation of tumor migratory and invasive attributes (Estrella et al., 2013; Daniel et al., 2013). Proton pumps, for example, (H+)-vacuolar-ATPase (V-ATPase), play a crucial role in promoting modification of the tumor cell pH. Moreover, V-ATPase can promote the pumping of H+ into the lumen of acidic vacuoles and/or into the extracellular space (Qi et al., 2007). Studies have shown that the expression of this proton pump is elevated in many cancers (Sun-Wada & Wada, 2013; Fogarty et al., 2014). TM9SF4 is a novel V-ATPase-activating protein that was reported to be involved in abnormal constitutive V-ATPase activation and also in the development of cancer cells bearing malignant phenotype (Lozupone et al., 2015).

Chemotherapy Agent and Chemoresistance

Elevated Drug Efflux As a Resistance Mechanism

Drug resistance to CT drugs is mainly driven by lower drug accumulation, which is brought about by increased efflux of CT drugs from tumor cells (Alfarouk et al., 2015; Krishna Vadlapatla et al., 2013; Wu et al., 2014; Amawi et al., 2019). Efflux pumps, a kind of drug efflux transporters, are crucial for the development of MDR in cancer cells (Scarborough, 1995; Sharom, 1998; Ruth et al., 2001; Sharom, 2006). Efflux transporters fall under the ABC superfamily of transporters. With the help of ATP hydrolysis-generated energy, ABC transporters move solutes into and out of the cell membrane. In particular, ABCC1, ABCB1, and ABCG2 transporters have a role in the development of MDR to cancer chemotherapeutics (Schmitt & Tampé, 2002; Vasiliou et al., 2009; Ford & Beis, 2019).

Novel Strategies to Overcome Chemotherapy Resistance in Breast Cancer

Novel Drug Delivery Systems

ET is currently the main therapy for treating receptor-positive or hormone-responsive BC. However, conventional therapies for BC have many challenges, especially in the treatment of TNBC. These challenges comprise of development of chemoresistance, deficient intracellular transport within tumor cells, and poor solubility and bioavailability (Ji et al., 2019; Xia & Xu, 2015). Therefore, the development and exploration of novel drug delivery systems as alternative methods for treating BC is imperative (Cao et al., 2021). Nanocarriers such as nanoscale, liposomes, and nanoparticles have been reported to have benefits such as prolonged blood circulation, targeted drug release, superior biocompatibility, and enhanced synergies (Pérez-Herrero & Fernández-Medarde, 2015). Zhang and colleagues created a core-shell nanocarrier that was coated with cationic albumin. This nanocarrier was used to deliver docetaxel, a CT drug, and miRNA-34a into BC cells, simultaneously. The authors reported that these co-delivery nanocarriers enhanced tumor cargo accumulation inside the tumor and prolonged docetaxel blood circulation. Furthermore, it markedly inhibited tumor growth and metastasis, in vitro and in vivo (Zhang et al., 2017). Similarly, Bose and colleagues investigated a nanoplatform based on extracellular vesicles produced from tumor cells. This platform was utilized for phototherapy and multimodal miRNA delivery. The authors reported that this platform reduced doxorubicin resistance in BC cells and also showed a threefold increase in cell-killing capability compared to cells exposed to doxorubicin alone (Jc Bose et al., 2018). Gong and colleagues developed a nanoscale target-specific Exo that can be used to co-deliver chemotherapeutic drugs and cholesterol-modified miRNA to BC cells. The authors reported that this platform demonstrated enhanced anticancer efficacies without any adverse effects (Gong et al., 2019). The ability of macrophages to target tumor cells via extracellular vesicles as drug-delivery vehicles is another alternative method for combating chemoresistance (Cao et al., 2021). Haney and colleagues showed that extracellular vesicles loaded with drugs can target TNBC in vivo and abolish cancer growth (Haney et al., 2020). On the other hand, the feasibility of a liposomal drug delivery system for treating HER2/MDR double-positive BC cells was assessed. This system combines chemotherapy and bevacizumab. In this study, tumor size steadily decreased within 60 days in multidrug-resistant and HER2-positive BC cell mouse models (Tang et al., 2017). Nanomedicine assists in bringing significant advances in metastasis and chemoresistance in BC. Therefore, nanomedicine which combines anticancer-targeted therapy and multifunctional nanocarriers is a promising alternative treatment method for BC. Nanomedicine can also advance personalized medicine and help in overcoming chemoresistance in BC (Cao et al., 2021).

Exosome-Based Drug Delivery Systems

Exosome-based drug delivery systems have more advantages compared to conventional drug delivery systems, as they demonstrate high stability in the physiological systems. Since exosomes have a hydrophobic core, they can store water-soluble drugs and are also separated from the patient's cells. Therefore, exosomes do not have adverse immunological effects compared to polymers and liposomes. Exosomes have a high capacity to pass through different biological barriers since they are nano-sized and can also carry cell surface molecules. In addition, there is less possibility of exomes being picked up by the host immune system because they have a natural targeting ability. Exomes provide a more stable environment for chemotherapeutic drugs. Furthermore, they can change the conditions to increase cell-specific targeting. Lastly, exosomes can directly enter the targeted cell by interacting with plasma cells during CT (Ha et al., 2016). Studies have been carried out on the use of exosome-based drug delivery systems for BC treatment. Tian and colleagues showed that exosomes can be used to deliver chemotherapeutic drugs such as doxorubicin to tumor tissue in BALB/c nude mice resulting in the inhibition of tumorigenesis without any evidence of toxicity (Tian et al., 2014). Eskiler and colleagues investigated the effect of solid lipid nanoparticles (SLNs) loaded with tamoxifen (Tam) on MCF7 Tam-resistant BC cells (MCF7-TamR). The authors reported that Tam-SLNs increased Tam efficacy and reversed Tam resistance through apoptosis induction without harming the control cells, in vitro. The authors concluded that SLNs can potentially be used as a chemotherapeutic strategy to combat Tam-resistance in BC for clinical utilization (Eskiler et al., 2018).

Gene Therapy

There is growing interest in using gene therapy as a mechanism for treating chemoresistant BC through correcting aberrant genes and regulation of gene expression (Bottai et al., 2017). There is substantial evidence that MDR1 antisense oligonucleotides can decrease chemoresistance in tumor cells. Jekerle and colleagues demonstrated that double-stranded antisense oligonucleotides can inhibit P-gp protein expression more efficiently in contrast to single-stranded antisense oligonucleotides. The subsequent result is the amelioration of tumor sensitivity to CT (Jekerle et al., 2005). On the other hand, ribozymes can decrease pathogenic gene expression by attaching to the target RNA and catalyzing RNA splicing reactions. Notably, anti-mdr-1 ribozyme plasmid transfection into BC cell line MCF7/ADR can efficiently depress MDR gene expression and can persistently reverse its chemoresistance (Gao et al., 2006). RNA interference (RNAi) is a crucial posttranslational method for regulating gene expression. Therefore, RNAi-based interventions may play a significant role in targeted therapeutics for cancer treatment (Ozpolat et al., 2014). The siRNAs and short hairpin RNAs (shRNAs) function by matching to the target gene transcript and subsequently inhibiting protein translation. Kaszubiak and colleagues demonstrated that adenoviral-mediated delivery of anti-MDR1/P-gp shRNAs can reverse MDR by depressing MDR1/P-gp mRNA and protein expression (Kaszubiak et al., 2007). Besides therapeutic attributes, numerous genes can be utilized as potential biomarkers for BC diagnosis. For example, DNA (ctDNA) is a potential BC biomarker that can be utilized for predicting efficacy, monitoring chemoresistance, and prognostically evaluating ET (Liu et al., 2017). Studies reported that patterns of ctDNA gene mutation are unique between HR/HER2 subtypes in metastatic BC patients. Therefore, cDNA can be utilized for monitoring resistance to anti-HER2 treatment (Hu et al., 2018; Ma et al., 2016).

Combination Therapy

Combination treatment strategies may provide a more efficient solution for combating chemoresistance in BC, compared to a single-agent regimen (Cao et al., 2021). For instance, trastuzumab, abemaciclib, and fulvestrant regimens were reported to ameliorate prognosis and PFS in patients suffering from advanced BC (Tolaney et al., 2020). On the other hand, CDK4/6 and PI3Kα combined inhibition was reported to be synergistically efficacious against multiple TNBC models. It does this by inducing immunogenic cell death as well as increasing cell-cycle arrest, tumor immunogenicity, and apoptosis (Teo et al., 2017). In another study, a cohort of patients were exposed to Palbociclib between days 1 and 19 of a 28-day cycle. The patients were also alternating with paclitaxel every week. The authors reported that the Palbociclib and paclitaxel regimen was safe and feasible. Additionally, there was no toxicity observed in advanced BC patients in this study (Clark et al., 2019). On the other hand, the nab-paclitaxel and atezolizumab combination regimen was reported to enhance PFS in patients with metastatic TNBC (Schmid et al., 2018). Moreover, trastuzumab, capecitabine, and tucatinib combination were reported to ameliorate OS and PFS in patients with HER2-positive metastatic BC (Murthy et al., 2020). Therefore, immunotherapy emerges as an efficacious novel strategy for treating TNBC. Nevertheless, more research needs to be carried out to determine the safety and efficacy of these immunotherapies to determine the most efficacious combination regimens, specifically for TNBC treatment (Cao et al., 2021).

The Use of Immunotherapy

Immune Checkpoint Inhibitors (ICIs)

Immunotherapy is a treatment method that can potentially be used to treat multiple solid tumors. It does this by utilizing the immune system of the patient to target and remove neoplastic cells directly (Cao et al., 2021). Studies have shown that immune checkpoint inhibitors (ICIs) primarily target cytotoxic T lymphocyte-associated protein 4 (CTLA-4) and programmed cell death protein 1 (PD-1) in few patients with metastatic BC (Emens, 2018; Jia et al., 2017). PD-1 is an ICI expressed on the surfaces of the immune effector cells. The function of PD-1 is to restrict the T-cell effector function in the tissues. A study involving PD-L1-positive advanced TNBC was carried out to assess the antitumor activity and safety of a PD-1 inhibitor called pembrolizumab. The authors reported a median duration of response of 10.4 months. On the other hand, they reported a median progression-free survival (PFS) of 2.1 months (95% CI 2.0–2.2) and an OS median of 18.0 months (95% CI 12.9–23.0) (Adams et al., 2019). In another study, safety and clinical activity were linked with exposure to a single-agent atezolizumab in metastatic TNBC patients. Atezolizumab is an anti-programmed cell death ligand 1 (PD-L1) drug. The authors reported a median PFS of 1.4 months (95% CI, 1.3–1.6 months) and an OS median of

17.6 months (95% CI, 10.2 months and above). Based on these findings, PD-1 antagonists have controllable safety attributes and also harbor durable antitumor activity as a first-line therapeutic intervention for PD-L1-positive BC patients (Emens et al., 2019).

CTLA-4 is a T-cell inhibitory receptor expressed on activated CD4+ regulatory T cells and CD8+ T cells which express FOXP3 and CD25. Therefore, inhibitors of CTLA-4 mediate antitumor immunity by inhibiting FOXP3+ Treg cells, and this culminates in the extensive blocking of tumor cells (Rowshanravan et al., 2018). Two anti-CTLA-4 antibodies called tremelimumab and ipilimumab were administered in TNBC clinical trials (Wang et al., 2019). On the other hand, a CTLA-4 inhibitor and a nanoparticle-based mRNA vaccine were suggested as potential treatment strategies for TNBC (Liu et al., 2018). Lastly, Pai and colleagues created a dual variable domain immunoglobulin of anti-CTLA4 antibody that can assist in the depletion of tumor infiltration and not tissue-resident Tregs. In return, this preserves antitumor activities while also minimizing toxicity (Pai et al., 2019).

Cyclin-Dependent Kinase 4/6 Inhibitors

The cyclin D/cyclin-dependent kinases 4 and 6 (CDK4/6)-retinoblastoma pathway plays a crucial role in the proliferation of BC cells and healthy breast epithelium (Pernas et al., 2018). Regarding CDK4/6 inhibitors, abemaciclib is the most potent inhibitor and it also shows potential clinical activity in metastatic BC (Fig. 6.5). For instance, the safety and single-agent activity of abemaciclib were evaluated in HR^+/HER^- metastatic BC patients. The authors reported a 42.4% clinical benefit rate, a 19.7% objective response rate, 6.0 months of median PFS, and 17.7 months of OS. These findings confirmed that abemaciclib has a significant activity as a single antitumor agent (Dickler et al., 2017). Palbociclib is another CDK4/6 inhibitor that was reported to overcome intrinsic endocrine resistance in primary BC. Patients in a neoadjuvant phase II study with clinical stage II/III ER+/HER2 BC were involved in this study (Ma et al., 2017). Letrozole is an aromatase inhibitor administered in women with BC who have undergone menopause. Finn and colleagues evaluated the safety and efficacy of the combined administration of letrozole and palbociclib in women with ER+ advanced BC. The authors reported a significant extension of PFS compared to monotherapy in advanced BC patients (Finn et al., 2016).

Breast Cancer Stem Cell-Directed Therapy

There is substantial evidence implicating CSCs in cancer chemoresistance, metastasis, and recurrence (Cao et al., 2021). There are BC patients' clinical trials currently taking place for novel anti-BC CSCs drugs that target hedgehog, notch, and Wnt/Fizzled/β-catenin signaling pathways (Palomeras et al., 2018). Notch signaling inhibition using gamma-secretase inhibitors (GSIs) is the most clinically advanced

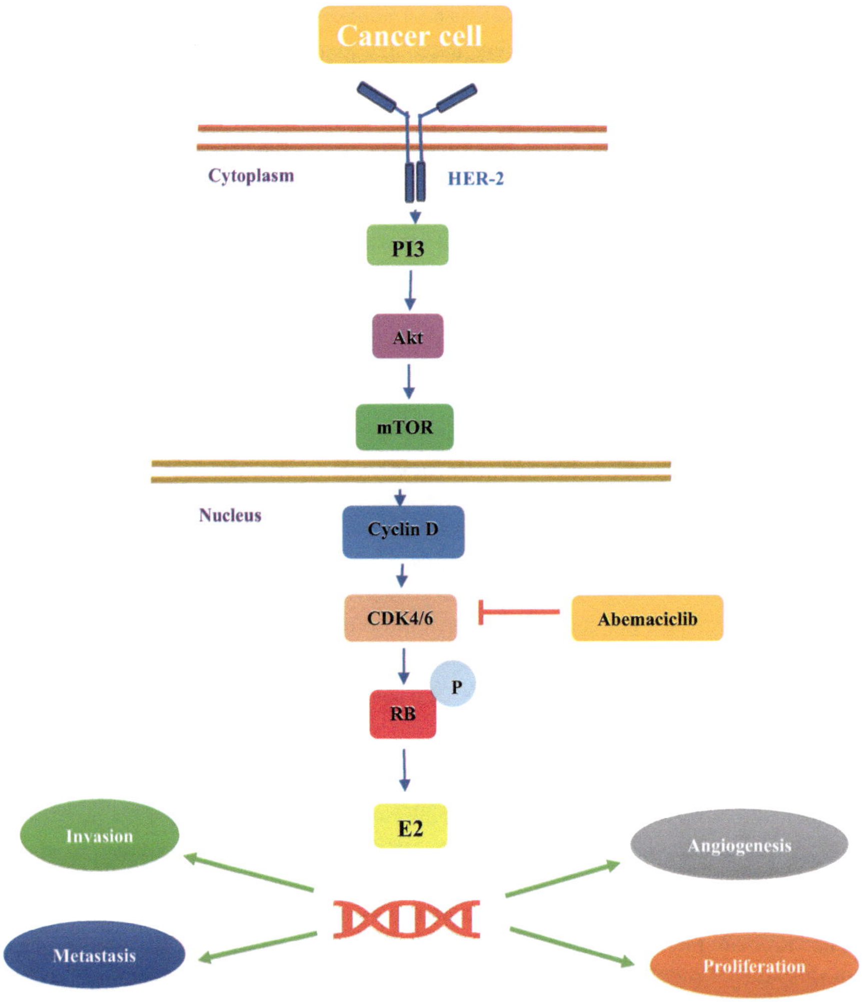

Fig. 6.5 *Mechanism of action of abemaciclib which is a CDK4/6 inhibitor used to treat metastatic BC.* The CDK4/6 signaling pathway is involved in BC metastasis, angiogenesis, invasion, and proliferation. Therefore, abemaciclib inhibits CDK4/6 consequently blocking these crucial processes involved in BC carcinogenesis. *BC* breast cancer, *HER2* human epidermal growth factor receptor 2, *CDK4/6* cyclin-dependent kinase 4/6, *PI3K* phosphatidylinositol 3-kinase, *Akt* Ser/Thr kinase, *mTOR* mammalian target of rapamycin, *RB* retinoblastoma

BC treatment approach. Studies have reported the inhibition of BC carcinogenesis in a process involving the induction of IL6. Therefore, this approach might be a novel treatment strategy for treating BC patients (Lehal et al., 2020; Wang et al., 2015). Other notch signaling inhibitors like CB-103 are currently in phase I/II clinical trials for the treatment of metastatic or advanced BC (Palomeras et al., 2018). The Wnt/Frizzled/b-catenin signaling pathway is overactivated in TNBC and several other cancer types. Wnt signaling inhibitors can eradicate chemoresistant CSCs and therefore, they can be used to combat chemoresistant to conventional CT (Krishnamurthy & Kurzrock, 2018). An anti-leprotic drug called clofazimine was reported to be efficacious against TNBC. It does this by distinctly inhibiting the canonical Wnt signaling (Ahmed et al., 2019). Hedgehog pathway inhibitors were tested in BC using both in vitro and in vivo experiments, but their effectiveness was not satisfactory (Bhateja et al., 2019). Overall, substantial evidence has shown that targeting CSCs in BC is a potentially efficacious approach for reversing chemoresistance both in vivo and in vitro (Cao et al., 2021). However, most clinical studies are still in the initial stages. Therefore, more research into clinically relevant biomarkers for BC treatment needs to be carried out to translate accumulated laboratory knowledge into clinical practice (Cao et al., 2021).

Autophagy Modulation

Autophagy is a constricted catabolic mechanism that mediates the recycling of nutrients from organelles and other cellular components. This process occurs via lysosomal degradation, and it also supplies energy and macromolecular precursors (Pérez-Hernández et al., 2019). There is substantial evidence indicating that autophagy modulates chemoresistance in patients with cancer in two ways: either by (1) elevating drug sensitivity or (2) mediating drug resistance (Levy et al., 2017; Liao et al., 2019). So far, hydroxychloroquine (HCQ) is the only autophagy inhibitor that is clinically approved and can increase tumor cell death either alone or in combination with targeted agents or cytotoxic CT (Levy et al., 2017; Liao et al., 2019). In 2014, Cook and colleagues showed that HCQ can increase responsiveness toward antiestrogen in ER-positive BC via autophagy inhibition. In the same study, tamoxifen demonstrated positive results for current neoadjuvant clinical trials (Cook et al., 2014). Nanomaterials can also regulate autophagy and thus, they have been utilized as therapeutic agents for cancer treatment (Cordani & Somoza, 2019). Autophagy has previously been reported as a potential method for overcoming chemoresistance in BC. However, the use of autophagy-linked kinase activators/inhibitors can result in uncontrolled side effects due to deficient organ specificity. Therefore, the utilization of these autophagy regulation agents in clinical settings requires further investigation (Cao et al., 2021).

Limitations of Exosome-Based Drug Delivery Systems

Exosomes have many advantages as vehicles for targeted drug delivery. However, they have several limitations that need to be addressed before they can be used in clinical settings (Allahverdiyev et al., 2018). Natural exosomes are complicated structures and this makes it difficult for pharmaceuticals to characterize them (Xu et al., 2016). Moreover, exosomes play a crucial role in diseases that are not yet fully elucidated. Furthermore, biological fluids carry different cell types from extracellular vesicles. Therefore, this makes it difficult to purify single cell-specific vesicular populations such as cancer cell-derived exosomes. Although exosome purification can be carried out from exosome-secreting cell lines, there are no exosomal signals and this can result in adverse immune responses. The mass synthesis of exosomes for medical use presents another obstacle (van der Meel et al., 2014). Rapid purification has been recommended as a method to circumvent this problem (Lamparski et al., 2002). However, this method still needs furthermore testing using various cell types. Therefore, it is critically important to understand the structure and functions of exosomes so that they can be optimized and applied in clinical settings as novel therapeutic mechanisms for cancer treatment (Luan et al., 2017).

Conclusion and Future Perspectives

Mechanisms underlying chemoresistance in BC are complex and thus, several factors need to be taken into consideration during therapeutic processes. These include cancer stage, cellular target, and tumor subtype, among others. The utilization of gene therapy and biologics is a highly active area of research into reversing chemoresistance. Significant advancements have been made in gene therapy as an approach to overcome chemoresistance in BC. Despite these advancements, many challenges remain to be solved such as gene expression controllability, target gene selection, and treatment dosage. Importantly, the efficacy of gene therapy and biologics is limited to animal models and in vitro experimental studies. Therefore, a broader research spectrum is still needed before results can be translated into clinical evidence. Novel drug delivery systems are prospective strategies for combination treatment, and they have a wide range of antitumor agents. These include chemotherapeutic drugs and nucleic acid. Novel drug delivery systems such as nanocarriers can specifically deliver chemotherapeutic drugs into the targeted tumors. In addition, the rate of drug release in these systems is controllable and they also serve as a potential approach for improving the efficacy of the already existing chemotherapeutic drugs (Ji et al., 2019).

The discovery of ICIs provided novel and effective treatments for chemoresistant tumors. Nevertheless, the main challenge with immunotherapies is the progression into secondary or acquired chemoresistance. Therefore, extensive research into various underlying chemoresistance mechanisms needs to be conducted. The possible chemoresistance mechanisms include deficient expression of tumor antigens on cancer cells or failure of T-cells to recognize cancer cells because of the absence of high-affinity T-cell receptors (Jenkins et al., 2018; Gajewski et al., 2013). In addition, alteration or silencing of some of the signal transduction pathways in some tumor cells can promote chemoresistance. Lastly, a single immunotherapy approach may be inadequate due to low responses, and thus, combination immunotherapy is more efficacious. A substantial number of novel agents for BC treatment have been developed. However, there are limited options for novel agents that are truly efficacious and with fewer adverse effects. Combination immunotherapy that targets a vast array of pathways is efficacious since there are several underlying mechanisms mediating chemoresistance in BC. Therefore, combination immunotherapy results in higher synergisms and effectiveness of the treatment. Notably, individualized administration strategies can potentially combat chemoresistance in BC. Yet, modes of drug-to-drug interaction and high toxicity are key challenges in combination immunotherapy. Therefore, more research needs to be carried out to optimize therapeutic combination approaches as they are a promising therapeutic solution to chemoresistance, recurrence, and relapse in BC (Ji et al., 2019).

References

Achinger-Kawecka, J., Valdes-Mora, F., Luu, P.-L., Giles, K. A., Caldon, C. E., Qu, W., et al. (2020). Epigenetic reprogramming at estrogen-receptor binding sites alters the 3D chromatin landscape in endocrine-resistant breast cancer. *Nature Communications, 11*, 320.

Adams, S., Loi, S., Toppmeyer, D., Cescon, D., De Laurentiis, M., Nanda, R., et al. (2019). Pembrolizumab monotherapy for previously untreated, PD-L1-positive, metastatic triple-negative breast cancer: Cohort B of the phase II KEYNOTE-086 study. *Annals of Oncology, 30*, 405–411.

Ahmed, K., Koval, A., Xu, J., Bodmer, A., & Katanaev, V. L. (2019). Towards the first targeted therapy for triple-negative breast cancer: Repositioning of clofazimine as a chemotherapy-compatible selective Wnt pathway inhibitor. *Cancer Letters, 449*, 45–55.

Alfarouk, K. O., Stock, C.-M., Taylor, S., Walsh, M., Muddathir, A. K., Verduzco, D., et al. (2015). Resistance to cancer chemotherapy: Failure in drug response from ADME to P-gp. *Cancer Cell International, 15*, 1–13.

Allahverdiyev, A. M., Parlar, E., Dinparvar, S., Bagirova, M., & Abamor, E. Ş. (2018). Current aspects in treatment of breast cancer based of nanodrug delivery systems and future prospects. *Artificial Cells, Nanomedicine, and Biotechnology, 46*, 755–762.

Amawi, H., Sim, H.-M., Tiwari, A. K., Ambudkar, S. V., & Shukla, S. (2019). ABC transporter-mediated multidrug-resistant cancer. *Drug Transporters in Drug Disposition, Effects and Toxicity, 1141*, 549–580.

Bhateja, P., Cherian, M., Majumder, S., & Ramaswamy, B. (2019). The hedgehog signaling pathway: A viable target in breast cancer? *Cancers, 11*, 1126.

Blows, F. M., Driver, K. E., Schmidt, M. K., Broeks, A., van Leeuwen, F. E., Wesseling, J., et al. (2010). Subtyping of breast cancer by immunohistochemistry to investigate a relationship between subtype and short and long term survival: A collaborative analysis of data for 10,159 cases from 12 studies. *PLoS Medicine, 7*, e1000279.

Bocca, C., Ievolella, M., Autelli, R., Motta, M., Mosso, L., Torchio, B., et al. (2014). Expression of Cox-2 in human breast cancer cells as a critical determinant of epithelial-to-mesenchymal transition and invasiveness. *Expert Opinion on Therapeutic Targets, 18*, 121–135.

Bottai, G., Truffi, M., Corsi, F., & Santarpia, L. (2017). Progress in nonviral gene therapy for breast cancer and what comes next? *Expert Opinion on Biological Therapy, 17*, 595–611.

Cao, J., Zhang, M., Wang, B., Zhang, L., Zhou, F., & Fang, M. (2021). Chemoresistance and metastasis in breast cancer molecular mechanisms and novel clinical strategies. *Frontiers in Oncology, 11*, 658552.

Cardoso, F., Kyriakides, S., Ohno, S., Penault-Llorca, F., Poortmans, P., Rubio, I., et al. (2019). Early breast cancer: ESMO clinical practice guidelines for diagnosis, treatment and follow-up. *Annals of Oncology, 30*, 1194–1220.

Chen, J., Imanaka, N., & Griffin, J. D. (2010). Hypoxia potentiates notch signaling in breast cancer leading to decreased E-cadherin expression and increased cell migration and invasion. *British Journal of Cancer, 102*, 351–360.

Clark, A. S., Mcandrew, N. P., Troxel, A., Feldman, M., Lal, P., Rosen, M., et al. (2019). Combination paclitaxel and palbociclib: Results of a phase I trial in advanced breast cancer. *Clinical Cancer Research, 25*, 2072–2079.

Cochrane, D. R., Spoelstra, N. S., Howe, E. N., Nordeen, S. K., & Richer, J. K. (2009). MicroRNA-200c mitigates invasiveness and restores sensitivity to microtubule-targeting chemotherapeutic agents. *Molecular Cancer Therapeutics, 8*, 1055–1066.

Cohen, B., Shimizu, M., Izrailit, J., Ng, N. F., Buchman, Y., Pan, J. G., et al. (2010). Cyclin D1 is a direct target of JAG1-mediated notch signaling in breast cancer. *Breast Cancer Research and Treatment, 123*, 113–124.

Cook, K. L., Wärri, A., Soto-Pantoja, D. R., Clarke, P. A., Cruz, M. I., Zwart, A., et al. (2014). Chloroquine inhibits autophagy to potentiate antiestrogen responsiveness in ER+ breast cancer. *Clinical Cancer Research, 20*, 3222–3232.

Cordani, M., & Somoza, Á. (2019). Targeting autophagy using metallic nanoparticles: A promising strategy for cancer treatment. *Cellular and Molecular Life Sciences, 76*, 1215–1242.

Daniel, C., Bell, C., Burton, C., Harguindey, S., Reshkin, S. J., & Rauch, C. (2013). The role of proton dynamics in the development and maintenance of multidrug resistance in cancer. *Biochimica et Biophysica Acta (BBA)-Molecular Basis of Disease, 1832*, 606–617.

Das, S., Mukherjee, P., Chatterjee, R., Jamal, Z., & Chatterji, U. (2019). Enhancing chemosensitivity of breast cancer stem cells by downregulating SOX2 and ABCG2 using wedelolactone-encapsulated nanoparticles. *Molecular Cancer Therapeutics, 18*, 680–692.

Dickler, M. N., Tolaney, S. M., Rugo, H. S., Cortés, J., Diéras, V., Patt, D., et al. (2017). MONARCH 1, a phase II study of abemaciclib, a CDK4 and CDK6 inhibitor, as a single agent, in patients with refractory HR+/HER2− metastatic breast cancer. *Clinical Cancer Research, 23*, 5218–5224.

Dittmer, J. (2018). *Breast cancer stem cells: Features, key drivers and treatment options. Seminars in cancer biology* (pp. 59–74). Elsevier.

Drago, J. Z., Formisano, L., Juric, D., Niemierko, A., Servetto, A., Wander, S. A., et al. (2019). FGFR1 amplification mediates endocrine resistance but retains TORC sensitivity in metastatic hormone receptor–positive (HR+) breast cancer. *Clinical Cancer Research, 25*, 6443–6451.

Emens, L. A. (2018). Breast cancer immunotherapy: Facts and hopes. *Clinical Cancer Research, 24*, 511–520.

Emens, L. A., Cruz, C., Eder, J. P., Braiteh, F., Chung, C., Tolaney, S. M., et al. (2019). Long-term clinical outcomes and biomarker analyses of atezolizumab therapy for patients with metastatic triple-negative breast cancer: A phase 1 study. *JAMA Oncology, 5*, 74–82.

Eskiler, G. G., Cecener, G., Dikmen, G., Egeli, U., & Tunca, B. (2018). Solid lipid nanoparticles: Reversal of tamoxifen resistance in breast cancer. *European Journal of Pharmaceutical Sciences, 120*, 73–88.

Estrella, V., Chen, T., Lloyd, M., Wojtkowiak, J., Cornnell, H. H., Ibrahim-Hashim, A., et al. (2013). Acidity generated by the tumor microenvironment drives local invasion. *Cancer Research, 73*, 1524–1535.

Finn, R. S., Martin, M., Rugo, H. S., Jones, S., Im, S.-A., Gelmon, K., et al. (2016). Palbociclib and letrozole in advanced breast cancer. *New England Journal of Medicine, 375*, 1925–1936.

Fogarty, F., O'keeffe, J., Zhadanov, A., Papkovsky, D., Ayllon, V., & O'connor, R. (2014). HRG-1 enhances cancer cell invasive potential and couples glucose metabolism to cytosolic/extracellular pH gradient regulation by the vacuolar-H+ ATPase. *Oncogene, 33*, 4653–4663.

Fontes-Sousa, M., Amorim, M., Salta, S., Palma De Sousa, S., Henrique, R., & Jerónimo, C. (2019). Predicting resistance to endocrine therapy in breast cancer: It's time for epigenetic biomarkers. *Oncology Reports, 41*, 1431–1438.

Ford, R. C., & Beis, K. (2019). Learning the ABCs one at a time: Structure and mechanism of ABC transporters. *Biochemical Society Transactions, 47*, 23–36.

Fragomeni, S. M., Sciallis, A., & Jeruss, J. S. (2018). Molecular subtypes and local-regional control of breast cancer. *Surgical Oncology Clinics, 27*, 95–120.

Gajewski, T. F., Schreiber, H., & Fu, Y.-X. (2013). Innate and adaptive immune cells in the tumor microenvironment. *Nature Immunology, 14*, 1014–1022.

Gao, P., Zhou, G., Zhang, Q., Li, H., Mu, K., Yuan, Y., et al. (2006). Reversal MDR in breast carcinoma cells by transfection of ribozyme designed according the secondary structure of mdr1 mRNA. *Chinese Journal of Physiology, 49*, 96.

Gao, A.-M., Ke, Z.-P., Shi, F., Sun, G.-C., & Chen, H. (2013a). Chrysin enhances sensitivity of BEL-7402/ADM cells to doxorubicin by suppressing PI3K/Akt/Nrf2 and ERK/Nrf2 pathway. *Chemico-Biological Interactions, 206*, 100–108.

Gao, L., Yang, Y., Song, S., Hong, H., Zhao, X., & Li, D. (2013b). The association between genetic variant of MDR1 gene and breast cancer risk factors in Chinese women. *International Immunopharmacology, 17*, 88–91.

Gao, D., Qi, X., Zhang, X., Fang, K., Guo, Z., & Li, L. (2019). hsa_circRNA_0006528 as a competing endogenous RNA promotes human breast cancer progression by sponging miR-7-5p and activating the MAPK/ERK signaling pathway. *Molecular Carcinogenesis, 58*, 554–564.

Giuliano, A. E., Connolly, J. L., Edge, S. B., Mittendorf, E. A., Rugo, H. S., Solin, L. J., et al. (2017). Breast cancer—Major changes in the American joint committee on cancer eighth edition cancer staging manual. *CA: a Cancer Journal for Clinicians, 67*, 290–303.

Gong, C., Tian, J., Wang, Z., Gao, Y., Wu, X., Ding, X., et al. (2019). Functional exosome-mediated co-delivery of doxorubicin and hydrophobically modified microRNA 159 for triple-negative breast cancer therapy. *Journal of Nanobiotechnology, 17*, 1–18.

Gottesman, M. M. (2002). Mechanisms of cancer drug resistance. *Annual Review of Medicine, 53*, 615–627.

Ha, D., Yang, N., & Nadithe, V. (2016). Exosomes as therapeutic drug carriers and delivery vehicles across biological membranes: Current perspectives and future challenges. *Acta Pharmaceutica Sinica B, 6*, 287–296.

Haney, M. J., Zhao, Y., Jin, Y. S., Li, S. M., Bago, J. R., Klyachko, N. L., et al. (2020). Macrophage-derived extracellular vesicles as drug delivery systems for triple negative breast cancer (TNBC) therapy. *Journal of Neuroimmune Pharmacology, 15*, 487–500.

Harbeck, N., Penault-Llorca, F., Cortes, J., Gnant, M., Houssami, N., Poortmans, P., et al. (2019). Breast cancer. *Nature Reviews. Disease Primers, 5*, 66.

He, Y. J., Wu, J. Z., Ji, M. H., Ma, T., Qiao, E. Q., Ma, R., et al. (2013). miR-342 is associated with estrogen receptor-α expression and response to tamoxifen in breast cancer. *Experimental and Therapeutic Medicine, 5*, 813–818.

He, X., Xiao, X., Dong, L., Wan, N., Zhou, Z., Deng, H., et al. (2015). MiR-218 regulates cisplatin chemosensitivity in breast cancer by targeting BRCA1. *Tumor Biology, 36*, 2065–2075.

Hu, Y., Qiu, Y., Yagüe, E., Ji, W., Liu, J., & Zhang, J. (2016). miRNA-205 targets VEGFA and FGF2 and regulates resistance to chemotherapeutics in breast cancer. *Cell Death & Disease, 7*, e2291–e2291.

Hu, Z.-Y., Xie, N., Tian, C., Yang, X., Liu, L., Li, J., et al. (2018). Identifying circulating tumor DNA mutation profiles in metastatic breast cancer patients with multiline resistance. *eBioMedicine, 32*, 111–118.

Huber, M. A., Azoitei, N., Baumann, B., Grünert, S., Sommer, A., Pehamberger, H., et al. (2004). NF-κB is essential for epithelial-mesenchymal transition and metastasis in a model of breast cancer progression. *The Journal of Clinical Investigation, 114*, 569–581.

Jc Bose, R., Uday Kumar, S., Zeng, Y., Afjei, R., Robinson, E., Lau, K., et al. (2018). Tumor cell-derived extracellular vesicle-coated nanocarriers: An efficient theranostic platform for the cancer-specific delivery of anti-miR-21 and imaging agents. *ACS Nano, 12*, 10817–10832.

Jekerle, V., Kassack, M. U., Reilly, R. M., & Piquette-Miller, M. W. M. (2005). Functional comparison of single-and double-stranded mdr1 antisense oligodeoxynucleotides in human ovarian cancer cell lines. *Therapy, 6*, 9–11.

Jenkins, R. W., Barbie, D. A., & Flaherty, K. T. (2018). Mechanisms of resistance to immune checkpoint inhibitors. *British Journal of Cancer, 118*, 9–16.

Ji, X., Lu, Y., Tian, H., Meng, X., Wei, M., & Cho, W. C. (2019). Chemoresistance mechanisms of breast cancer and their countermeasures. *Biomedicine & Pharmacotherapy, 114*, 108800.

Jia, H., Truica, C. I., Wang, B., Wang, Y., Ren, X., Harvey, H. A., et al. (2017). Immunotherapy for triple-negative breast cancer: Existing challenges and exciting prospects. *Drug Resistance Updates, 32*, 1–15.

Johnson, K. S., Conant, E. F., & Soo, M. S. (2021). Molecular subtypes of breast cancer: A review for breast radiologists. *Journal of Breast Imaging, 3*, 12–24.

Kalluri, R., & Weinberg, R. A. (2009). The basics of epithelial-mesenchymal transition. *The Journal of Clinical Investigation, 119*, 1420–1428.

Kang, Y., & Massagué, J. (2004). Epithelial-mesenchymal transitions: Twist in development and metastasis. *Cell, 118*, 277–279.

Kaszubiak, A., Holm, P. S., & Lage, H. (2007). Overcoming the classical multidrug resistance phenotype by adenoviral delivery of anti-MDR1 short hairpin RNAs and ribozymes. *International Journal of Oncology, 31*, 419–430.

Kim, R.-K., Kaushik, N., Suh, Y., Yoo, K.-C., Cui, Y.-H., Kim, M.-J., et al. (2016). Radiation driven epithelial-mesenchymal transition is mediated by notch signaling in breast cancer. *Oncotarget, 7*, 53430.

Km, C. (2002). Hypoxia-inducible factor-1-dependent regulation of the multidrug resistance (MDR1) gene. *Cancer Research, 62*, 3387–3394.

Kokudo, T., Suzuki, Y., Yoshimatsu, Y., Yamazaki, T., Watabe, T., & Miyazono, K. (2008). Snail is required for TGFβ-induced endothelial-mesenchymal transition of embryonic stem cell-derived endothelial cells. *Journal of Cell Science, 121*, 3317–3324.

Kovalchuk, O., Filkowski, J., Meservy, J., Ilnytskyy, Y., Tryndyak, V. P., Chekhun, V. F., et al. (2008). Involvement of microRNA-451 in resistance of the MCF-7 breast cancer cells to chemotherapeutic drug doxorubicin. *Molecular Cancer Therapeutics, 7*, 2152–2159.

Krishna Vadlapatla, R., Dutt Vadlapudi, A., Pal, D., & Kmitra, A. (2013). Mechanisms of drug resistance in cancer chemotherapy: Coordinated role and regulation of efflux transporters and metabolizing enzymes. *Current Pharmaceutical Design, 19*, 7126–7140.

Krishnamurthy, N., & Kurzrock, R. (2018). Targeting the Wnt/beta-catenin pathway in cancer: Update on effectors and inhibitors. *Cancer Treatment Reviews, 62*, 50–60.

Kuo, M. T. (2007). Roles of multidrug resistance genes in breast cancer chemoresistance. *Breast Cancer Chemosensitivity*, 23–30.

Lainetti, P. D. F., Leis-Filho, A. F., Laufer-Amorim, R., Battazza, A., & Fonseca-Alves, C. E. (2020). Mechanisms of resistance to chemotherapy in breast cancer and possible targets in drug delivery systems. *Pharmaceutics, 12*, 1193.

Lamparski, H. G., Metha-Damani, A., Yao, J.-Y., Patel, S., Hsu, D.-H., Ruegg, C., et al. (2002). Production and characterization of clinical grade exosomes derived from dendritic cells. *Journal of Immunological Methods, 270*, 211–226.

Lapidus, R. G., Ferguson, A. T., Ottaviano, Y. L., Parl, F. F., Smith, H. S., Weitzman, S. A., et al. (1996). Methylation of estrogen and progesterone receptor gene 5'CpG islands correlates with lack of estrogen and progesterone receptor gene expression in breast tumors. *Clinical Cancer Research: An Official Journal of the American Association for Cancer Research, 2*, 805–810.

Lehal, R., Zaric, J., Vigolo, M., Urech, C., Frismantas, V., Zangger, N., et al. (2020). Pharmacological disruption of the notch transcription factor complex. *Proceedings of the National Academy of Sciences, 117*, 16292–16301.

Levin, E. R. (2014). Extranuclear estrogen receptor's roles in physiology: Lessons from mouse models. *American Journal of Physiology-Endocrinology and Metabolism, 307*, E133–E140.

Levy, J. M. M., Towers, C. G., & Thorburn, A. (2017). Targeting autophagy in cancer. *Nature Reviews Cancer, 17*, 528–542.

Li, C.-W., Xia, W., Huo, L., Lim, S.-O., Wu, Y., Hsu, J. L., et al. (2012). Epithelial–mesenchymal transition induced by TNF-α requires NF-κB–mediated transcriptional upregulation of Twist1. *Cancer Research, 72*, 1290–1300.

Li, L., Zhao, F., Lu, J., Li, T., Yang, H., Wu, C., et al. (2014). Notch-1 signaling promotes the malignant features of human breast cancer through NF-κB activation. *PLoS One, 9*, e95912.

Li, S., Payne, S., Wang, F., Claus, P., Su, Z., Groth, J., et al. (2015). Nuclear basic fibroblast growth factor regulates triple-negative breast cancer chemo-resistance. *Breast Cancer Research, 17*, 1–16.

Li, L., Zhang, J., Xiong, N., Li, S., Chen, Y., Yang, H., et al. (2016). Notch-1 signaling activates NF-κB in human breast carcinoma MDA-MB-231 cells via PP2A-dependent AKT pathway. *Medical Oncology, 33*, 1–11.

Li, W., Ma, H., Zhang, J., Zhu, L., Wang, C., & Yang, Y. (2017a). Unraveling the roles of CD44/CD24 and ALDH1 as cancer stem cell markers in tumorigenesis and metastasis. *Scientific Reports, 7*, 13856.

Li, Z.-H., Weng, X., Xiong, Q.-Y., Tu, J.-H., Xiao, A., Qiu, W., et al. (2017b). miR-34a expression in human breast cancer is associated with drug resistance. *Oncotarget, 8*, 106270.

Liang, Z., Wu, H., Xia, J., Li, Y., Zhang, Y., Huang, K., et al. (2010). Involvement of miR-326 in chemotherapy resistance of breast cancer through modulating expression of multidrug resistance-associated protein 1. *Biochemical Pharmacology, 79*, 817–824.

Liao, Y. X., Yu, H. Y., Lv, J. Y., Cai, Y. R., Liu, F., He, Z. M., et al. (2019). Targeting autophagy is a promising therapeutic strategy to overcome chemoresistance and reduce metastasis in osteosarcoma. *International Journal of Oncology, 55*, 1213–1222.

Liu, S., Cong, Y., Wang, D., Sun, Y., Deng, L., Liu, Y., et al. (2014). Breast cancer stem cells transition between epithelial and mesenchymal states reflective of their normal counterparts. *Stem Cell Reports, 2*, 78–91.

Liu, B., Yang, Y., Yi, Z., Guan, X., & Ma, F. (2017). The application of estrogen receptor-1 mutations' detection through circulating tumor DNA in breast cancer. *Cancer Translational Medicine, 3*, 46–52.

Liu, L., Wang, Y., Miao, L., Liu, Q., Musetti, S., Li, J., et al. (2018). Combination immunotherapy of MUC1 mRNA nano-vaccine and CTLA-4 blockade effectively inhibits growth of triple negative breast cancer. *Molecular Therapy, 26*, 45–55.

Lo, H.-W., Hsu, S.-C., Xia, W., Cao, X., Shih, J.-Y., Wei, Y., et al. (2007). Epidermal growth factor receptor cooperates with signal transducer and activator of transcription 3 to induce epithelial-mesenchymal transition in cancer cells via up-regulation of TWIST gene expression. *Cancer Research, 67*, 9066–9076.

Lozupone, F., Borghi, M., Marzoli, F., Azzarito, T., Matarrese, P., Iessi, E., et al. (2015). TM9SF4 is a novel V-ATPase-interacting protein that modulates tumor pH alterations associated with drug resistance and invasiveness of colon cancer cells. *Oncogene, 34*, 5163–5174.

Luan, Q.-X., Zhang, B.-G., Li, X.-J., & Guo, M.-Y. (2016). MiR-129-5p is downregulated in breast cancer cells partly due to promoter H3K27m3 modification and regulates epithelial-mesenchymal transition and multi-drug resistance. *European Review for Medical & Pharmacological Sciences, 20*, 4257–4265.

Luan, X., Sansanaphongpricha, K., Myers, I., Chen, H., Yuan, H., & Sun, D. (2017). Engineering exosomes as refined biological nanoplatforms for drug delivery. *Acta Pharmacologica Sinica, 38*, 754–763.

Lustberg, M., & Ramaswamy, B. (2009). Epigenetic targeting in breast cancer: Therapeutic impact and future direction. *Drug News & Perspectives, 22*, 369.

Ma, F., Zhu, W., Guan, Y., Yang, L., Xia, X., Chen, S., et al. (2016). ctDNA dynamics: A novel indicator to track resistance in metastatic breast cancer treated with anti-HER2 therapy. *Oncotarget, 7*, 66020.

Ma, C. X., Gao, F., Luo, J., Northfelt, D. W., Goetz, M., Forero, A., et al. (2017). NeoPalAna: Neoadjuvant palbociclib, a cyclin-dependent kinase 4/6 inhibitor, and anastrozole for clinical stage 2 or 3 estrogen receptor–positive breast cancer. *Clinical Cancer Research, 23*, 4055–4065.

Magnani, L., Brunelle, M., Gevry, N., & Lupien, M. (2012). Chromatin landscape and endocrine response in breast cancer. *Epigenomics, 4*, 675–683.

Mani, S. A., Guo, W., Liao, M.-J., Eaton, E. N., Ayyanan, A., Zhou, A. Y., et al. (2008). The epithelial-mesenchymal transition generates cells with properties of stem cells. *Cell, 133*, 704–715.

Mansoori, B., Mohammadi, A., Davudian, S., Shirjang, S., & Baradaran, B. (2017). The different mechanisms of cancer drug resistance: A brief review. *Advanced pharmaceutical bulletin, 7*, 339.

Martin, C. M., Ferdous, A., Gallardo, T., Humphries, C., Sadek, H., Caprioli, A., et al. (2008). Hypoxia-inducible factor-2α transactivates Abcg2 and promotes cytoprotection in cardiac side population cells. *Circulation Research, 102*, 1075–1081.

Muluhngwi, P., & Klinge, C. M. (2015). Roles for miRNAs in endocrine resistance in breast cancer. *Endocrine-Related Cancer, 22*, R279.

Murthy, R. K., Loi, S., Okines, A., Paplomata, E., Hamilton, E., Hurvitz, S. A., et al. (2020). Tucatinib, trastuzumab, and capecitabine for HER2-positive metastatic breast cancer. *New England Journal of Medicine, 382*, 597–609.

Nassar, Z. D., Mah, C. Y., Centenera, M. M., Irani, S., Sadowski, M. C., Scott, J. S., et al. (2020). Fatty acid oxidation is an adaptive survival pathway induced in prostate tumors by HSP90 inhibition. *Molecular Cancer Research, 18*, 1500–1511.

Nedeljković, M., & Damjanović, A. (2019). Mechanisms of chemotherapy resistance in triple-negative breast cancer—How we can rise to the challenge. *Cell, 8*, 957.

Nikolaou, M., Pavlopoulou, A., Georgakilas, A. G., & Kyrodimos, E. (2018). The challenge of drug resistance in cancer treatment: A current overview. *Clinical & Experimental Metastasis, 35*, 309–318.

Ozpolat, B., Sood, A. K., & Lopez-Berestein, G. (2014). Liposomal siRNA nanocarriers for cancer therapy. *Advanced Drug Delivery Reviews, 66*, 110–116.

Pai, C.-C. S., Simons, D. M., Lu, X., Evans, M., Wei, J., Wang, Y.-H., et al. (2019). Tumor-conditional anti-CTLA4 uncouples antitumor efficacy from immunotherapy-related toxicity. *The Journal of Clinical Investigation, 129*, 349–363.

Palomeras, S., Ruiz-Martínez, S., & Puig, T. (2018). Targeting breast cancer stem cells to overcome treatment resistance. *Molecules, 23*, 2193.

Pavitra, E., Kancharla, J., Gupta, V. K., Prasad, K., Sung, J. Y., Kim, J., et al. (2023). The role of NF-κB in breast cancer initiation, growth, metastasis, and resistance to chemotherapy. *Biomedicine & Pharmacotherapy, 163*, 114822.

Pérez-Hernández, M., Arias, A., Martínez-García, D., Pérez-Tomás, R., Quesada, R., & Soto-Cerrato, V. (2019). Targeting autophagy for cancer treatment and tumor chemosensitization. *Cancers, 11*, 1599.

Pérez-Herrero, E., & Fernández-Medarde, A. (2015). Advanced targeted therapies in cancer: Drug nanocarriers, the future of chemotherapy. *European Journal of Pharmaceutics and Biopharmaceutics, 93*, 52–79.

Pernas, S., Tolaney, S. M., Winer, E. P., & Goel, S. (2018). CDK4/6 inhibition in breast cancer: Current practice and future directions. *Therapeutic Advances in Medical Oncology, 10*, 1758835918786451.

Pham, C. G., Bubici, C., Zazzeroni, F., Knabb, J. R., Papa, S., Kuntzen, C., et al. (2007). Upregulation of Twist-1 by NF-κB blocks cytotoxicity induced by chemotherapeutic drugs. *Molecular and Cellular Biology, 27*, 3920–3935.

Qi, J., Wang, Y., & Forgac, M. (2007). The vacuolar (H+)-ATPase: Subunit arrangement and in vivo regulation. *Journal of Bioenergetics and Biomembranes, 39*, 423–426.

Rowshanravan, B., Halliday, N., & Sansom, D. M. (2018). CTLA-4: A moving target in immunotherapy. *Blood, The Journal of the American Society of Hematology, 131*, 58–67.

Ruddy, K. J., & Ganz, P. A. (2019). Treatment of nonmetastatic breast cancer. *JAMA, 321*, 1716–1717.

Ruth, A., Stein, W. D., Rose, E., & Roninson, I. B. (2001). Coordinate changes in drug resistance and drug-induced conformational transitions in altered-function mutants of the multidrug transporter P-glycoprotein. *Biochemistry, 40*, 4332–4339.

Scarborough, G. A. (1995). Drug-stimulated ATPase activity of the human P-glycoprotein. *Journal of Bioenergetics and Biomembranes, 27*, 37–41.

Schmid, P., Adams, S., Rugo, H. S., Schneeweiss, A., Barrios, C. H., Iwata, H., et al. (2018). Atezolizumab and nab-paclitaxel in advanced triple-negative breast cancer. *New England Journal of Medicine, 379*, 2108–2121.
Schmitt, L., & Tampé, R. (2002). Structure and mechanism of ABC transporters. *Current Opinion in Structural Biology, 12*, 754–760.
Ściskalska, M., & Milnerowicz, H. (2020). The role of GSTπ isoform in the cells signalling and anticancer therapy. *European Review for Medical & Pharmacological Sciences, 24*, 8537–8550.
Shah, N., Mohammad, A. S., Saralkar, P., Sprowls, S. A., Vickers, S. D., John, D., et al. (2018). Investigational chemotherapy and novel pharmacokinetic mechanisms for the treatment of breast cancer brain metastases. *Pharmacological Research, 132*, 47–68.
Shannon, A. M., Bouchier-Hayes, D. J., Condron, C. M., & Toomey, D. (2003). Tumour hypoxia, chemotherapeutic resistance and hypoxia-related therapies. *Cancer Treatment Reviews, 29*, 297–307.
Sharom, F. (1998). The P-glycoprotein efflux pump: How does it transport drugs. *The Journal of Membrane Biology, 166*, 71–73.
Sharom, F. J. (2006). Shedding light on drug transport: Structure and function of the P-glycoprotein multidrug transporter (ABCB1). *Biochemistry and Cell Biology, 84*, 979–992.
Sherlach, K. S., & Roepe, P. D. (2014). *Drug resistance associated membrane proteins*. Frontiers Media SA.
Society, A. C. 2022. *American Cancer Society. Treatment of Triple Negative Breast Cancer. Treating Breast Cancer.* [Online]. Cancer.org. Available: https://www.cancer.org/cancer/breast-cancer/treatment/treatment-of-triple-negative.html. Accessed 11 August 2023 2023.
Stone, A., Zotenko, E., Locke, W. J., Korbie, D., Millar, E. K., Pidsley, R., et al. (2015). DNA methylation of oestrogen-regulated enhancers defines endocrine sensitivity in breast cancer. *Nature Communications, 6*, 7758.
Su, S., Chen, J., Yao, H., Liu, J., Yu, S., Lao, L., et al. (2018). CD10+ GPR77+ cancer-associated fibroblasts promote cancer formation and chemoresistance by sustaining cancer stemness. *Cell, 172*, 841–856.e16.
Sun-Wada, G.-H., & Wada, Y. (2013). Vacuolar-type proton pump ATPases: Acidification and pathological relationships. *Histology and Histopathology, 28*(7), 805–815.
Synold, T. W., Dussault, I., & Forman, B. M. (2001). The orphan nuclear receptor SXR coordinately regulates drug metabolism and efflux. *Nature Medicine, 7*, 584–590.
Tang, Y., Soroush, F., Tong, Z., Kiani, M. F., & Wang, B. (2017). Targeted multidrug delivery system to overcome chemoresistance in breast cancer. *International Journal of Nanomedicine, 12*, 671–681.
Teo, Z. L., Versaci, S., Dushyanthen, S., Caramia, F., Savas, P., Mintoff, C. P., et al. (2017). Combined CDK4/6 and PI3Kα inhibition is synergistic and immunogenic in triple-negative breast cancer. *Cancer Research, 77*, 6340–6352.
Tian, Y., Li, S., Song, J., Ji, T., Zhu, M., Anderson, G. J., et al. (2014). A doxorubicin delivery platform using engineered natural membrane vesicle exosomes for targeted tumor therapy. *Biomaterials, 35*, 2383–2390.
Tolaney, S. M., Wardley, A. M., Zambelli, S., Hilton, J. F., Troso-Sandoval, T. A., Ricci, F., et al. (2020). Abemaciclib plus trastuzumab with or without fulvestrant versus trastuzumab plus standard-of-care chemotherapy in women with hormone receptor-positive, HER2-positive advanced breast cancer (monarcHER): A randomised, open-label, phase 2 trial. *The Lancet Oncology, 21*, 763–775.
Tsuruo, T., Naito, M., Tomida, A., Fujita, N., Mashima, T., Sakamoto, H., et al. (2003). Molecular targeting therapy of cancer: Drug resistance, apoptosis and survival signal. *Cancer Science, 94*, 15–21.
Van Der Meel, R., Fens, M. H., Vader, P., Van Solinge, W. W., Eniola Adefeso, O., & Schiffelers, R. M. (2014). Extracellular vesicles as drug delivery systems: Lessons from the liposome field. *Journal of Controlled Release, 195*, 72–85.

Vannini, I., Zoli, W., Tesei, A., Rosetti, M., Sansone, P., Storci, G., et al. (2008). Role of p53 codon 72 arginine allele in cell survival in vitro and in the clinical outcome of patients with advanced breast cancer. *Tumor Biology, 29*, 145–151.

Vasiliou, V., Vasiliou, K., & Nebert, D. W. (2009). Human ATP-binding cassette (ABC) transporter family. *Human Genomics, 3*, 1–10.

Verde, G., Llobet, L. I. D., Wright, R. H., Quilez, J., Peiró, S., Dily, F. L., et al. (2018). Unliganded progesterone receptor governs estrogen receptor gene expression by regulating DNA methylation in breast cancer cells. *Cancers, 10*, 371.

Vesuna, F., Lisok, A., Kimble, B., Domek, J., Kato, Y., Van Der Groep, P., et al. (2012). Twist contributes to hormone resistance in breast cancer by downregulating estrogen receptor-α. *Oncogene, 31*, 3223–3234.

Wang, K., Zhang, Q., Li, D., Ching, K., Zhang, C., Zheng, X., et al. (2015). PEST domain mutations in notch receptors comprise an oncogenic driver segment in triple-negative breast cancer sensitive to a γ-secretase inhibitor. *Clinical Cancer Research, 21*, 1487–1496.

Wang, X., Qi, Y., Kong, X., Zhai, J., Li, Y., Song, Y., et al. (2019). Immunological therapy: A novel thriving area for triple-negative breast cancer treatment. *Cancer Letters, 442*, 409–428.

Wu, Q., Yang, Z., Nie, Y., Shi, Y., & Fan, D. (2014). Multi-drug resistance in cancer chemotherapeutics: Mechanisms and lab approaches. *Cancer Letters, 347*, 159–166.

Wu, Q., Wu, W., Fu, B., Shi, L., Wang, X., & Kuca, K. (2019). JNK signaling in cancer cell survival. *Medicinal Research Reviews, 39*, 2082–2104.

Xia, P., & Xu, X.-Y. (2015). PI3K/Akt/mTOR signaling pathway in cancer stem cells: From basic research to clinical application. *American Journal of Cancer Research, 5*, 1602.

Xiang, H., Zhang, J., Lin, C., Zhang, L., Liu, B., & Ouyang, L. (2020). Targeting autophagy-related protein kinases for potential therapeutic purpose. *Acta Pharmaceutica Sinica B, 10*, 569–581.

Xu, R.-H., Pelicano, H., Zhou, Y., Carew, J. S., Feng, L., Bhalla, K. N., et al. (2005). Inhibition of glycolysis in cancer cells: A novel strategy to overcome drug resistance associated with mitochondrial respiratory defect and hypoxia. *Cancer Research, 65*, 613–621.

Xu, R., Greening, D. W., Zhu, H.-J., Takahashi, N., & Simpson, R. J. (2016). Extracellular vesicle isolation and characterization: Toward clinical application. *The Journal of Clinical Investigation, 126*, 1152–1162.

Yang, F., Xu, J., Tang, L., & Guan, X. (2017). Breast cancer stem cell: The roles and therapeutic implications. *Cellular and Molecular Life Sciences, 74*, 951–966.

Yeldag, G., Rice, A., & Del Río Hernández, A. (2018). Chemoresistance and the self-maintaining tumor microenvironment. *Cancers, 10*, 471.

Yu, Y., Luo, W., Yang, Z.-J., Chi, J.-R., Li, Y.-R., Ding, Y., et al. (2018). miR-190 suppresses breast cancer metastasis by regulation of TGF-β-induced epithelial–mesenchymal transition. *Molecular Cancer, 17*, 1–12.

Zhang, L., Yang, X., Lv, Y., Xin, X., Qin, C., Han, X., et al. (2017). Cytosolic co-delivery of miRNA-34a and docetaxel with core-shell nanocarriers via caveolae-mediated pathway for the treatment of metastatic breast cancer. *Scientific Reports, 7*, 46186.

Zhou, M., Liu, Z., Zhao, Y., Ding, Y., Liu, H., Xi, Y., et al. (2010). MicroRNA-125b confers the resistance of breast cancer cells to paclitaxel through suppression of pro-apoptotic Bcl-2 antagonist killer 1 (Bak1) expression. *Journal of Biological Chemistry, 285*, 21496–21507.

Part III
Innovative Approaches and Strategies to Overcome Drug Resistance

Unraveling the Impact of Aberrant Splicing Machinery on Drug Resistance in Breast Cancer: Identifying Targets for Innovative Counteractive Strategies

Rodney Hull, Bahoueli Gaudji, David O. Bates, and Zodwa Dlamini

Abstract The alternative splicing of pre-mRNA is an important process that increases the number of proteins a genome can code for and is important for nearly all biological processes within a cell. Alternative splicing has been found to be dysregulated in cancers including breast cancer, where it contributes to the development and progression of the disease. Alternative splicing can also contribute to the development of drug resistance. This is due to either new isoform not being targeted by drugs or being able to bypass the inhibitory activity of drugs. These splicing events can alter the expression of proteins targeted by drugs, alter the expression of proteins involved in signaling pathways up or downstream of drug targets or they can occur in the components of the splicing machinery, resulting in broad changes in splicing of many other proteins. This can change the whole splicing pattern of a cell. This has resulted in alternative splicing becoming a viable target in the attempt to reverse drug resistance by targeting the new isoforms that can result in drug resistance. This can be done by targeting the mRNA coding for these new isoforms, targeting the pre-mRNA to correct or alter splicing, and targeting the protein isoforms through small molecular inhibitors that can bind to or specially act upon

R. Hull (✉) · Z. Dlamini
SAMRC Precision Oncology Research Unit (PORU), DSI/NRF SARChI Chair in Precision Oncology and Cancer Prevention (POCP), Pan African Cancer Research Institute (PACRI), University of Pretoria, Pretoria, South Africa
e-mail: rodney.hull@up.ac.za; zodwa.dlamini@up.ac.za

B. Gaudji
Department of Urology, Level 7, Bridge C, Steve Biko Academic Hospital, Faculty of Health Sciences, University of Pretoria, Pretoria, South Africa
e-mail: guy.gaudji@up.ac.za

D. O. Bates
SAMRC Precision Oncology Research Unit (PORU), DSI/NRF SARChI Chair in Precision Oncology and Cancer Prevention (POCP), Pan African Cancer Research Institute (PACRI), University of Pretoria, Hatfield, South Africa

Centre for Cancer Sciences, School of Medicine, Biodiscovery Institute, University of Nottingham, Nottingham, UK
e-mail: David.Bates@nottingham.ac.uk

Z. Dlamini (ed.), *Overcoming Breast Cancer Therapy Resistance*,
https://doi.org/10.1007/978-3-031-52860-6_7

certain isoforms. Finally, the splicing machinery and splicing factors can be targeted in order to prevent the switch to pro-oncogenic splice variants. This chapter will explore the different splicing events that occur in individual genes, components of signaling pathways, or components of the splicing machinery, which can result in breast cancer developing resistance to specific treatments. It will then discuss mechanisms and strategies for targeting these transcripts, proteins, and regulators of splicing in order to switch splicing to favor the expression of anti, or non- carcinogenic splice variants.

Keywords Tamoxifen · Taxanes · Cytotoxic agents · Splice-switching oligonucleotides · Splicing switches · Estrogen receptor · Splicing machinery · Splicing factors

Introduction

The aberrant or dysregulation of alternative splicing gives rise to abnormal splicing patterns that have been linked to a wide variety of human diseases (Ibáñez-Costa et al., 2022). This includes breast cancer (Yang et al., 2019) where aberrant splicing, splicing processes, and the abnormal expression of alternate protein isoforms are not only associated with the development and progression of breast cancer but also with chemo/radiotherapeutic resistance (Yang et al., 2019). This is due to the altered expression of protein isoforms with different or even opposite functions since the cellular proteome plays a major role in the response of tumor cells to chemotherapy. The manipulation of the normal process of alternative splicing can be manipulated by cancer cells to promote survival following treatment with chemotherapeutic drugs.

This chapter will focus on the role played by alternative splicing in the development of drug resistance in breast cancer. It will discuss the pathways and individual genes that are altered through the process of alternative splicing. Entire signaling pathways can be altered through the splicing of components within the pathway while the isoforms of individual genes can change the response of a cell to a specific drug by being less sensitive to a drug that targets the "normal" isoform. The review will then go on to discuss the role played by changes in the expression of splicing factors in breast cancer. Finally, it will discuss the targeting of specific isoforms, alternative splicing processes, and splicing machinery to reverse drug resistance and the limitations of this strategy.

A Summary of Splicing Alterations in Breast Cancer

Breast cancer sequence related data from the Cancer Genome Atlas have been analyzed in order to identify splicing vents. This analysis showed that 45,421 splicing events were present in this data from 1098 patients. These events took place in

21,232 genes and demonstrated that alternative splicing is a common process in breast cancer. Of these splicing events 2802 events in 1878 genes were the result of intron retention, 233 events in 227 genes were due to mutually exclusive exons, 17,702 events in 6812 genes were the result of exon skipping, 8595 events in 3755 genes were due to alternate termination sites, 9112 events in 3654 genes were due to alternate promoter sites, and finally 6977 events in 4906 genes were the result of alternate donor or acceptor sites (Han et al., 2021).

A univariate Cox analysis of these splicing events identified that 1121 AS events in 931 genes could be correlated with prognostic outcomes of breast cancer patients. An examination of splicing factors showed that splicing factors were significantly correlated with AS events and these various splicing factor and splicing events can also be associated with prognostic outcomes (Steensma et al., 2019). Gene ontogeny analysis revealed that these splicing events are enriched in pathways associated with cancer. These include pathways such as MAPK signaling pathway, cell cycle regulation, and cell–matrix adhesion (Steensma et al., 2019).

A meta-analysis of pharmacological data from large-scale drug screening datasets including data related to breast cancer shows that there were 1723 alternative splicing events involved in the response of breast cancer to drug treatment. There were also 41 splicing factors whose regulation, expression, and splicing were altered in the acquired resistance of breast cancer cells to doxorubicin (Tanaka et al., 2020). This implies that the expression of various isoforms and the occurrence of various splicing events can be used as biomarkers for drug resistance. For instance, changes in the alternative splicing of IGF2BP2 are associated with the development of resistance to AZD6244 in breast cancers. The same is true of splicing events in NECTIN4 and resistance to Lapatinib, ITGB6 splicing events and resistance to Erlotinib, and finally splicing events within KLHDC9 and resistance to Paclitaxel on breast cancers (Tanaka et al., 2020).

Pathways Involved in Drug Resistance Affected By Aberrant Splicing

Multiple pathways are deregulated in breast cancer development and progression. These pathways control processes such as cell cycle control, proliferation, and apoptosis. And the loss or deregulation of these pathways can result in resistance to apoptosis and acquired rug resistance.

Splicing Events in Pathways Involved in Anti-estrogen Therapy

Estrogen receptor (ER)-driven signaling initiates or is involved in pathways that contribute to the development and progression of ER + ve breast cancer. Nearly 70% of breast cancers are (ER + ve). An obvious therapeutic strategy for these cancers is the suppression of ER-mediated signaling. This can be done using compounds such as tamoxifen (TAM), which is an antagonist of ER. TAM binds to the ligand-binding domain of ER and prevents the binding of the actual ligand, blocking ER activation and signaling (Tsoi et al., 2023). Tam is actually an agonist of ER and will only partially activate the receptor. This means it has different inhibitory abilities in different tissues. However, in breast cancer it predominantly behaves like an inhibitor of ER signaling.

The ER alpha (*ERα*) gene produces two important splice variants (Fig. 7.1a) that play a role in drug resistance in breast cancer. The splicing of ERα varies in different tissues and in different diseases (Herynk & Fuqua, 2004; Taylor et al., 2010). Full-length ERα66 contains all eight exons and codes for a protein with three domains and a flexible hinge region. These domains include an activation domain, a DNA binding domain, and a ligand-binding domain. The DNA binding domain is a Zinc finger binding domain. The ligand-binding domain is a specialized ligand-binding

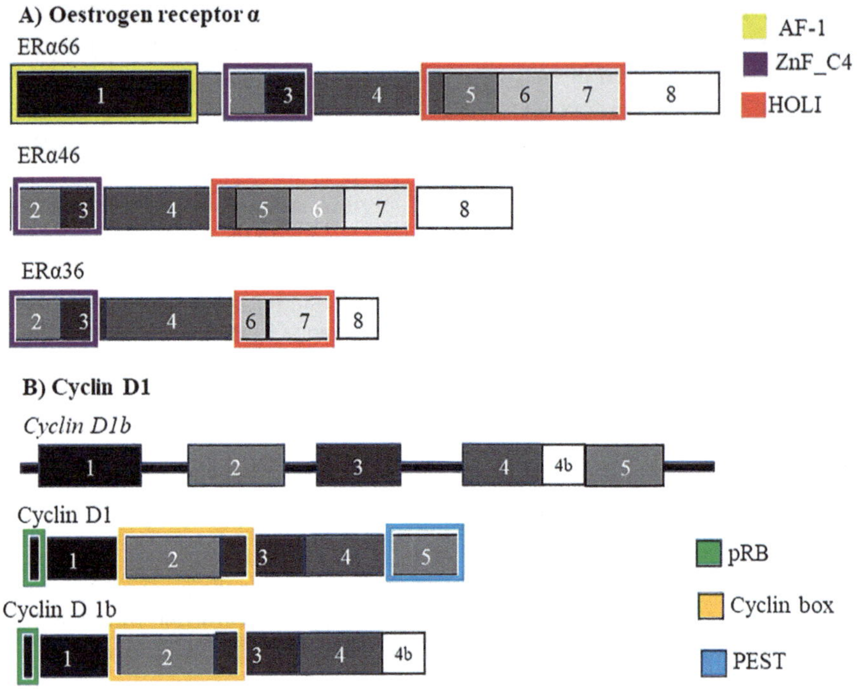

Fig. 7.1 Splicing variants involved in the development of resistance to anti-estrogen therapy. (**a**) Estrogen receptor alpha is alternatively spliced by use of a differential transcriptional start sites to give rise to two truncated isoforms which lack the AF-1 domain and, by exon skipping of exon 5, the isoform Erα36 which has a truncated HOLI domain. This shorter form promotes resistance to tamoxifen. (**b**) The drug-resistant Cyclin D1 isoform, cyclin D1b lacks the PEST domain, which is normally associated with intracellular signaling and contains a phosphorylation target which acts as a signal for nuclear export. The shorter form is therefore retained in the nucleus. AF-1, Activation function; HOLI domain, ligand-binding domain of hormone receptors; PEST domain, proline (P), glutamic acid (E), serine (S) and threonine (T); pRB, retinoblastoma protein; ZMF, zinc finger

domain found in hormone receptors and is known as a HOLI domain (Fig. 7.1a). The two isoforms ERα36 and Erα46 contribute to TAM resistance.

ERα36 lacks the activation domain and a large section of the ligand-binding domain, which changes its ligand affinities and means TAM does not bind to it as well as its own ligand, Erα46 lacks the activation domain (Chantalat et al., 2016; Inoue & Fry, 2015). The expression of ERα46 in breast cancer cells leads to decreased proliferation and cell survival. Overexpression of this isoform also sensitizes TAM-resistant breast cancer cells to TAM. This is due to this isoform acting as an antagonist to the function of the full-length ERα66 (Fig. 7.2; Huber-Keener, 2022). In addition, ER-α46 has also been reported to be involved in breast cancer development and drug resistance (Klinge et al., 2010; Li et al., 2003).

It has been found that ER-α36 is overexpressed in breast cancer cells that are resistant to TAM. This increased expression is accompanied by high levels of ERK phosphorylation. Previous studies have suggested that the AF1 domain of ER-α66 plays a role in the agonist action of TAM (Fig. 7.2; Reddy & Glaros, 2007). Increased expression of this isoform on TAM-sensitive breast cancer cells led to TAM resistance (Reddy & Glaros, 2007). Therefore ER-α36 seems to have the ability to mediate both E2- and TAM-induced activation of the MAPK/ERK and AKT pathways. In this way this isoform can not only decrease the anti-proliferative activity of TAM, but TAM may induce phosphorylation of MAPK, ERK, and AKT, leading to increased proliferation and cell survival. This is further evidenced by the increased expression of c-Myc oncoprotein observed in breast cancer cells overexpressing this isoform, following treatment of these cells with TAM (McNeil et al., 2006). Not only does ERα act as a transcription factor, following hormone binding, but it also functions as a noncanonical RNA-binding protein. In this case it acts to mediate the splicing of genes such as XBP1. This activity is associated with breast cancer progression and TAM resistance (Xu et al., 2021).

Cyclin D1 mediates appropriate cell cycle regulation and is aberrantly regulated in cancers including breast cancer (Knudsen et al., 2006; Bartkova et al., 1994). It fulfills this function by regulating cyclin-dependent kinase 4 (CDK4) (Matsushime et al., 1994) and phosphorylates RB inhibiting it to promote cell cycle progression (Ewen et al., 1993). Cyclin D1 can also act as a transcriptional modulator stimulating transcription factors like the estrogen receptor (Neuman et al., 1997; Zwijsen et al., 1997). Cyclin D1 is alternatively spliced by intron retention, to give rise to an isoform named cyclin D1b (Knudsen, 2006) which lacks exon 5 and includes sequences from intron four (Hosokawa et al., 1997) since CyclinD1 is normally regulated by phosphorylation at T286, leading to its nuclear export, that is absent in cyclinD1b (Alt et al., 2000; Lu et al., 2003). Anti-estrogen therapy results in cell cycle arrest and overexpression of cyclin D1b prevents the cell cycle arrest induced by anti-estrogen therapy (Wang et al., 2008).

The nuclear receptor co-repressor 2 (NCOR2) is a transcriptional coregulatory protein and acts to repress the activity of multiple transcription factors. It is able to achieve this by recruiting histone deacetylases to the promoter regions bound by multiple transcription factors. In this way NCOR2 functions to repress the activity of pathways activated by receptors such as ERα. The multiple interaction domains

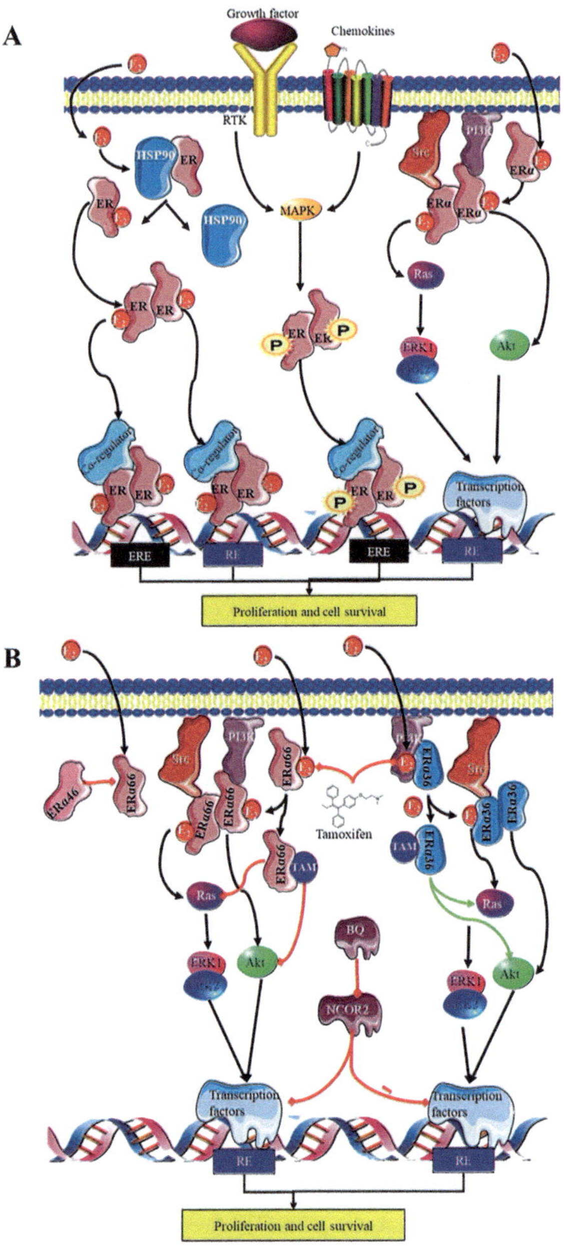

Fig. 7.2 *Estrogen signaling pathways and the role played by ER alpha and NCOR2 isoforms in acquired drug resistance.* (**a**) Estrogen signaling pathways, with the canonical ER alpha signaling pathway furthest to the right. (**b**) The shorter ER alpha isoforms are either able to inhibit the pathway, promoting drug sensitivity or continue to activate downstream signaling cascades regardless of tamoxifen binding, thereby increasing drug resistance. NCOR2 represses transcriptional activation by ER alpha; however, the CQ splice variant inhibits this activity

within NCOR2 allow it to achieve its function. NCOR2 is alternatively spliced by exon skipping to give rise to an isoform lacking exon 11. This isoform is known as BQ323636.1 (BQ) (Zhang et al., 2013). The expression of BQ is higher in estrogen receptor-positive breast cancer patients who have developed resistance to TAM. And it is now known that BQ expression is one of the mechanisms behind TAM resistance (Tsoi et al., 2023). The expression of BQ depends on the activity of SRSF5 with higher levels of SRSF5 leading to lower levels of BQ and a reversal of TAM resistance (Tsoi et al., 2023).

Inflammation

Stress can be defined as an actual or perceived threat which causes the central nervous system to alter hormonal and neuronal secretions (Harbuz & Lightman, 1992). It is estimated that 50% of breast cancer originates through genetic, physiologic, or behavioral factors (Madigan et al., 1995). However, only about a tenth to a fifth of these cases is thought to arise due to genetic risk factors (Tonin, 2000). The rest are attributed to physiological and behavioral factors including early menarche, late menopause, conceiving and giving birth to their first child later in life, being overweight, hormone replacement therapy, alcohol use, diet, a sedentary lifestyle, and benign breast diseases (Hankinson et al., 2004). One of these factors which is commonly overlooked is the contribution of stress, both physical and psychological (Gerber et al., 2003). Epidemiological and physiological studies have demonstrated a clear link between stress and breast cancer development and progression. There are common molecules and signaling pathways shared between stress response pathways and pro-tumorigenic pathways (Antonova et al., 2011). Humans respond to stress via hypothalamic–pituitary–adrenal (HPA) axis (Harbuz & Lightman, 1992). This axis is initiated by the production of corticotropin-releasing hormone in the hypothalamus which in turn stimulates the release of adrenocorticotropic hormone. Adrenocorticotropic hormone is released from the anterior pituitary and leads to the production and release of cortisol from the adrenal cortex. Cortisol is known as the stress hormone (Noureddine et al., 2021) and leads to the breakdown of protein, lipid, and carbohydrate, as well as the transcription of specific genes, in response to stress through signaling pathways initiated by its receptor, the glucocorticoid receptor (GR) (Homo-Delarche et al., 1991).

Glucocorticoids such as cortisol are steroid hormones that act as anti-inflammatory agents as well as playing a role as immunosuppressors (Hunt et al., 2017). The GR is encoded by the NR3C1 gene which is alternatively spliced by mutually exclusive exon selection to produce two families of transcripts coding for two separate isoforms, namely GRα and GRβ (Fig. 7.3; Kadmiel & Cidlowski, 2013; Weikum et al., 2017). GR is found in the cytoplasm in an inactive state, where it is also bound to proteins such as heat shock proteins. Once the glucocorticoid binds to the GR, GR complexes are transported to the nucleus Here, they act as transcription factors to initiate the expression of genes such as MAPK1 and PI3K

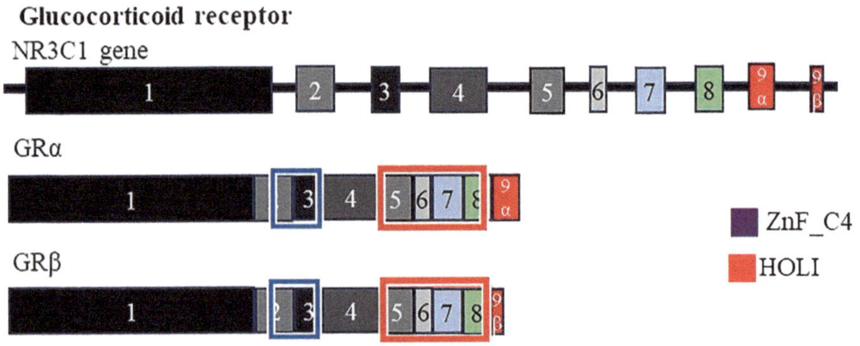

Fig. 7.3 *Glucocorticoid receptor splicing*. The longer GR alpha isoform promotes endocrine therapy resistance

(Kadmiel & Cidlowski, 2013). However, the mouse GR was also found to be expressed as a membrane bound isoform containing exon 1A (Chen et al., 1999). The interaction of glucocorticoids leads to a rapid response not involving transcription activation, rather the activated membrane bound GR interacts with proteins in other signaling pathways. These pathways include the MAPK pathway, activator Protein 1 (AP-1), and Nuclear Factor-kappa B (NFκB) (Herr et al., 2007; Kadmiel & Cidlowski, 2013; Strehl & Buttgereit, 2013). The glucocorticoid receptor isoform-α is the most commonly expressed isoform and is associated with endocrine therapy resistance which is involved in the expression of C kinase 1, promoting cell migration (Buoso et al., 2019). Expression of this isoform is connected to the SRSF3 splicing factor and this pathway is induced by cortisol (Read & Natrajan, 2018).

Receptor Tyrosine Kinase Pathways

Aggressive, metastasis of cancer cells occurs in response to a multitude of signals including growth factors and extracellular matrix (ECM) proteins. The migration of cancer cells requires continuous, coordinated cytoskeletal remodeling and changes in cell adhesion both cell–matrix and cell–cell adhesion (Bear & Haugh, 2014). This requires the activation of various receptor tyrosine kinases (RTKs) including the epidermal growth factor receptor (EGFR) pathway (Nürnberg et al., 2011; Roussos et al., 2011). This pathway requires the Mena protein to facilitate invasion, metastasis, actin polymerization, and changes in adhesion (Gertler & Condeelis, 2011). This protein is a member of a family of proteins that promote F-actin elongation, increasing elongation rates and delaying the termination of filament growth (Bear & Gertler, 2009; Breitsprecher et al., 2011).

Mena and other family members contain an N-terminal Ena/VASP homology (EVH) 1 domain and a C-terminal EVH2 domain, separated by a polyproline-rich center and an LERER repeat region. The EVH1 and 2 domains promote protein–protein interactions (Ball et al., 2002). Mena attenuates RTK signaling through interactions with PTP1B and SHIP2. Mena is overexpressed in breast cancer (Gertler & Condeelis, 2011), with Mena deficiencies leading to decreased progression and invasion (Roussos et al., 2010). Mena is alternatively spliced to give rise to multiple isoforms (Fig. 7.4). One of these isoforms Mena^{INV} is generated by alternative 3′ (acceptor) splicing of exon 3a which promotes migration and invasion (Fig. 7.4a) (Gertler et al., 1996) by increasing the potency of EGF signaling

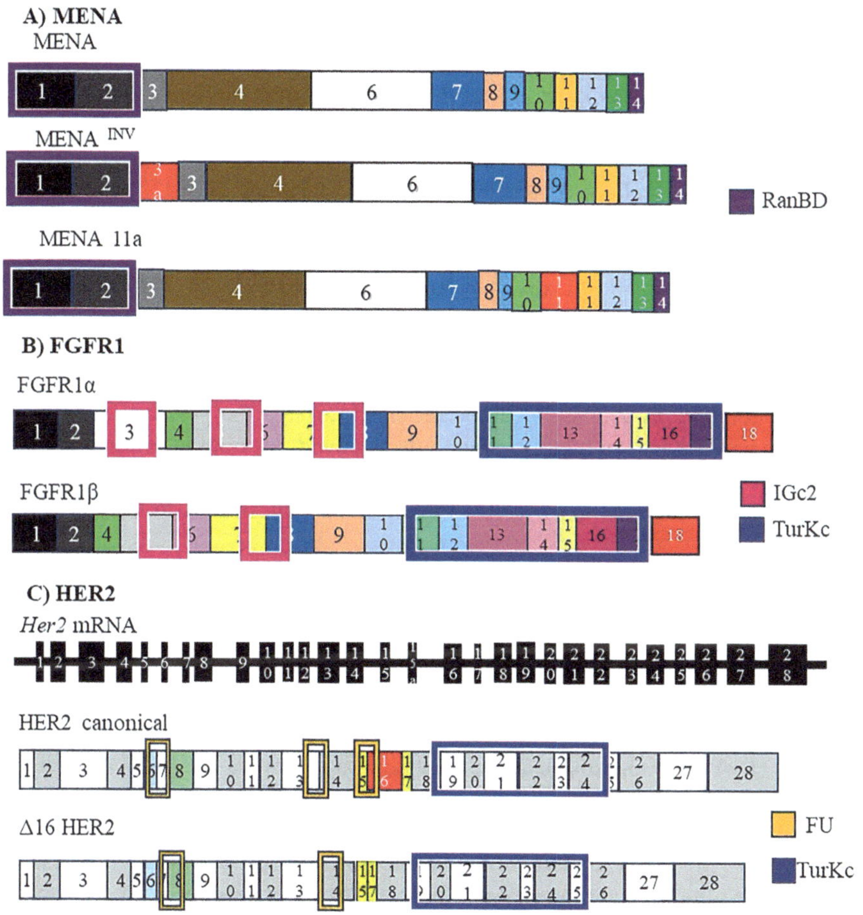

Fig. 7.4 *The alternative splicing of genes involved in RTK signaling contributes to drug resistance in breast cancer*. (**a**) The Mena invasion isoform promotes EGFR signaling resulting in increased invasion and migration and increased resistance to RTK inhibitors (**b**) FGFR1 splicing results in transcripts lacking exon 2. This isoform is missing one of the Immunoglobulin type c domains, resulting in altered FGF ligand binding (**c**) HER2 splicing leads to the expression of the truncated isoform lacking the first furin domain coded for by exon 17. This increases the ability of the receptor to bind its ligand, increasing signaling

(Philippar et al., 2008). Mena^{INV} is able to accomplish this by disrupting the interactions of "normal" Mena with PTP1B and SHIP, increasing RTK signaling. The expression of this isoform also leads to decreased sensitivity to targeted RTK inhibitors (Hughes et al., 2015).

The fibroblast growth factor receptor contains three Ig-like domains in its extracellular region. These domains dictate ligand binding and specificity (Kalinina et al., 2012). FGFR mRNA is alternatively spliced by exon skipping to give rise to transcripts that either include (FGFR1α) or lack (FGFR1β) exon 3 (Fig. 7.4b). This exon codes for the IgC and AB linker region (Wang et al., 1995). These isoforms differ in their binding of FGF ligands, with FGFR1β binding these ligands with a higher affinity and this isoform is associated with cancer development and progression and poor survival in breast cancer (Luqmani et al., 1995; Wendt et al., 2014). The ratio of the expression of these two isoforms influenced sensitivity to FGFR inhibitors such as BGJ-398. Those cells that expressed higher levels of FGFR1β leading to a higher FGFR1β/FGFR1α ratio were more sensitive to this inhibitor. In ER+ cells estrogen treatment led to higher FGFR1β levels (Zhao et al., 2019).

Taxanes are a family of compounds used to treat breast cancer and include drugs such as paclitaxel and docetaxel. They function by inducing apoptosis by triggering the spindle assembly checkpoint through the disruption of microtubule assembly (Yasuhira et al., 2016). Taxane resistance in breast cancer can be mediated by increased efflux pump activity or by the modification of the microtubule targets. This microtubule modification can be achieved through the presence of different isoforms and isotypes of tubulin, which affects how drugs bind to and interact with them (Orr et al., 2003). Human epidermal growth factor receptor 2 (HER2) expression levels are linked with the sensitivity of breast cancer cells to taxanes (Perez et al., 2005).

HER2 is a tyrosine kinase receptor whose overexpression defines the HER2-positive breast cancer phenotype (Hart et al., 2020). HER2 is overexpressed in many breast cancers (20–30%) (Wahler & Suh, 2015) and as such its expression is used as a biomarker for taxane response, with increased expression of HER2 correlating with increased resistance to taxanes (Yu et al., 1996). However, some studies have shown increased expression of HER2 being associated with a better response to taxanes (Di Leo et al., 2004). These contradictions may be the result of complex genetic interactions in HER2-positive breast cancer, or these studies not distinguishing between the different isoforms of HER2.

The *Her2* mRNA is alternatively spliced to form at least seven isoforms, some of which have important clinical roles in breast cancer. These isoforms include Δ16HER2, Δ15HER2, Herstatin, p100HER2, X5-HER2, HER2-PI9, and HER2-I12 (Hart et al., 2020). Exon 16 (Fig. 7.4c) encodes a small extracellular region rich in cysteine residues, and this is skipped in the splice variant, Δ16HER2. This leads to an extracellular domain that promotes homodimerization, leading to a conformational change in the receptor that allows it to activate oncogenic signaling (Inoue & Fry, 2015). These signals are able to promote drug resistance (Jackson et al., 2013). Another splice variant is p100HER2, which retains intron 15 resulting in a premature stop codon, and a protein that lacks the intracellular domain, but the RNA encoding it is not targeted for nonsense mediated decay. This isoform can also be secreted and its presence results in reduced downstream, ERK1/2 and HER4 phosphorylation signaling (Aigner et al., 2001). However, p100HER2 reduces the efficacy of monoclonal antibodies targeting HER2 by reducing antibody binding.

Unfolded Protein Response

Studies have demonstrated a link between the unfolded protein response (UPR), taking place within the endoplasmic reticulum and increased drug resistance in breast cancer. This relationship has been shown to involve alternative splicing of genes involved in this response. In particular, a noncanonical form of alternative splicing of the human X-box binding protein-1 (XBP1) gives rise to two isoforms. A 26-nucleotide section of exon 4 can be excised by the endonuclease IRE1 under stress. XBP1 is a transcription factor and controls the expression of genes involved in the UPR, in particular it controls the splicing of some of these genes (Davies et al., 2008). The overexpression of the XBP1s isoform, which contains the full-length exon4, in ER-positive breast cancer cells stimulates estrogen-independent cell growth. The overexpression of this isoform also results in increased resistance to TAM in these cells (Ding et al., 2003; Fang et al., 2004). As such a drug named STF-080310 has been developed that targets and inhibits IRE1α/XBP1. This inhibitor has demonstrated the ability to sensitize TAM-resistant MCF-7 breast cancer cells to TAM treatment by disrupting noncanonical XBP1 splicing and reducing the expression of XBP1s (Papandreou et al., 2011; Ming et al., 2015; Fig. 7.5).

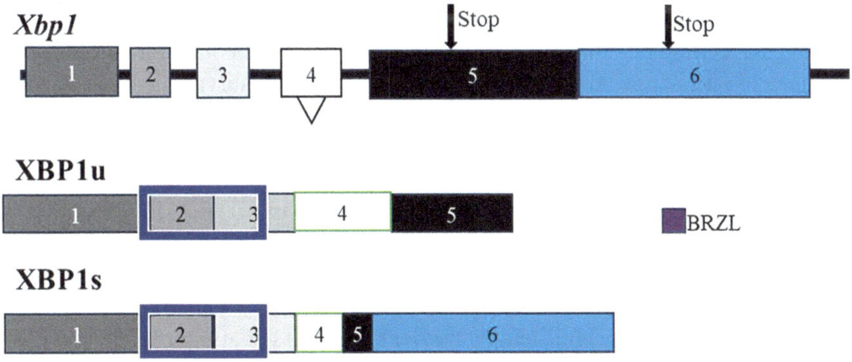

Fig. 7.5 *XBP1 splicing*. Noncanonical splicing by excision of a 26nt section of exon 4 of the X-box binding protein-1 results in the XBP1u transcript with a truncated exon 4. The expression of this isoform results in cells that are more sensitive to tamoxifen. The expression of the s isoform results in increased tamoxifen resistance

Metabolic Pathways

The epithelial splicing regulatory protein 1 (ESRP1) is known to regulate the splicing of genes involved in epithelial-to-mesenchymal transition (EMT) in cancers. This splicing regulator also plays a role in promoting the growth of endocrine-resistant ER+ breast cancer. High levels of this protein are also associated with a poor prognosis in these cancers. The protein also plays a role in TAM resistance, by upregulating the expression of (FASN), stearoyl-CoA desaturase 1 (SCD1), and phosphoglycerate dehydrogenase (PHGDH). This leads to an alteration in cell metabolism characterized by a decrease in the basal respiration and spare respiration capacity. These metabolic changes are likely due to splicing changes initiated by ESRP1 and as such this splicing regulator could be targeted to reverse TAM resistance (Gökmen-Polar et al., 2019). In addition.

Apoptosis Pathways

Apoptotic pathways are deregulated through the expression of anti-apoptotic proteins, including Survivin. This is a member of the Inhibitors of Apoptosis Protein (IAP) family of proteins. Survivin is encoded by the *Baculoviral IAP repeat containing 5 (BIRC5)* gene, which is alternatively spliced to give rise to six survivin splice variants: full-length survivin, survivin 2B, survivin 2α, survivin 3B, survivin ΔEx3, and survivin 3α (Coumar et al., 2013). Full-length survivin 3B, survivin ΔEx3, and survivin 3α are all anti-apoptotic and show increased expression associated with drug resistance (Fig. 7.6; Végran et al., 2007). The expression of Survivin and some of its splice variants is also regulated by p53 Mutations in p53 can lead to the expression of anti-apoptotic splice variants survivin-DeltaEx3, which lacks exon 3, and survivin-3B, which contains the extra exon 3b. These isoforms are therefore the result of exon skipping and the use of an alternate splice site. This means that certain p64 mutations will lead to the expression of anti-apoptotic splice variants of surviving and may increase breast cancer cell survival and resistance to therapy (Végran et al., 2007). Arsenic trioxide has shown promise as a viable treatment for breast cancer (Liu et al., 2015; Hoffman et al., 2015). As_2O_3 inhibited MCF-7 breast cancer cell growth, by induing a G2/M cell cycle arrest and promoting caspase-dependent apoptosis. As_2O_3 accomplishes this by inducing apoptosis by downregulating survivin expression, activating p38 and c-Jun N-terminal kinases (JNK) pathways (Cheng et al., 2006) and inhibiting Phosphoinositide 3-Kinase (PI3K) or extracellular signal-regulated kinases (ERK) signaling (Cheng et al., 2006). Before treatment, full-length survivin is expressed at high levels in MCF-7 cells and expression decreased following treatment, with low levels in As_2O_3-induced G2/M cell cycle arrest and apoptosis. The pro-apoptotic variant Survivin 2B, not expressed during treatment, increased expression following treatment

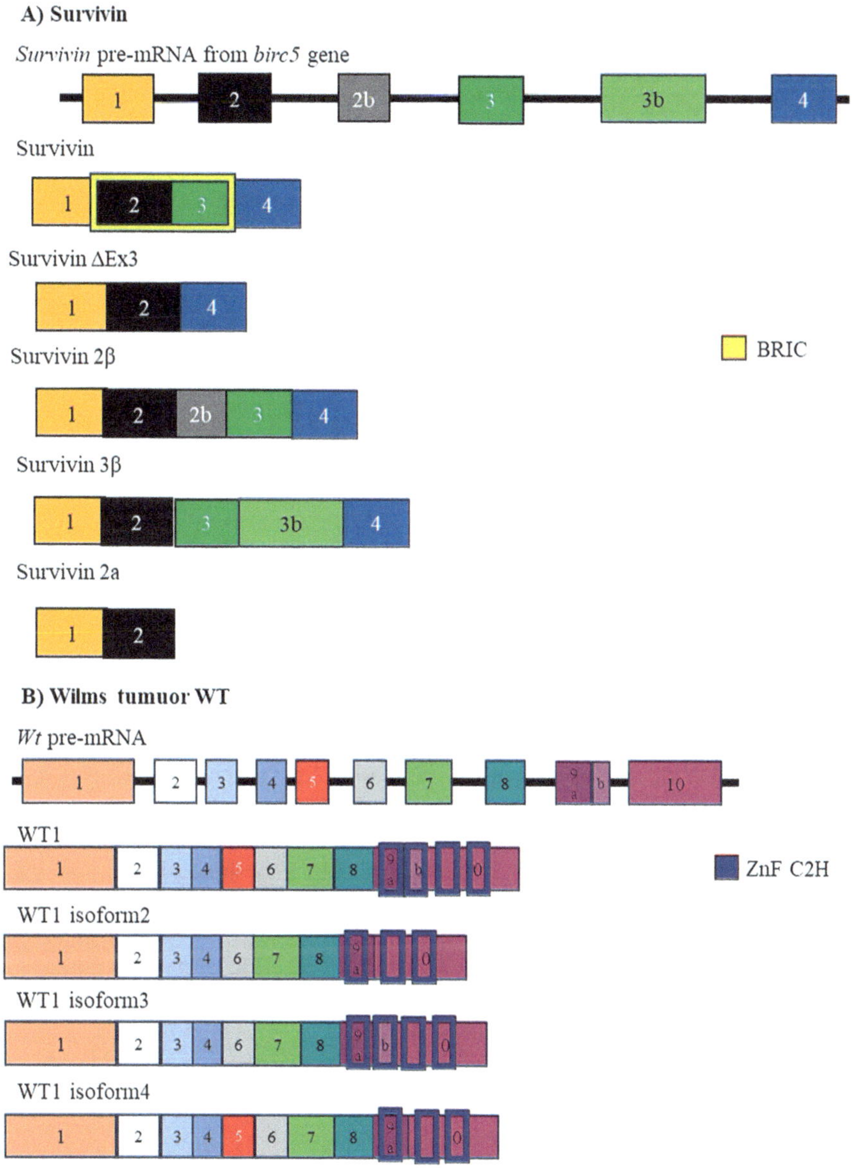

Fig. 7.6 *The splicing of genes involved in increased drug resistance I breast cancer due to altering apoptotic pathways*. (**a**) Different isoforms of survivin alter the ability of these isoforms to inhibit apoptosis and promote survival, while others promote apoptosis. (**b**) The splicing of the Wilms Tumor pre-mRNA results in their retention of exon 5 and a section of the intron following exon 9 due to a 3′ splice site within this intron. The inclusion of exon 5 leads to an isoform that promotes cell survival and resistance to genotoxic agents

leading to a higher expression during cell cycle arrest, followed by increased apoptosis and downregulated survivin expression (Laka et al., 2019). This means that the expression of the pro-apoptotic variant is induced by arsenic trioxide and may prove to be a useful therapeutic target.

Increased expression of the Wilms' tumor gene (WT1) is associated with breast cancer development and progression due to its inhibition of the apoptotic pathways. High levels of WT1 are found in tumors with a poor prognosis. Increased WT1 expression also occurs following the treatment of drug resistant breast cancer cells with cytotoxic agents. WT1 is alternatively spliced to give rise to four major isoforms (Fig. 7.6b). The splicing events around exon 5 give rise to isoforms associated with this resistance to cytotoxic agents. These isoforms appear to have a pro-apoptotic function compared to the anti-apoptotic full-length form (Renshaw et al., 2004).

The Cell Cycle ECT

Alterations in the function of two splicing factors were found to be associated with doxorubicin, a genotoxic agent, resistance in breast cancer cells. Increased expression of these splicing factors was associated with an increase in the resistance of breast cancer cells to doxorubicin (Millour et al., 2011). These splicing factors were found to regulate the splicing of the epithelial cell-transforming sequence 2 oncogene, ECT2, which is involved in the cytokinesis phase of the cell cycle (Zou et al., 2014; Tanaka et al., 2020). The increase of these splicing factors favors the expression of the ECT2 variant that includes exon 5 (ECT2-Ex5+). This exon encodes an ERCT domain which is normally found in proteins that play a role in the response of cells to DNA damage (Zou et al., 2014). The canonical shorter ECT2 was found to play a role in the induction of cell death in response to DNA damage. The expression of this isoform is also related to the sensitivity of cells to an inhibitor of ATR. The inhibition of ATR reduces the ability of a cell to respond to replication stress (He et al., 2016). Since this shorter isoform also contains BRCT domains and the addition of another of these domains may make the ECT2-Ex5+ isoform a more effective checkpoint, enabling the cell to have more time to repair DNA damage and prevent cell death (Manic et al., 2018; Wang & Lee, 2018).

DNA Damage Repair BRCA1

Breast cancer type 1 susceptibility protein, encoded by the *BRCA1* gene, acts as a tumor suppressor protein that plays a role in repairing DNA (Duncan et al., 1998). In performing its homologous recombination DNA repair function BRCA1 interacts with different partners. *BRCA1* mutations are common in breast cancer, being the most common genomic alteration in hereditary-related breast cancer (Semmler et al., 2019). Seven splice variants have been identified in normal and tumoral tissues and dysregulated alternative splicing of *BRCA1* is involved in the development of breast cancer (Orban & Olah, 2003). The full-length BRCA and the two splice variants BRCA1-Δ11 and BRCA1-Δ11q are the most important in breast cancer. Exon 11 encodes the nuclear localization signal, which is responsible for the translocation of the protein to the nucleus (Martínez-Montiel et al., 2017). BRCA1-Δ11 lacks exon 11 and BRCA1-Δ11q only contains a partial sequence of exon 11 (Fig. 7.7) due to the use of an alternative 5′ donor splice site. This results in both these isoforms remaining in the cytoplasm and cannot bind to RAD51 and function in the repair of DNA. However, BRCA1-Δ11q can translocate to the nucleus in a noncanonical way. As such BRCA1-Δ11 acts as a tumor suppressor and mice lacking BRCA1-Δ11 develop gynecological related cancers.

The ability of BRCA1-Δ11q to translocate to the nucleus means that it can partially compensate when full-length BRCA1 is absent. The expression of this isoform is not only associated with a decrease in the repair of DNA, but BRCA1-Δ11 binds inefficiently to RAD51 which further decreases the DNA repair activity (Hube et al., 2006). The exclusive expression of BRCA1-Δ11q promotes cancer cell growth with this splicing variant being associated with tumorigenesis and drug resistance in breast cancer (Nielsen et al., 2016). The increased expression of the BRCA1-Δ11q isoform also increases resistance of breast cancer cells to the PARP inhibitor Olaparib and the increased expression of this isoform can be caused by germline mutations in the *BRCA1* gene (Paschalis et al., 2018; Siegfried & Karni, 2018).

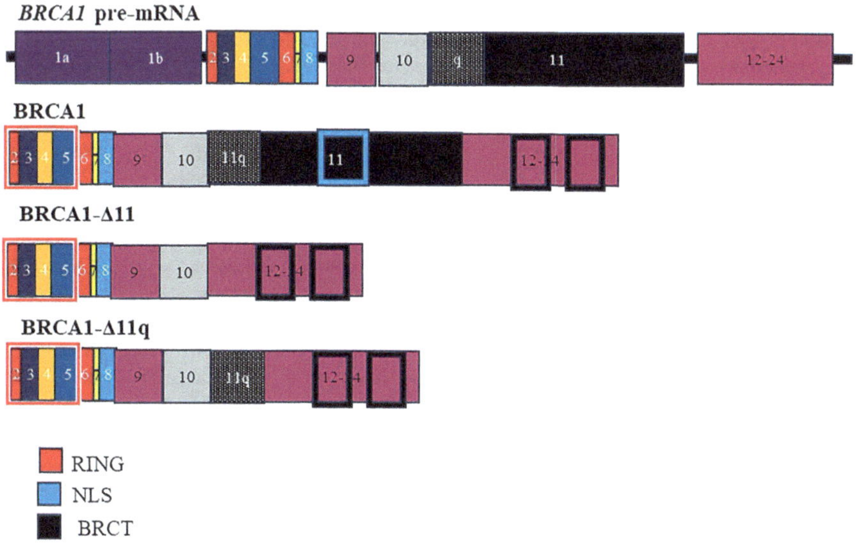

Fig. 7.7 *Splicing of the BRRCA1 pre-mRNA*. Exon 11 is the longest in the NRCA1 mRNA. A portion of this exon encodes the nuclear localization signal. Two isoforms of BRCA1 linked to drug resistance in breast cancer have altered expression of this exon. One isoform, BRCA1-Δ11, lacks this exon while BRCA1- Δ11q only contains a short segment of this exon, denoted as 11q. As a result, both these isoforms lack the signal to be translocated to the nucleus

CDK4/6 Inhibitors

CDK4, a target of both of the licensed breast cancer treatments palbociclib and ribociclib, is a cell cycle regulator thar controls the G_1/S phase transition (Baker & Reddy, 2012). An alternative transcript of CDK4, lacking exons 1, 2, and 7, is referred to as ENST00000547281. Li et al. have shown that in breast cancer, sensitivity to the CDK4/6 inhibitors palbociclib and ribociclib correlates with ENST00000547281 expression more so than the CDK4 gene. They further went on to show that ENST00000547281 significantly increased ribociclib resistance in cell culture, showing that the correlation seen in patients is likely to be mechanistic in nature.

Table 7.1 shows alternatively spliced transcripts and their role in treatment resistance.

Table 7.1 Alternatively spliced transcripts and their role in treatment resistance

Gene	Isoforms	Splicing effect	Effect	Reference
SRPK splicing factor kinases	BARD1, BCL2L1, and MCL-1	Various	Resistance to treatment	Lin et al. (2014)
Cyclin D1	Cyclin D1b	Exon skipping	Anti-estrogen therapy	Wang et al. (2008)
Ncor2 nuclear receptor co-repressor 2	BQ323636.1	ETSS, exon skipping	Tamoxifen	Tsoi et al. (2023)
ERα estrogen receptor alpha	ERα66, ERα46, and ERα36	Alternate promoter and exon skipping	Tamoxifen	Huber-Keener et al. (2012)
NR3C1 glucocorticoid receptor	GRα and GRβ	Noncanonical exon	Endocrine therapy resistance	Read and Natrajan (2018)
Mena	Mena^{INV}	Noncanonical exon	RTK inhibitors	Hughes et al. (2015)
FGFR1 fibroblast growth factor Receptor1	FGFR1β/FGFR1α skipping/inclusion of exon 3	Exon skipping	Resistance to treatment	Zhao et al. (2019)
Her2	Δ16HER2, Δ15HER2, Herstatin, p100HER2, X5-HER2, HER2-PI9, and HER2-I12	Exon skipping in Δ16HER2	Taxane resistance	Aigner et al. (2001)
Xbp1	XBP1s, XBP1u	Alternative 3′ and 5; splice sites and noncanonical exon	Tamoxifen	Ming et al. (2015)
BIRC5 baculoviral IAP repeat containing 5, Survivin	Survivin 2B, survivin 2α, survivin 3B, survivin ΔEx3, and survivin 3α	Exon skipping, noncanonical exon and alternate termination site	Arsenic trioxide and other cytotoxic compounds	Laka et al. (2019)

(continued)

Table 1 (continued)

Gene	Isoforms	Splicing effect	Effect	Reference
Wt1 Wilms tumor 1	Isoforms 1–4	Exon skipping and alternate 3; splice site	Cytotoxic compounds	Renshaw et al. (2004)
RSRC2 (Arginine and serine-rich coiled coil protein 2)	RSRC2s to RSRC2	Alternative promoter	Paclitaxel resistance	
ECT2 MYB-like transcription factor ETC2	ECT2-Ex5+ inclusion of exon 5	Mutually exclusive exon	Doxorubicin resistance	Tanaka et al. (2020)
BRCA1	BRCA as well as the two spice variants BRCA1-Δ11 and BRCA1-Δ11q	Exon skipping and alternate splice sites	PARP inhibitors	Paschalis et al. (2018)

Dysregulation of Splicing Machinery in Drug-Resistant Breast Cancer

Mutations, alterations in the expression of or the expression of isoforms of components of the spliceosome are common in breast cancer. In addition to these splicing factors, splicing regulators or associated proteins may also be dysregulated. All this can result in disruptions to the canonical splicing mechanisms.

SF3b

The splicing factor SF3B3 is overexpressed in aggressive ER+ breast cancers and is associated with tamoxifen resistance. This protein is a member of the SF3B complex in the larger U2 complex (Gökmen-Polar et al., 2015) and can alter pre-mRNA splicing and alter gene expression (Garcia-Blanco et al., 2004). The overexpression of SF3B3 observed in basal-like breast cancers (Srihari et al., 2016) and is thought to lead to aberrant splicing in these cells. For instance, the Enhancer of zeste homolog 2, a histone-lysine N-methyltransferase, undergoes alternate splicing to give rise to 2 isoforms. One full-length and the other a shorter isoform which is more commonly expressed in healthy tissue. The full-length EZH2 promotes proliferation and is the isoform found overexpressed in cancer tissue. The shorter EZH2Δ14 from normal tissue does not promote proliferation (Chen et al., 2017).

HnRNP

The hnRNP K and the hnRNP F/H family of splicing factors regulate the splicing of the Myeloid cell leukemia-1 (Mcl −1) protein. This protein is a member of the Bcl-2 family and is involved in the control of the intrinsic apoptotic pathway. MCL-1 is frequently overexpressed in breast cancer where it is associated with poor prognosis and drug resistance. *Mcl-1* mRNA undergoes alternative splicing to generate two transcripts coding for two proteins. These isoforms are functionally distinct, an anti-apoptotic isoform named Mcl-1_L and the pro-apoptotic isoform named Mcl-1_S. These isoforms differ in the retention of exon 2 which is included in Mcl-1_L and excluded in Mcl-1. Decreased or knocked down expression of hnRNP K and hnRNP F/H leads to a splicing switch to the pro-apoptotic Mcl-1_S (Tyson-Capper & Gautrey, 2018).

PRP4K

The pre-mRNA processing factor 4 kinase (PRP4K) protein is a Clk/Sty kinase family member that is a component of the spliceosome where it is involved in pre-mRNA splicing and phosphorylates SF2/ASF. This protein is encoded by the *PRPF4B* gene (Corkery et al., 2015a), and was discovered as a mutation in *Schizosaccharomyces pombe* associated with splicing defects (Rosenberg et al., 1991; Alimonti et al., 2010).

The protein consists of an N-terminal domain that is rich in lysine and histidine (KKHK), arginine serine (RS)-rich protein domains, and a C-terminal dual-specificity kinase domain (Dellaire et al., 2002). Breast cancers with reduced levels of PRP4K are associated with decreased rates of overall survival (Cho et al., 2018; Corkery et al., 2015b; Corkery et al., 2018).

PRP4K expression is regulated by HER2 in breast cancer, with increased levels of PRP4K being associated with increased sensitivity of breast cancer cells to paclitaxel (Corkery et al., 2015a). PRP4K expression can also be regulated by estrogen, as a study demonstrated a reduction in the levels of PRP4K occurred when MCF7 breast cancer cells were treated with tamoxifen. This treatment not only reduced the levels of PRP4K but also increased the resistance of the cells to multiple taxanes (Lahsaee et al., 2016). The role played by PRP4K in regulating SAC means that decreased expression or inhibition of PRP4K can prevent mitotic arrest on cells treated with anti-mitotic agents (Montembault et al., 2007). Breast cancer cell lines with decreased levels of PRP4K did not undergo cell cycle arrest in metaphase and showed signs of "mitotic slippage" by entering interphase without the preceding cell division (Corkery et al., 2015a).

TRA2α

Paclitaxel resistance in triple-negative breast cancer (TNBC) may also be associated with aberrant alternative splicing regulated by the *Transformer-2 protein homolog. There are two separate gene paralogs of this gene, named alpha and beta* (TRA2α and TRA2β). The expression of TRA2B is upregulated in TNBC cells where it promotes cancer cell survival and is associated with paclitaxel-sensitive tumors. TRA2B is less commonly expressed and is associated with cancer cell proliferation, survival, migration, and invasion. However, this paralog promotes paclitaxel resistance in TNBC through its regulation of cancer-related splicing such as the splicing of genes such as CALU, PALM, and RSRC2 (Liu et al., 2017). The Arginine and serine-rich coiled coil protein 2 (RSRC2) is normally expressed as the RSRC2s isoform. This isoform of RSRC2 has been found to inhibit proliferation in esophageal cancer cells (Kurehara et al., 2007). The increased presence of TRA2A leads to a shift to the RSRC2 isoform to the RSRC2l isoform as a result of TRA2A binding to the upstream intronic sequence of exon4. Overexpression of TRA2β in TNBC cell lines leads to an increase in the expression of cancer promoting isoforms that also promote resistance to TAM (Liu et al., 2017).

Counteractive Strategies

The presence or abundance of specific isoforms can be targeted by targeting these isoforms using specific small oligonucleotides to decrease the expression of these isoforms or the proteins can themselves be targeted using inhibitors specific for certain isoforms. In addition to this the splicing factors or those proteins that regulate them can be targeted to change the alternate splicing patterns within a cancer cell (Lee & Abdel-Wahab, 2016).

Small molecules capable of modulating splicing are a source of great interest as potential therapies to treat breast cancer. These include natural products and their synthetic derivatives which can bind to spliceosome components. This includes pladienolide and its derivative E7107, meyamycins and pladienolide, all of which target the SF3b1 subunit. Other small molecule inhibitors can target splicing factors. Examples of this type include Spliceostatin A, which once again functions by targeting SF3b (Kaida et al., 2007). The targets of these drugs include protein arginine *N*-methyltransferase 5 (PRMT5). These include molecules such as JNJ-64619178, GSK3326595 (Siu et al., 2019), and PF-06939999. For example, caspase 9 is alternatively spliced to give rise to multiple isoforms. Some of these isoforms have opposing functions to the wild-type caspase 9 and can act to inhibit apoptosis (Schwerk & Schulze-Osthoff, 2005). Small molecules such as ceramide and emetine can inhibit the synthesis of the pro-apoptotic isoform of caspase9 (Chalfant et al., 2002; Grollman, 1968).

Another strategy involves the use of Splice-Switching Oligonucleotides (SSOs) which can be used to alter splicing by selective splice site usage (Fig. 7.8). SSOs are synthetic oligonucleotides that range between 15 and 30 nucleotides in length which may also contain nucleotide analogs. They are designed to be complementary to a target complementary pre-mRNA sequence where they create a steric block preventing splicing factors from binding. This alters the ability of the spliceosome components to recognize splice sites, altering or switching splicing from one transcript to another (Havens & Hastings, 2016). Nuclease-resistant antisense

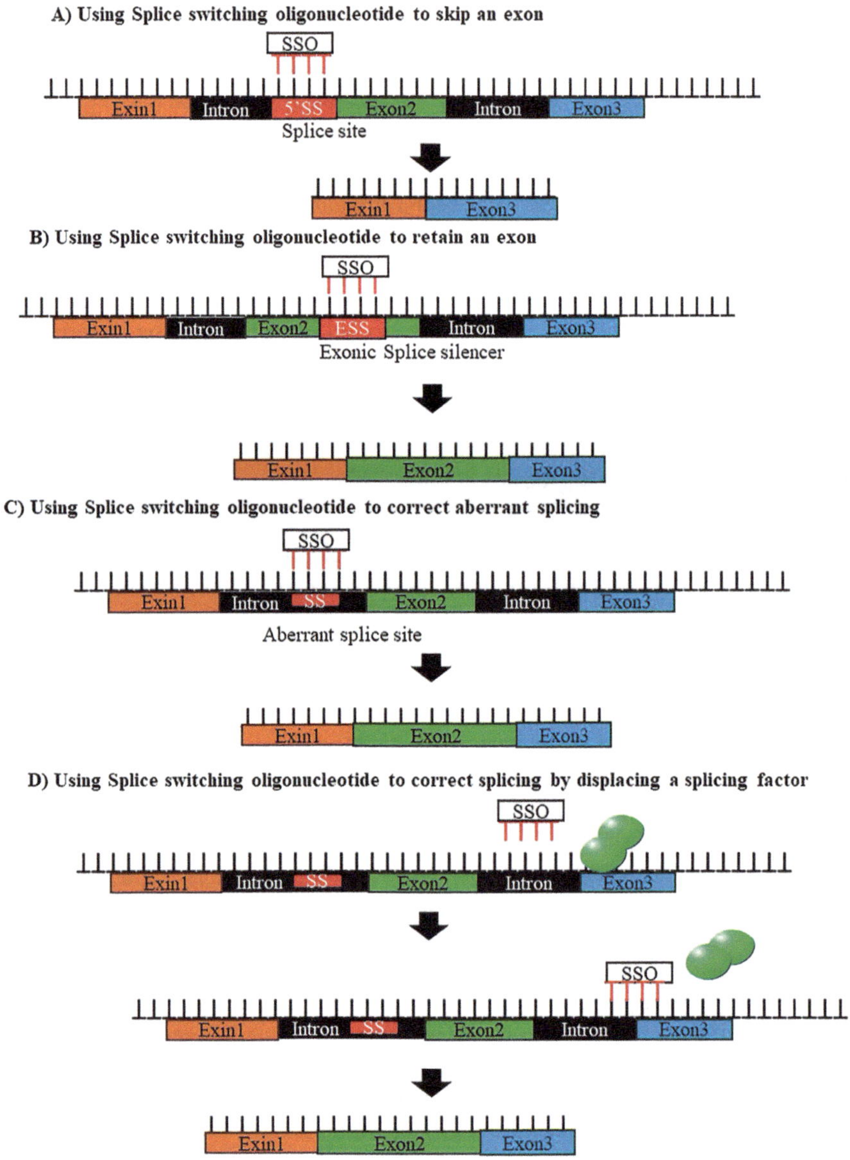

Fig. 7.8 *Splice-switching oligonucleotides as therapeutic strategy to favor the expression of drug-sensitive isoforms*. The oligonucleotide function is due to the presence of multiple splicing splice sites which can be either blocked using oligonucleotides with a sequence complementary to these sites. This can be used to (**a**) block splice sites to slip the inclusion of an exon (**b**) block splice silencing sites to include an exon (**c**) Block a mutation site that can lead to aberrant splicing or (**d**) prevent the binding of a splicing factor

oligonucleotide targeting isoforms of the *WT1* mRNA containing exon 5 resulted in increased levels of cell death in cytotoxic drug-resistant cells following treatment with cytotoxic agents (Renshaw et al., 2004).

Therapeutic Strategies Targeting the Spliceosome

Disruption of spliceosome proteins is an attractive target for the treatment of breast cancer. Examples of this are the inhibitors spliceostatin A, pladienolides (E7107), and meyamycin analogs. These are all SF3B-specific inhibitors (Lee & Abdel-Wahab, 2016) that inhibit canonical splicing (Kaida et al., 2007). Knockdown of SF3B3 in *sfb3* mutants that lead to SF3B3-overexpression reduced tumor growth (Chen et al., 2017). Sensitivity to spliceosomal inhibitors is increased in cells with *Sf3b1* mutants (Maguire et al., 2015; Obeng et al., 2016). SF3b inhibition in cells with *SF3B1* mutations which change the function of SF3b leads to changes in the pattern of splicing events (Maguire et al., 2015). This means that mutations in various spliceosomal components can be targeted using inhibitors for therapeutic interventions. Apart from SF3b mutations other splicing component mutations that can be targeted by spliceosomal inhibitors include SRSF2 mutations (Lee & Abdel-Wahab, 2016) and U2AF1 mutations (Shirai et al., 2015). The compound H3B-8800 inhibits the SF3b complex and was undergoing preclinical studies in 2018 to assess its effectiveness as an inhibitor of cancer growth and survival in tumors harbouring mutations in spliceosome components (Seiler et al., 2018). The results of this clinical trial demonstrated that the drug was able to bind to its target in a dose-dependent manner and alter splicing. The drug also demonstrated a high degree of safety (Steensma et al., 2019).

SRSF protein kinase 1 (SRPK1) regulates SRSF5 and SRSF1 activity through phosphorylation, thereby inhibiting SSF5. Decreased expression and activity of SRSF5 is linked to TAM resistance and increased metastasis. As such SRPK1 can be targeted for therapeutic intervention using molecules of the SPHINX family (Batson et al) or derivatives of Alectinib such as SRPKIN-1, a small SRPK1 inhibitor, both of which decrease the phosphorylation of both SRSF5 and SRSF1. This allows the splicing factor to perform its function, such as increasing the expression of the full-length NCOR2 isoform in breast cancer and reversing TAM resistance associated with the expression of the BQ isoform (Tsoi et al., 2023).

Aberrant alternative splicing can also be induced through the treatment of cancers with chemotherapeutic drugs, leading to the expression of isoforms that promote cancer cell survival. These genes could be involved in processes such as apoptosis, DNA damage, and drug metabolism (Lu & Chao, 2012; Siegfried & Karni, 2018). An example of this is cisplatin treatment altering the splicing events mediated by SRSF4, to induce apoptosis (Gabriel et al., 2015).

Limitations to Targeting Splicing for Therapeutic Interventions or As Biomarkers

Despite the promise offered by targeting alternative splicing in breast cancer for drug resistance strategies, there are limitations to these approaches. The major limitation to targeting core spliceosome components is the non-specific and toxic effects that the targeting of these components can result in. This is due to the disruption of the early stages of spliceosome assembly that some of these approaches result in. These toxic effects can be overcome by focusing on more specific splicing factors or targets (Bashari et al., 2023). The anti-cancer drug E7107 targets the SF3b complex, preventing duplex formation between the branch point-binding region of the U2 component of the spliceosome and the mRNA, preventing splicing. However, clinical trials have shown that unexpected toxicity resulted in the treatment of solid tumors despite the drug being on target and disrupting splicing. This toxicity manifested as bilateral optic neuritis (Eskens et al., 2013; Hong et al., 2014).

Conclusion

The prevalence of splicing alterations in breast cancer have been shown in multiple studies. The fact that these splice variants can not only promote the development and progression of cancer, but also promote resistance to various treatments, highlights splicing switches as a potential avenue for the development of new therapies. These therapies can be based on either reversing these splicing switches, targeting these new isoforms or even inhibiting components of the splicing machinery to cause a large-scale change in the splicing pattern of breast cancers. However due to the vital role played by mRNA splicing in the normal functioning of the cell, non-specific or extreme alterations or inhibition of the splicing machinery will result in these therapies being toxic or preventing the normal splicing of mRNA. Despite this as the study of splicing events advances through the use of new technologies such as next generation sequencing, more specific small molecule inhibitors, splice switching oligonucleotides and inhibitors of specific splicing factors can be developed. This will lessen any non-specific toxic effects these treatments will have.

References

Aigner, A., Juhl, H., Malerczyk, C., Tkybusch, A., Benz, C. C., & Czubayko, F. (2001). Expression of a truncated 100 kDa HER2 splice variant acts as an endogenous inhibitor of tumour cell proliferation. *Oncogene, 20*, 2101–2111.

Alimonti, A., Carracedo, A., Clohessy, J. G., Trotman, L. C., Nardella, C., Egia, A., et al. (2010). Subtle variations in Pten dose determine cancer susceptibility. *Nature Genetics, 42*, 454–458.

Alt, J. R., Cleveland, J. L., Hannink, M., & Diehl, J. A. (2000). Phosphorylation-dependent regulation of cyclin D1 nuclear export and cyclin D1-dependent cellular transformation. *Genes & Development, 14*, 3102–3114.

Antonova, L., Aronson, K., & Mueller, C. R. (2011). Stress and breast cancer: From epidemiology to molecular biology. *Breast Cancer Research, 13*, 208.

Baker, S. J., & Reddy, E. P. (2012). CDK4: A key player in the cell cycle, development, and cancer. *Genes & Cancer, 3*, 658–669.

Ball, L. J., Jarchau, T., Oschkinat, H., & Walter, U. (2002). EVH1 domains: Structure, function and interactions. *FEBS Letters, 513*, 45–52.

Bartkova, J., Lukas, J., Müller, H., Lützhøft, D., Strauss, M., & Bartek, J. (1994). Cyclin D1 protein expression and function in human breast cancer. *International Journal of Cancer, 57*, 353–361.

Bashari, A., Siegfried, Z., & Karni, R. J. R. (2023). Targeting splicing factors for cancer therapy. *RNA, 29*, 506–515.

Bear, J. E., & Gertler, F. B. (2009). Ena/VASP: Towards resolving a pointed controversy at the barbed end. *Journal of Cell Science, 122*, 1947–1953.

Bear, J. E., & Haugh, J. M. (2014). Directed migration of mesenchymal cells: Where signaling and the cytoskeleton meet. *Current Opinion in Cell Biology, 30*, 74–82.

Breitsprecher, D., Kiesewetter, A. K., Linkner, J., Vinzenz, M., Stradal, T. E., Small, J. V., et al. (2011). Molecular mechanism of Ena/VASP-mediated actin-filament elongation. *The EMBO Journal, 30*, 456–467.

Buoso, E., Ronfani, M., Galasso, M., Ventura, D., Corsini, E., & Racchi, M. (2019). Cortisol-induced SRSF3 expression promotes GR splicing, RACK1 expression and breast cancer cells migration. *Pharmacological Research, 143*, 17–26.

Chalfant, C. E., Rathman, K., Pinkerman, R. L., Wood, R. E., Obeid, L. M., Ogretmen, B., et al. (2002). De novo ceramide regulates the alternative splicing of caspase 9 and Bcl-x in A549 lung adenocarcinoma cells: DEPENDENCE ON PROTEIN PHOSPHATASE-1∗. *Mechanisms of Signal Transduction, 277*, 12587–12595.

Chantalat, E., Boudou, F., Laurell, H., Palierne, G., Houtman, R., Melchers, D., et al. (2016). The AF-1-deficient estrogen receptor ERα46 isoform is frequently expressed in human breast tumors. *Breast Cancer Research, 18*, 123.

Chen, F., Watson, C. S., & Gametchu, B. (1999). Association of the glucocorticoid receptor alternatively-spliced transcript 1A with the presence of the high molecular weight membrane glucocorticoid receptor in mouse lymphoma cells. *Journal of Cellular Biochemistry, 74*, 430–446.

Chen, K., Xiao, H., Zeng, J., Yu, G., Zhou, H., Huang, C., et al. (2017). Alternative splicing of EZH2 pre-mRNA by SF3B3 contributes to the tumorigenic potential of renal cancer. *Clinical Cancer Research, 23*, 3428–3441.

Cheng, Y., Chang, L. W., & Tsou, T. C. (2006). Mitogen-activated protein kinases mediate arsenic-induced down-regulation of survivin in human lung adenocarcinoma cells. *Archives of Toxicology, 80*, 310–318.

Cho, Y. S., Zhu, J., Li, S., Wang, B., Han, Y., & Jiang, J. (2018). Regulation of Yki/Yap subcellular localization and Hpo signaling by a nuclear kinase PRP4K. *Nature Communications, 9*, 1657.

Corkery, D. P., Holly, A. C., Lahsaee, S., & Dellaire, G. (2015a). Connecting the speckles: Splicing kinases and their role in tumorigenesis and treatment response. *Nucleus, 6*, 279–288.

Corkery, D. P., Le Page, C., Meunier, L., Provencher, D., Mes-Masson, A. M., & Dellaire, G. (2015b). PRP4K is a HER2-regulated modifier of taxane sensitivity. *Cell Cycle, 14*, 1059–1069.

Corkery, D. P., Clarke, L. E., Gebremeskel, S., Salsman, J., Pinder, J., Le Page, C., et al. (2018). Loss of PRP4K drives anoikis resistance in part by dysregulation of epidermal growth factor receptor endosomal trafficking. *Oncogene, 37*, 174–184.

Coumar, M. S., Tsai, F. Y., Kanwar, J. R., Sarvagalla, S., & Cheung, C. H. (2013). Treat cancers by targeting survivin: Just a dream or future reality? *Cancer Treatment Reviews, 39*, 802–811.

Davies, M. P., Barraclough, D. L., Stewart, C., Joyce, K. A., Eccles, R. M., Barraclough, R., et al. (2008). Expression and splicing of the unfolded protein response gene XBP-1 are significantly associated with clinical outcome of endocrine-treated breast cancer. *International Journal of Cancer, 123*, 85–88.

Dellaire, G., Makarov, E. M., Cowger, J. J., Longman, D., Sutherland, H. G., Lührmann, R., et al. (2002). Mammalian PRP4 kinase copurifies and interacts with components of both the U5 snRNP and the N-CoR deacetylase complexes. *Molecular and Cellular Biology, 22*, 5141–5156.

Di Leo, A., Chan, S., Paesmans, M., Friedrichs, K., Pinter, T., Cocquyt, V., et al. (2004). HER-2/neu as a predictive marker in a population of advanced breast cancer patients randomly treated either with single-agent doxorubicin or single-agent docetaxel. *Breast Cancer Research and Treatment, 86*, 197–206.

Ding, L., Yan, J., Zhu, J., Zhong, H., Lu, Q., Wang, Z., Huang, C., & Ye, Q. (2003). Ligand-independent activation of estrogen receptor alpha by XBP-1. *Nucleic Acids Research, 31*, 5266–5274.

Duncan, J. A., Reeves, J. R., & Cooke, T. G. (1998). BRCA1 and BRCA2 proteins: Roles in health and disease. *Molecular Pathology, 51*, 237–247.

Eskens, F. A., Ramos, F. J., Burger, H., O'brien, J. P., Piera, A., De Jonge, M. J., et al. (2013). Phase I pharmacokinetic and pharmacodynamic study of the first-in-class spliceosome inhibitor E7107 in patients with advanced solid tumors. *Clinical Cancer Research, 19*, 6296–6304.

Ewen, M. E., Sluss, H. K., Sherr, C. J., Matsushime, H., Kato, J., & Livingston, D. M. (1993). Functional interactions of the retinoblastoma protein with mammalian D-type cyclins. *Cell, 73*, 487–497.

Fang, Y., Yan, J., Ding, L., Liu, Y., Zhu, J., Huang, C., Zhao, H., et al. (2004). XBP-1 increases ERalpha transcriptional activity through regulation of large-scale chromatin unfolding. *Biochemical and Biophysical Research Communications, 323*, 269–274.

Gabriel, M., Delforge, Y., Deward, A., Habraken, Y., Hennuy, B., Piette, J., Klinck, R., Chabot, B., et al. (2015). Role of the splicing factor SRSF4 in cisplatin-induced modifications of pre-mRNA splicing and apoptosis. *BMC Cancer, 15*, 227.

Garcia-Blanco, M. A., Baraniak, A. P., & Lasda, E. L. (2004). Alternative splicing in disease and therapy. *Nature Biotechnology, 22*, 535–546.

Gerber, B., Müller, H., Reimer, T., Krause, A., & Friese, K. (2003). Nutrition and lifestyle factors on the risk of developing breast cancer. *Breast Cancer Research and Treatment, 79*, 265–276.

Gertler, F., & Condeelis, J. (2011). Metastasis: Tumor cells becoming MENAcing. *Trends in Cell Biology, 21*, 81–90.

Gertler, F. B., Niebuhr, K., Reinhard, M., Wehland, J., & Soriano, P. (1996). Mena, a relative of VASP and drosophila enabled, is implicated in the control of microfilament dynamics. *Cell, 87*, 227–239.

Gökmen-Polar, Y., Neelamraju, Y., Goswami, C. P., Gu, X., Nallamothu, G., Janga, S. C., & Badve, S. (2015). Expression levels of SF3B3 correlate with prognosis and endocrine resistance in estrogen receptor-positive breast cancer. *Modern Pathology, 28*, 677–685.

Gökmen-Polar, Y., Neelamraju, Y., Goswami, C. P., Gu, Y., Gu, X., Nallamothu, G., et al. (2019). Splicing factor ESRP1 controls ER-positive breast cancer by altering metabolic pathways. *EMBO Reports, 20*, e46078.

Grollman, A. P. (1968). Inhibitors of protein biosynthesis. V. Effects of emetine on protein and nucleic acid biosynthesis in HeLa cells. *The Journal of Biological Chemistry, 243*, 4089–4094.

Han, P., Zhu, J., Feng, G., Wang, Z., & Ding, Y. (2021). Characterization of alternative splicing events and prognostic signatures in breast cancer. *BMC Cancer, 21*, 587.

Hankinson, S. E., Colditz, G. A., & Willett, W. C. (2004). Towards an integrated model for breast cancer etiology: The lifelong interplay of genes, lifestyle, and hormones. *Breast Cancer Research, 6*, 1–6.

Harbuz, M. S., & Lightman, S. L. (1992). Stress and the hypothalamo-pituitary-adrenal axis: Acute, chronic and immunological activation. *The Journal of Endocrinology, 134*, 327–339.

Hart, V., Gautrey, H., Kirby, J., & Tyson-Capper, A. (2020). HER2 splice variants in breast cancer: investigating their impact on diagnosis and treatment outcomes. *Oncotarget, 11*, 4338–4357.

Havens, M. A., & Hastings, M. L. (2016). Splice-switching antisense oligonucleotides as therapeutic drugs. *Nucleic Acids Research, 44*, 6549–6563.

He, D., Xiang, J., Li, B., & Liu, H. (2016). The dynamic behavior of Ect2 in response to DNA damage. *Scientific Reports, 6*, 24504.

Herr, I., Gassler, N., Friess, H., & Büchler, M. W. (2007). Regulation of differential pro- and anti-apoptotic signaling by glucocorticoids. *Apoptosis, 12*, 271–291.

Herynk, M. H., & Fuqua, S. A. (2004). Estrogen receptor mutations in human disease. *Endocrine Reviews, 25*, 869–898.

Hoffman, E. A., Gizelska, K., Mirowski, M., & Mielicki, W. (2015). Arsenic trioxide downregulates cancer procoagulant activity in MCF-7 and WM-115 cell lines in vitro. *Contemp Oncol (Pozn), 19*, 108–112.

Homo-Delarche, F., Fitzpatrick, F., Christeff, N., Nunez, E. A., Bach, J. F., & Dardenne, M. (1991). Sex steroids, glucocorticoids, stress and autoimmunity. *The Journal of Steroid Biochemistry and Molecular Biology, 40*, 619–637.

Hong, D. S., Kurzrock, R., Naing, A., Wheler, J. J., Falchook, G. S., Schiffman, J. S., et al. (2014). A phase I, open-label, single-arm, dose-escalation study of E7107, a precursor messenger ribonucleic acid (pre-mRNA) splicesome inhibitor administered intravenously on days 1 and 8 every 21 days to patients with solid tumors. *Investigational New Drugs, 32*, 436–444.

Hosokawa, Y., Gadd, M., Smith, A. P., Koerner, F. C., Schmidt, E. V., & Arnold, A. (1997). Cyclin D1 (PRAD1) alternative transcript b: Full-length cDNA cloning and expression in breast cancers. *Cancer Letters, 113*, 123–130.

Hube, F., Guo, J., Chooniedass-Kothari, S., Cooper, C., Hamedani, M., Dibrov, A., et al. (2006). Alternative splicing of the first intron of the steroid receptor RNA activator (SRA) participates in the generation of coding and noncoding RNA isoforms in breast cancer cell lines. *DNA Cell Biol, 25*, 418–428.

Huber-Keener, K. J. (2022). Cancer genetics and breast cancer. *Best Practice & Research. Clinical Obstetrics & Gynaecology, 82*, 3–11.

Huber-Keener, K. J., Liu, X., Wang, Z., Wang, Y., Freeman, W., Wu, S., et al. (2012). Differential gene expression in tamoxifen-resistant breast cancer cells revealed by a new analytical model of RNA-Seq data. *PLoS One, 7*, e41333.

Hughes, S. K., Oudin, M. J., Tadros, J., Neil, J., Del Rosario, A., Joughin, B. A., et al. (2015). PTP1B-dependent regulation of receptor tyrosine kinase signaling by the actin-binding protein Mena. *Molecular Biology of the Cell, 26*, 3867–3878.

Hunt, H. J., Belanoff, J. K., Walters, I., Gourdet, B., Thomas, J., Barton, N., et al. (2017). Identification of the clinical candidate (R)-(1-(4-fluorophenyl)-6-((1-methyl-1H-pyrazol-4-yl) sulfonyl)-4,4a,5,6,7,8-hexahydro-1H-pyrazolo[3,4-g]isoquinolin-4a-yl)(4-(trifluoromethyl) pyridin-2-yl)methanone (CORT125134): A selective glucocorticoid receptor (GR) antagonist. *Journal of Medicinal Chemistry, 60*, 3405–3421.

Ibáñez-Costa, A., Perez-Sanchez, C., Patiño-Trives, A., Luque-Tevar, M., Font, P., Arias De La Rosa, I., et al. (2022). Splicing machinery is impaired in rheumatoid arthritis, associated with disease activity and modulated by anti-TNF therapy. *Annals of the Rheumatic Diseases, 81*, 56–67.

Inoue, K., & Fry, E. (2015). Aberrant splicing of estrogen receptor, HER2, and CD44 genes in breast cancer. *Genetics & Epigenetics, 7*, 19–32.

Jackson, C., Browell, D., Gautrey, H., & Tyson-Capper, A. (2013). Clinical significance of HER-2 splice variants in breast cancer progression and drug resistance. *International Journal of Cell Biology, 2013*, 973584.

Kadmiel, M., & Cidlowski, J. A. (2013). Glucocorticoid receptor signaling in health and disease. *Trends in Pharmacological Sciences, 34*, 518–530.

Kaida, D., Motoyoshi, H., Tashiro, E., Nojima, T., Hagiwara, M., Ishigami, K., et al. (2007). Spliceostatin a targets SF3b and inhibits both splicing and nuclear retention of pre-mRNA. *Nature Chemical Biology, 3*, 576–583.

Kalinina, J., Dutta, K., Ilghari, D., Beenken, A., Goetz, R., Eliseenkova, A. V., Cowburn, D., & Mohammadi, M. (2012). The alternatively spliced acid box region plays a key role in FGF receptor autoinhibition. *Structure, 20*, 77–88.

Klinge, C. M., Riggs, K. A., Wickramasinghe, N. S., Emberts, C. G., Mcconda, D. B., Barry, P. N., & Magnusen, J. E. (2010). Estrogen receptor alpha 46 is reduced in tamoxifen resistant breast cancer cells and re-expression inhibits cell proliferation and estrogen receptor alpha 66-regulated target gene transcription. *Molecular and Cellular Endocrinology, 323*, 268–276.

Knudsen, K. E. (2006). The cyclin D1b splice variant: An old oncogene learns new tricks. *Cell Div, 1*, 15.

Knudsen, K. E., Diehl, J. A., Haiman, C. A., & Knudsen, E. S. (2006). Cyclin D1: Polymorphism, aberrant splicing and cancer risk. *Oncogene, 25*, 1620–1628.

Kurehara, H., Ishiguro, H., Kimura, M., Mitsui, A., Ando, T., Sugito, N., et al. (2007). A novel gene, RSRC2, inhibits cell proliferation and affects survival in esophageal cancer patients. *International Journal of Oncology, 30*, 421–428.

Lahsaee, S., Corkery, D. P., Anthes, L. E., Holly, A., & Dellaire, G. (2016). Estrogen receptor alpha (ESR1)-signaling regulates the expression of the taxane-response biomarker PRP4K. *Experimental Cell Research, 340*, 125–131.

Laka, K., Makgoo, L., & Mbita, Z. (2019). Survivin splice variants in arsenic trioxide (As_2O_3)-induced deactivation of PI3K and MAPK cell signalling pathways in MCF-7 cells. *Genes (Basel), 10*, 41.

Lee, S. C., & Abdel-Wahab, O. (2016). Therapeutic targeting of splicing in cancer. *Nature Medicine, 22*, 976–986.

Li, L., Haynes, M. P., & Bender, J. R. (2003). Plasma membrane localization and function of the estrogen receptor alpha variant (ER46) in human endothelial cells. *Proceedings of the National Academy of Sciences of the United States of America, 100*, 4807–4812.

Lin, J. C., Lin, C. Y., Tarn, W. Y., & Li, F. Y. (2014). Elevated SRPK1 lessens apoptosis in breast cancer cells through RBM4-regulated splicing events. *RNA, 20*, 1621–1631.

Liu, Z. M., Tseng, H. Y., Cheng, Y. L., Yeh, B. W., Wu, W. J., & Huang, H. S. (2015). TG-interacting factor transcriptionally induced by AKT/FOXO3A is a negative regulator that antagonizes arsenic trioxide-induced cancer cell apoptosis. *Toxicology and Applied Pharmacology, 285*, 41–50.

Liu, T., Sun, H., Zhu, D., Dong, X., Liu, F., Liang, X., et al. (2017). TRA2A promoted paclitaxel resistance and tumor progression in triple-negative breast cancers via regulating alternative splicing. *Molecular Cancer Therapeutics, 16*, 1377–1388.

Lu, H. P., & Chao, C. C. (2012). Cancer cells acquire resistance to anticancer drugs: An update. *Biomedical Journal, 35*, 464–472.

Lu, F., Gladden, A. B., & Diehl, J. A. (2003). An alternatively spliced cyclin D1 isoform, cyclin D1b, is a nuclear oncogene. *Cancer Research, 63*, 7056–7061.

Luqmani, Y. A., Mortimer, C., Yiangou, C., Johnston, C. L., Bansal, G. S., Sinnett, D., et al. (1995). Expression of 2 variant forms of fibroblast growth factor receptor 1 in human breast. *International Journal of Cancer, 64*, 274–279.

Madigan, M. P., Ziegler, R. G., Benichou, J., Byrne, C., & Hoover, R. N. (1995). Proportion of breast cancer cases in the United States explained by well-established risk factors. *Journal of the National Cancer Institute, 87*, 1681–1685.

Maguire, S. L., Leonidou, A., Wai, P., Marchiò, C., Ng, C. K., Sapino, A., et al. (2015). SF3B1 mutations constitute a novel therapeutic target in breast cancer. *The Journal of Pathology, 235*, 571–580.

Manic, G., Sistigu, A., Corradi, F., Musella, M., De Maria, R., & Vitale, I. (2018). Replication stress response in cancer stem cells as a target for chemotherapy. *Seminars in Cancer Biology, 53*, 31–41.

Martínez-Montiel, N., Anaya-Ruiz, M., Pérez-Santos, M., & Martínez-Contreras, R. (2017). Alternative splicing in breast cancer and the potential development of therapeutic tools. *Genes (Basel), 8*, 217.

Matsushime, H., Quelle, D. E., Shurtleff, S. A., Shibuya, M., Sherr, C. J., & Kato, J. Y. (1994). D-type cyclin-dependent kinase activity in mammalian cells. *Molecular and Cellular Biology, 14*, 2066–2076.

Mcneil, C. M., Sergio, C. M., Anderson, L. R., Inman, C. K., Eggleton, S. A., Murphy, N. C., et al. (2006). C-Myc overexpression and endocrine resistance in breast cancer. *The Journal of Steroid Biochemistry and Molecular Biology, 102*, 147–155.

Millour, J., De Olano, N., Horimoto, Y., Monteiro, L. J., Langer, J. K., Aligue, R., Hajji, N., & Lam, E. W. (2011). ATM and p53 regulate FOXM1 expression via E2F in breast cancer epirubicin treatment and resistance. *Molecular Cancer Therapeutics, 10*, 1046–1058.

Ming, J., Ruan, S., Wang, M., Ye, D., Fan, N., Meng, Q., et al. (2015). A novel chemical, STF-083010, reverses tamoxifen-related drug resistance in breast cancer by inhibiting IRE1/XBP1. *Oncotarget, 6*, 40692–40703.

Montembault, E., Dutertre, S., Prigent, C., & Giet, R. (2007). PRP4 is a spindle assembly checkpoint protein required for MPS1, MAD1, and MAD2 localization to the kinetochores. *The Journal of Cell Biology, 179*, 601–609.

Neuman, E., Ladha, M. H., Lin, N., Upton, T. M., Miller, S. J., Direnzo, J., et al. (1997). Cyclin D1 stimulation of estrogen receptor transcriptional activity independent of cdk4. *Molecular and Cellular Biology, 17*, 5338–5347.

Nielsen, F., Van Overeem Hansen, T., & Sørensen, C. (2016). Hereditary breast and ovarian cancer: New genes in confined pathways. *Nature Reviews. Cancer, 16*, 599–612.

Noureddine, L. M., Trédan, O., Hussein, N., Badran, B., Le Romancer, M., & Poulard, C. (2021). Glucocorticoid receptor: A multifaceted actor in breast cancer. *International Journal of Molecular Sciences, 22*, 446.

Nürnberg, A., Kitzing, T., & Grosse, R. (2011). Nucleating actin for invasion. *Nature Reviews. Cancer, 11*, 177–187.

Obeng, E. A., Chappell, R. J., Seiler, M., Chen, M. C., Campagna, D. R., Schmidt, P. J., et al. (2016). Physiologic expression of Sf3b1(K700E) causes impaired erythropoiesis, aberrant splicing, and sensitivity to therapeutic spliceosome modulation. *Cancer Cell, 30*, 404–417.

Orban, T., & Olah, E. (2003). Emerging roles of BRCA1 alternative splicing. *Molecular Pathology, 56*, 191–197.

Orr, G. A., Verdier-Pinard, P., Mcdaid, H., & Horwitz, S. B. (2003). Mechanisms of Taxol resistance related to microtubules. *Oncogene, 22*, 7280–7295.

Papandreou, I., Denko, N. C., Olson, M., Van Melckebeke, H., Lust, S., Tam, A., Solow-Cordero, D. E., et al. (2011). Identification of an Ire1alpha endonuclease specific inhibitor with cytotoxic activity against human multiple myeloma. *Blood, 117*, 1311–1314.

Paschalis, A., Sharp, A., Welti, J. C., Neeb, A., Raj, G. V., Luo, J., Plymate, S. R., et al. (2018). Alternative splicing in prostate cancer. *Nature Reviews. Clinical Oncology, 15*, 663–675.

Perez, E. A., Suman, V. J., Rowland, K. M., Ingle, J. N., Salim, M., Loprinzi, C. L., et al. (2005). Two concurrent phase II trials of paclitaxel/carboplatin/trastuzumab (weekly or every-3-week schedule) as first-line therapy in women with HER2-overexpressing metastatic breast cancer: NCCTG study 983252. *Clinical Breast Cancer, 6*, 425–432.

Philippar, U., Roussos, E. T., Oser, M., Yamaguchi, H., Kim, H. D., Giampieri, S., et al. (2008). A Mena invasion isoform potentiates EGF-induced carcinoma cell invasion and metastasis. *Developmental Cell, 15*, 813–828.

Read, A., & Natrajan, R. (2018). Splicing dysregulation as a driver of breast cancer. *Endocrine-Related Cancer, 25*, R467–r478.

Reddy, K., & Glaros, S. (2007). AF-1 domain of ER α regulates the agonistic and antagonistic actions of tamoxifen. *Cancer Research, 67*, 997–997.

Renshaw, J., Orr, R. M., Walton, M. I., Te Poele, R., Williams, R. D., Wancewicz, E. V., et al. (2004). Disruption of WT1 gene expression and exon 5 splicing following cytotoxic drug treatment: Antisense down-regulation of exon 5 alters target gene expression and inhibits cell survival. *Molecular Cancer Therapeutics, 3*, 1467–1484.

Rosenberg, G. H., Alahari, S. K., & Käufer, N. F. (1991). prp4 from Schizosaccharomyces pombe, a mutant deficient in pre-mRNA splicing isolated using genes containing artificial introns. *Molecular & General Genetics, 226*, 305–309.

Roussos, E. T., Wang, Y., Wyckoff, J. B., Sellers, R. S., Wang, W., Li, J., et al. (2010). Mena deficiency delays tumor progression and decreases metastasis in polyoma middle-T transgenic mouse mammary tumors. *Breast Cancer Research, 12*, R101.

Roussos, E. T., Condeelis, J. S., & Patsialou, A. (2011). Chemotaxis in cancer. *Nature Reviews. Cancer, 11*, 573–587.

Schwerk, C., & Schulze-Osthoff, K. (2005). Regulation of apoptosis by alternative pre-mRNA splicing. *Molecular Cell, 19*, 1–13.

Seiler, M., Yoshimi, A., Darman, R., Chan, B., Keaney, G., & Thomas, M. (2018). H3B-8800, an orally available small-molecule splicing modulator, induces lethality in spliceosome-mutant cancers. *Nature Medicine, 24*, 497–504.

Semmler, L., Reiter-Brennan, C., & Klein, A. (2019). BRCA1 and breast cancer: A review of the underlying mechanisms resulting in the tissue-specific tumorigenesis in mutation carriers. *Journal of Breast Cancer, 22*, 1–14.

Shirai, C. L., Tripathi, M., Ley, J. N., Ndonwi, M., White, B. S., Tapia, R., Saez, B., et al. (2015). Preclinical activity of splicing modulators in U2AF1 mutant MDS/AML. *Blood, 126*, 1653.

Siegfried, Z., & Karni, R. (2018). The role of alternative splicing in cancer drug resistance. *Current Opinion in Genetics & Development, 48*, 16–21.

Siu, L. L., Rasco, D. W., Vinay, S. P., Romano, P. M., Menis, J., Opdam, F. L., et al. (2019). METEOR-1: A phase I study of GSK3326595, a first-in-class protein arginine methyltransferase 5 (PRMT5) inhibitor, in advanced solid tumours. *Annals of Oncology, 30*, v159.

Srihari, S., Kalimutho, M., Lal, S., Singla, J., Patel, D., Simpson, P. T., Khanna, K. K., et al. (2016). Understanding the functional impact of copy number alterations in breast cancer using a network modeling approach. *Molecular BioSystems, 12*, 963–972.

Steensma, D. P., Wermke, M., Klimek, V. M., Greenberg, P. L., Font, P., & Komrokji, R. S. (2019). Results of a clinical trial of H3B-8800, a splicing modulator, in patients with myelodysplastic syndromes (MDS), acute myeloid Leukemia (AML) or chronic myelomonocytic Leukemia (CMML). *Blood, 134*, 673–673.

Strehl, C., & Buttgereit, F. (2013). Optimized glucocorticoid therapy: Teaching old drugs new tricks. *Molecular and Cellular Endocrinology, 380*, 32–40.

Tanaka, I., Chakraborty, A., Saulnier, O., Benoit-Pilven, C., Vacher, S., & Labiod, D. (2020). ZRANB2 and SYF2-mediated splicing programs converging on ECT2 are involved in breast cancer cell resistance to doxorubicin. *Nucleic Acids Research, 48*, 2676–2693.

Taylor, S. E., Martin-Hirsch, P. L., & Martin, F. L. (2010). Oestrogen receptor splice variants in the pathogenesis of disease. *Cancer Letters, 288*, 133–148.

Tonin, P. N. (2000). Genes implicated in hereditary breast cancer syndromes. *Seminars in Surgical Oncology, 18*, 281–286.

Tsoi, H., Fung, N. N., Man, E. P. S., Leung, M. H., You, C. P., & Chan, W. L. (2023). SRSF5 regulates the expression of BQ323636.1 to modulate tamoxifen resistance in ER-positive breast cancer. *Cancers (Basel), 15*, 2271.

Tyson-Capper, A., & Gautrey, H. (2018). Regulation of mcl-1 alternative splicing by hnRNP F, H1 and K in breast cancer cells. *RNA Biology, 15*, 1448–1457.

Végran, F., Boidot, R., Oudin, C., Defrain, C., Rebucci, M., & Lizard-Nacol, S. (2007). Association of p53 gene alterations with the expression of antiapoptotic survivin splice variants in breast cancer. *Oncogene, 26*, 290–297.

Wahler, J., & Suh, N. (2015). Targeting HER2 positive breast cancer with Chemopreventive agents. *Curr Pharmacol Rep, 1*, 324–335.

Wang, B. D., & Lee, N. H. (2018). Aberrant RNA splicing in cancer and drug resistance. *Cancers (Basel), 10*, 458.

Wang, F., Kan, M., Yan, G., Xu, J., & Mckeehan, W. L. (1995). Alternately spliced NH2-terminal immunoglobulin-like loop I in the ectodomain of the fibroblast growth factor (FGF) receptor 1 lowers affinity for both heparin and FGF-1. *The Journal of Biological Chemistry, 270*, 10231–10235.

Wang, Y., Dean, J. L., Millar, E. K., Tran, T. H., Mcneil, C. M., & Burd, C. J. (2008). Cyclin D1b is aberrantly regulated in response to therapeutic challenge and promotes resistance to estrogen antagonists. *Cancer Research, 68*, 5628–5638.

Weikum, E. R., Knuesel, M. T., Ortlund, E. A., & Yamamoto, K. R. (2017). Glucocorticoid receptor control of transcription: Precision and plasticity via allostery. *Nature Reviews. Molecular Cell Biology, 18*, 159–174.

Wendt, M. K., Taylor, M. A., Schiemann, B. J., Sossey-Alaoui, K., & Schiemann, W. P. (2014). Fibroblast growth factor receptor splice variants are stable markers of oncogenic transforming growth factor β1 signaling in metastatic breast cancers. *Breast Cancer Research, 16*, R24.

Xu, Y., Huangyang, P., Wang, Y., Xue, L., Devericks, E., & Nguyen, H. G. (2021). ERα is an RNA-binding protein sustaining tumor cell survival and drug resistance. *Cell, 184*, 5215–5229.e17.

Yang, Q., Zhao, J., Zhang, W., Chen, D., & Wang, Y. (2019). Aberrant alternative splicing in breast cancer. *Journal of Molecular Cell Biology, 11*, 920–929.

Yasuhira, S., Shibazaki, M., Nishiya, M., & Maesawa, C. (2016). Paclitaxel-induced aberrant mitosis and mitotic slippage efficiently lead to proliferative death irrespective of canonical apoptosis and p53. *Cell Cycle, 15*, 3268–3277.

Yu, D., Liu, B., Tan, M., Li, J., Wang, S. S., & Hung, M. C. (1996). Overexpression of c-erbB-2/neu in breast cancer cells confers increased resistance to Taxol via mdr-1-independent mechanisms. *Oncogene, 13*, 1359–1365.

Zhang, L., Gong, C., Lau, S. L., Yang, N., Wong, O. G., Cheung, A. N., Tsang, J. W., et al. (2013). SpliceArray profiling of breast cancer reveals a novel variant of NCOR2/SMRT that is associated with tamoxifen resistance and control of ERα transcriptional activity. *Cancer Research, 73*, 246–255.

Zhao, M., Zhuo, M. L., Zheng, X., Su, X., & Meric-Bernstam, F. (2019). FGFR1β is a driver isoform of FGFR1 alternative splicing in breast cancer cells. *Oncotarget, 10*, 30–44.

Zou, Y., Shao, Z., Peng, J., Li, F., Gong, D., & Wang, C. (2014). Crystal structure of triple-BRCT-domain of ECT2 and insights into the binding characteristics to CYK-4. *FEBS Letters, 588*, 2911–2920.

Zwijsen, R. M., Wientjens, E., Klompmaker, R., Van Der Sman, J., Bernards, R., & Michalides, R. J. (1997). CDK-independent activation of estrogen receptor by cyclin D1. *Cell, 88*, 405–415.

Unveiling Strategies to Conquer Virus-Induced Breast Cancer Drug Resistance

Boitumelo Phakathi, Benny Mosoane, Prashti Harichunder, Ruvashni Naidoo, Nondumiso Mabaso, Shenaaz Ismail, Sumayyah Ebrahim, Thabiso Victor Miya, Andreas Martin Kaufmann, Rodney Hull, and Zodwa Dlamini

---

B. Phakathi (✉) · R. Naidoo
Department of Surgery, College of Health Sciences, University of KwaZulu Natal, Durban, South Africa

King Edward VIII Hospital, Sydney Road, Durban, South Africa
e-mail: PhakathiB@ukzn.ac.za; naidoor@ukzn.ac.za

B. Mosoane
Department of Anatomical Pathology, National Health Laboratory Services (NHLS), University of Pretoria, Pretoria, South Africa
e-mail: Benny.Mosoane@nhls.ac.za

P. Harichunder
Department of Surgery, College of Health Sciences, University of KwaZulu Natal, Durban, South Africa

Dr Pixley Ka Isaka Seme Memorial Hospital, KwaMashu, South Africa
e-mail: prashtiharichunder@kznhealth.gov.za

N. Mabaso
Department of Surgery, College of Health Sciences, University of KwaZulu Natal, Durban, South Africa

Harry Gwala Regional Hospital, Pietermaritzburg, South Africa
e-mail: Nondumiso.Mabaso2@kznhealth.gov.za

S. Ismail
Department of Surgery, College of Health Sciences, University of KwaZulu Natal, Durban, South Africa

Inkosi Albert Luthuli Central Hospital, Durban, South Africa
e-mail: Ismaill@ialch.co.za

S. Ebrahim
Department of Surgery, College of Health Sciences, University of KwaZulu Natal, Durban, South Africa

Z. Dlamini (ed.), *Overcoming Breast Cancer Therapy Resistance*,
https://doi.org/10.1007/978-3-031-52860-6_8

Health Systems Research Unit, South African Medical Research Council,
Cape Town, South Africa
e-mail: Ebrahims@ukzn.ac.za

T. V. Miya · R. Hull · Z. Dlamini
SAMRC Precision Oncology Research Unit (PORU), DSI/NRF SARChI Chair in Precision Oncology and Cancer Prevention (POCP), Pan African Cancer Research Institute (PACRI), University of Pretoria, Pretoria, South Africa
e-mail: thabiso.miya@up.ac.za; rodney.hull@up.ac.za; Zodwa.Dlamini@up.ac.za

A. M. Kaufmann
Charité – Universitätsmedizin Berlin, corporate member of Freie Universität Berlin and Humboldt, Universität zu Berlin, Berlin, Germany
e-mail: Andreas.kaufmann@charite.de

Abstract One of the primary causes of cancer-related deaths among women worldwide is breast cancer (BC). Conventional medical approaches to treating breast cancer have been tried and failed in some cases. As a result of cancer resistance to current therapeutic regimens and their related negative effects, research is progressing toward a new era of virus-based cancer treatment. Due to the variety of applications it has, virotherapy is one of the unique strategies that has received a lot of research. Live oncolytic viruses or viruses that have undergone genetic modification are used in viral therapy to specifically target and infect tumor cells, which then multiply and kill cancerous cells. These viruses also trigger the host's immune system's antitumor response, which is how they exert their anticancer effects. To address this issue, this chapter covers the part that viruses play in BC treatment resistance (chemoresistance) as well as cutting-edge techniques including virotherapy and immunotherapies.

Keywords Breast cancer · Chemoresistance · Oncolytic viruses · Virotherapy tumor · Immunotherapy

Introduction

Nearly 18% of all malignancies in humans are caused by infectious agents, with viral infections accounting for approximately 12% of all infections (Carrillo–Infante et al., 2007). Viral oncogenesis can occur in several ways, such as direct viral gene impact, viruses that weaken the host's immune system, or viruses that provide a persistent inflammatory state that facilitates the process of neoplastic transformation (Akhter et al., 2014; Gannon et al., 2018). The role of viral infection carcinogenesis in breast cancer (BC) has drawn the interest of reseachers since the discovery of the Mouse Mammary Tumor Virus (MMTV) in the 1930s (Bittner, 1936). Furthermore, the literature's conclusions about the causal role of viruses in the development of BC are contradictory since there is a discrepancy in the tissue types used, sample preparation, and virus detection techniques (in situ hybridization, PCR, etc.) (Akhter et al., 2014; Gannon et al., 2018). Carcinogenesis induced by viruses is a complicated, multi-step process that depends on the interaction of various host and virus components (Akhter et al., 2014). This process begins with a viral infection-induced acute inflammatory phase, which if left untreated may progress to a chronic inflammatory condition. Various inflammatory cells are activated during this process, which causes the production of cytokines and other substances. These compounds can then disrupt the cell cycle, damage the host DNA, and increase cell differentiation, and proliferation, all of which can lead to cell malignancy (Carrillo–Infante et al., 2007). Some viruses that have been linked to breast oncogenesis include the Human Papilloma Virus (HPV), MMTV, Epstein-Barr Virus, Bovine Leukemia Virus, Mouse Mammary Tumor-Like Viruses, Cytomegalovirus, and Measles Virus (Fig. 8.1; Akhter et al., 2014; Gannon et al., 2018).

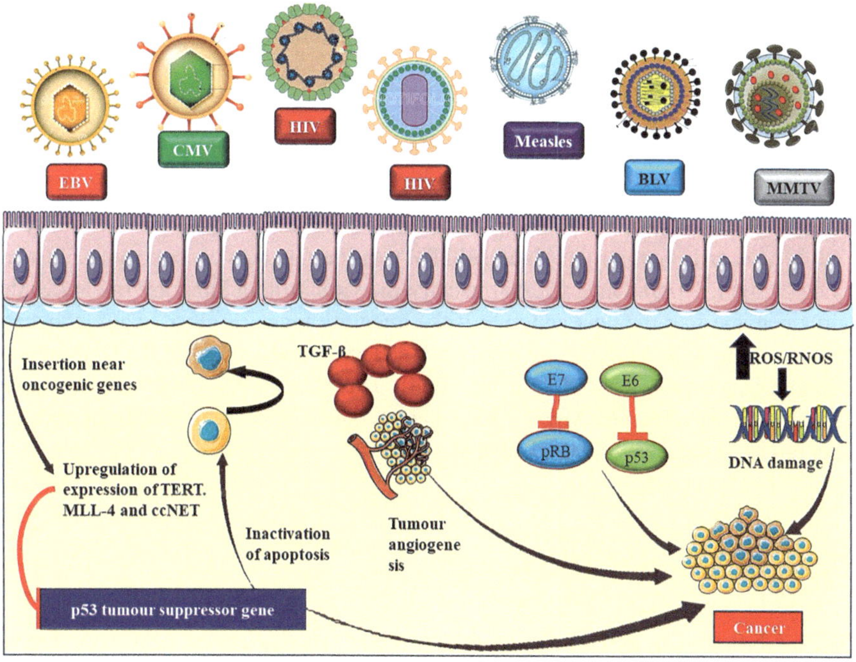

Fig. 8.1 *A schematic diagram demonstrating the role of viruses in cancer development.* The insertion of viruses near tumor-promoting genes including TERT, CCNA2, and CCNE1 increases their expression, which inactivates p53 and the apoptosis mediated by that gene. Furthermore, viruses may induce the growth of tumors by promoting and maintaining tumor angiogenesis by raising the expression of certain proteins, such as TGF-β. Additionally, these viruses alter ROS production and produce oxidative stress (OS), resulting in DNA damage and therefore raising the chance of mutagenesis and tumorigenesis. *HPV* Human Papillomavirus, *EBV* Epstein-Barr Virus, *MMTV* Mouse Mammary Tumor-Like Viruses, *BLV* Bovine Leukemia Virus, *CMV* Cytomegalovirus, *RNOS* Reactive nitrogen oxide species, *TERT* Telomerase reverse transcriptase, *CCNA2* Cyclin A2, and *CCNE1* Cyclin E1, *ROS* Reactive oxygen species

Human Papillomavirus (HPV)

Numerous studies have produced conflicting findings regarding the causality of HPV in the development of BC, so this issue is still up for debate. It is hypothesized that HPV may enter the breast through physical contact or homogenously and that the reported prevalence of HPV-positive BC ranges between 4% and 86% depending on geography and race (Akhter et al., 2014). The viral genes E6 and E7, which inhibit tumor suppressor genes p53 and the retinoblastoma gene product, are expressed when HPV directly infects tissue stem cells. When the normal cell cycle is aberrant, unrepaired mutations may be retained, the genome may become unstable, and eventually, the condition may turn cancerous. The precise carcinogenic mechanism of HPV in BC is still unknown. However, based on its carcinogenic effect in cervical cancer, it can be inferred (Yugawa & Kiyono, 2009). The need to assess HPV mRNA expression rather than merely HPV DNA presence is highlighted by the fact that some studies have revealed that there is a possibility that the HPV found in BC specimens was merely a contaminant and not a cause (Baltzell et al., 2012).

The Mammary Tumor Viruses (MMTV)

Animal model research has been carried out to investigate the virus's ability to induce cancer in human BC since MMTV was identified as an oncogenic virus in mice (Bittner, 1936). Once within the cells, the viral protein integrase integrates the virus genome into the host genome. If the integration occurs close to an oncogene, the oncogene will then become overexpressed, potentially causing the host cells to become cancerous (Ross SR, et al. 2008). The Human Mammary Tumor Virus (HMTV), a provirus with MMTV-like characteristics, was discovered in human BC specimens in the early 2000s (Liu et al., 2001).

Cytomegalovirus (CMV)

The inhibition of apoptosis, disruption of cellular processes in the tumor microenvironment, and interference with normal cell cycle control are just a few of the ways that CMV infection may contribute to BC carcinogenesis (Katz et al., 1989).

Epstein-Barr Virus (EBV)

BC has a five-fold higher prevalence of Epstein-Barr virus (EBV) than healthy and benign breast tissue controls (Lawson & Glenn, 2021). Saliva is the main method of transmission of the virus. Human epidermal growth factor receptor (HER2/HER3) signaling cascade activation by EBV makes breast epithelial cells more susceptible to developing into cancer (Akhter et al., 2014; Gannon et al., 2018). EBV produces various transforming growth factors at various periods of latency, including EBNA, LMP1, and LMP2. These factors deregulate cell growth, differentiation, and proliferation, resulting in carcinogenesis (Richardson et al., 2020).

Measles Virus

Despite the discovery of measles virus antigens in BC specimens, its etiopathogenesis has not yet been determined (Ariad et al., 2011).

HIV

HIV is a permissive virus, none oncogenic, and it weakens the host immune system, rendering it more susceptible to the reactivation of dormant oncogenes, lowering immune monitoring for tumor cells, and increasing the risk of developing new opportunistic infections (Akhter et al., 2014). Its precise function in the development and progression of BC has not yet been established. However, research has shown that HIV-positive women present with BC disease at an advanced stage were more frequently compared to women without HIV (Brandão et al., 2021; Cubasch et al., 2017; Phakathi et al., 2019). In addition, the studies revealed that HIV infection was linked to poor disease-free survival (DFS) and overall survival (OS) in patients suffering from BC, and the worst results occurred in patients with HIV and were not receiving the anti-retroviral therapy (ART) (Brandão et al., 2021, Cubasch et al., 2017, Phakathi et al., 2019).

Overview of Drug Chemoresistance in Virus-Associated Cancers

The most common modalities of therapy for virus-associated carcinogenesis include immunotherapy, cytotoxic chemotherapy, targeted therapy, antiviral medicines, highly active antiretroviral medications, radiotherapy, and specialized cytotoxic T cells (Chang et al., 2017; Ghosh et al., 2012; Sadri Nahand et al., 2021). In virus-associated cancers, chemoresistance to the more popular cytotoxic and conventional chemotherapy is becoming a growing problem. The resistance is frequently connected to intrinsic proteins and viral components (Sadrı Nahand et al., 2021). One method that demonstrated tumor growth suppression in EBV-associated nasopharyngeal cancer was targeting EBNA1 and inhibiting the DNA binding capability (Wang et al., 2020).

The development of resistance seen in the treatment of infectious illnesses (ID) and chemotherapy (CT) resistance in virus-associated cancers is fairly similar. Resistance to treatment in ID and malignancy includes the growth of internal and/or extrinsic triggers that cause relapse soon after remission (Mesri et al., 2010). Genetic mutations induce intrinsic mechanisms (acquired before therapy), which prevent cancer cells from becoming sensitive to their targets (Vasan et al., 2019). A real-world example is the triple-negative BC (TNBC), which has an innate resistance to targeted therapy and CT. Extrinsic (acquired) resistance can be brought on by mechanisms like the development of a new driver gene or another proto-oncogene. As a result, the new mutation may have other effects, such as dysregulation in the expression of the therapeutic targets. Acquired resistance can result from both treatment-induced alterations in the tumor microenvironment (TME) and a new infection that dysregulates cell death signaling pathways that were previously triggered by CT (Baselga et al., 2010; Kinnel et al., 2023; Lu et al., 2015; Wang et al., 2019).

Mechanisms of Chemoresistance in Virus-Associated Breast Cancer

Drug Efflux-Mediated Chemoresistance in Virus-Associated Cancer

Reduced intracellular drug accumulation in BC is the basis of drug efflux mechanisms of resistance, which are carried out by an ATP-binding cassette (ABC) transporter system (Kinnel et al., 2023). A multidrug resistance (MDR) mechanism that responds to cancer-specific medications and other treatment agents can make CT ineffective. BC resistance protein (BCRP)/ABCC2, P-glycoprotein (Pgp), and multidrug resistance protein 1 (MDR1)/ABCC1 are the three most significant ABC transporters in the emergence of MDR (Fig. 8.2; Boumendjel et al., 2009; Dean et al., 2001; Vasiliou et al., 2009). Cytotoxic chemicals are known to be actively pumped out of the cytoplasm by functional MDR1 (Sun et al., 2012).

Pgp and MDR1 reduce drug accumulation in tumor cells, which causes cell lines to develop chemoresistance to 5 fluorouracil (5 FU) (Zhang, 2021; Zhu et al., 2013a). Chemoresistance in T cells with EBV infection has been connected to the Pgp pathway (Yoshimori et al., 2015).

Virus-Mediated Chemoresistance by Regulation of Apoptosis

Cancer cell lines may become resistant to radiotherapy and CT if they learn to avoid apoptosis. (Hanahan & Weinberg, 2000). The tumor suppressor genes Rb and p53 are inactivated by high-risk HPV genotype E6 and E7 oncoproteins, which

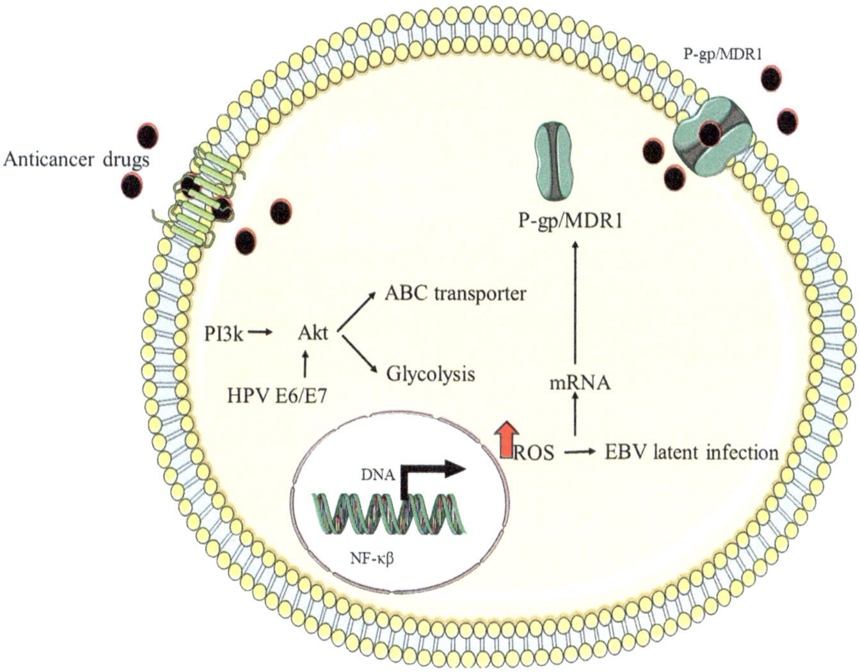

Fig. 8.2 *Drug efflux pump-mediated mechanisms leading to chemotherapy resistance in viral infection.* Viruses obstruct many signaling pathways that mediate the hazardous drug export from cancer cells. They may affect protein phosphorylation, which in turn interacts with viral oncoproteins to activate transporters, or they may change the cellular redox balance, which results in a compensatory response of transporter upregulation. *NF-kB* nuclear factor *kappa* B, *HPV E6/E7* Human Papillomavirus oncoprotein E6 and E7, *ROS* reactive oxygen species

are known to induce carcinogenesis in the uterine cervix (Lowe et al., 1993). Research has shown that HPV16 promotes apoptosis resistance and resistance to CT medicines, which block apoptotic pathways and cause cell immortality and transformation. Promotion of BCL2 family members and other anti-apoptotic drugs, as well as p53 suppression, have all been linked to chemoresistance in HPV-driven tumor cells for the intrinsic apoptotic pathway (Sugimoto et al., 1999). The extrinsic apoptotic pathway is affected by decreased CD95/fas activation (Yuan et al., 2005).

Notably, head and neck tumors with HPV tend to have a more favorable prognosis and respond better to CT and radiotherapy (Faraji et al., 2017) than their counterparts who are HPV-negative. This is due to the fact that whereas p53 in HPV-negative head and neck tumors is phenotypically reduced by the E6, p53 in HPV-positive head and neck cancers is modified to permanently become inactive. Apoptosis and a stronger response to genotoxic therapy than in the case of mutant p53 occur when p53 is high and cannot be totally depleted by E6 under genotoxic stress. For BC, comparable statistics are lacking.

Virus-Mediated Cancer Chemoresistance Through Upregulation of the Glycolysis Pathway

Cancer development has been linked to anaerobic glycolysis and several metabolic intermediates. For instance, higher glycolytic overactivity in HPV-positive cervical cancer cells has been associated with increased lactate dehydrogenase (LDH) activity (Hoppe–Seyler et al., 2017; Zhao et al., 2013). The altered glycolytic activity is thought to be induced by HPV E6/E7 stimulation of the oncogenic AKT/mTOR pathways. According to data, the HPV E6/E7 glycolysis axis either contributes to or is a direct cause of 5FU resistance in cervical cancer cells (Ma et al., 2019).

Exosome and Autophagy-Mediated Cancer Chemoresistance

Mitophagy, microautophagy, macroautophagy, and chaperone-mediated autophagy (CMA) are four types of autophagy. Autophagy, which results in the breakdown and recycling of cell fragments, fatty acids, damaged organelles, and amino acids, can be triggered by cell deprivation, hypoxia, lipopolysaccharides, and chemotherapeutic drugs.

CMA has been associated with the growth of tumors, their metastases, and their chemoresistance. Shock cognate protein in CMA recognizes cytosolic proteins that have pentapeptide patterns linked to KFERQ, allowing for easier transport to the lysosomal membranes and translocation thereby lysosome-associated membrane protein 2a (Lam2a) (Catarino et al., 2017). In BC cells, Lam2a-controlled CMA contributes to the extension of cell survival (Boumendjel et al., 2009). Thus, it has been shown that BC can potentially benefit from the therapeutic use of inhibiting CMA activity in BC cells (Saha, 2012).

Exosomes are microvesicles produced by cells that contain cellular materials like DNA fragments, mRNA, and miRNA. According to reports, therapeutic drugs are aggressively broken down by BC cell-derived exosomes through MDR1 and Pgp shuttling, leading to drug resistance (Wang et al., 2016). Paclitaxel-treated BC cells generate surviving-bearing exosomes that boost cell survival in BC cells and fibroblasts that are serum-starved (Wang et al., 2017). Increased chemoresistance in cancer cells is correlated with the intercellular transfer of certain types of miRNAs (Wang et al., 2017).

Oncogenic Signaling Pathways

Carcinogenesis involves signaling pathways, with oncogenic pathways being upregulated and tumor-suppressive pathways being downregulated. Mitogen-activated protein kinase (MAPK), phosphoinositide 3 kinase (PI3K), and several other pathways play a role in the extension of cell survival and promote cell proliferation (Chen et al., 2014). Chemoresistance may develop when these pathways are upregulated in altered cells, either as a result of mutation or pharmacological activation.

Chemotherapeutic medications like paclitaxel target BCL2 as well as the MAPK and PI3K pathway genes. Drugs targeting the MAPK pathway as well as its MEK1/2 components typically do not reach their full efficacy due to resistance to CT that develops throughout therapy (Mendoza et al., 2011). Nuclear factor kappa B (NF-κB), a regulatory molecule, can increase pro-survival and proliferative proteins' expression in altered cells, opening up new anti-apoptotic pathways (Zhao, 2016).

Attenuation of the measles vaccine strain Edmonston B (MV Edm), according to a study that offers a treatment option for CT-resistant BC, can re-sensitize BC cells to radiation and doxorubicin (Godwin et al., 2013). By reducing the amounts of p53 binding protein 1's mRNA and protein expression and dismantling the nonhomologous end joining (NHEJ) complex, MV Edm reduces the efficacy of DNA double-strand repair (Yang et al., 2020).

Mutagenic Role of Antiviral Factors in Breast Cancer

The host frequently triggers an immunological response against BC cells, which are typically invaded by immune cells, either within the tumor or in the microenvironment (Friedenson, 2013). Mutations in immune cells can lead to a weakened immune response to cancer cells, accelerating the development and progression of BC. These mutations may have an impact on the immune response, cytokine production, autophagy, and specific genes involved in innate immunity. Certain viruses (for example, influenza, herpes viruses, and HIV-1) have been shown to disrupt the autophagic pathway, a key mechanism in the innate immune response, to increase their own replication (García–Sastre, 2013). In addition, certain mutations limit the synthesis of chemokines and other cytokines (for example, NF-κB and interferon-gamma), resulting in tumorigenesis (Campbell et al., 2005; Hiscott et al., 2001; Porter et al., 2003). Viruses or other innate immune system mediators generally induce these alterations (Hiscott et al., 2001).

Oncolytic Viruses in Breast Cancer Treatment (Viral Oncotherapy)

The term "oncolytic therapy" refers to the utilization of altered viruses, either naturally occurring or created intentionally, to specifically target and eradicate tumor cells while avoiding healthy cells (Jin et al., 2021). Notably, oncolytic viruses (OVs) were first identified in leukemia patients whose clinical outcomes improved after an influenza infection (Kelly & Russell, 2007). This sparked a more, in-depth investigation into the types, functions, and mechanisms of oncolytic viruses in the management of a variety of solid tumors. The OVs that supposedly achieved positive results in preclinical testing for BC are in Table 8.1 below.

Combination therapy strategy has been a recurring topic that has gained popularity in the field during the development of oncolytic BC virotherapy. Each virus used in oncolytic therapy has a different mode of entry into the cell and a different mode of replication. Human Coxsackievirus and adenovirus receptors, which are largely utilized by adenovirus serotype constructions to target the cell, are present in most human cells. Adenovirus then engages in cellular endocytosis after attaching to the receptor, which involves moving the viral genome into the host cell's nucleus for transcription and replication to create viral protein. By altering the physical features of the virion and including therapeutic and targeted transgenes, the engineering of oncolytic ads makes use of the aforementioned lifecycle. The introduction of tumor-specific promoters, which only allow replication in cells that are expressing those genes, is another modification that has been seen in numerous oncolytic advertisements. Because the adenovirus and human Coxsackievirus receptors employed by the Ads vector were reported to be expressed at low levels in breast tumor cells, altering the Ads fiber protein's role in binding the receptor was shown to boost the infectivity of cancer cells. (Sm & Mathis, 2018).

The herpes simplex virus type 1 (HSV1) is a sizable double-stranded DNA (dsDNA) virus that is enveloped. To release its naked virion, HSV1 fuses its envelope into the host cells. The majority of HSV oncolytic vectors introduce additional therapeutic and targeted strategies, as well as viral gene alterations.

The vaccinia virus (VV) is the most distinctive dsDNA virus because it replicates outside of the cell's nucleus, in the cytoplasm. Since there is no longer a chance that the oncolytic virus will integrate its genome, this special characteristic is promoted as being safer. Additionally, VV exhibits a natural affinity for tumors, making it the ideal choice for an oncolytic virus. Due to the oncolytic VV's strong tumor cell infectivity and effective replication in BC, tumors have been demonstrated to regress after treatment (Sm & Mathis, 2018).

Another dsRNA virus that is still being studied in terms of its lifecycle mechanics is reovirus. The virus has been used as an oncolytic virus since it is generally recognized as being non-pathogenic to people. The oncolytic effects of the strain in BC cells have been investigated in several studies. According to a study that examined a variety of BC cell lines, the healthy breast epithelial cells were not vulnerable to reovirus infection independent of the hormone receptor status of the investigated cell lines. Ras protein mutation and activated Ras pathway in cancer cells were thought to be the causes of the wide infection potential (Sm & Mathis, 2018).

The Coxsackievirus A21 (CVA21) strain, a minimally pathogenic strain of Coxsackievirus for humans, uses the Intercellular Adhesion Molecule 1 (ICAM) and Decay-Accelerating Factor (DAF) complex to enter the cell via receptor-mediated infection. In several malignancies, including BC, the DAF and ICAM-1 receptor complex is shown to be overexpressed. According to a study by SM and Mathis, CVA21 effectively eliminated BC cells in vivo and in vitro models of xenograft and orthotopic metastatic BC in severe combined immunodeficient mice (Sm

Table 8.1 A summary of OVs that reportedly had good outcomes in preclinical testing in BC

Oncolytic virus (OVs)	Vector	Mechanism	Reference
Adenovirus	CNHK600-IL24	Activates TNBC apoptosis	Zhu et al. (2012)
	p55-Htert-HRE-TRAIL	Targets TNBC and activates apoptosis	Zhu et al. (2013b)
	OBP-401 adenovirus	Upregulates the targeting of tumor cells	Yano et al. (2016)
	Ad5-10miR145T	Targets miR-145-5P	Shayestehpour et al. (2017)
	Ad.DCN	Upregulates decorin expression	Zhao et al. (2019)
	SG400-E2F/IL-15	Targets E2F and mediates IL-15 expression	Yan et al. (2019)
Herpes simplex virus	G47Δ	Increases cytotoxicity to tumor cells	Wang et al. (2012) and Peters and Rabkin (2015)
	GD116	Increases the replication and virulence	Cheng et al. (2018)
	G47Δ-mIL12	Increases antitumor immune response	Ghouse et al. (2020)
Vaccinia virus	VV40L	Targets CD40	Governa et al. (2019)
	VG9-IL-24	Induce apoptosis	Deng et al. (2020)
Reovirus	Reo-dox	Increases cytotoxicity	Berry et al. (2020)
Vesicular stomatitis virus	VSVd51	Increases tropism for a vast array of cancers	Niavarani et al. (2020)
Measles virus	rMV-SLAMblind	Entry of cancer cells via the nectin-4 receptor	Fujiyuki et al. (2020)
	rMV-BNiP3	Increases the ability of apoptosis activation	Lal and Rajala (2019)
Newcastle disease virus	rAF-IL12	Increases anti-tumor immune response	Mohamed Amin et al. (2019)
Maraba virus	MG1	Ameliorates virulence and decreases the ability to kill healthy cells	Brun et al. (2010) and Bourgeois–Daigneault et al. (2016)
Coxsackievirus	CVA21	Has the ability to lytically infect BC cells	Skelding et al. (2009)

BC breast cancer, *TNBC* Triple-negative breast cancer cells

& Mathis, 2018). The introduction of transcriptionally controlled miRNA sequences into the coxsackievirus B3 strain has boosted safety. In the study, TNBC was treated both in vivo and in vitro, and the outcomes showed greater safety and decreased tumor growth (Sagara et al., 2016). These findings introduce coxsackievirus strains to BC oncolytic virotherapy and set the stage for subsequent safety investigations of both single agents and medication combinations thanks to their promising outcomes (Sm & Mathis, 2018).

For entrance, the poliovirus employs the CD155 receptor that is present in almost all malignancies. As a result, oncolytic therapy is ideally suited for the poliovirus.

PVSRIPO caused cell lysis and delayed tumor growth when tested on BC cells in vitro and in vivo xenografts in this study. The most intriguing finding was that PVSRIPO therapy significantly increased neutrophil infiltration in tumors and immunological activation, underlining its potential as an immunotherapeutic vector.

In BC, studies on the negative-sense single-stranded RNA (−ssRNA) virus family have been carried out. This category of viruses has frequently been utilized to treat various malignancies. The use of the—ssRNA category of viruses has recently been investigated in BC. Measles virus (MV), vesicular stomatitis virus (VSV), Maraba virus, and Newcastle disease virus (NDV) have all been studied both in vivo and in vitro (Sm & Mathis, 2018).

VSV is comparatively new to BC viral treatment. Although preliminary research has shown that VSV has oncolytic potential, there are still issues that need more engineering and testing. The accumulation of genetic abnormalities in cancer cells, along with potential antiviral mechanisms, allows VSV to replicate in human cancer cells even though it cannot do so in normal human cells. One distinctive safety feature that is sought in cancer virotherapy is the low pathogenicity of VSV in humans. In a previous study using the oncolytic VSV mutant rM51RM, the injection of IL-12 was not successful in inhibiting tumorigenesis completely in an in vivo model of BC (Sm & Mathis, 2018).

The attenuated measles virus vaccination strain's offspring, the oncolytic measles virus (oMV), has been tried in numerous trials for a variety of human tumors. In BC, oMV has recently been investigated. MV uses receptors such as CD46, which is widely expressed on all nucleated cells, SLAM, which is frequently overexpressed in several cancer cells, and PVRL4, which is a receptor related to the poliovirus (Dörig et al., 1993). Utilizing reduced oMV in cancer cells prevents cancer cells specifically from reproducing oncogenic cells (Sm & Mathis, 2018).

Another relatively recent addition to oncolytic virotherapy vectors that has found its way into BC research is the Maraba virus. A recombinant Maraba, MG1 was created in a study that investigated the −ssRNA virus as a VSV-related rhabdovirus with high oncolytic activity. Its oncolytic potential was increased while its capacity to reproduce in healthy cells was diminished (Brun et al., 2010; Sm & Mathis, 2018). Maraba MG1 has shown complete tumor regression in human cancer models when delivered safely in repeated dosages (Brun et al., 2010).

The final vector from the −ssRNA group discovered in BC is the Newcastle Disease Virus (NDV). NDV was recently evaluated as an oncolytic vector in British Columbia, even though the virus had previously been investigated as an oncolytic vector. A recent study that looked at the pro-inflammatory response to NDV in a variety of tumor lines, such as BC, discovered that NDV is a potent inducer of type I and II interferon responses, as well as IL-6 production (Ginting et al., 2017; Sm & Mathis, 2018).

As depicted in Fig. 8.3, several pathways have been revealed by which oncolytic viruses destroy cancer cells (Jin et al., 2021).

- *Direct lysis of cancer cells by the virus*: When the virus infects a tumor, it replicates and induces autolysis of tumor cells.

- *Destruction of the blood vessels by the virus*: Endothelial cells (ECs) that are directly damaged by the virus can interfere with blood flow to the tumor and deprive cancer cells of the nutrients and oxygen they need to develop.
- *Tropism*: Selective viral replication within cancer cells is one of the most crucial factors to consider in OV therapy. To get to and affect their target, viruses must overcome several obstacles, including selective attachment to cell membranes, internalization of viral particles, and efficient viral protein synthesis in the host cell. In certain cases, genetic alterations can be created to boost a virus's selectivity for tumor cells, whereas in other cases, some viruses have an innate affinity for cancer cells. Since they are deficient in an antiviral response mechanism that needs the expression of interferon (IFN)-related proteins, tumor cells, in general, encourage the development of viruses. Notably, protein kinase R (PKR) in healthy cells may identify dsRNA viruses that stimulate the production of the IFN gene. Tumor cells, which have lower PKR levels and phosphorylation, can be an exception to this rule. Additionally, abnormally active oncogenic pathways and the vast number of nucleotides found in cancer cells create the ideal conditions for viral replication, especially for those OVs that have been purposefully inhibited. (Cejalvo et al., 2022).
- *Induction of innate immunity*: Through immunogenic cell death (ICD), virus-induced lysis can trigger a potent anti-tumor immune response. The virus-induced lysis, which might involve pyroptosis, apoptosis, necrosis, or autophagy, not only reduces tumor size but also induces a powerful antitumor immune response via the previously stated immunogenic cell death (ICD). ICD causes the release of soluble tumor-associated antigens and neoantigens (TAAs and TANs), damage-associated molecular patterns (DAMPs) like ATP, and release high mobility group box 1 protein (HMGB1), pathogen-associated molecular patterns (PAMPs), viral components like proteins, nucleic acids (dsRNA, ssRNA, and DNA), and capsid components, activation of Annexin I, ectoexpression of calreticulin (an ER-associated chaperone) and exposure of F-actin and heat-shock proteins (HSP70, HSP90). All of these mechanisms recruit innate immune cells such as natural killer cells (NK), dendritic cells (DCs), and other antigen-presenting cells (APCs) to launch a specific anti-tumor response. These cells are recruited in the TME, where they aid in clearing the viruses as well as anticancer action. DAMPs and PAMPs can bind to pattern recognition receptors (PRR), also known as Toll-like receptors (TLR), on DCs, causing them to mature and produce cytokines (e.g., IL-12, IL-6, and TNF), as well as promote migration to nearby lymph nodes for T cell priming. MHC class I and class II expression as well as co-stimulatory molecules on DCs, such as CD40, CD80, CD83, and CD86, can also activate innate immunity and trigger the adaptive immune response (Cejalvo et al., 2022).
- *Induction of adaptive immunity*: An anti-tumor response will be initiated by the activation of a T cell response, which will also increase T cell recruitment. DCs stimulate and activate antigen-specific effector T cell responses by presenting antigens to CD4+ and CD8+ T cells via MHC class II and I molecules, respectively. Chemokines cause activated T lymphocytes to move to the tumor after

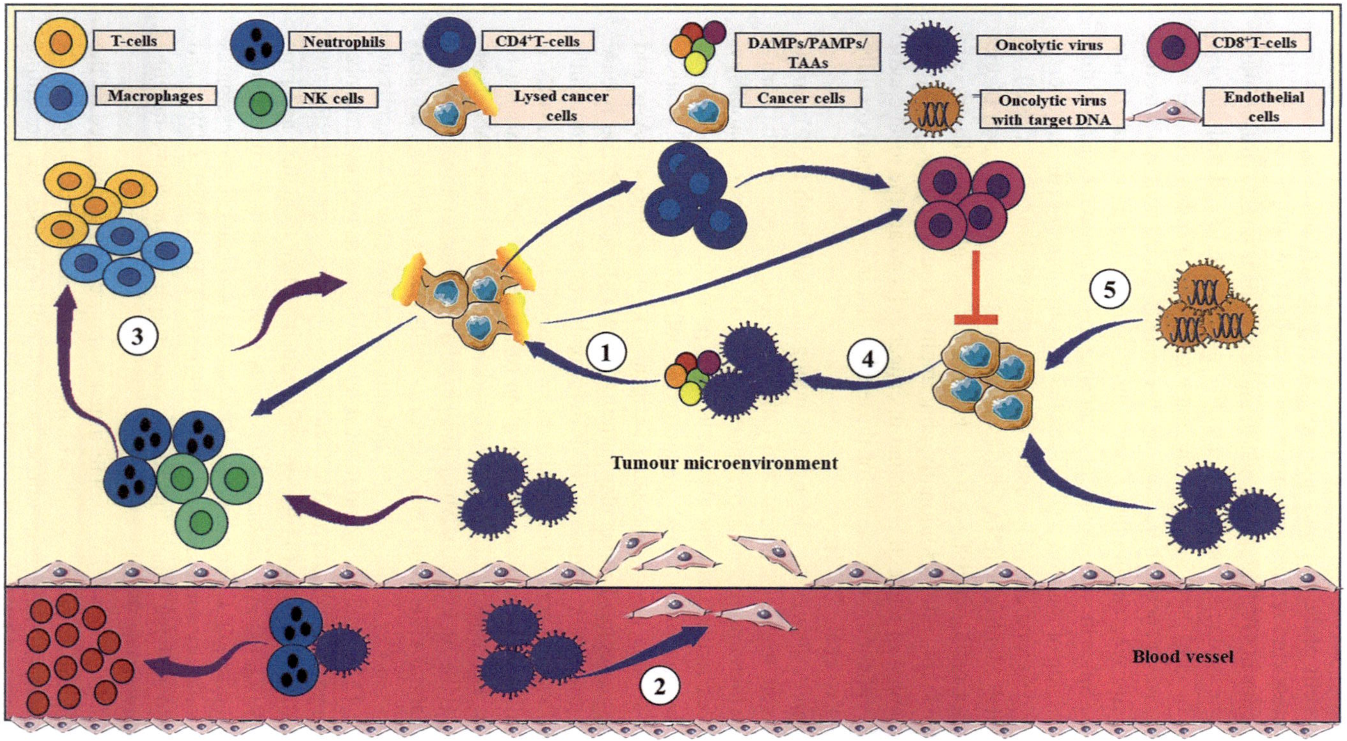

Fig. 8.3 *A schematic diagram showing how OVs exert antitumor effects*. This occurs in the following ways: (1) Cancer cells can be directly infected by OVs and lysed. (2) Vascular endothelial cells are infected by OVs, which lyse them and attract neutrophils. These cells then stimulate coagulation and thrombosis to obliterate blood arteries and stop angiogenesis. (3) "Cold" tumors become "hot" tumors as a result of OVs attracting DCs, macrophages, neutrophils, and T lymphocytes into the tumor microenvironment. (4) Cancer cells that have been lysed generate TAAs, DAMPs, and PAMPs that are identified by DCs and induce stimulation of CD4+ T and CD8+ T cells which subsequently kill tumor cells. (5) OVs can express transgenic targets, which strengthens the anticancer impact. *OVs* Oncolytic viruses, *DCs* Dendritic cells, *DAMPs* Damage-associated molecular patterns, *PAMPs* Pathogen-associated molecular patterns, *TAAs* Tumor-associated antigens

being clonally amplified in the local lymph node. The viral response and cross-presentation of tumor antigens are both components of T-cell responses. Viral antigens are potent immunogens that boost the recruitment of T cells to start a powerful antitumor response, that is diminished in many tumors. Notably, upon inducing tumor cell lysis, followed by the release and dissemination of soluble tumor antigens, OVs also enhance the cross-presentation of TAAs and TANs. Antitumor action is considerably aided by this cross-presentation. (Cejalvo et al., 2022).

Research has focused on the aggressive triple-negative BC (TNBC) subtype, which makes up 15% of all BC subtypes and has few systemic therapeutic options for chemoresistant breast tumors (Jin et al., 2021). Numerous oncolytic viruses have been studied in a pre-clinical setting for utilization in TNBC subtypes.

The most extensively studied oncolytic viruses in BC are adenoviruses, which are altered by recombination with genes that have anticancer or immune mediating effects (Jin et al., 2021). The IL24 gene was recombined to create a type 5 adenovirus (CNHK600 – IL24), which was tested in a mouse model and showed better anti-tumor activity and overall outcome of TNBC, in vivo (Kelly & Russell, 2007). A well-known immune regulator and an oncolytic drug, IL 24 stops the development of cancer cells and induces their death (Sm & Mathis, 2018). Other recombinants, such as IL – 15, have also been investigated in vivo with encouraging outcomes since they play a substantial role in triggering the immune response and limiting the proliferation of BC cells (Zhu et al., 2012). Coxsackievirus, Herpes simplex virus (HSV), Vaccinia virus, Reovirus, and Measles virus (MV), to mention a few, are a few additional oncolytic viruses being investigated for usage in vivo and in vitro in patients with TNBC (Jin et al., 2021).

Oncolytic Viruses As Immunotherapeutics

BC has not benefited from immunotherapy as much as other cancers, although it has been a game changer in the treatment of some malignancies. Triple-negative breast tumors have shown some promise for treatment, whereas luminal BCs have had less success. This is explained by its comparatively minimal inflammation and immune quiescence. Oncolytic viruses have been introduced as a potential novel immunotherapy strategy to improve the effectiveness of immunotherapy in BC. Viruses are small molecules that employ the host cell's molecular machinery to proliferate. The pathogenic activity of viruses and their ability to cause inflammation are typically linked to viral infection. Due to inherent anomalies in the signaling pathways, cancer cells constitute a favorable environment for virus multiplication. The virus should only infect and spread throughout the cancer cells, ultimately causing tumor lysis. This lysis can subsequently trigger the host's powerful anti-tumor immune response.

Oncolytic viral therapy research holds promise, but it has not yet achieved therapeutic success. The virus replicates upon introduction; therefore, the dose may be unpredictable and subject to limitations such as targeted virus delivery into the tumor and potential genome inclusion. The immune system of the host is necessary for the removal of viruses from the body since they are not eliminated by simple cell metabolism. Although oncolytic viruses might enhance immunotherapy as a treatment for BC, particularly the luminal forms, more research is required to fully understand the biology of the tumor and its microenvironment. To identify the ideal patient, viral vector, and delivery mechanism, research is still ongoing (Cejalvo et al., 2022).

Combination of Virotherapy and Immunotherapy

One therapeutic treatment is insufficient for completely eradicating cancer considering the disease is typically complex. Therefore, for cancer attacks with multiple fronts, a combination of two or more medicines is more successful. One of the most frequently researched methods to increase the efficacy of virotherapy is the combination of virotherapy and immunotherapy. Viruses can be genetically modified to code for immunotherapeutic components, which can serve as both virotherapy and immunotherapy, or immunotherapy can be paired with virotherapy as a stand-alone process. To treat BC, numerous replicating and non-replicating viruses have been altered to encode cytokines (Chaurasiya & Fong, 2020). Ghouse and colleagues, for instance, altered an oncolytic HSV to encode cytokine IL-12 and investigated its antitumor efficiency in TNBC murine models. According to the authors, HSV boosted CD8+ and CD45 cell tumor invasion. HSV also produced local and systemic antitumor effects in a syngeneic TNBC murine model (Ghouse et al., 2020). Likewise, Zhu and colleagues showed that an oncolytic adenovirus containing the cytokine IL-24 can prevent the formation of BC cells in mice in an in vitro setting (Zhu et al., 2012). Bramante and colleagues discovered that a low-dose cyclophosphamide regimen combined with an oncolytic adenovirus expressing GM-CSF exerts antitumor effectiveness in both human patients and a mouse model with TNBC (Bramante et al., 2016). Given that OVs may induce tumors that are immunologically "cold" to become "hot," combining OVs with treatments that call for "hot" TME might produce synergistic antitumor effects (Chaurasiya & Fong, 2020). Numerous research studies have demonstrated that cancer cells can increase their expression of PD-L1 in response to OV therapy, even though OVs can encourage tumor infiltration via cytotoxic T cells and other immune cells (Liu et al., 2017; Chaurasiya et al., 2020b). Instead of destroying cancer cells, this gatekeeper protein prevents cytotoxic T cells from doing so. To achieve the greatest antitumor effects, immune checkpoint inhibitors (ICIs) must be taken. As a result, research combining OVs and ICIs to treat different malignancies has been conducted. To ascertain if OVs could make TNBC more sensitive to ICIs, Bourgeois–Daigneault and associates investigated this combination in BC. According to the scientists, the oncolytic

Maraba inhibited disease relapse in the majority of the treated mice and was able to make TNBC more sensitive to ICIs (Bourgeois–Daigneault et al., 2018). Likewise, Mostafa and colleagues looked into the relationship between an oncolytic reovirus and an anti-PD-1 antibody in BC models. Reovirus, according to the authors, increased PD-L1 levels in tumor cells and immune cell infiltration in tumors (Mostafa et al., 2018). In comparison either monotherapy or combination therapy exhibited a significantly higher anti-tumor efficacy. By increasing the expression of PD-L1 on BC cells in mice, both in vivo and in vitro, Chaurasiya and colleagues showed that an oncolytic chimeric poxvirus changes immunologically "cold" TME into "hot." Additionally, the inclusion of an anti-PD-L1 antibody improved the virus's overall antitumor effectiveness (Chaurasiya et al., 2020b).

Effective Strategies to Overcome Virus-Induced Drug Resistance

Ongoing and Future Research

Next-Generation Sequencing Technology with Pathogen Discovery

Next-generation sequencing (NGS) is a form of DNA sequencing technology that determines the sequence by running parallel reads on several small bits of DNA. "High-throughput" technology has revolutionized the classification of genetic mutations and aberrations in a complete cancer genome, and it has also significantly boosted (while getting less expensive) the rate at which a person's genome can be sequenced. According to several research, EBV, Human Herpes Virus 6 (HHV-6), and HPV2 (a cutaneous wart HPV type) are the main viruses that cause BC due to the expression of their early and late genes. According to certain findings, BC may be linked to the bovine leukemia virus. However, numerous large-scale, case-controlled NGS studies conducted across multiple centers with various patient cohorts have been unable to identify any viral pathogens in BCs, despite demonstrating sensitivity and specificity in the identification of viruses in common cancers that are induced by viruses (Reis–Filho, 2009; Sturgill et al., 2021).

Limitations of Virotherapy for Breast Cancer Treatment

While virotherapy has the potential to significantly improve BC treatment, various obstacles need to be removed before patients can fully take advantage of this cutting-edge therapeutic approach. The majority of the restrictions associated with virotherapy for BC are related to therapeutic efficacy, unchecked viral spread, and appropriate delivery, all of which are frequent in other solid tumors (Chaurasiya & Fong, 2020). Oncolytic viruses have been reported to be safe for humans in clinical research; however, their ability to produce tumors has only been somewhat effective. Moreover, due to manufacturing-related limitations, dose-limiting toxicity has not been reached in most of the cases (Chaurasiya et al., 2020a). One strategy to get around these restrictions is to develop oncolytic viruses that are more effective in eliminating tumors, allowing for great antitumor efficacy with a low viral dosage. Choi and colleagues recombined multiple poxvirus species/strains to produce a chimeric poxvirus (CF33) in this regard. Comparing this CF33 virus to its parental viruses in vitro, it showed a strong ability to kill tumor cells. In contrast to other oncolytic poxviruses, the scientists claim that the CF33 poxvirus totally controlled the growth of TNBC xenografts at doses 100 to 1000 times lower (Choi et al., 2018). Similarly, by chimerizing several vaccinia virus strains, Ricordel and colleagues produced a chimeric poxvirus with ameliorated oncolytic effectiveness (Ricordel et al., 2018).

It can be difficult to ensure the best virus delivery to the targeted tumor, which is particularly difficult with metastatic disease. To target certain tumors, local or regional viral administration has been used in the majority of preclinical studies. This is a rudimentary approach, though, and it might not be effective for metastatic lesions that are challenging to inject. The distribution of the virus is hampered by several mechanisms, including virus sequestration in the spleen and liver, virus neutralization via serum factors, and virus incapacity to pass the endothelial cells lining tumor vasculature (Russell et al., 2012). A phase I clinical experiment using the oncolytic vaccinia virus called JX594 revealed that the viremic threshold dose of 109 infectious units was necessary to recover the virus from tumors following systemic injection (Breitbach et al., 2011). Despite the study's exclusion of BC patients, it offers a critical demonstration of the large amount of virus required for systemic administration for the virus to reach tumors. Utilizing such huge dosages is impractical for numerous types of OVs due to manufacturing restrictions. Furthermore, the extracellular matrix and other dense stromal components impede viral propagation inside the tumor (Wojton & Kaur, 2010). Numerous methods have been researched to get past these barriers and induce virus propagation in the tumors (Martinez-Quintanilla et al., 2019). Even though these methods led to hopeful preclinical research results, it is still unknown whether they will be effective in clinical settings (Chaurasiya & Fong, 2020).

Conclusion and Recommendations

Viruses have the potential to have a role in the development of CT in both cellular mechanisms and the TME. Drug resistance can be caused by both inherent tumor features and acquired perturbations from treatment. Viral oncoproteins alter the signaling pathways involved in responses to drug-mediated cell death, affect cellular drug transporters and the efflux of chemotherapeutics from cancer cells, dysregulate the cellular targets of the medications, and produce treatment resistance. The viral oncoproteins not only promote cancer but also escape chemotherapeutics, which are used to treat cancer. The present knowledge is derived from in vitro studies, which are also applicable in vivo; nevertheless, additional research is required to corroborate the findings in real patients. The use of numerous oncolytic viruses to attack the same disease in various mechanisms is a revolutionary approach to oncolytic virotherapy.

References

Akhter, J., Ali Aziz, M. A., Al Ajlan, A., Tulbah, A., & Akhtar, M. (2014). Breast cancer: Is there a viral connection? *Advances in Anatomic Pathology, 21*, 373–381.

Ariad, S., Milk, N., Bolotin, A., Gopas, J., Sion–Vardy, N., & Benharoch, D. (2011). Measles virus antigens in breast cancer. *Anticancer Research, 31*, 913–920.

Baltzell, K., Buehring, G. C., Krishnamurthy, S., Kuerer, H., Shen, H. M., & Sison, J. D. (2012). Limited evidence of human papillomavirus in [corrected] breast tissue using molecular in situ methods. *Cancer, 118*, 1212–1220.

Baselga, J., Gelmon, K. A., Verma, S., Wardley, A., Conte, P., Miles, D., et al. (2010). Phase ii trial of Pertuzumab and trastuzumab in patients with human epidermal growth factor receptor 2–positive metastatic breast cancer that progressed during prior trastuzumab therapy. *Journal of Clinical Oncology, 28*, 1138–1144.

Berry, J. T., Muñoz, L. E., Stewart, R. M. R., Selvaraj, P., & Mainou, B. A. (2020). Doxorubicin conjugation to reovirus improves oncolytic efficacy in triple–negative breast cancer. *Molecular Therapy–Oncolytics, 18*, 556–572.

Bittner, J. J. (1936). Some possible effects of nursing on the mammary gland tumor incidence in mice. *Science, 84*, 162.

Boumendjel, A., Florin, A., & Boutonnat, J. (2009). Reversal agents of multidrug resistance mediated by multidrug resistance-associated proteins (Mrps). In *Abc transporters and multidrug resistance* (pp. 261–288). Wiley.

Bourgeois–Daigneault, M. C., St–Germain, L. E., Roy, D. G., Pelin, A., Aitken, A. S., Arulanandam, R., et al. (2016). Combination of paclitaxel and Mg1 oncolytic virus as a successful strategy for breast cancer treatment. *Breast Cancer Research, 18*, 1–10.

Bourgeois–Daigneault, M. C., Roy, D. G., Aitken, A. S., El Sayes, N., Martin, N. T., Varette, O., et al. (2018). Neoadjuvant oncolytic virotherapy before surgery sensitizes triple–negative breast cancer to immune checkpoint therapy. *Science Translational Medicine, 10*, Eaao1641.

Bramante, S., Koski, A., Liikanen, I., Vassilev, L., Oksanen, M., Siurala, M., et al. (2016). Oncolytic virotherapy for the treatment of breast cancer, including triple–negative breast cancer. *Oncoimmunology, 5*, E1078057.

Brandão, M., Bruzzone, M., Franzoi, M. A., De Angelis, C., Eiger, D., Caparica, R., et al. (2021). Impact of Hiv infection on baseline characteristics and survival of women with breast cancer. *AIDS, 35*, 605–618.

Breitbach, C. J., Burke, J., Jonker, D., Stephenson, J., Haas, A. R., Chow, L. Q., et al. (2011). Intravenous delivery of a multi–mechanistic cancer–targeted oncolytic poxvirus in humans. *Nature, 477*, 99–102.

Brun, J., Mcmanus, D., Lefebvre, C., Hu, K., Falls, T., Atkins, H., et al. (2010). Identification of genetically modified Maraba virus as An oncolytic rhabdovirus. *Molecular Therapy, 18*, 1440–1449.

Campbell, M. J., Scott, J., Maecker, H. T., Park, J. W., & Esserman, L. J. (2005). Immune dysfunction and micrometastases in women with breast cancer. *Breast Cancer Research and Treatment, 91*, 163–171.

Carrillo–Infante, C., Abbadessa, G., Bagella, L., & Giordano, A. (2007). Viral infections as a cause of cancer (review). *International Journal of Oncology, 30*, 1521–1528.

Catarino, S., Pereira, P., & Girão, H. (2017). Molecular control of chaperone–mediated autophagy. *Essays in Biochemistry, 61*, 663–674.
Cejalvo, J. M., Falato, C., Villanueva, L., Tolosa, P., González, X., Pascal, M., et al. (2022). Oncolytic viruses: A new immunotherapeutic approach for breast cancer treatment? *Cancer Treatment Reviews, 106*, 102392.
Chang, Y., Moore, P. S., & Weiss, R. A. (2017). Human oncogenic viruses: Nature and discovery. *Philosophical Transactions of the Royal Society of London. Series B, Biological Sciences, 372*, 20160264.
Chaurasiya, S., & Fong, Y. (2020). Viroimmunotherapy for breast cancer: promises, problems and future directions [Published Online Ahead Of Print, 2020 Dec 2]. Cancer Gene Ther.
Chaurasiya, S., Fong, Y., & Warner, S. G. (2020a). Optimizing oncolytic viral design to enhance antitumor efficacy: Progress and challenges. *Cancers, 12*, 1699.
Chaurasiya, S., Yang, A., Kang, S., Lu, J., Kim, S. I., & Park, A. K. (2020b). Oncolytic poxvirus Cf33–Hnis–Δf14. 5 Favorably modulates tumor immune microenvironment and works synergistically with anti–pd–L1 antibody in a triple–negative breast cancer model. *Oncoimmunology, 9*, 1729300.
Chen, W. X., Cai, Y. Q., Lv, M. M., Chen, L., Zhong, S. L., Ma, T. F., Zhao, J. H., & Tang, J. H. (2014). Exosomes from docetaxel–resistant breast cancer cells Alter chemosensitivity by delivering Micrornas. *Tumor Biology, 35*, 9649–9659.
Cheng, L., Jiang, H., Fan, J., Wang, J., Hu, P., Ruan, Y., et al. (2018). A novel oncolytic herpes simplex virus armed with the carboxyl–terminus of murine Myd116 has enhanced anti–tumor efficacy against human breast cancer cells. *Oncology Letters, 15*, 7046–7052.
Choi, A. H., O'leary, M. P., Lu, J., Kim, S. I., Fong, Y., & Chen, N. G. (2018). Endogenous Akt activity promotes virus entry and predicts efficacy of novel chimeric Orthopoxvirus in triple–negative breast cancer. *Molecular Therapy–Oncolytics, 9*, 22–29.
Cubasch, H., Ruff, P., Joffe, M., Norris, S., Chirwa, T., Nietz, S., et al. (2017). South African breast cancer and Hiv outcomes study: Methods and baseline assessment. *J Glob Oncol, 3*, 114–124.
Dean, M., Hamon, Y., & Chimini, G. (2001). The human Atp–binding cassette (Abc) transporter superfamily. *Journal of Lipid Research, 42*, 1007–1017.
Deng, L., Fan, J., Ding, Y., Yang, X., Huang, B., & Hu, Z. (2020). Target therapy with vaccinia virus Harboring il–24 for human breast cancer. *Journal of Cancer, 11*, 1017.
Dörig, R. E., Marcil, A., Chopra, A., & Richardson, C. D. (1993). The human Cd46 molecule is a receptor for measles virus (Edmonston strain). *Cell, 75*, 295–305.
Faraji, F., Eisele, D. W., & Fakhry, C. (2017). Emerging insights into recurrent and metastatic human papillomavirus–related oropharyngeal squamous cell carcinoma. *Laryngoscope Investig Otolaryngol, 2*, 10–18.
Friedenson, B. (2013). Mutations in components of antiviral or microbial Defense as a basis for breast cancer. *Functional & Integrative Genomics, 13*, 411–424.
Fujiyuki, T., Amagai, Y., Shoji, K., Kuraishi, T., Sugai, A., Awano, M., et al. (2020). Recombinant Slamblind measles virus is a promising candidate for Nectin–4–positive triple negative breast cancer therapy. *Molecular Therapy–Oncolytics, 19*, 127–135.
Gannon, O. M., Antonsson, A., Bennett, I. C., & Saunders, N. A. (2018). Viral infections and breast cancer – a current perspective. *Cancer Letters, 420*, 182–189.
García–Sastre, A. (2013). Cell biology: Beneficial lessons from viruses. *Nature, 494*, 181–182.
Ghosh, S. K., Perrine, S. P., & Faller, D. V. (2012). Advances in virus–directed therapeutics against Epstein–Barr virus–associated malignancies. *Advances in Virology, 2012*, 509296.
Ghouse, S. M., Nguyen, H. M., Bommareddy, P. K., Guz–Montgomery, K., & Saha, D. (2020). Oncolytic herpes simplex virus encoding Il12 controls triple–negative breast cancer growth and metastasis. *Frontiers in Oncology, 10*, 384.
Ginting, T. E., Suryatenggara, J., Christian, S., & Mathew, G. (2017). Proinflammatory response induced by Newcastle disease virus in tumor and Normal cells. *Oncolytic Virother, 6*, 21–30.
Godwin, P., Baird, A. M., Heavey, S., Barr, M. P., O'byrne, K. J., & Gately, K. (2013). Targeting nuclear factor–kappa B to overcome resistance to chemotherapy. *Frontiers in Oncology, 3*, 120.

Governa, V., Brittoli, A., Mele, V., Pinamonti, M., Terracciano, L., Muenst, S., et al. (2019). A replication–incompetent Cd154/40l recombinant vaccinia virus induces direct and macrophage–mediated antitumor effects in vitro and in vivo. *Oncoimmunology, 8*, E1568162.
Hanahan, D., & Weinberg, R. A. (2000). The hallmarks of cancer. *Cell, 100*, 57–70.
Hiscott, J., Kwon, H., & Génin, P. (2001). Hostile takeovers: Viral appropriation of the Nf–Kappab pathway. *The Journal of Clinical Investigation, 107*, 143–151.
Hoppe–Seyler, K., Honegger, A., Bossler, F., Sponagel, J., Bulkescher, J., Lohrey, C., et al. (2017). Viral E6/E7 oncogene and cellular hexokinase 2 expression in Hpv–positive cancer cell lines. *Oncotarget, 8*, 106342–106351.
Jin, S., Wang, Q., Wu, H., Pang, D., & Xu, S. (2021). Oncolytic viruses for triple negative breast cancer and beyond. *Biomarker Research, 9*, 71.
Katz, B. Z., Raab–Traub, N., & Miller, G. (1989). Latent and replicating forms of Epstein–Barr virus Dna in lymphomas and lymphoproliferative diseases. *The Journal of Infectious Diseases, 160*, 589–598.
Kelly, E., & Russell, S. J. (2007). History of oncolytic viruses: Genesis to genetic engineering. *Molecular Therapy, 15*, 651–659.
Kinnel, B., Singh, S. K., Oprea–Ilies, G., & Singh, R. (2023). Targeted therapy and mechanisms of drug resistance in breast cancer. *Cancers (Basel)*, 15.
Lal, G., & Rajala, M. S. (2019). Combination of oncolytic measles virus armed with Bnip3, a pro–apoptotic gene and paclitaxel induces breast cancer cell death. *Frontiers in Oncology, 8*, 676.
Lawson, J. S., & Glenn, W. K. (2021). Catching viral breast cancer. *Infect Agent Cancer, 16*, 37.
Liu, B., Wang, Y., Melana, S. M., Pelisson, I., Najfeld, V., Holland, J. F., et al. (2001). Identification of a proviral structure in human breast cancer. *Cancer Research, 61*, 1754–1759.
Liu, Z., Ravindranathan, R., Kalinski, P., Guo, Z. S., & Bartlett, D. L. (2017). Rational combination of oncolytic vaccinia virus and pd–L1 blockade works synergistically to enhance therapeutic efficacy. *Nature Communications, 8*, 14754.
Lowe, S. W., Ruley, H. E., Jacks, T., & Housman, D. E. (1993). P53–dependent apoptosis modulates the cytotoxicity of anticancer agents. *Cell, 74*, 957–967.
Lu, L., Ju, F., Zhao, H., & Ma, X. (2015). Microrna–134 modulates resistance to doxorubicin in human breast cancer cells by downregulating Abcc1. *Biotechnology Letters, 37*, 2387–2394.
Ma, D., Huang, Y., & Song, S. (2019). Inhibiting the Hpv16 oncogene–mediated glycolysis sensitizes human cervical carcinoma cells to 5–fluorouracil. *Oncotargets and Therapy, 12*, 6711–6720.
Martinez–Quintanilla, J., Seah, I., Chua, M., & Shah, K. (2019). Oncolytic viruses: Overcoming translational challenges. *The Journal of Clinical Investigation, 129*, 1407–1418.
Mendoza, M. C., Er, E. E., & Blenis, J. (2011). The Ras–Erk and Pi3k–Mtor pathways: Cross–talk and compensation. *Trends in Biochemical Sciences, 36*, 320–328.
Mesri, E. A., Cesarman, E., & Boshoff, C. (2010). Kaposi's sarcoma and its associated herpesvirus. *Nature Reviews. Cancer, 10*, 707–719.
Mohamed Amin, Z., Che Ani, M. A., Tan, S. W., Yeap, S. K., Alitheen, N. B., Syed Najmuddin, S. U. F., et al. (2019). Evaluation of a recombinant Newcastle disease virus expressing human Il12 against human breast cancer. *Scientific Reports, 9*, 13999.
Mostafa, A. A., Meyers, D. E., Thirukkumaran, C. M., Liu, P. J., Gratton, K., Spurrell, J., et al. (2018). Oncolytic reovirus and immune checkpoint inhibition as a novel immunotherapeutic strategy for breast cancer. *Cancers, 10*, 205.
Niavarani, S. R., Lawson, C., Boudaud, M., Simard, C., & Tai, L. H. (2020). Oncolytic vesicular stomatitis virus–based cellular vaccine improves triple–negative breast cancer outcome by enhancing natural killer and Cd8+ T–cell functionality. *Journal for Immunotherapy of Cancer, 8*, e000465.
Peters, C., & Rabkin, S. D. (2015). Designing herpes viruses as Oncolytics. *Molecular Therapy–Oncolytics, 2*, 15010.
Phakathi, B., Cubasch, H., Nietz, S., Dickens, C., Dix–Peek, T., Joffe, M., et al. (2019). Clinico–pathological characteristics among south African women with breast cancer receiving anti–retroviral therapy for Hiv. *Breast, 43*, 123–129.

Porter, D., Lahti–Domenici, J., Keshaviah, A., Bae, Y. K., Argani, P., Marks, J., et al. (2003). Molecular markers in ductal carcinoma in situ of the breast. *Molecular Cancer Research, 1*, 362–375.

Reis–Filho, J. S. (2009). Next–generation sequencing. *Breast Cancer Research, 11*(Suppl 3), S12.

Richardson, A. K., Walker, L. C., Cox, B., Rollag, H., Robinson, B. A., Morrin, H., et al. (2020). Breast cancer and cytomegalovirus. *Clinical & Translational Oncology, 22*, 585–602.

Ricordel, M., Foloppe, J., Antoine, D., Findeli, A., Kempf, J., Cordier, P., et al. (2018). Vaccinia virus shuffling: Devv5, a novel chimeric poxvirus with improved oncolytic potency. *Cancers, 10*, 231.

Russell, S. J., Peng, K. W., & Bell, J. C. (2012). Oncolytic virotherapy. *Nature Biotechnology, 30*, 658–670.

Sadri Nahand, J., Rabiei, N., Fathazam, R., Taghizadieh, M., Ebrahimi, M. S., Mahjoubin–Tehran, M., et al. (2021). Oncogenic viruses and chemoresistance: What do we know? *Pharmacological Research, 170*, 105730.

Sagara, M., Takishima, Y., Miyamoto, S., Shimizu, H., Nakanishi, Y., & Tani, K. (2016). 409. Novel recombinant coxsackievirus B3 infection elicits robust oncolytic activity against human non–small lung cancer and triple–negative breast cancer. *Molecular Therapy, 24*, S162.

Saha, T. (2012). Lamp2a overexpression in breast Tumors promotes cancer cell survival via chaperone–mediated autophagy. *Autophagy, 8*, 1643–1656.

Shayestehpour, M., Moghim, S., Salimi, V., Jalilvand, S., Yavarian, J., Romani, B., et al. (2017). Targeting human breast cancer cells by An oncolytic adenovirus using Microrna–targeting strategy. *Virus Research, 240*, 207–214.

Skelding, K. A., Barry, R. D., & Shafren, D. R. (2009). Systemic targeting of metastatic human breast tumor xenografts by coxsackievirus A21. *Breast Cancer Research and Treatment, 113*, 21–30.

Sm, O. B., & Mathis, J. M. (2018). Oncolytic virotherapy for breast cancer treatment. *Current Gene Therapy, 18*, 192–205.

Sturgill, E. G., Misch, A., Lachs, R., Jones, C. C., Schlauch, D., Jones, S. F., et al. (2021). Next–generation sequencing of patients with breast cancer in community oncology clinics. *JCO Precision Oncology, 5*, 1297–1311.

Sugimoto, C., Fujieda, S., Seki, M., Sunaga, H., Fan, G. K., Tsuzuki, H., et al. (1999). Apoptosis–promoting gene (Bax) transfer potentiates sensitivity of squamous cell carcinoma to cisplatin in vitro and in vivo. *International Journal of Cancer, 82*, 860–867.

Sun, Y. L., Patel, A., Kumar, P., & Chen, Z. S. (2012). Role of Abc transporters in cancer chemotherapy. *Chinese Journal of Cancer, 31*, 51–57.

Vasan, N., Baselga, J., & Hyman, D. M. (2019). A view on drug resistance in cancer. *Nature, 575*, 299–309.

Vasiliou, V., Vasiliou, K., & Nebert, D. W. (2009). Human Atp–binding cassette (Abc) transporter family. *Human Genomics, 3*, 281–290.

Wang, J., Hu, P., Zeng, M., Rabkin, S. D., & Liu, R. (2012). Oncolytic herpes simplex virus treatment of metastatic breast cancer. *International Journal of Oncology, 40*, 757–763.

Wang, Z., Chen, J. Q., Liu, J. L., & Tian, L. (2016). Exosomes in tumor microenvironment: Novel transporters and biomarkers. *Journal of Translational Medicine, 14*, 297.

Wang, T., Ning, K., Lu, T. X., Sun, X., Jin, L., Qi, X., Jin, J., & Hua, D. (2017). Increasing circulating exosomes–carrying Trpc5 predicts chemoresistance in metastatic breast cancer patients. *Cancer Science, 108*, 448–454.

Wang, D., Bao, F., Teng, Y., Li, Q., & Li, J. (2019). Microrna–506–3p initiates mesenchymal–to–epithelial transition and suppresses autophagy in osteosarcoma cells by directly targeting Sphk1. *Bioscience, Biotechnology, and Biochemistry, 83*, 836–844.

Wang, L., Laing, J., Yan, B., Zhou, H., Ke, L., Wang, C., et al. (2020). Epstein–Barr virus episome physically interacts with active regions of the host genome in lymphoblastoid cells. *Journal of Virology, 94*, e01390–e01320.

Wojton, J., & Kaur, B. (2010). Impact of tumor microenvironment on oncolytic viral therapy. *Cytokine & Growth Factor Reviews, 21*, 127–134.

Yan, Y., Xu, H., Wang, J., Wu, X., Wen, W., Liang, Y., et al. (2019). Inhibition of breast cancer cells by targeting E2f−1 gene and expressing Il15 oncolytic adenovirus. *Bioscience Reports, 39*, Bsr20190384.

Yang, B., Shi, J., Sun, Z., Zhu, D., & Xu, X. (2020). Attenuated measles virus overcomes radio-and chemoresistance in human breast cancer cells by inhibiting the non-homologous end joining pathway. *Oncology Reports, 44*, 2253–2264.

Yano, S., Takehara, K., Kishimoto, H., Tazawa, H., Urata, Y., Kagawa, S., et al. (2016). Tumor−targeting adenovirus Obp−401 inhibits primary and metastatic tumor growth of triple−negative breast cancer in orthotopic nude−mouse models. *Oncotarget, 7*, 85273.

Yoshimori, M., Takada, H., Imadome, K., Kurata, M., Yamamoto, K., Koyama, T., et al. (2015). P−glycoprotein is expressed and causes resistance to chemotherapy in Ebv−positive T−cell lymphoproliferative diseases. *Cancer Medicine, 4*, 1494–1504.

Yuan, H., Fu, F., Zhuo, J., Wang, W., Nishitani, J., An, D. S., et al. (2005). Human papillomavirus type 16 E6 and E7 oncoproteins upregulate C−Iap2 gene expression and confer resistance to apoptosis. *Oncogene, 24*, 5069–5078.

Yugawa, T., & Kiyono, T. (2009). Molecular mechanisms of cervical carcinogenesis by high−risk human papillomaviruses: Novel functions of E6 and E7 oncoproteins. *Reviews in Medical Virology, 19*, 97–113.

Zhang, Y. (2021). The root cause of drug resistance in Her2−positive breast cancer and the therapeutic approaches to overcoming the resistance. *Pharmacology & Therapeutics, 218*, 107677.

Zhao, J. (2016). Cancer stem cells and chemoresistance: The smartest survives the raid. *Pharmacology & Therapeutics, 160*, 145–158.

Zhao, Y., Butler, E. B., & Tan, M. (2013). Targeting cellular metabolism to improve cancer therapeutics. *Cell Death & Disease, 4*, E532.

Zhao, H., Wang, H., Kong, F., Xu, W., Wang, T., Xiao, F., et al. (2019). Oncolytic adenovirus rad. Dcn inhibits breast tumor growth and lung metastasis in An immune−competent orthotopic xenograft model. *Human Gene Therapy, 30*, 197–210.

Zhu, W., Wei, L., Zhang, H., Chen, J., & Qin, X. (2012). Oncolytic adenovirus armed with il−24 inhibits the growth of breast cancer in vitro and in vivo. *Journal of Experimental & Clinical Cancer Research, 31*, 1–10.

Zhu, C. Y., Lv, Y. P., Yan, D. F., & Gao, F. L. (2013a). Knockdown of Mdr1 increases the sensitivity to Adriamycin in drug resistant gastric cancer cells. *Asian Pacific Journal of Cancer Prevention, 14*, 6757–6760.

Zhu, W., Zhang, H., Shi, Y., Song, M., Zhu, B., & Wei, L. (2013b). Oncolytic adenovirus encoding tumor necrosis factor−related apoptosis inducing ligand (trail) inhibits the growth and metastasis of triple−negative breast cancer. *Cancer Biology & Therapy, 14*, 1016–1023.

Harnessing the Power of Natural Products in Overcoming Drug Resistance in Breast Cancer

Nkhensani Y. Chauke-Malinga, Alaouna Mohammed, Kgomotso Poopedi, Nqobile Bundwini, Rodney Hull, Daniel Sambili, Sylvester L. Lyantagaye, and Zodwa Dlamini

Abstract This chapter explores the use of substances, including cannabis, curcumin, resveratrol, and green tea polyphenols, in the fight against drug resistance in breast cancer treatment. As traditional therapies face increasing resistance, scientists are turning to nature's resources for solutions. The chapter provides an analysis of compounds derived from various natural sources like plants, fungi, and marine organisms. It investigates how these compounds can overcome drug resistance mechanisms observed in breast cancer by targeting pathways such as apoptosis (cell death), cell cycle regulation, inhibition of efflux pumps (which remove drugs from cells), and angiogenesis (formation of blood vessels). Additionally, it highlights how these natural products can modify drug pathways to enhance the effectiveness of existing treatments. Through a

N. Y. Chauke-Malinga (✉) · D. Sambili
Department of Plastic and Reconstructive Surgery, Faculty of Health Sciences, Steve Biko Academic Hospital, University of Pretoria, Hatfield, Pretoria, South Africa
e-mail: ny.chauke-malinga@up.ac.za

A. Mohammed · R. Hull · Z. Dlamini
SAMRC Precision Oncology Research Unit (PORU), DSI/NRF SARChI Chair in Precision Oncology and Cancer Prevention (POCP), Pan African Cancer Research Institute (PACRI), University of Pretoria, Pretoria, South Africa
e-mail: 321814@students.wits.ac.za; rodney.hull@up.ac.za; zodwa.dlamini@up.ac.za

K. Poopedi
Department of Biochemistry, Microbiology and Biotechnology, University of Limpopo, Polokwane, South Africa
e-mail: kgomotso.poopedi@ul.ac.za

N. Bundwini
School on Management studies, Marketing section, University of Cape Town, Rondebosch, South Africa
e-mail: Nqobile.bundwini@uct.ac.za

S. L. Lyantagaye
Department of Molecular Biology and Biotechnology, College of Natural and Applied Sciences, University of Dar es Salaam, Dar es Salaam, Tanzania
e-mail: slyantagaye@udsm.ac.tz

Z. Dlamini (ed.), *Overcoming Breast Cancer Therapy Resistance*,
https://doi.org/10.1007/978-3-031-52860-6_9

review of research findings, this chapter explores the potential benefits of using natural products as complementary therapies to address drug resistance. Examples such as cannabis demonstrate the effectiveness of phytocannabinoids; curcumin's anti-inflammatory properties and resveratrol's impact on metabolic pathways are also discussed in detail. Furthermore, this chapter examines the limitations associated with using products, including side effects, variability in potency levels between different sources or batches, and challenges related to standardization and regulation.

This chapter provides valuable insights into the changing landscape of breast cancer treatment and the role that natural products play in addressing one of the urgent challenges in cancer therapy today. By presenting perspectives and showcasing a range of natural compounds, it offers a comprehensive understanding of this important topic.

Keywords South Africa · Sub-Saharan Africa · Socioeconomic conditions · Health education · Screening programs · Cultural beliefs · Toxicity · Cancer stem cells · Clinical translation · Bioavailability

Introduction

Breast cancer continues to be a pressing issue for women around the globe, drawing attention from scientists due to its societal impact. Despite advancements in the field of cancer research and treatment, the emergence of drug resistance remains a hurdle, resulting in reduced effectiveness of chemotherapy and an increased risk of disease recurrence (Adhikari et al., 2019; Braman et al., 2022). In response to this challenge, researchers are exploring an avenue of investigation into bioactive natural compounds with properties derived from various sources, such as plants, marine organisms, and microorganisms.

There has been a rise in the occurrence of breast cancer in sub-Saharan Africa, as indicated by recent studies and statistical analysis. This increase is also linked to mortality rates. These findings emphasize the need to comprehend the factors driving this trend and develop interventions to tackle this growing public health issue in the region (Anyigba, Awandare and Paemka, 2021). Outdated methods in the treatment of breast cancer, such as relying on chemotherapy and lacking targeted therapies, insufficient screening of patients, and delayed diagnoses, contribute to mortality rates from breast cancer caused by resistance to multiple drugs (Amjad, Chidharla and Kasi 2023). This chapter will delve into these challenges while emphasizing the necessity for precisely targeted interventions to combat drug resistance.

Particular interest is given to compounds derived from sources that have shown effectiveness in combating drug resistance in different strains of human breast carcinoma, such as MCF-7/ADR (Wang et al., 2015), MCF-7 (Catalano, 2019), MDA-MB-468 (Akogo et al., 2018), and T47D (Chaudhry et al., 2022).

Mechanisms of Action Exhibited By Natural Products in Overcoming Drug Resistance

The fight against breast cancer has encountered a hurdle in the form of drug resistance. To overcome this challenge, scientists are now exploring the benefits of natural products. In this section, we delve into the ways these compounds combat drug resistance in breast cancer treatment. By studying their effects on breast cancer cell lines like MCF-7, T47D, and MDA-MB-231, we gain insights into the exciting potential of natural therapeutic agents.

The modulation of pathways is a strategy used by natural products. A recent study focused on the MCF-7 cell line showed that specific compounds derived from plants can trigger apoptosis, effectively halting the growth of cancer cells (Dehelean et al., 2021). By encouraging programmed cell death in drug-resistant cancer cells, these compounds have the potential to make tumors more responsive to treatments, revitalizing their effectiveness.

Moreover, the utilization of substances is of significance in suppressing drug efflux pumps, which are frequently found to be expressed highly in cancer cells that are resistant to drugs. Studies conducted on the MDA-MB 231 cell line have uncovered that certain compounds derived from sources possess the ability to impede these pumps, thereby reinstating the sensitivity of drugs (Housman et al., 2014). By bypassing mechanisms that cause drug resistance, these products open doors for chemotherapy approaches.

Moreover, these compounds demonstrate the capability to alter signaling pathways that are often disrupted in cancer. Research conducted on the T47D cell line has indicated that specific compounds derived from microorganisms can effectively regulate these pathways, potentially diminishing the proliferation of cancer cells (Einarsdóttir et al., 2010). By focusing on signaling pathways associated with cancer growth, these compounds offer novel prospects for precise therapeutic interventions.

There is another strategy that focuses on using substances to target cancer stem cells. These cells are believed to be a contributor to the recurrence of cancer and resistance to therapy. Ongoing studies are working toward finding compounds that can effectively target these cells in different types of breast cancer cell lines (Wu et al., 2015). The hope is that by eliminating these cells, natural products can help prevent the return of the disease and enhance long-term treatment results.

In conclusion, the study of how products can help overcome drug resistance in breast cancer provides hope for personalized treatment options. These compounds show potential as medicines in breast cancer treatment by affecting cell death pathways, blocking drug removal pumps, adjusting abnormal signaling pathways, and targeting cancer stem cells. This section highlights the importance of agents in our ongoing battle against drug-resistant breast cancer through recent research findings and supporting evidence from scientific literature. By exploring these mechanisms and incorporating them into our practices, we can advance toward stronger and more successful treatment strategies for patients with breast cancer.

Modulation of Apoptosis Pathways

Apoptosis, which is the process of programmed cell death, plays a role in maintaining the balance of tissues by eliminating cells that are damaged or abnormal. In cancer, disruptions in these pathways can lead to drug resistance, allowing cancer cells to evade cell death induced by chemotherapy. The family of Bcl-2 proteins (BCL-2, BCL-XL, and BCLw) plays a central role in the regulation of apoptosis (Hardwick and Soane 2013). Bak, Bax, and Bid are the promoters of the induction of apoptosis, while the Bcl-2 proteins are the inhibitors of apoptosis (Adams and Cory, 2007). Apoptotic pathways can be divided into intrinsic and extrinsic pathways. This will be based on whether the stimulus originates from inside the cell or outside and is facilitated by caspases (Fulda & Debatin, 2006). In the extrinsic apoptotic pathway, a death domain transmits a signal from the outside to the interior of the cell. This is done by binding a ligand to the receptors, which recruits death domains to bind to the receptors (Muzio, 1998). As a result, pro-caspase-8 is activated by caspase-8, triggering the process of apoptosis (Elmore, 2007).

Under normal circumstances, the anti-apoptotic proteins Bcl-2 and Bcl-xL bind to and inhibit Bax and Bak to block the occurrence of apoptosis unless there is an absolute need or signal (Shamas-Din et al., 2013). The intrinsic pathway, or mitochondrial pathway, is triggered in the event of extensive DNA damage. The p53 gene initiates a cascade of processes to execute cell death by rendering the mitochondrion porous and eventually releasing cytochrome c. Some studies have also indicated the clinical utility of the anti-apoptotic protein Bcl-2 as a prediction marker for sensitivity to chemotherapy in breast cancer (Buchholz et al., 2003, Kasiri et al., 2020). Tumor cells have thus mastered the process of survival by evading the normal regulation of the anti-apoptotic and pro-apoptotic proteins, thus marking apoptosis as a vital target for natural compounds.

This section explores how natural substances offer hope for promoting apoptosis in breast cancer cells and countering the advantage that drug resistance mechanisms provide. We will focus on compounds derived from plants, like quercetin, curcumin, resveratrol, and epigallocatechin gallate (EGCG), exploring their effectiveness and understanding how they work.

Quercetin is a phytochemical classified under flavonoids, which are a group of secondary plant metabolites with a polyphenolic structure that are extensively present in fruits, vegetables, and some drinks. They exhibit many beneficial antioxidant, anti-inflammatory, and anti-cancer properties (Panche, Diwan and Chandra, 2016). Studies have shown quercetin-induced apoptosis via mitochondrial-mediated apoptosis in MCF-7 cells (Dhumale, Waghela and Pathak, 2015), the caspase-mediated death pathway in BT-474 breast cancer cells (Seo et al., 2016), and the enhancement of Bax and reduction of Bcl-2 (Khorsandi et al., 2017). This indicates the potential use of quercetin in sensitizing breast cancer cells to chemotherapeutic treatment by inhibiting the expression of Bcl-2.

Curcumin, a compound that is derived from turmeric (Curcuma longa), has gained attention for its potential as a cancer agent. Research conducted on breast cancer cell lines such as MCF-7 and MDA-MB-231 has demonstrated that curcumin can induce apoptosis by targeting signaling pathways (Tomeh et al., 2019). It is important to note that curcumin impacts the NF-B pathway, which regulates cell survival and inflammation. This characteristic leads to its efficacy in inducing apoptosis in breast cancer cells (Mansouri et al., 2020).

Resveratrol, a compound found in grapes (*Vitis vinifera*), shows promise in its ability to combat cancer by affecting pathways related to cell survival and the regulation of apoptosis. Research conducted on the MDA-MB-231 breast cancer cell line has demonstrated that resveratrol decreases the presence of proteins that inhibit apoptosis while promoting the release of factors that support apoptosis, ultimately leading to programmed cell death (Özdemi̇ et al., 2021, Jiang et al., 2022).

Harnessing the potential of tea is epigallocatechin gallate (EGCG), a polyphenol found in Camellia sinensis. It shows promise in stimulating apoptosis (cell death) in breast cancer cells by targeting signaling pathways like the PI3K/Akt pathway, which plays a role in cell survival and apoptosis regulation. Research indicates that EGCG boosts sensitivity to signals that trigger apoptosis, offering hope as a solution to drug resistance during breast cancer treatment (Puig et al., 2008; Qin et al., 2007; Shimizu et al., 2008).

Utilizing the modulation of apoptosis for treating breast cancer: By studying the ways in which these natural substances work and interact, researchers strive to develop therapies that can combat drug resistance in breast cancer. The capacity of substances like curcumin, resveratrol, and EGCG to regulate apoptosis pathways presents possibilities for cancer treatments. As scientists delve deeper into their understanding of these substances, incorporating them into treatment approaches may yield improved outcomes and management of drug-resistant breast cancer. The potential of utilizing products to modulate apoptosis holds promise for transforming the landscape of breast cancer treatment and providing patients with more effective and personalized therapeutic choices (Fig. 9.1).

Inhibition of Drug Efflux Pumps

Overcoming multidrug resistance (MDR) is an obstacle in the treatment of breast cancer as it reduces the effectiveness of chemotherapy and often leads to treatment failure. In this section, we delve into the potential of natural compounds as agents that can sensitize cancer cells, thus reversing MDR. These compounds work by inhibiting drug efflux pumps like P-glycoprotein (P-gp), which actively remove chemotherapy drugs from cancer cells, resulting in a decrease in their concentration inside the cells. Natural compounds such as plant-derived phytochemicals have demonstrated their ability to inhibit these drug efflux pumps, sensitizing cancer cells to chemotherapy and potentially overcoming MDR (Flint et al., 2022). This

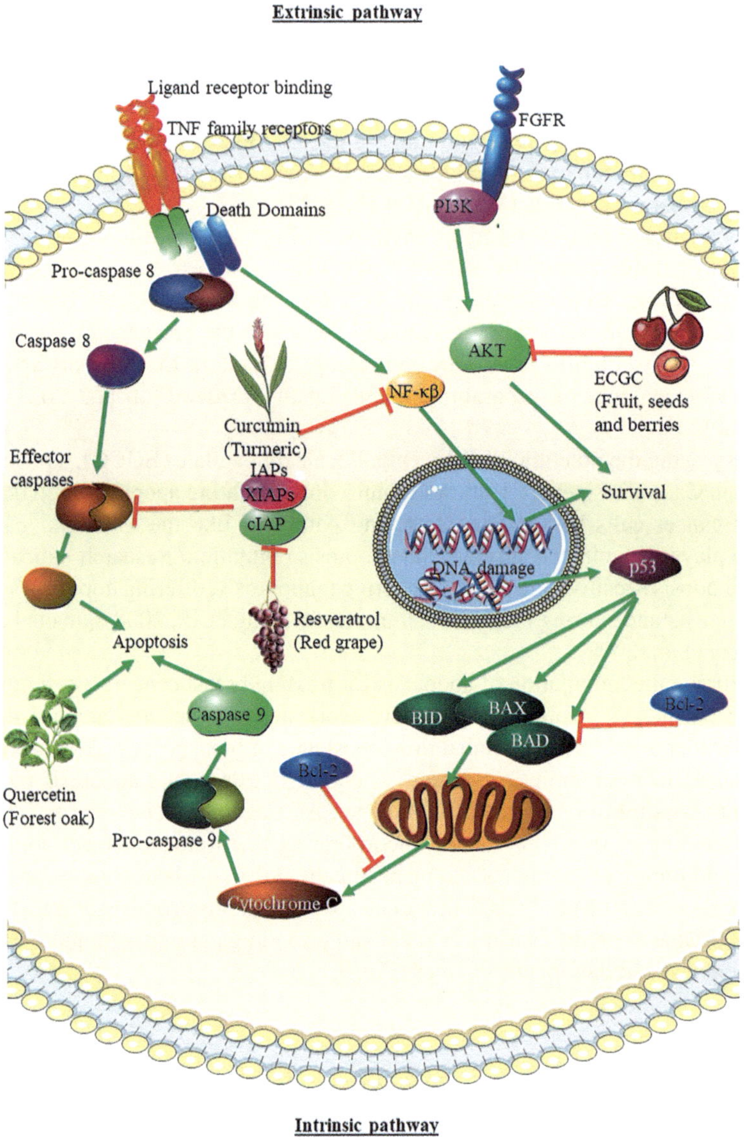

Fig. 9.1 *Breast Cancer Treatment*. This diagram portrays the interaction between the intrinsic and extrinsic apoptosis pathways in relation to breast cancer. The intrinsic pathway is set in motion by damage, while the extrinsic pathway is triggered by external signals. Essential proteins like Bcl-2 proteins, Bak, Bax, and Bid control apoptosis by utilizing mechanisms such as Death Domain and Caspase Activation that contribute to the pathway. The diagram also highlights how natural substances like quercetin, curcumin, resveratrol, and EGCG (derived from plants) can potentially influence these pathways and their impact on apoptosis in breast cancer cells. It provides an account of the actions of these substances on apoptosis pathways, including targets and induction. This underscores the exploration of compounds as potential therapeutic agents for overcoming drug resistance in breast cancer

offers an approach to improving the sensitivity of cancer cells to chemotherapy and overcoming drug resistance.

A compound found in fruits and vegetables, Quercetin, has shown promise for boosting the effectiveness of chemotherapy. It has been observed to inhibit drug efflux pumps such as P-gp. Studies conducted on MCF-7/DOX indicated that quercetin enhanced the antitumor activities of doxorubicin, paclitaxel, and vincristine via inhibition of the expression of P-gp and also eliminated cancer stem cells (Li et al., 2018). This flavonoid, at a concentration of 0.7 μM also raised the intracellular concentration of doxorubicin in MCF-7/DOX cells by suppressing the expression of P-gp (Li et al., 2013). The treatment of MDA-MB-231/MDR1 cells with quercetin sensitized the cells to treatment with doxorubicin (Liu et al., 2020). This ability of quercetin to sensitize drug-resistant cancer cells makes it an exciting potential addition to chemotherapy regimens.

Studies have shown that curcumin, a turmeric extract, can sensitize breast cancer drug-resistant cells to chemotherapy by inhibiting P-gp and other ABC transporters (Kong et al., 2021). A study by Wen et al., (2019) showed that curcumin significantly enhanced the effect of doxorubicin in doxorubicin-resistant breast cancer cells (MCF/DOX). *Curcumina wenyujin* and *Chrysanthemum indicum* are Chinese medicinal herbs. The fractionated extracts of those herbs, consisting, among others, of curcuminol, curcumin, curcumenone, and jasmolin, enhanced the accumulation levels of doxorubicin in the MCF/ADR cells by inhibiting the expression of P-gp (Yang et al., 2011). Schisandra chinensis is an Asian medicinal herb and supplement. Schisandrin A is a component of the herb that suppresses the expression of P-gp in MCF-7/DOX cells by blocking P-gp, NF-B, and Stat3 signaling (Zhang, Jiang and Wang, 2018).

Several flavonoids, including baicalein, have been found to improve the sensitivity of breast cancer cells to doxorubicin. The ability of baicalein and other phytochemicals to overcome drug resistance provides prospects for the development of novel treatment approaches (Table 9.1).

Pterostilbene, a compound present in blueberries and grapes, has been discovered to have the potential to enhance the effectiveness of chemotherapy. Research suggests that it can inhibit the expression of P-glycoprotein (P-gp) and make breast cancer cells more receptive to chemotherapy medications. In a study conducted by Bozorgi et al. (2020) and Obrador, Salvador-Palmer et al. (2021), it was found that pterostilbene can suppress MDR1 expression, a protein for multidrug resistance in cancer cells. Additionally, it triggers apoptotic mechanisms in cisplatin-treated human oral cancer CAR cells through AKT signaling. Other studies have also shed light on pterostilbene's role in promoting apoptosis in multidrug-resistant human breast cancer cells through the AKT/mTOR pathway (Hsu et al., 2020; Obrador, Salvador-Palmer et al., 2021); improving chemotherapy's effectiveness by reversing multidrug resistance in breast cancer cells (Bozorgi et al., 2020, Obrador, Salvador- Palmer et al., 2021); and reducing the expression of multidrug resistance proteins in breast cancer cells (Chang et al., 2018). These findings collectively emphasize the potential of pterostilbene as an agent for overcoming multidrug resistance during breast cancer treatment. As scientists delve deeper into

Table 9.1 Flavonoids enhancing sensitivity to doxorubicin in breast cancer cells

Flavonoid	Source	Mechanism of action	References
Baicalein	*Scutellaria baicalensis*	Inhibits P-gp, enhances sensitivity to doxorubicin	Meng et al. (2016) and Lin et al. (2021)
Glabridin	Licorice root	Inhibits migration, invasion, and angiogenesis	Mu et al. (2017)
Myricetin	Various plants and herbs	Suppresses breast cancer metastasis	Ci et al. (2018)
Daidzein	Various plants and herbs	Effects on breast cancer growth	de Lemos (2001)
Quercetin	Various sources	MicroRNA targeting, inhibits proliferation and invasion	Tao, He and Chen (2015) and Kim et al. (2019)

understanding how it works and its safety profile, pterostilbene offers hope for treatment strategies.

The effectiveness of plant phytochemicals in targeting drug efflux pumps is promising. Compounds such as curcumin, quercetin, and pterostilbene have shown their potential for circumventing drug resistance in breast cancer cells, thus making them more receptive to chemotherapy. However, there are still challenges to delivering the right amount of medication to breast cancer sites. It is important to explore strategies like using nanotechnology-based drug delivery systems and combination therapies to improve the effectiveness and availability of these remedies (Calixto et al., 2016; Parhi et al., 2012; Suri et al., 2007). This integration has the ability to significantly enhance the effectiveness of breast cancer treatment and open doors for new strategies. By targeting drug efflux pumps with plant phytochemicals, we can make progress in combating drug resistance and improving the quality of life for breast cancer patients (Fig. 9.2).

Modulation of Signaling Pathways

In this section, the potential of substances to target the irregularities in signaling pathways are observed in cancer cells. These irregularities contribute to the survival, proliferation, and resistance to treatment of these cells. One notable compound found in grapes is resveratrol, which has shown promise in modulating signaling pathways, including the PI3K/Akt pathway. This pathway plays a role in the survival of cancer cells and their resistance to drugs (Fulda & Debatin, 2006; Gupta et al., 2011; He et al., 2011). For instance, resveratrol, a polyphenol commonly found in grapes, has been discovered to suppress the activation of the PI3K/Akt pathway. This pathway is crucial for cancer cell survival and their ability to resist therapies (Jang et al., 2022). By disrupting this pathway, resveratrol can make drug-resistant breast cancer cells more susceptible to treatment, offering a strategy against MDR.

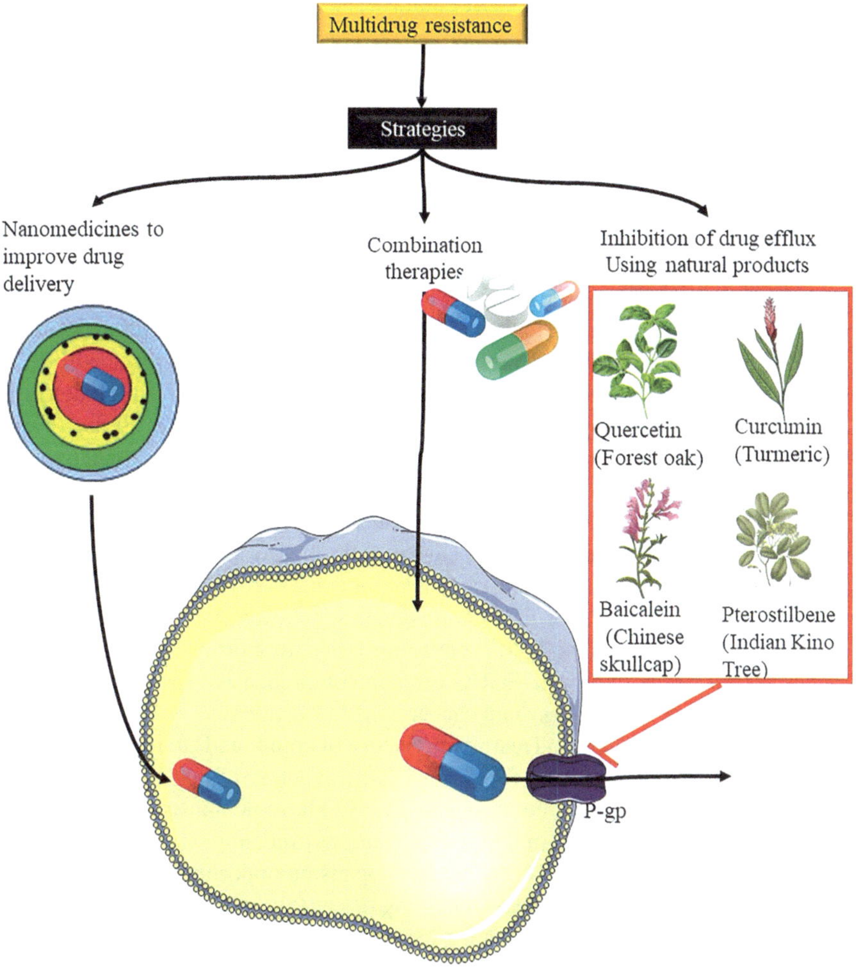

Fig. 9.2 *Breast cancer. Overcoming drug resistance***.** This diagram depicts the process of addressing multidrug resistance (MDR) in breast cancer by targeting drug efflux pumps, such as P-glycoprotein (P-gp). The main focus is on compounds like quercetin, curcumin, baicalein, and pterostilbene, which have shown promise in inhibiting these pumps and enhancing the effectiveness of chemotherapy. The diagram also explores the pathways through which these compounds work, including the AKT/mTOR pathway. It also delves into strategies like nanotechnology-based drug delivery and combination therapies to further improve treatment outcomes. The interconnected nodes represent an approach to combating drug resistance in breast cancer while highlighting the benefits of plant-derived phytochemicals in improving patients' quality of life

Similarly, quercetin, found in fruits and vegetables, has demonstrated its capability to inhibit the NF-B signaling pathway associated with both drug resistance and cancer cell survival (Khan et al., 2016). By modulating this pathway, quercetin presents a means to enhance the susceptibility of breast cancer cells to apoptosis and improve their response to chemotherapy. Resveratrol is known for its ability to inhibit the activation of the PI3K/Akt pathway, which plays a role in controlling cellular processes such as cell growth, proliferation, and survival. It is commonly observed that dysregulation of this pathway contributes to tumor formation and resistance to cancer treatments. In the case of resveratrol, it has shown promising outcomes by arresting the cell cycle and inducing apoptosis in cancer cells. This mechanism makes resveratrol an agent for sensitizing drug-resistant cancer cells and improving the efficacy of chemotherapy treatments (Cal et al., 2003; Jazirehi & Bonavida, 2004; Kweon et al., 2010).

Curcumin, which is a compound extracted from turmeric, has shown potential for hindering the NF-B signaling pathway. This particular pathway plays a role in supporting the survival of cells affected by inflammation and making cancer cells resistant to apoptosis (Shanmugam et al., 2015). Through its interference with NF-B activity, curcumin enhances the responsiveness of cancer cells to signals that trigger apoptosis, thus improving the effectiveness of chemotherapy. The ability of curcumin to combat drug resistance further highlights its value as a treatment, alongside chemotherapy, for breast cancer.

Epigallocatechin gallate (EGCG), a polyphenol present in tea, has the ability to influence signaling pathways within cancer cells. It can modulate pathways like PI3K/Akt and Wnt/ catenin, which are crucial for cancer progression (Pozo-Guisado et al., 2002). These effects of EGCG on signaling pathways not only contribute to its cancer properties but also hold promise for combating drug resistance in breast cancer. By targeting pathways, EGCG offers a comprehensive strategy to enhance the responsiveness of drug-resistant cancer cells to treatment.

Promising Approaches for Treatment: The use of compounds to influence signaling pathways shows potential for developing treatment strategies against drug-resistant cancer. Resveratrol, curcumin, and EGCG have demonstrated their ability to disrupt signaling processes, making them additions to chemotherapy. Incorporating these compounds into combination therapies opens up opportunities for enhancing treatment outcomes in breast cancer. Ongoing research continues to reveal the interactions and mechanisms underlying the impacts of these substances. By harnessing the power of these compounds in combination treatments, we may be able to devise approaches to overcome drug resistance and advance breast cancer treatment (Fig. 9.3).

Targeting Cancer Stem Cells

In recent years, the identification of cancer stem cells (CSCs) within tumors has provided insights into an important factor that contributes to drug resistance and the recurrence of breast cancer. This section explores the features of CSCs and their involvement in promoting tumor growth and resistance to treatments. Researchers are actively investigating methods to target CSCs as a way of overcoming drug resistance and minimizing the risk of tumor recurrence. Natural products have

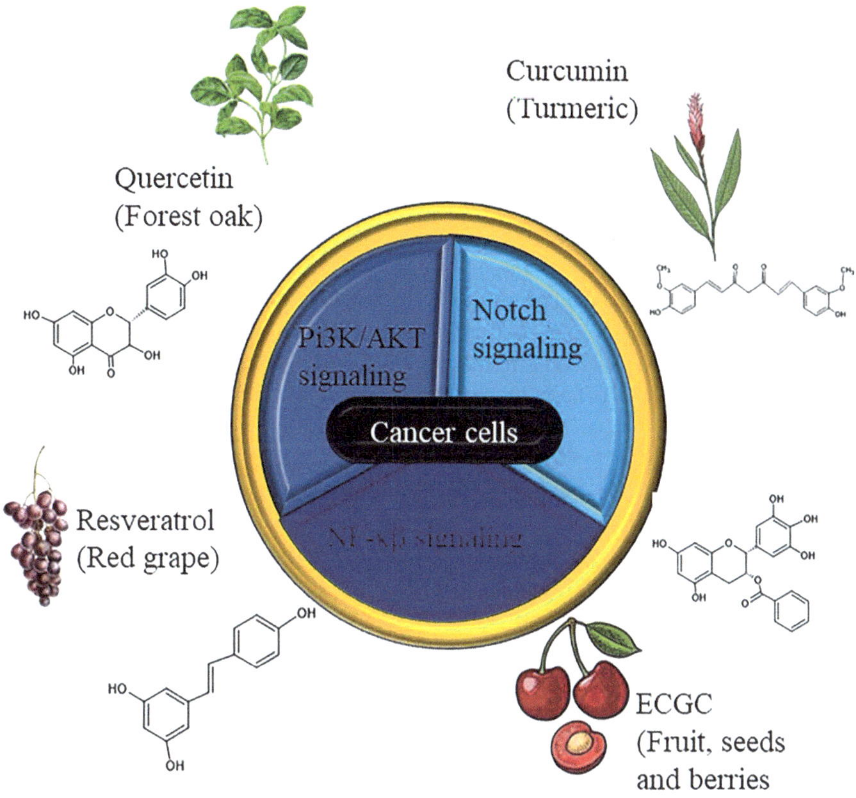

Fig. 9.3 *Modulating signaling pathways in the treatment of cancer*. "Exploring the potential of compounds to target abnormalities" delves into the use of substances such as resveratrol, a polyphenol found in grapes that suppresses the PI3K/Akt pathway vital for cancer cell survival; quercetin, present in fruits and vegetables, which inhibits the NF-κB signaling pathway and enhances susceptibility to apoptosis; curcumin, extracted from turmeric, that hinders the NF-B signaling pathway and improves the effectiveness of chemotherapy; and Epigallocatechin Gallate (EGCG) a polyphenol found in tea that modulates pathways like PI3K/Akt and Wnt/catenin, enhancing responsiveness to treatment. These compounds collectively offer promising approaches to address irregularities in signaling pathways observed in cancer cells. They provide strategies against drug cancer. Contribute to advancements in breast cancer treatment

emerged as contenders for targeting CSCs and presenting avenues for improving outcomes in breast cancer treatment.

Salinomycin, a compound derived from *Streptomyces albus*, has garnered attention due to its ability to target cancer stem cells (CSCs). Numerous studies have demonstrated that salinomycin exhibits efficacy in eliminating CSCs found in cancer types, including well-known breast cancer cell lines such as MCF-7 and MDA-MB-231 (Zhou et al., 2013). Its mechanism of action involves disrupting the pathways for CSC self-renewal and survival. Additionally, salinomycin enhances the sensitivity of CSCs toward therapies, thereby improving the effectiveness of chemotherapy and reducing the risk of drug resistance.

Sulforaphane, which is present in vegetables such as broccoli and cauliflower, has been the subject of research regarding its ability to target CSCs (cancer stem cells). Studies have shown that sulforaphane can effectively hinder the growth of CSCs while encouraging their transformation into stem cells. The sulforaphane metabolite enhances the responsiveness of CSCs to chemotherapy medications. Consequently, it aids in preventing tumor reappearance and metastasis (Coutinho et al., 2023).

Apart from salinomycin and sulforaphane, several other natural substances have shown promising outcomes in targeting cancer stem cells (CSCs) and overcoming drug resistance in breast cancer. Curcumin, for instance, has displayed the ability to specifically target CSCs in breast cancer, resulting in reduced tumor growth and increased responsiveness to chemotherapy (Zoi et al., 2021). Additionally, honokiol derived from Magnolia officinalis has demonstrated its potential for targeting CSCs not only in breast cancer but in other types of malignancies (Wang, Zhang, & Chen, 2019a)

In conclusion, there is potential for researching ways to target CSCs for breast cancer treatment outcomes and overcoming drug resistance. Natural substances such as salinomycin, sulforaphane, curcumin, and honokiol have shown promise in eliminating CSCs and making them more responsive to therapies. By studying how these natural compounds affect CSCs, we can explore the possibility of incorporating them into combination treatments, which could lead to effective approaches for patients dealing with drug-resistant forms of breast cancer (Fig. 9.4).

The Role of Natural Products As Chemosensitizers in Reversing Multidrug Resistance in Breast Cancer

Natural products have shown promise not in inhibiting drug efflux pumps but in targeting signaling pathways linked to drug resistance. This creates opportunities for tackling multidrug resistance (MDR) and improving the effectiveness of chemotherapy.

Scientists have been investigating the potential of substances to target cancer stem cells (CSCs), a small group of cells within tumors that contribute to drug resistance and tumor recurrence. By focusing on CSCs' natural compounds, they hold promise for combating multidrug resistance (MDR), reducing the likelihood of tumor reoccurrence (Phi et al., 2018). One such compound is salinomycin, an antibiotic derived from *Streptomyces albus*. Studies have shown its effectiveness in eliminating CSCs in breast cancer (Qi et al., 2022). By targeting CSCs, salinomycin offers potential for overcoming MDR and decreasing the chances of tumor reoccurrence.

Another natural compound called sulforaphane, which is found in vegetables, has demonstrated its ability to hinder the proliferation of CSCs and induce their differentiation. This leads to reduced tumor growth. Increased sensitivity to

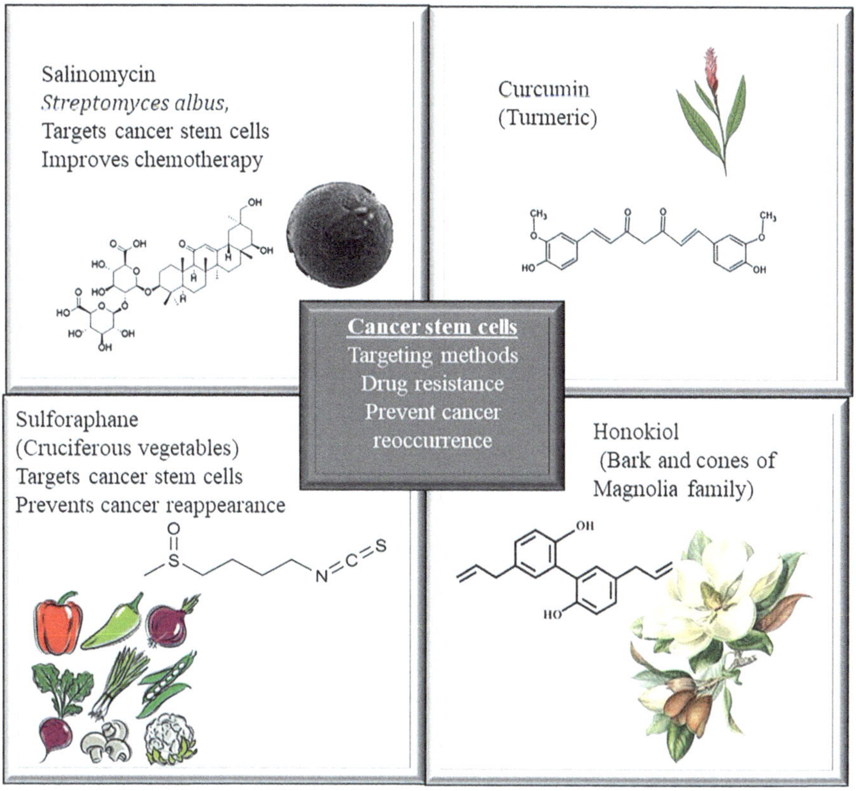

Fig. 9.4 *Strategies and Natural Compounds for Targeting Cancer Stem Cells.* In this diagram, we can see the advancements in combating drug resistance and recurrence in breast cancer by focusing on cancer stem cells (CSCs). The diagram emphasizes the role of CSCs in promoting tumor growth and the ongoing research efforts to target them. It showcases natural compounds such as salinomycin, sulforaphane, curcumin, and honokiol that have shown promise in effectively targeting CSCs. Salinomycin disrupts the self-renewal process of CSCs. Sulforaphane inhibits CSC growth. Curcumin specifically targets CSCs in breast cancer cases, while Honokiol exhibits potential across types of malignancies. Together, these substances offer avenues for enhancing breast cancer treatment outcomes and exploring combination therapies to address drug-resistant forms of the disease

chemotherapy drugs in breast cancer patients (Li et al., 2010). In conclusion, natural products show potential as chemosensitizers for reversing multidrug resistance in breast cancer. Compounds like curcumin, resveratrol, quercetin, salinomycin, and sulforaphane offer mechanisms that inhibit drug efflux pumps, modulate signaling pathways, and target cancer stem cells. Integrating these products into combination therapies could lead to targeted treatments for breast cancer patients facing multidrug-resistant malignancies. As research progresses further into these compounds, they hold promise for enhancing the effectiveness of chemotherapy and overcoming drug resistance in breast cancer treatment.

The Transition of Natural Compounds from the Laboratory to Clinical Settings in Breast Cancer Treatment

In the field of breast cancer research, natural products have been used since ancient times. Some of these substances, like curcumin, quercetin, and genistein, have shown promise in fighting drug resistance during breast cancer treatment. This section delves into their potential. Discusses the challenges that need to be overcome to effectively apply these findings in clinical settings and improve patient care.

Bioavailability Challenges

A major hurdle in bringing advancements to reality is the problem of bioavailability. Numerous natural substances encounter difficulties in getting absorbed and distributed properly within the body, which consequently impacts their effectiveness in treating breast cancer. Scientists are actively investigating techniques such as nanoformulations or drug delivery systems to boost the bioavailability of these substances (Date et al., 2016). The objective of these approaches is to enhance the efficacy of products in medical scenarios by improving their absorption and distribution.

The bioavailability of the most studied phytochemicals, such as curcumin, quercetin, and epigallocatechin, was improved by conjugation with different delivery systems, as summarized in this study (Cas and Ghidoni, 2019, Manzoor et al., 2021).

Interaction with Conventional Therapies

Given that individuals with breast cancer receive treatments such as chemotherapy, hormonal therapy, and targeted therapies, it is crucial to comprehend the potential interactions between natural compounds and these treatments. The simultaneous use of products alongside therapies may influence how these therapies are processed in the body or how they exert their effects, which can potentially impact the effectiveness and safety of treatment (Ekor, 2014). It is vital to evaluate these interactions to successfully incorporate products into breast cancer treatment plans. Verapamil, a medication that blocks calcium channels, has attracted interest due to its potential to address drug resistance in breast cancer. Research has shown that verapamil can hinder P-gp activity, making cancer cells more responsive to chemotherapy (Belpomme et al., 2000; Dönmez et al., 2011; Wang et al., 2011). This discovery has opened up possibilities for combination treatments, where verapamil is used in conjunction with phytochemical compounds to enhance the efficacy of the treatment. The most studied natural compound, paclitaxel, which is used as conventional medicine in the treatment of different types of cancer, has issues with chemoresistance in breast cancer patients (Rivera, 2010). To improve the efficacy and sensitivity of paclitaxel to MCF-7/ADR cells, it was combined with verapamil (Li, Zhong and Gong, 2019). Other studies indicated that the combination of paclitaxel with other phytochemical compounds such as the green tea polyphenol epigallocatechin gallate (EGCG) (Scandlyn et al., 2008; Luo et al., 2010), allicin (Vemuri et al., 2017), thymoquinone (Mosalam et al., 2020), and piperine (Khamisi et al., 2018) sensitized the breast cancer cells to paclitaxel treatment. A study by Talib et al. (2022) extensively reviews the combination of anti-cancer therapies with phytochemicals.

Clinical Trials and Effectiveness

Several ongoing clinical trials are currently studying the efficacy of interventions utilizing products in patients with drug-resistant breast cancer (Table 9.2). The objective of these trials is to assess whether natural products can enhance the sensitivity of drug-resistant breast cancer cells to therapies, ultimately resulting in improved treatment outcomes and patient survival (Wang, Zhang & Chen, 2019b). Furthermore, these trials aim to investigate the effects that may arise from combining interventions derived from natural products with traditional treatments. The potential of using products in the treatment of breast cancer is promising, especially when it comes to tackling drug resistance and improving the effectiveness of treatments. However, it is important to address challenges related to how these products are absorbed by the body, their potential for toxicity, and their interactions with therapies. Ongoing clinical trials are providing knowledge about the capabilities of compounds in treating breast cancer. If these findings can be successfully applied, they may lead to effective treatment strategies for patients with breast cancer.

Cannabis As a Natural Cancer Therapy

Following the recent changes in laws pertaining to the medicinal use of cannabis globally, there has been increased interest in the role of cannabis in treating various ailments. Cannabis is a natural product extracted from the *Cannabis sativa* plant and has been used extensively for medicinal purposes for multiple centuries (Bowles et al., 2012). Cannabinoids are the chemical compounds that make up the plant, and tetrahydrocannabinol (THC) is the cannabinoid that produces its psychoactive and physiological effects, while cannabidiol (CBD) is non-psychoactive but also known for its pharmacological properties (Heider et al., 2022).

Some studies have found evidence of the anti-cancer effects of cannabinoids in lung cancer as early as the 1970s (Munson et al., 1975) and, more recently, their

Table 9.2 List of phytochemicals currently in clinical trials on breast cancer

Phytochemical	Curcumin	Epigallocatehin (EGCG)	Resveratrol	Baicalin
Botanical name	*Curcuma longa*	*Camellia sinensis*	*Polygonum cuspidatum*	*Scutellaria baicalensis*
Mechanism	NF-κB signaling pathway: ↓ P-g expression ↓ BCRP ↓ MRP1 ↓ MDR1 mRNA ↓ ABCG2 and ABCC1 ↓ PKC-α and –ζ ↓ GSTπ ↓ Topo IIα	Cell proliferation on and apoptosis ↓ P-g expression ↓ MDR1 ↓ ATPase activity	↓ BCRP ↓ P-gp expression ↓ HIF-1α ↓ GST mRNA	↓ P-gp expression ↓ MRP1
Clinical trials	A randomized, double-blind, placebo-controlled phase 2/3 trial of 150 women with advanced and metastatic breast cancer	Randomized, double-blinded, placebo-controlled phase II clinical trial involving 1075 healthy	A randomized, double-blinded, placebo-controlled trial	A randomized, double-blinded, placebo-controlled trial Multicenter, open-label, dose-escalation phase 1B clinical trial with 27 women diagnosed with
Assessment	Efficacy and safety of curcumin in combination with paclitaxel in advanced and metastatic breast cancer patients	Investigate whether supplementation with green tea extract modifies mammographic density as a potential	Efficacy of a phenolic compound, trans-resveratrol, to decrease methylation	Safety and efficacy of *Scutellaria baicalensis* (BZL101)
Outcomes	Curcumin was safe and tolerable in humans. Its combination with paclitaxel was superior to the paclitaxel, Placebo-combination	EGCG significantly reduced the percent mammographic density of younger women	Trans-resveratrol decreased methylation of tumor	Oral administration of BZL101 was safe, well tolerated, and showed promising
References	Bharti and Aggarwal (2002), Saghatelyan et al. (2020) and Bashmail et al. (2020)	Michalak and Wesolowska (2012), Nabekura (2010) and Samavat et al. (2017)	Zhu et al. (2012)	Talib et al. (2021) and Perez et al. (2010)

inhibitive properties for tumor growth in breast, thyroid, and prostate cancer (Pisanti et al., 2009). The manner in which this effect occurs is believed to involve the suppression of proliferative cell signaling pathways, the inhibition of angiogenesis and cell migration, the stimulation of apoptosis, and/or the induction of autophagy (Salazar et al., 2009). Similarly, other research found that cannabinoids may exert their anti-cancer effects primarily by binding to a group of cannabinoid receptors, which can exert anti-inflammatory, pro-apoptotic, and antiproliferative effects, thereby helping fight against cancer (Pertwee, 2008).

Although research on cannabis use in cancer is limited, there have been other documented medicinal effects of cannabis. It has been known to stimulate appetite in anorexic patients (Ben Amar 2006) and to treat anxiety and insomnia. Cannabis has been found to have palliative effects, reducing pain associated with various cancer therapies (Bar-Sela et al., 2013), as well as antinausea effects in patients undergoing chemotherapy. Tramèrl et al. (2001) found cannabinoids to be significantly more effective antiemetics than other pharmacological products such as prochlorperazine, metoclopramide, chlorpromazine, thiethylperazine, haloperidol, domperidone, or alizapride.

Given the rising popularity of cannabis as an alternative or supplement to established cancer treatments as well as the aforementioned challenges of these treatments, due attention should be given to researching cannabis as a natural product in cancer treatment. Cannabinoids have the ability to palliate some symptoms, but their effectiveness is not certain in comparison to or in combination with conventional treatments. The future involvement of cannabis in cancer will be largely affected by law, politics, and social sentiment; however, scientific research should carefully investigate both the potential benefits and risks to society.

Conclusion

To sum up, tackling the obstacles posed by drug resistance in breast cancer treatment demands an approach that considers trends, possible contributing factors, and innovative therapeutic methods. The occurrence and prevalence of breast cancer in South Africa and sub-Saharan Africa have been shaped by circumstances such as restricted healthcare access, insufficient health education, ineffective screening programs, and cultural beliefs. These aspects underscore the significance of implementing comprehensive public health initiatives to enhance breast cancer outcomes in the region.

Outdated methods of treating breast cancer, which often come with side effects and issues like toxicity and drug resistance, pose obstacles to effective therapy. To address these challenges, natural products have emerged as an avenue for solutions. These products offer a range of mechanisms to combat drug-resistant breast cancer, including regulating apoptosis, inhibiting drug efflux pumps, influencing signaling pathways, and targeting cancer stem cells.

Experts in biochemistry, molecular biology, and cell biology have an advantage when it comes to delving into the possibilities of using natural products for treating breast cancer. With their expertise, they can create customized treatment plans that cater specifically to each patient's needs, increasing the likelihood of results.

As natural substances progress from testing to trials, they hold the promise of transforming breast cancer treatments. Compounds such as curcumin have shown their capacity to make drug-resistant breast cancer cells more receptive to chemotherapy, paving the way for innovative and impactful combination therapies. By combining remedies with treatment approaches, we have the potential to greatly boost the efficiency of chemotherapy, conquer drug resistance, and enhance patient results. Ongoing exploration and analysis in this field offer hope for a future where breast cancer treatments are customized to each individual and yield outcomes that instill optimism in patients and push forward in the battle against breast cancer. In this chapter, we have presented evidence from the literature that supports the use of products in breast cancer research. If these compounds are properly integrated into practice, they could bring about advancements in the treatment of breast cancer, benefiting patients all over the world. By continuing research, fostering collaborations, and receiving commitment from the community, we can further harness the potential of natural products to combat drug resistance and improve outcomes for those with breast cancer.

References

Adams, J. M., & Cory, S. (2007). The Bcl-2 apoptotic switch in cancer development and therapy. *Oncogene, 26*(9), 1324–1337.

Adhikari, P., Nagesh, P. K. B., Alharthi, F., Chauhan, S. C., Jaggi, M., Yallapu, M. M., & Pradhan, P. (2019). Optical detection of the structural properties of tumor tissue generated by xenografting of drug-sensitive and drug-resistant cancer cells using partial wave spectroscopy (PWS). *Biomedical Optics Express, 10*, 6422–6431.

Akogo, D. A., Appiah, V. & Palmer, X.-L. (2018). CellLineNet: end-to-end learning and transfer learning for multiclass epithelial breast cell line classification via a convolutional neural network. arXiv preprint arXiv:1808.06041.

Amjad, M. T., Chidharla, A., & Kasi, A. (2023). Cancer Chemotherapy. In *StatPearls [Internet]*. StatPearls Publishing. 2024 Jan–. PMID: 33232037.

Anyigba, C. A., Awandare, G. A., & Paemka, L. (2021). Breast cancer in sub-Saharan Africa: The current state and uncertain future. *Experimental Biology and Medicine, 246*(12), 1377–1387.

Bar-Sela, G., Vorobeichik, M., Drawsheh, S., Omer, A., Goldberg, V., & Muller, E. (2013). The medical necessity for medicinal cannabis: Prospective observational study evaluating the treatment in cancer patients on supportive or palliative care. *Evidence-based Complementary and Alternative Medicine, 2013*, 510392.

Bashmail, H. A., Alamoudi, A. A., Noorwali, A., Hegazy, G. A., Ajabnoor, G. M., & Al-Abd, A. M. (2020). Thymoquinone enhances paclitaxel anti-breast cancer activity via inhibiting tumor-associated stem cells despite apparent mathematical antagonism. *Molecules, 25*(2), 426.

Belpomme, D., Gauthier, S., Pujade-Lauraine, E., Facchini, T., Goudier, M. J., Krakowski, I., et al. (2000). Verapamil increases the survival of patients with anthracycline-resistant metastatic breast carcinoma. *Annals of Oncology, 11*, 1471–1476.

Bharti, A. C., & Aggarwal, B. B. (2002). Nuclear factor-kappa B and cancer: Its role in prevention and therapy. *Biochemical Pharmacology, 64*(5-6), 883–888.
Bowles, D. W., O'Bryant, C. L., Camidge, D. R., & Jimeno, A. (2012). The intersection between cannabis and cancer in the United States. *Critical Reviews in Oncology/Hematology, 83*(1), 1–10.
Bozorgı, A., Khazaei, S., Khademi, A., & Khazaei, M. (2020). Natural and herbal compounds targeting breast cancer, a review based on cancer stem cells. *Iranian Journal of Basic Medical Sciences, 23*, 970–983.
Braman, N., Prasanna, P., Bera, K., Alilou, M., Khorrami, M., Leo, P., et al. (2022). Novel radiomic measurements of tumor-associated vasculature morphology on clinical imaging as a biomarker of treatment response in multiple cancers. *Clinical Cancer Research, 28*, 4410–4424.
Buchholz, T. A., Davis, D. W., McConkey, D. J., Symmans, W. F., Valero, V., Jhingran, A., Tucker, S. L., Pusztai, L., Cristofanilli, M., Esteva, F. J., Hortobagyi, G. N., & Sahin, A. A. (2003). Chemotherapy-induced apoptosis and Bcl-2 levels correlate with breast cancer response to chemotherapy. *The Cancer Journal, 9*(1), 33–41.
Cal, C., Garban, H., Jazirehi, A., Yeh, C., Mizutani, Y., & Bonavida, B. (2003). Resveratrol and cancer: Chemoprevention, apoptosis, and Chemoimmunosensitizing activities. *Current Medicinal Chemistry-Anti-Cancer Agents, 3*, 77–93.
Calixto, G. M. F., Bernegossi, J., De Freitas, L. M., Fontana, C. R., & Chorilli, M. (2016). Nanotechnology-based drug delivery systems for photodynamic therapy of cancer: A review. *Molecules, 21*, 342.
Cas, M. D., & Ghidoni, R. (2019). Dietary curcumin: Correlation between bioavailability and health potential. *Nutrients, 11*(9), 2147.
Catalano, E. (2019). Superparamagnetic iron oxide nanoparticles conjugated with doxorubicin for targeting breast cancer. arXiv preprint arXiv:1911.05378.
Chang, H. P., Lu, C. C., Chiang, J. H., Tsai, F. J., Juan, Y. N., Tsao, J. W., et al. (2018). Pterostilbene modulates the suppression of multidrug resistance protein 1 and triggers autophagic and apoptotic mechanisms in cisplatin-resistant human oral cancer CAR cells via AKT signaling. *International Journal of Oncology, 52*, 1504–1514.
Chaudhry, G. E., Md Akim, A., Sung, Y. Y., & Sifzizul, T. M. T. (2022). Cancer and apoptosis: The apoptotic activity of plant and marine natural products and their potential as targeted cancer therapeutics. *Frontiers in Pharmacology, 13*, 842376.
Ci, Y., Zhang, Y., Liu, Y., Lu, S., Cao, J., Li, H., Zhang, J., Huang, Z., Zhu, X., Gao, J., & Han, M. (2018). Myricetin suppresses breast cancer metastasis through down-regulating the activity of matrix metalloproteinase (MMP)-2/9. *Phytotherapy Research, 32*(7), 1373–1381.
Coutinho, L. L., Junior, T. C. T., & Rangel, M. C. (2023). Sulforaphane: An emergent anti-cancer stem cell agent. *Frontiers in Oncology, 13*, 1089115.
Date, A. A., Hanes, J., & Ensign, L. M. (2016). Nanoparticles for oral delivery: Design, evaluation and state-of-the-art. *Journal of Controlled Release, 240*, 504–526.
Dehelean, C. A., Marcovici, I., Soica, C., Mioc, M., Coricovac, D., Iurciuc, S., Cretu, O. M., et al. (2021). Plant-derived anticancer compounds as new perspectives in drug discovery and alternative therapy. *Molecules, 26*, 1109.
de Lemos, M. L. (2001). Effects of soy phytoestrogens genistein and daidzein on breast cancer growth. *Annals of Pharmacotherapy, 35*(9), 1118–1121.
Dhumale, S. S., Waghela, B. N., & Pathak, C. (2015). Quercetin protects necrotic insult and promotes apoptosis by attenuating the expression of RAGE and its ligand HMGB1 in human breast adenocarcinoma cells. *IUBMB Life, 67*(5), 361–373.
Dönmez, Y., Akhmetova, L., Işeri, Ö. D., Kars, M. D., & Gündüz, U. (2011). Effect of MDR modulators verapamil and promethazine on gene expression levels of MDR1 and MRP1 in doxorubicin-resistant MCF-7 cells. *Cancer Chemotherapy and Pharmacology, 67*, 823–828.
Einarsdóttir, E., Groeneweg, J., Björnsdóttir, G. G., Harðardottir, G., Omarsdóttir, S., Ingólfsdóttir, K., et al. (2010). Cellular mechanisms of the anticancer effects of the lichen compound Usnic acid. *Planta Medica, 76*, 969–974.
Ekor, M. (2014). The growing use of herbal medicines: Issues relating to adverse reactions and challenges in monitoring safety. *Frontiers in Pharmacology, 4*, 177.

Elmore, S. (2007). Apoptosis: A review of programmed cell death. *Toxicologic Pathology, 35*(4), 495–516.

Flint, A. L., Hansen, D. W., Brown, L. D., Stewart, L. E., Ortiz, E., & Panda, S. S. (2022). Modified curcumins as potential drug candidates for breast cancer: An overview. *Molecules, 27*, 8891.

Fulda, S., & Debatin, K.-M. (2006). Resveratrol modulation of signal transduction in apoptosis and cell survival: A mini-review. *Cancer Detection and Prevention, 30*, 217–223.

Fulda, S., & Debatin, K. M. (2006). Extrinsic versus intrinsic apoptosis pathways in anticancer chemotherapy. *Oncogene, 25*(34), 4798–4811.

Gupta, S. C., Kannappan, R., Reuter, S., Kim, J. H., & Aggarwal, B. B. (2011). Chemosensitization of tumors by resveratrol. *Annals of the New York Academy of Sciences, 1215*, 150–160.

Hardwick, J. M., & Soane, L. (2013). Multiple functions of BCL-2 family proteins. *Cold Spring Harbor Perspectives in Biology, 5*(2), a008722–a008722.

He, X., Wang, Y., Zhu, J., Orloff, M., & Eng, C. (2011). Resveratrol enhances the anti- tumor activity of the mTOR inhibitor rapamycin in multiple breast cancer cell lines mainly by suppressing rapamycin-induced AKT signaling. *Cancer Letters, 301*, 168–176.

Heider, C. G., Itenberg, S. A., Rao, J., Ma, H., & Wu, X. (2022). Mechanisms of cannabidiol (CBD) in cancer treatment: A review. *Biology, 11*(6), 817. https://doi.org/10.3390/biology11060817

Housman, G., Byler, S., Heerboth, S., Lapinska, K., Longacre, M., Snyder, N., et al. (2014). Drug resistance in cancer: An overview. *Cancers (Basel), 6*, 1769–1792.

Hsu, Y-H., Chen, S-Y., Wang, S-Y., Lin, J-A., & Yen, G-C. (2020). Pterostilbene enhances cytotoxicity and chemosensitivity in human pancreatic cancer cells. *Biomolecules, 10*(5), 709. https://doi.org/10.3390/biom10050709

Jang, J. Y., Im, E., & Kim, N. D. (2022). Mechanism of resveratrol-induced programmed cell death and new drug discovery against cancer: A review. *International Journal of Molecular Sciences, 23*, 13689.

Jazirehi, A. R., & Bonavida, B. (2004). Resveratrol modifies the expression of apoptotic regulatory proteins and sensitizes non-Hodgkin's lymphoma and multiple myeloma cell lines to paclitaxel-induced apoptosis. *Molecular Cancer Therapeutics, 3*, 71–84.

Jiang, L., Yu, H., Wang, C., He, F., Shi, Z., Tu, H., et al. (2022). The anti-cancer effects of mitochondrial-targeted Triphenylphosphonium-resveratrol conjugate on breast cancer cells. *Pharmaceuticals (Basel), 15*, 1271.

Kasiri, N., Rahmati, M., Ahmadi, L., Eskandari, N., & Motedayyen, H. (2020). Therapeutic potential of quercetin on human breast cancer in different dimensions. *Inflammopharmacology, 28*(1), 39–62.

Khamis, A. A. A., Ali, E. M. M., El-Moneim, M. A. A., Abd-Alhaseeb, M. M., El-Magd, M. A., & Salim, E. I. (2018). Hesperidin piperine and bee venom synergistically potentiate the anticancer effect of tamoxifen against breast cancer cells. *Biomedicine & Pharmacotherapy, 105*, 1335–1343.

Khan, F., Niaz, K., Maqbool, F., Ismail Hassan, F., Abdollahi, M., Nagulapalli Venkata, K. C., et al. (2016). Molecular targets underlying the anticancer effects of quercetin: An update. *Nutrients, 8*, 529.

Khorsandi, L., Orazizadeh, M., Niazvand, F., Abbaspour, M. R., Mansouri, E., & Khodadadi, A. (2017). Quercetin induces apoptosis and necroptosis in MCF-7 breast cancer cells. *Bratislava Medical Journal, 118*(02), 123–128.

Kim, D. H., Khan, H., Ullah, H., Hassan, S. T. S., Šmejkal, K., Efferth, T., Mahomoodally, M. F., Xu, S., Habtemariam, S., Filosa, R., Lagoa, R., & Rengasamy, K. R. (2019). MicroRNA targeting by quercetin in cancer treatment and chemoprotection. *Pharmacological Research, 147*, 104346-10.

Kong, W. Y., Ngai, S. C., Goh, B. H., Lee, L. H., Htar, T. T., & Chuah, L. H. (2021). Is curcumin the answer to future chemotherapy cocktail? *Molecules, 26*, 4329.

Kweon, S. H., Song, J. H., & Kim, T. S. (2010). Resveratrol-mediated reversal of doxorubicin resistance in acute myeloid leukemia cells via downregulation of MRP1 expression. *Biochemical and Biophysical Research Communications, 395*, 104–110.

Li, Y., Zhang, T., Korkaya, H., Liu, S., Lee, H. F., Newman, B., et al. (2010). Sulforaphane, a dietary component of broccoli/broccoli sprouts, inhibits breast cancer stem cells. *Clinical Cancer Research, 16*, 2580–2590.

Li, S., Li, K., Zhang, J., & Dong, Z. (2013). The effect of quercetin on doxorubicin cytotoxicity in human breast cancer cells. *Anti-Cancer Agents in Medicinal Chemistry, 13*(2), 352–355.

Li, S., Yuan, S., Zhao, Q., Wang, B., Wang, X., & Li, K. (2018). Quercetin enhances chemotherapeutic effect of doxorubicin against human breast cancer cells while reducing toxic side effects of it. *Biomedicine & Pharmacotherapy, 100*, 441–447.

Li, P., Zhong, D., Gong, P., & yao. (2019). Synergistic effect of paclitaxel and verapamil to overcome multi-drug resistance in breast cancer cells. *Biochemical and Biophysical Research Communications, 516*(1), 183–188.

Lin, M. Y., Cheng, W. T., Cheng, H. C., Chou, W. C., Chen, H. I., Ou, H. C., et al. (2021). Baicalin enhances chemosensitivity to doxorubicin in breast cancer cells via upregulation of oxidative stress-mediated mitochondria-dependent apoptosis. *Antioxidants, 10*(10), 1506–1510.

Liu, S., Li, R., Qian, J., Sun, J., Li, G., Shen, J., et al. (2020). Combination therapy of doxorubicin and quercetin on multidrug-resistant breast cancer and their sequential delivery by reduction-sensitive hyaluronic acid-based conjugate/ d -α-Tocopheryl poly(ethylene glycol) 1000 succinate mixed micelles. *Molecular Pharmaceutics, 17*(4), 1415–1427.

Luo, T., Wang, J., Yin, Y., Hua, H., Jing, J., Sun, X., Li, M., Zhang, Y., & Jiang., Y. (2010). (-)-Epigallocatechin gallate sensitizes breast cancer cells to paclitaxel in a murine model of breast carcinoma. *Breast Cancer Research, 12*(1), R8.

Mansouri, K., Rasoulpoor, S., Daneshkhah, A., Abolfathi, S., Salari, N., Mohammadi, M., et al. (2020). Clinical effects of curcumin in enhancing cancer therapy: A systematic review. *BMC Cancer, 20*, 791.

Manzoor, M. F., Hussain, A., Sameen, A., Sahar, A., Khan, S., Siddique, R., Aadil, R. M., & Xu, B. (2021). Novel extraction, rapid assessment and bioavailability improvement of quercetin: A review. *Ultrasonics Sonochemistry, 78*, 105686.

Meng, L., Xia, X., Yang, Y., Ye, J., Dong, W., Ma, P., Jin, Y., & Liu, Y. (2016). Co-encapsulation of paclitaxel and baicalein in nanoemulsions to overcome multidrug resistance via oxidative stress augmentation and P-glycoprotein inhibition. *International Journal of Pharmaceutics, 513*(1-2), 8–16.

Michalak, K. W., & Wesolowska, O. (2012). Polyphenols counteract tumor cell chemoresistance conferred by multidrug resistance proteins. *AntiCancer Agents in Medicinal Chemistry, 12*(8), 880–890.

Mosalam, E. M., Zidan, A. A. A., Mehanna, E. T., Mesbah, N. M., & Abo-Elmatty, D. M. (2020). Thymoquinone and pentoxifylline enhance the chemotherapeutic effect of cisplatin by targeting Notch signaling pathway in mice. *Life Sciences, 244*, 117299-10.

Mu, J., Zhu, D., Shen, Z., Ning, S., Liu, Y., Chen, J., Li, Y., & Li, Z. (2017). The repressive effect of miR-148a on Wnt/β-catenin signaling involved in Glabridin-induced anti-angiogenesis in human breast cancer cells BMC. *Cancer, 17*(1). https://doi.org/10.1186/s12885-017-3298-1

Munson, A. E., Harris, L. S., Friedman, M. A., Dewey, W. L., & Carchman, R. A. (1975). Antineoplastic activity of cannabinoids. *Journal of the National Cancer Institute, 55*(3), 597–602.

Muzio, M., Stockwell, B. R., Stennicke, H. R., Salvesen, G. S., & Dixit, V. M. (1998). An induced proximity model for caspase-8 activation. *Journal of Biological Chemistry, 273*(5), 2926–2930.

Nabekura, T. (2010). Overcoming multidrug resistance in human cancer cells by natural compounds. *Toxins, 2*(6), 1207–1224.

Obrador, E., Salvador-Palmer, R., Jihad-Jebbar, A., López-Blanch, R., Dellinger, T. H., Dellinger, R. W., & Estrela, J. M. (2021). Pterostilbene in cancer therapy. *Antioxidants, 10*(3), 492–410.

Özdemi, R. F., Sever, A., Keçeci, Y., & Incesu, Z. (2021). Resveratrol increases the sensitivity of breast cancer MDA-MB-231 cell line to cisplatin by regulating intrinsic apoptosis. *Iranian Journal of Basic Medical Sciences, 24*, 66–72.

Panche, A. N., Diwan, A. D., & Chandra, S. R. (2016). Flavonoids: An overview. *Journal of Nutritional Science, 29*(5), e47.

Parhi, P., Mohanty, C., & Sahoo, S. K. (2012). Nanotechnology-based combinational drug delivery: An emerging approach for cancer therapy. *Drug Discovery Today, 17*, 1044–1052.

Perez, A. T., Arun, B., Tripathy, D., Tagliaferri, M. A., Shaw, H. S., Kimmick, G. G., Cohen, I., Shtivelman, E., Caygill, K. A., Grady, D., Schactman, M., & Shapiro, C. L. (2010). A phase 1B dose escalation trial of Scutellaria barbata (BZL101) for patients with metastatic breast cancer. *Breast Cancer Research and Treatment, 120*(1), 111–118.

Pertwee, R. G. (2008). The diverse CB 1 and CB 2 receptor pharmacology of three plant cannabinoids: Δ 9 -tetrahydrocannabinol cannabidiol and Δ 9 -tetrahydrocannabivarin. *British Journal of Pharmacology, 153*(2), 199–215.

Phi, L. T. H., Sari, I. N., Yang, Y. G., Lee, S. H., Jun, N., Kim, K. S., et al. (2018). Cancer stem cells (CSCs) in drug resistance and their therapeutic implications in cancer treatment. *Stem Cells International, 2018*, 5416923.

Pisanti, S., Malfitano, A. M., Grimaldi, C., Santoro, A., Gazzerro, P., Laezza, C., & Bifulco, M. (2009). Use of cannabinoid receptor agonists in cancer therapy as palliative and curative agents. *Best Practice & Research Clinical Endocrinology & Metabolism, 23*(1), 117–131.

Pozo-Guisado, E., Alvarez-Barrientos, A., Mulero-Navarro, S., Santiago-Josefat, B., & Fernandez-Salguero, P. M. (2002). The antiproliferative activity of resveratrol results in apoptosis in MCF-7 but not in MDA-MB-231 human breast cancer cells: Cell-specific alteration of the cell cycle. *Biochemical Pharmacology, 64*, 1375–1386.

Puig, T., Vázquez-Martín, A., Relat, J., Pétriz, J., Menéndez, J. A., Porta, R., et al. (2008). Fatty acid metabolism in breast cancer cells: Differential inhibitory effects of epigallocatechin gallate (EGCG) and C75. *Breast Cancer Research and Treatment, 109*, 471–479.

Qi, D., Liu, Y., Li, J., Huang, J. H., Hu, X., & Wu, E. (2022). Salinomycin as a potent anticancer stem cell agent: State of the art and future directions. *Medicinal Research Reviews, 42*, 1037–1063.

Qin, J., Xie, L.-P., Zheng, X.-Y., Wang, Y.-B., Bai, Y., Shen, H.-F., et al. (2007). A component of green tea, (−)-epigallocatechin-3-gallate, promotes apoptosis in T24 human bladder cancer cells via modulation of the PI3K/Akt pathway and Bcl-2 family proteins. *Biochemical and Biophysical Research Communications, 354*, 852–857.

Talib, W. H., Awajan, D., Hamed, R. A., Azzam, A. O., Mahmod, A. I., & AL-Yasari, I. H. (2022). Combination anticancer therapies using selected phytochemicals. *Molecules, 27*(17), 5452–5410.

Rivera, E. G. (2010). Chemotherapy resistance in metastatic breast cancer: The evolving role of ixabepilone. *Breast Cancer Research, 12*(S2).

Saghatelyan, T., Tananyan, A., Janoyan, N., Tadevosyan, A., Petrosyan, H., Hovhannisyan, A., Hayrapetyan, L., Arustamyan, M., Arnhold, J., Rotmann, A. R., Hovhannisyan, A., & Panossian, A. (2020). Efficacy and safety of curcumin in combination with paclitaxel in patients with advanced metastatic breast cancer: A comparative randomized double-blind placebo-controlled clinical trial. *Phytomedicine, 70*, 153218.

Salazar, M., Carracedo, A., Salanueva, I. J., Hernández-Tiedra, S., Lorente, M., Egia, A., Vázquez, P., Blázquez, C., Torres, S., García, S., Nowak, J., Fimia, G. M., Piacentini, M., Cecconi, F., Pandolfi, P. P., González-Feria, L., Iovanna, J. L., Guzmán, M., Boya, P., & Velasco, G. (2009). Cannabinoid action induces autophagy-mediated cell death through stimulation of ER stress in human glioma cells. *Journal of Clinical Investigation, 119*(5), 1359–1372.

Samavat, H., Ursin, G., Emory, T. H., Lee, E., Wang, R., Torkelson, C. J., Dostal, A. M., Swenson, K., Le, C. T., Yang, C. S., Yu, M. C., Yee, D., Wu, A. H., Yuan, J. M., & Kurzer, M. S. (2017). A randomized controlled trial of green tea extract supplementation and mammographic density in postmenopausal women at increased risk of breast cancer. *Prevention Research, 10*(12), 710–718.

Scandlyn, M. J., Stuart, E. C., Somers-Edgar, T. J., Menzies, A. R., & Rosengren, R. J. (2008). A new role for tamoxifen in oestrogen receptor-negative breast cancer when it is combined with epigallocatechin gallate. *British Journal of Cancer, 99*(7), 1056–1063.

Seo, H., Ku, J. M., Choi, H., Choi, Y. K., Woo, J., Kim, M., Kim, I., Na, C. H., Hur, H., Jang, B., Shin, Y. C., & Ko, S. (2016). Quercetin induces caspase-dependent extrinsic apoptosis through inhibition of signal transducer and activator of transcription 3 signaling in HER2-overexpressing BT-474 breast cancer cells. *Oncology Reports, 36*(1), 31–42.

Shamas-Din, A., Kale, J., Leber, B., & Andrews, D. W. (2013). Mechanisms of action of Bcl-2 family proteins. *Cold Spring Harbor Perspectives in Biology, 5*(4), a008714–a008714.

Shanmugam, M. K., Rane, G., Kanchi, M. M., Arfuso, F., Chinnathambi, A., Zayed, M. E., et al. (2015). The multifaceted role of curcumin in cancer prevention and treatment. *Molecules, 20*, 2728–2769.

Shimizu, M., Shirakami, Y., & Moriwaki, H. (2008). Targeting receptor tyrosine kinases for chemoprevention by green tea catechin, EGCG. *International Journal of Molecular Sciences, 9*, 1034–1049.

Suri, S. S., Fenniri, H., & Singh, B. (2007). Nanotechnology-based drug delivery systems. *Journal of Occupational Medicine and Toxicology, 2*, 16.

Talib, W. H., Alsayed, A. R., Barakat, M., Abu-Taha, M. I., & Mahmod, A. I. (2021). Targeting drug chemo-resistance in cancer using natural products. *Biomedicines, 9*(10).

Tao, S. F., He, H. F., & Chen, Q. (2015). Quercetin inhibits proliferation and invasion acts by up-regulating miR-146a in human breast cancer cells. *Molecular and Cellular Biochemistry, 402*(1-2), 93–100.

Tomeh, M. A., Hadianamrei, R., & Zhao, X. (2019). A review of curcumin and its derivatives as anticancer agents. *International Journal of Molecular Sciences, 20*, 1033.

Tramèr, M. R., Carroll, D., Campbell, F. A., Reynolds, D. J., Moore, R. A., & McQuay, H. J. (2001). Cannabinoids for control of chemotherapy induced nausea and vomiting: Quantitative systematic review. *British Medical Journal, 323*(7303), 16–21.

Vemuri, S. K., Banala, R. R., Subbaiah, G. P. V., Srivastava, S. K., Reddy, A. V. G., & Malarvili, T. (2017). Anti-cancer potential of a mix of natural extracts of turmeric ginger and garlic: A cell-based study. *Egyptian Journal of Basic and Applied Sciences, 4*(4), 332–344.

Wang, F., Zhang, D., Zhang, Q., Chen, Y., Zheng, D., Hao, L., et al. (2011). Synergistic effect of folate-mediated targeting and verapamil- mediated P-gp inhibition with paclitaxel -polymer micelles to overcome multi-drug resistance. *Biomaterials, 32*, 9444–9456.

Wang, P., Yang, H. L., Yang, Y. J., Wang, L., & Lee, S. C. (2015). Overcome cancer cell drug resistance using natural products. *Evidence-Based Complementary and Alternative Medicine, 2015*, 1–14. https://doi.org/10.1155/2015/767136

Wang, W. D., Shang, Y., Li, Y., & Chen, S. Z. (2019a). Honokiol inhibits breast cancer cell metastasis by blocking EMT through modulation of snail/slug protein translation. *Acta Pharmacologica Sinica, 40*, 1219–1227.

Wang, X., Zhang, H., & Chen, X. (2019b). Drug resistance and combating drug resistance in cancer. *Cancer Drug Resist, 2*, 141–160.

Wen, C., Fu, L., Huang, J., Dai, Y., Wang, B., Xu, G., et al. (2019). Curcumin reverses doxorubicin resistance via inhibition the efflux function of ABCB4 in doxorubicin-resistant breast cancer cells. *Molecular Medicine Reports, 19*(6), 5162–5168.

Wu, C. H., Hong, B. H., Ho, C. T., & Yen, G. C. (2015). Targeting cancer stem cells in breast cancer: Potential anticancer properties of 6-shogaol and pterostilbene. *Journal of Agricultural and Food Chemistry, 63*, 2432–2441.

Yang, L., Wei, D. D., Chen, Z., Wang, J. S., & Kong, L. Y. (2011). Reversal of multidrug resistance in human breast cancer cells by Curcuma wenyujin and Chrysanthemum indicum. *Phytomedicine : International Journal of Phytotherapy and Phytopharmacology, 18*(8–9), 710–718.

Zhang, Z. L., Jiang, Q. C., & Wang, S. R. (2018). Schisandrin A reverses doxorubicin-resistant human breast cancer cell line by the inhibition of P65 and Stat3 phosphorylation. *Breast Cancer, 25*(2), 233–242.

Zhou, S., Wang, F., Wong, E. T., Fonkem, E., Hsieh, T. C., Wu, J. M., et al. (2013). Salinomycin: A novel anti-cancer agent with known anti-coccidial activities. *Current Medicinal Chemistry, 20*, 4095–4101.

Zhu, W., Qin, W., Zhang, K., Rottinghaus, G. E., Chen, Y. C., Kliethermes, B., & Saute, E. R. (2012). Trans -resveratrol alters mammary promoter hypermethylation in women at increased risk for breast cancer. *Nutrition and Cancer, 64*(3), 393–400.

Zoi, V., Galani, V., Lianos, G. D., Voulgaris, S., Kyritsis, A. P., & Alexiou, G. A. (2021). The role of curcumin in cancer treatment. *Biomedicine, 9*, 1086.

Revolutionizing Breast Cancer Treatment: Harnessing the Power of Artificial Intelligence in Overcoming Drug Resistance

Zilungile Mkhize-Kwitshana, Pragalathan Naidoo, Zamathombeni Duma, Kamal S. Saini, and Zodwa Dlamini

Abstract Drug resistance is one of the major challenges in the treatment of breast cancer (BC) and contributes to its high mortality rate. Detecting breast cancer at an early stage, before the cells have formed subpopulations which can reduce heterogeneous molecular features, could mitigate the development of drug resistance, and increase the efficacy of treatment. Several artificial intelligence (AI)-based models and tools that are integrated with multi-omics data (genomics, epigenetics, proteomics, and metabolomics) are available for drug discovery, drug design using AI-based database repositories and de novo drug design through AI-based algorithms, including deep reinforcement learning, variational auto-encoders, recurrent neural network, and generative adversarial network. As more data becomes available, the capacity of these algorithms improves to make them iteratively more accurate, timely, and precise. By integrating AI into predictive models, healthcare

Z. Mkhize-Kwitshana (✉) · P. Naidoo · Z. Duma
Department of Medical Microbiology, School of Laboratory Medicine & Medical Sciences, Medical School Campus, College of Health Sciences, University of KwaZulu-Natal-Natal, Durban, South Africa

SAMRC Research Capacity Development Division, South African Medical Research Council, Tygerberg, South Africa
e-mail: mkhizekwitshanaz@ukzn.ac.za; naidoop5@ukzn.ac.za; zamathombeni.duma@smu.ac.za

K. S. Saini
Fortrea Inc., Durham, USA

Addenbrooke's Hospital, Cambridge University Hospitals NHS Foundation Trust, Cambridge, UK
e-mail: kamal.saini@nhs.net

Z. Dlamini
SAMRC Precision Oncology Research Unit (PORU), DSI/NRF SARChI Chair in Precision Oncology and Cancer Prevention (POCP), Pan African Cancer Research Institute (PACRI), University of Pretoria, Pretoria, South Africa
e-mail: zodwa.dlamini@up.ac.za

Z. Dlamini (ed.), *Overcoming Breast Cancer Therapy Resistance*,
https://doi.org/10.1007/978-3-031-52860-6_10

professionals can gain valuable insights into the mechanisms of drug resistance and develop personalized treatment strategies to overcome treatment failure in BC. This chapter highlights the revolutionary impact of AI in addressing early detection of BC, drug discovery and design, overcoming drug resistance, improving treatment outcomes, and paving the way for precision medicine in BC.

Keywords Breast cancer · Drug resistance · Artifical intelligence · Precision medicine · Overcoming drug resistance

Introduction

Over 2 million new cases of breast cancer (BC) are diagnosed globally each year (Sung et al., 2021 Globocan), and their treatment is based on the expression of cell receptors such as human epidermal growth factor receptor-2 (HER-2), estrogen receptor (ER), and several other clinical and molecular features (Yersal & Barutca, 2014). The nature of BC is itself complex and so are the broad categories of mechanisms of resistance to BC treatment, which include, among others, genetic modifications, cell membranes acting as efflux pumps, enzyme systems metabolizing BC drugs, and hormone receptor quality/quantity affecting endocrine therapy. These negatively affect all forms of therapy, including chemo- and endocrine therapy, HER2-directed therapy, CDK4/6 inhibitors, immune checkpoint inhibitors, PARP inhibitors, TROP2-directed antibody-drug conjugates, and other mechanisms (Yersal & Barutca, 2014).

The past decade has witnessed an exponential growth in powerful, high-throughput molecular technologies ranging from genomics, transcriptomics, proteomics, and epigenomics, all of which are enhanced by bioinformatics (Chakraborty et al., 2018). Recently, another powerful arsenal in the form of artificial intelligence (AI) has been added. These combined advances will propel efforts to systematically address different aspects of cancer starting from easy, early, and accurate diagnosis to early prediction of metastasis or drug resistance as well as new therapeutic discoveries at scale (Paul et al., 2021; Khan et al., 2022).

The capability of AI to perform accurate, quantitative, consistent, and instantaneous analysis promises to lead to the generation of a more precise and personalized therapeutic plan and predict treatment outcomes for individual patients. This will assist in averting, or at least ameliorating, the occurrence of drug resistance. The need for alternative treatment strategies that exploit the power of AI for precision medicine is therefore more urgent and will be described below (Liao et al., 2022).

This chapter aims to explore AI-driven drug discovery and design with enhanced efficacy against drug-resistant BC, define the role of AI in minimizing the risk of drug resistance in personalized BC therapies and summarize

AI-enhanced predictive models and early detection of drug resistance for adapting treatment strategies to overcome drug resistance in BC. The chapter will also highlight the challenges and limitations associated with AI-driven efforts in overcoming BC drug resistance.

AI-Driven Drug Discovery and Design with Enhanced Efficacy Against Drug-Resistant Breast Cancer

AI plays a significant role in BC, including: (i) *Target identification:* by predicting the 3D structure of target protein and drug–protein interactions, in determining drug activity and in de novo drug design. (ii) *Drug design:* by designing biospecific and multitarget drug molecules. (iii) *Drug synthesis:* by predicting reaction yield and retrosynthesis pathways, developing insights into reaction mechanisms and in designing synthetic routes. (iv) *Drug repurposing:* by identifying therapeutic targets and predicting new therapeutic use. (v) *Drug screening*: by predicting toxicity, bioactivity, and physicochemical properties, and identifying and classifying target cells (Paul et al., 2021; You et al., 2022).

Several AI-based models and tools that are integrated with multi-omics data (genomics, epigenetics, proteomics, and metabolomics) are available to assist in BC drug discovery, drug design using AI-based database repositories, and de novo drug design through AI-based algorithms, including deep reinforcement learning, variational auto-encoders, recurrent neural network, and generative adversarial network (You et al., 2022) (Fig. 1).

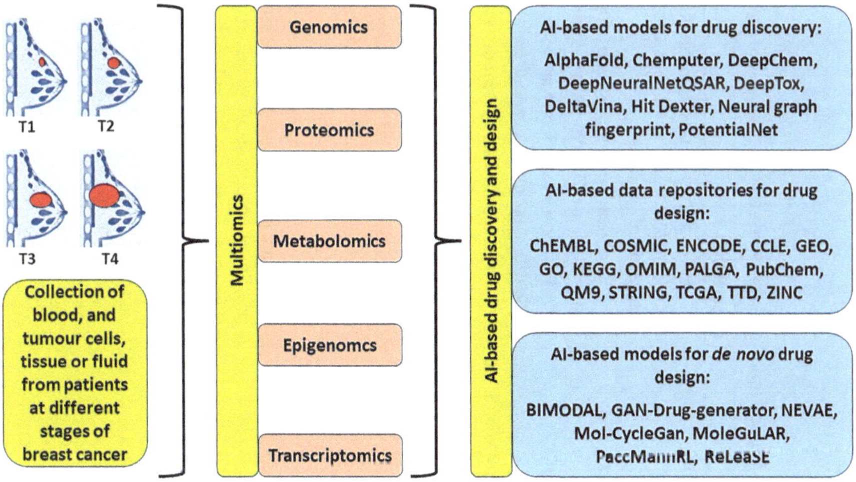

Fig. 1 Integration of AI-based models and multi-omics data for BC drug discovery and design

Table 1 AI-based tools used for breast cancer drug discovery

Model	Description	Website URL	References
AlphaFold	• Predicts a protein's 3D structure from its amino acid sequence. • Can determine how a mutation in a gene can alter the structure and function of proteins.	https://alphafold.ebi.ac.uk/	(Ren et al., 2023)
Chemputer	• Chemical computer system, together with a chemical programming language, used to synthesize organic molecules automatically.	https://github.com/croningp/ChemputerSoftware	(Gromski et al., 2020)
DeepChem	• Python-based AI system using machine learning and deep learning to identify a promising candidate in drug discovery.	https://github.com/deepchem/deepchem	(Ramsundar, 2018)
DeepNeuralNetQSAR	• Python-based AI system driven by quantitative structure-activity relationship (QSAR) computational models to predict the molecular and biological activities of compounds.	https://github.com/Merck/DeepNeuralNetQSAR	(Xu, 2022)
DeepTox	• AI-based computational software using deep learning to predict the toxic effects of over 12,000 drugs.	http://www.bioinf.jku.at/research/DeepTox	(Mayr et al., 2016)
DeltaVina	• Scoring function for rescoring protein-ligand binding affinity and stability.	https://github.com/chengwang88/deltavina	(Wang & Zhang, 2017)
Hit Dexter	• A machine learning tool to determine the probability of a small drug molecule triggering a positive response in biochemical assays. • Small drug molecules can act as "badly behaving compounds" or "nuisance compounds" and are typically aggregators, reactive compounds, and/or pan-assay interference compounds (PAINS).	https://nerdd.univie.ac.at/hitdexter/	(Stork et al., 2018)
Neural graph fingerprint	• Predicting core molecular properties of novel drug molecules. • Drug carcinogenicity prediction.	https://github.com/HIPS/neural-fingerprint	(Fradkin et al., 2022)
PotentialNet	• Uses neural networks to predict protein–ligand binding affinity and molecular properties.	https://pubs.acs.org/doi/full/10.1021/acscentsci.8b00507	(Feinberg et al., 2018)

The different types of AI-based BC drug discovery and design models and tools available are: *(i) Drug discovery:* AlphaFold, Chemputer, DeepChem, DeepNeuralNetQSAR, DeepTox, DeltaVina, Hit Dexter, Neural graph fingerprint, and PotentialNet (Table 1). *(ii) Drug design using AI-based database repositories:* Cancer Cell Line Encyclopedia (CCLE), ChEMBL, Catalogue Of Somatic Mutations in Cancer (COSMIC), DrugBank, Encyclopedia of DNA Elements (ENCODE), Gene Expression Omnibus (GEO), Gene Ontology (GO), Kyoto Encyclopedia of Genes and Genomes (KEGG), Online Mendelian Inheritance in Man (OMIM), Pathologisch Anatomisch Landelijk Geautomatiseerd Archief (PALGA), PubChem, Quantum Machines 9 (QM9), Search Tool for the Retrieval of Interacting Genes/Proteins (STRING), The Cancer Genome Atlas (TCGA), Therapeutic Targets Database (TTD), and ZINC (Table 2). *(iii)* De novo *drug design through AI-based algorithms, including deep reinforcement learning, variational auto-encoders, recurrent neural network, and generative adversarial network:* BIMODAL, GAN-Drug-generator, Mol-CycleGAN, MoleGuLAR, NEVAE, PaccMannRL and ReLeaSE (Paul et al., 2021; Wang et al., 2023; You et al., 2022) (Table 3).

The Role of AI in Minimizing the Risk of Drug Resistance in Personalized Breast Cancer Therapies

Along with cardiovascular disease, neurodegenerative disease, and metabolic syndrome, cancer is a serious threat to human health, with a high burden of morbidity and mortality (Bray et al., 2013). BC is now the most common type of cancer occurring in women worldwide (Arnold et al., 2022). Clinical outcomes can be significantly improved if cancer is detected and treated early (Torre et al., 2016). However, most tumors lack effective screening methods, and consequently patients are often diagnosed at more advanced stages. Furthermore, tumor heterogeneity often increases in advanced stages of cancer, which can pose significant challenges in treatment (ICGC/TCGA Pan-Cancer Analysis of Whole Genomes Consortium, 2020).

New treatment and diagnostic strategies that are personalized for each patient are required (MacEachern & Forkert, 2021). Precision medicine and AI appear to be an appealing strategy that focuses on clarifying, identifying, and treating diseases to create a personalized therapy for patients by obtaining multi-omics or multi-mode data from individuals (Gore, 2020). Cancer research and personalized clinical care are being rapidly reshaped by AI. The availability of high-dimensionality datasets, combined with advances in high-performance computing and novel deep learning architectures, has resulted in an explosion of AI use in various aspects of oncology research (Zhou et al., 2020). Deployment of AI-based algorithms may help some patients avoid the serious side effects of chemotherapy while also making it easier to identify patients who would benefit from it. In addition, AI-based decision-support tools could predict whether a patient is likely to respond to a given

Table 2 AI-based database repositories used for breast cancer drug design

Tools	Description	Website URL	References
CCLE	• Compilation of chromosomal copy Number, gene expression, and sequencing data from 947 human cancer cell lines.	https://sites.broadinstitute.org/ccle	(Barretina et al., 2012; You et al., 2022)
ChEMBL	• Database of bioactivity data that correlates drug-like compounds to their biological targets.	https://www.ebi.ac.uk/chembldb	(Gaulton et al., 2012; You et al., 2022)
COSMIC	• Gathers in-depth and comprehensive information on somatic mutations in human cancers.	http://www.sanger.ac.uk/cosmic	(Forbes et al., 2011; You et al., 2022)
DrugBank	• Curates comprehensive molecular information on the mechanisms, interactions, and targets of drugs.	https://www.drugbank.ca/	(Wishart et al., 2018; You et al., 2022)
ENCODE	• Contains systematically mapped regions of transcription, transcription factor association, histone modification, and chromatin structure.	https://www.encodeproject.org/	The ENCODE Project Consortium (2012, You et al., 2022)
GEO	• Public functional genomics data repository. • Archives comprehensive sets of next-generation sequencing, microarray, and other high-throughput functional genomic data.	https://www.ncbi.nlm.nih.gov/geo/	(Edgar et al., 2002; You et al., 2022)
GO	• World's largest source of information on the molecular, cellular component, and biological process functions of genes.	http://www.geneontology.org/	(Consortium, 2004; You et al., 2022)
KEGG	• Collection of databases dealing with chemical substances, drugs, genomes, biological pathways, and diseases.	http://www.genome.jp/kegg/	(Kanehisa & Goto, 2000; You et al., 2022)
OMIM	• A comprehensive knowledge base on human genes and genetic disorders, particularly on the gene–phenotype relationship.	http://www.omim.org/	(Hamosh et al., 2005; You et al., 2022)
PALGA	• Pathology database containing cytopathology and histopathology data.	https://www.palga.nl/	(Casparie et al., 2007; You et al., 2022)
PubChem	• Database of chemical molecules and their activities against biological assays.	http://pubchem.ncbi.nlm.nih.gov/	(Wang et al., 2009; You et al., 2022)

(continued)

Table 2 (continued)

Tools	Description	Website URL	References
QM9	• Provides quantum chemical properties for small organic molecules and drugs. • Provides the foundational basis for hybrid quantum mechanics/ machine learning, and systematic identification of structure–property relationships of molecules and drugs.	https://www.kaggle.com/datasets/zaharch/quantum-machine-9-aka-qm9 https://paperswithcode.com/dataset/qm9	(Pinheiro et al., 2020; You et al., 2022)
STRING	• Biological database of known and predicted protein–protein interactions.	http://string-db.org/	(Szklarczyk et al., 2021; You et al., 2022)
TCGA	• Contains genomic, epigenomic, proteomic, and transcriptomic clinical data of several human cancers (genomic mutations, miRNA expression, mRNA expression, DNA/RNA methylation profiles, etc.).	https://www.cancer.gov/about-nci/organization/ccg/research/structural-genomics/tcga	(Ma & Ellis, 2013; You et al., 2022)
TTD	• Database containing information on the known and explored therapeutic nucleic acid and protein targets, the cancer targeted, biological pathway information, and the parallel drugs directed at each of these targets.	http://db.idrblab.net/ttd/	(Wang et al., 2019; You et al., 2022)
ZINC	• Database of commercially available molecular compounds for ligand discovery and virtual screening. • Used to identify the biological targets for a compound.	https://zinc.docking.org/	(Irwin et al., 2020; You et al., 2022)

treatment, providing clinicians with additional information to optimize a personalized treatment plan for individual patients (Tai et al., 2023).

AI-Based Models That May Be Employed for Personalized Breast Cancer Therapy

Mammography has been shown to reduce mortality from BC by identifying early signs of disease (Broeders et al., 2012; Independent UK Panel on Breast Cancer Screening, 2012). Such population-wide screening methods generate a large number of mammograms that must be read by radiologists. In low-prevalence conditions, radiologist readings are more likely to miss subtle signs of disease, resulting in false-negative test results (Evans et al., 2013; Nordenskjöld and Rutqvist, 2002).

Table 3 AI-based models used for breast cancer de novo drug design

Model	Description	Website URL	References
BIMODAL	• Proposes a bidirectional strategy for molecular SMILES strings generation. • Combines a forward and a backward recurrent neural network to predict a joint probability distribution of bioactive molecules. • Uses the ChEMBL data source repositories.	https://github.com/ETHmodlab/BIMODAL	(Fang et al., 2023; Grisoni et al., 2020)
GAN-drug-generator	• Generation of novel molecular structures with desired properties, including high binding affinity to a target protein or low toxicity. • Stereochemical information generated with high accuracy. • Uses the ChEMBL and ZINC data source repositories.	https://github.com/larngroup/GAN-Drug-Generator	(Abbasi et al., 2022)
Mol-CycleGAN	• A CycleGAN-based model (used to map the distribution of molecular images to another or to transfer a molecule's image characteristic to another) that generates optimized compounds with high structural similarity to the original ones. • Uses the ChEMBL and ZINC data source repositories.	https://github.com/ardigen/mol-cycle-gan	(Maziarka et al., 2020)
MoleGuLAR	• A deep generative model with recurrent neural networks for the generation of molecules with desired properties, including high binding affinities to specified targets. • Uses the ChEMBL and ZINC data source repositories.	https://github.com/devalab/MoleGuLAR	(Goel et al., 2021)
NEVAE	• A deep generative gradient-based algorithm model for molecular graphs. • Provides the spatial coordinates and bond features of the atoms of the molecules it generates. • Able to optimize the spatial configuration of molecular atoms for greater stability. • Identify molecule's solubility in water. • Uses the QM9 and ZINC data source repositories.	https://github.com/Networks-Learning/nevae	(Samanta et al., 2020)

(continued)

Table 3 (continued)

Model	Description	Website URL	References
PaccMannRL	• Generation of hit-like anticancer molecules from transcriptomic data and gene expression profiles via reinforcement learning. • Generates cancer-type-specific candidate drugs similar to currently available cancer drugs in terms of drug-likeness, synthesizability, and solubility. • Cancer drugs generated exhibit the highest structural similarity to compounds with known efficacy against a particular cancer. • Assess drug toxicity. • Uses the TCGA, ChEMBL, and CCLE data source repositories.	https://github.com/PaccMann/	(Born et al., 2021)
ReLeaSE	• Integrates two deep neural networks (generative and predictive) that are trained separately but are used jointly to generate and design novel targeted chemical libraries through SMILES strings generation. • Chemical libraries contain compounds with minimal, maximal, or specific range of physical properties, including melting point or hydrophobicity, or toward compounds with inhibitory activity against Janus protein kinase 2. • Uses the ChEMBL and ZINC data source repositories.	https://github.com/isayev/ReLeaSE	(Popova et al., 2018)

AI-based mammogram support systems, sometimes regarded as a second set of eyes for radiologists, could: (i) Pick up subtle signs of early disease, triaging suspicious scans for human review and interpretation, and thereby reducing false-negative results; and (ii) Detect patterns that are too subtle for the human eye to detect (DePolo, 2023).

A team from the Massachusetts Institute of Technology (MIT) Computer Science and Artificial Intelligence Laboratory (CSAIL) and Massachusetts General Hospital (MGH) have developed a deep learning model that can predict whether a patient is likely to develop BC more than 5 years in the future based on a mammogram. According to the study's findings, the model was significantly better at predicting BC risk than existing approaches. Essentially, this model learns the subtle patterns in breast tissue that are precursors to malignant tumors (Conner-Simons & Gordon, 2019). Instead of radiologists manually identifying the patterns in a mammogram that lead to future cancer, it is suggested that AI-based screening be considered, which could detect normal, moderate risk, and suspicious mammograms in a BC

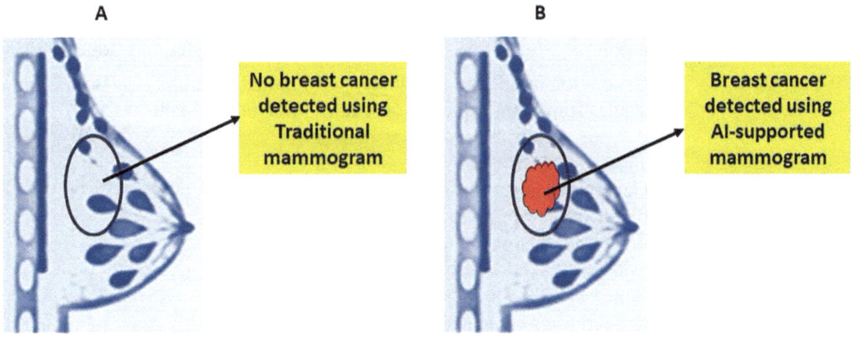

Fig. 2 Traditional mammography screening was compared to AI-supported mammography screening for breast cancer in the same patient. With traditional mammography screening, the patient's scan was found to be normal (**a**). AI-supported mammography screening detected breast cancer (**b**)

screening program, potentially reducing radiologist workload (Lauritzen et al., 2022).

In another study, researchers evaluated the scans of 80,000 Swedish women who had a mammogram between April 2021 and July 2022. They discovered that the group whose mammogram scans were read by two radiologists with additional technical assistance had 20% more cancers detected as opposed to the other group whose mammogram scans were read by two radiologists without additional technical assistance (Christensen, 2023). The advantages of early detection of BC include reduced heterogeneity of cancerous cells, reduced drug resistance, and increased chances of successful treatment (Wang et al., 2019). Figure 2 shows that AI-supported mammography screening has a higher accuracy for early detection of BC than traditional mammography screening.

AI and Anticancer Drug Development (Machine Learning and Deep Learning in Anticancer Drug Development)

One of the greatest obstacles in effective cancer therapy is the development of drug resistance, which occurs because of the cancer adapting, evolving, and becoming resistant to treatment (Wang et al., 2019; The Institute of Cancer Research, 2023). Chemotherapy fails to result in long-term cures in the vast majority of patients because tumor cells develop resistance to the anticancer agent (Goodman et al., 1946; Emran et al., 2022). To design the precisely targeted cancer drugs of the future, researchers must combine expertise in drug discovery, AI, and experimental cancer models and platforms in a new program (The Institute of Cancer Research, 2023). Here, AI can be used to predict anticancer drug activity or to aid in the development of anticancer drugs. Lind and Anderson (2019) designed a random forest model that combined screening data and machine learning, which could predict the

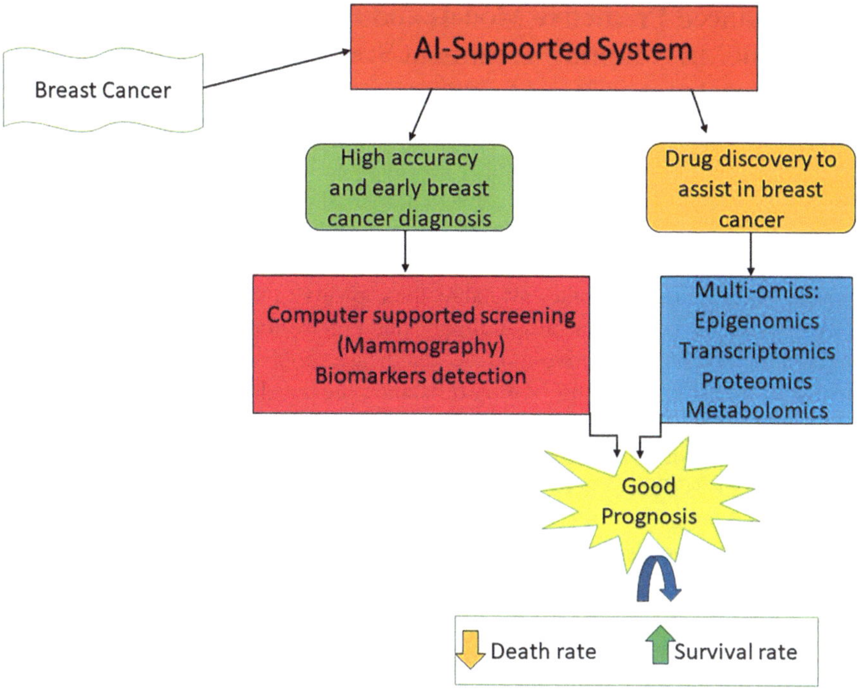

Fig. 3 A summary of AI-supported systems for assisting in the early detection of breast cancer and lowering the risk of drug resistance in personalized breast cancer therapies

activity of anticancer drugs based on the mutation state of the cancer cell genome (Lind & Anderson, 2019). In another study, Wang et al. (2018) created a drug sensitivity model based on a machine learning method known as elastic net regression (Wang et al., 2018), which successfully predicted drug sensitivity in ovarian cancer, gastric cancer, and endometrial cancer patients. Furthermore, the results of the model indicate that AI has a higher potential for predicting anticancer sensitivity (Beck et al., 2020; Goldenberg et al., 2019; Leventakos et al., 2019). AI-based tools can help us understand how cancer cells become resistant to cancer drugs by learning and analyzing data from large drug-resistant cancers, which can help improve drug development and drug use, including proposed drug combinations and sequencing (Liang et al., 2020). To summarize, AI could be a helpful aid to clinicians seeking to ameliorate the emergence of drug resistance in their patients (Fig. 3).

AI-Enhanced Predictive Models and Early Detection of Drug Resistance in Adapting Treatment Strategies to Overcome Drug Resistance in Breast Cancer

Machine learning and AI algorithms can analyze large amounts of patient data, including clinical, demographic, and genomic information to identify patterns. These algorithms can learn from historical data and interpret the emerging patterns that translate to diagnosis of diseases such as cancer and predict treatment outcomes. As more data becomes available, the capacity of these algorithms improves to make them even more accurate, timely, and precise for a variety of patients. By integrating AI into predictive models, healthcare professionals can gain valuable insights into the mechanisms of drug resistance and develop personalized treatment strategies. AI models and algorithms have been integrated into different BC patient features to predict therapy resistance. The availability of extensive cancer genomic studies, such as The Cancer Genome Atlas (TCGA), provide the opportunity to evaluate the predictive capability of genome-wide molecular data association with clinical drug responses in a wide range of cancer types (Wang et al., 2011).

Integration of AI-Enhanced Technology and Clinicopathological Features to Predict Breast Cancer Recurrence

Drug resistance is one of the key causes of treatment failure that can lead to recurrence therefore the latter can be a proxy for chemoresistance (Prihantono, 2021). A majority of patients with advanced BC patients will experience recurrence/progression within 5 years after initial diagnosis and treatment (Ahmad, 2023). Harnessing the power of AI for the prediction of recurrence and hence prevention of treatment failure can contribute toward effective, personalized precision medicine for breast cancer treatment.

Zeng et al. (2023) integrated AI to analyze data for the recurrence risk of postoperative BC patients. They extracted data from electronic health records (EHR) to collect integrated pathological and clinical information. The large datasets from each patient were accurately (95%) processed and digitized to simplify the machine learning process. Using a BC cohort of 1841 patients who had undergone surgical treatment, the authors developed a machine learning model to predict recurrence risk. Of the total 1841 patient record data, 1289 were used to train and develop the machine learning algorithm and 552 cohort datasets were used to test the predictive capability of the model. The model further confirmed a strong correlation between a high risk of recurrence and resistance to chemotherapy after surgery among BC patients (Zeng et al., 2023). The data provides valuable AI-enhanced insight for adapting treatment strategies to overcome drug resistance in BC.

A literature review of 31 research articles that have investigated the use of AI for the prediction of BC recurrence revealed that a variety of techniques were used (Mazo et al., 2022). These varied from traditional versus deep learning methods, with the former being more widely used. In addition, differences were noted in performance characteristics of the different machine learning methods and algorithms, with the Support Vector Method (SVM) being superior in predictive capability (96% accuracy, 97% sensitivity, and 95% specificity) while others performed far below this threshold. The Decision Tree and Naïve Bayes were the next two methods with high prediction accuracy (Mazo et al., 2022).

Another important feature that can affect the performance of training models is the type of input data used. The broad categories of the input information identified in the literature are: (i) patient medical history and demographic profile; (ii) anatomic (clinicopathological staging; imaging data and post-therapy staging) information; and (iii) prognostic (tumor grade, type and invasion status, receptor type, oncogenes, and molecular markers) information (Mazo et al., 2022). Some of the key findings on the capability of different patient data types to predict BC recurrence, based on the frequency of use in the reviewed literature are summarized in Table 4 as modified by Mazo and colleagues (2022), noting that only key performing ones are highlighted in this section. The table lists the main features in the order of their predictive performance. Some of the molecular markers (tumor-infiltrating lymphocytes, CD44, ABCC 4 and 11, N- Cadherin, Pan Cadherin, cytokeratin 5/6, and epidermal growth factor receptor) all rated below 5% in frequency of use as predictors of BC recurrence in the cited literature (Mazo et al., 2022).

Table 4 Summary of the key effective features for prediction of breast cancer recurrence used in AI models (Mazo et al., 2022)

Type of feature used	Most discriminant features in descending order
Patient medical history	1.Age at diagnosis 2.Menopausal status 3.Family history of breast cancer
Anatomic /pathologic staging-TNM	1.Nodal status 2.Tumor size 3.Metastasis
Medical imaging	1.Magnetic resonance imaging 2.Fine needle aspirate and/or histopathological images 3.Tissue microarray images
Prognostic stage	1.Tumor grade 2.Hormone receptor status 3.Tumor invasion
Post-therapy staging	1.Radiation 2.Hormone therapy 3.Chemotherapy

TNM (T: the size of the tumor and any spread of cancer into nearby tissue; N: spread of cancer to nearby lymph nodes; M: metastasis)

Integration of AI with Immunohistopathological Records Datasets to Predict Metastasis

Since metastatic BC is well known to be refractory to treatment (Darby et al., 2005; Chica-Parrado et al., 2020), early prediction of metastasis, particularly of triple-negative BC, will strengthen early adaption of tailored treatment strategies toward precision medicine.

Verghese et al. (2023) developed a deep learning, multiscale convolutional neural network (CNN) model to retrospectively characterize the morphological and immunological changes in 5224, hematoxylin and eosin stained and digitized lymph nodes from 345 patients from two independent cohorts to predict metastatic (secondary) BC. A remarkable advancement in the model developed by these authors included the modification of the deep learning from a single-scale CNN to a multiscale, to optimally replicate the pathologist's viewing at different magnifications and different parts of the whole slide. Previous machine learning algorithms were trained on a single-scale basis. The model quantified lymph node germinal centers and sinuses of triple-negative BC patients. The results showed that the model effectively predicted metastatic potential from the immunomorphological features of lymph nodes for prognostication of triple-negative BC patients using AI multiscale features that accurately mimic pathologist's multifield and multi-magnification assessments. These results show that integration of AI into digitized immunohistopathological lymph node datasets can effectively and timeously predict metastatic potential and thus plan effective, personalized treatment strategies, particularly for triple-negative BC patients (Verghese et al., 2023). Triple-negative BC is the most aggressive form of BC, even though responsive to treatment, it has a poor prognosis and a higher potential for metastasis. The integration of AI to predict triple negative BC metastasis bears significant value for BC patients and saves resources as well as healthcare provider time.

Integration of AI with Biomarkers Signatures to Predict Drug Resistance in Breast Cancer

Another major development in clinical research is the advances in molecular techniques able to identify molecular genetic signatures that can be associated with a variety of functions, including response to therapy. In this sense, the availability of molecular profiles of breast cancer tumors before treatment initiation, provides sources of large datasets that can be exploited through integration of AI and multiomics plus bioinformatic technologies to enable the goal of precision oncology.

The association between gene alterations and response to treatment has been well established and explains the heterogenous drug treatment efficacy in different patients or within the same patient as drug-induced mutations accumulate. This has led to the identification of several molecular biomarkers associated with drug sensitivity or resistance (Ogunleye et al., 2022). In most instances, single-gene mutations have been used as predictors of drug response markers. Challenges with this approach have been identified, for example, issues of interplay between biological and technical effects, epistatic effects, or low prevalence of single point mutations-induced functional changes or drug responses have been highlighted (Ogunleye et al., 2022). Essentially, single-gene markers of response may not be able to achieve a significant clinical application impact (Nguyen et al., 2021). To avoid these, a new approach to harness the combined power of AI, machine deep learning, and increased availability of molecular biomarkers, has been used. Integration of AI algorithms and multiple biomarker signatures have been developed to predict BC resistance. Several studies have reported that the use of multiple gene alterations and a machine deep learning approach is more predictive (Nguyen et al., 2021; Ogunleye et al., 2022).

Multiple characteristics, including patient and tumor features, rather than single-gene alterations, are thus critically needed to guide personalized BC therapy (Gehrmann et al., 2008). Therefore, precision oncology requires characterization of specific patients and specific tumor features of this highly heterogenous malignancy before treatment initiation. Machine learning and large datasets of molecular profiles provide this prerequisite basis to timeously predict specific tumor responses for individualized therapy. Ding et al. (2016) obtained drug treatment information from TCGA to evaluate molecular predictive performance for the four cancer drugs (paclitaxel, cisplatin, fluorouracil, and carboplatin) based on 180 clinical response records. The training and testing models across different cancer types showed, among other findings, that miRNA and mRNA expression had superior predictive performance compared to copy number alterations (CNA) and methylation data to predict cisplatin and carboplatin responses. In addition, mRNA expression performed better in predicting cisplatin responses in bladder cancer and cervical cancer squamous carcinoma. On the other hand, miRNA expression showed superior predictive capacity for breast and cervical squamous carcinoma responses to paclitaxel (Ding et al., 2016). This work paved the way for more evaluation studies using molecular-based AI-enhanced prediction models specific to BC.

Bomane et al. (2019) generated ten machine learning algorithms to evaluate 6 molecular profiles (60 classifiers) of BC patient tumors from the US National Cancer Institute's Genomic Data Commons to evaluate their capacity to predict responses to paclitaxel. Their work further confirmed the superior performance of miRNA plus DNA methylation profiles as predictors of paclitaxel sensitivity or resistance (Bomane et al., 2019).

Likewise, another group (Ogunleye et al., 2022) generated 16 machine learning configured algorithms and 6 molecular profiles to predict resistance to another drug, doxorubicin. These were evaluated against preexisting doxorubicin clinical response data. The authors showed that only 2 of the 128 classifiers were highly predictive in discriminating responders and non-responders, with the best model having highest performance on miRNA and miRNA isoforms.

These studies on the two most commonly used drugs against BC (paclitaxel and doxorubicin) aptly demonstrate the value of integrating AI with molecular markers for predicting BC resistance for precise, personalized BC treatment, one of the most problematic cancers regarding therapeutic outcomes. These two studies, (Bomane et al., 2019; Ogunleye et al., 2022) together with work by Ding and colleagues (2016), have consistently revealed that mRNA and epigenetic markers (miRNA and DNA methylation) are good candidates for AI-enhanced molecular predictors of BC drug resistance. As more data from high-throughput molecular technologies and advances in AI/ machine learning algorithms advance, the many challenges of BC drug resistance will be met and accelerate the efforts toward effective personalized BC treatment regimens. This approach will prevent overtreatment, save resources, and also avert unnecessary patient exposure to side effects of drugs such as doxorubicin, which sometimes causes life-threatening side effects (Ogunleye et al., 2022).

Challenges and Limitations of Harnessing the Power of AI in Drug Design, Early Detection, and Overcoming Drug Resistance in Breast Cancer

Corti et al. (2022) conducted a systematic review of design, reporting standards, and bias associated with AI for prediction of anticancer drug and treatment outcomes in women with BC. The authors found access to AI-based datasets and codes was severely restricted (unavailable in 77% and 88% of studies, respectively). On request, data and codes were only made available in 28% and 18% of cases, respectively. Ethnicity and AI model calibration were underreported in 81% and 99% of studies, respectively. The risk of bias was also very high in 72% of the studies, especially analysis bias (Corti et al., 2022).

Although AI-based machine learning algorithms are useful in drug target identification and drug development, they also have several limitations. Firstly, there is a significant lack of reliable and consistent biomedical data for the validation of deep learning models despite the recent advances in biotechnologies which enabled the rapid generation of huge data. In addition, there is a great dependence on biomedical data and a restricted explanation of what the data means. Secondly, there is a major challenge in the integration of heterogenous data information despite deep learning models having the ability to integrate multimodal biological data. As a result, this poses a major challenge in building up a universal deep learning model since there is a deficit of biological domain knowledge. Thirdly, it is difficult to provide interpretability of deep learning models which makes it extremely hard to troubleshoot when the model unexpectedly fails on new and unseen datasets (You et al., 2022; Vamathevan et al., 2019).

Another challenge is the high cost associated with attaining accurate, high-quality, and curated data in big quantities to train and develop machine learning models. Also, data curation is important to the provision of trustworthy and reusable data and can be expensive with regard to skills and time required (Vamathevan et al.,

2019). Lastly, scientists are unable to use algorithms for hypothesis validation and data mining due to the "black box" nature of existing AI models making it difficult to predict the underlying logical reason behind a model which is crucial in designing the correct drug molecules (Wang et al., 2023; Vamathevan et al., 2019).

Repeatability is a problem with neural networks as well because machine learning outputs are extremely dependent on the initial weights or values of the network parameters or even the sequence in which training examples are presented to the network, which is usually done with all of them being randomly selected. This raises important questions: (i) If the same expression data were used as input, would the network always choose the same disease target? and (ii) Would the drug structure suggested by the machine learning technique always be the same? As demonstrated by instances where various tools produced various prognostic biomarkers for BC based on molecular expression profiles, this lack of repeatability is particularly troublesome for biomarker identification (Vamathevan et al., 2019; Koscielny, 2010).

Another challenge is lack of uniformity in data collection and storage. The major source of data for predictive modelling of BC drug resistance will come from health facilities. To accelerate the use of AI retrospective analyses of large amounts of longitudinal datasets are needed for the development of DL algorithms. The data collected differs from facility to facility. In addition, these may not be uniformly structured and insufficiently large, therefore require at least some preorganization before input for training in Machine Deep Learning. Health personnel are already overstretched, particularly in public health facilities. This may require additional human resources who are clinically/medically trained to understand the medical terminology working together with a software engineer (Koh et al., 2022).

In addition, there is a lack of standardization of predictive AI techniques and appropriate longitudinal data. Consensus on different machine learning techniques and standardization of breast cancer characteristics to be used are needed in addition to availability of large numbers of longitudinal data for deep learning machine training. Heterogeneity of breast tumors between patient and within patients before and after treatment initiation, accumulation of genetic mutations with resultant changes in the downstream molecular features as cancer progresses, are some of the challenges that may require additional steps in curating input data for machine learning (Ogunleye et al.,2022).

Poor patient record file maintenance is another challenge. In many remote and poorly resourced health facilities, the data is not digitized, and loss of patient record files is a common occurrence. Collection of relevant data in these settings will also be limited by poor access to healthcare facilities, wherein patients will present, if at all, at the advanced stages of BC and opportunities for longitudinal data collection will be missed. There is also a slow-paced adoption of digital advances and incorporation of AI in healthcare in many poor countries. Even in well-resourced settings, AI has not been fully deployed into routine clinical practice/workflow. This could be partly attributed to reluctance by pathologists/ clinicians and other healthcare workers' concerns. These concerns range from mistrust in AI's performance, fear of losing their "touch" as they rely more and more on technology or even becoming redundant. In 2023, a literature review shows no clinical implementation of AI-enhanced predictive models for BC drug resistance, only theoretical applications (Verghese et al., 2023).

Lastly, the ethics of data ownership and usage rights remain a contentious issue that needs to be resolved by all stakeholders including patient advocates, national governments, and civil society to enable an optimal beneficence of the advances of the digital phase for better patient outcomes.

Concluding Remarks

There are several AI-based models and tools with the potential to revolutionize early detection, drug discovery, and design, as well as prediction of BC drug resistance. These advances have been accelerated by the rapid development of multi-omics technology, clinical biomarkers, and bioinformatics, complemented by the revolutionary power of AI. There are definite progressive achievements in AI-enhanced systems that far outperform traditional techniques. AI improves medical decision-making regarding the therapeutic benefits of personalized precision medicine, prevents side effects of therapy for better patient outcomes, and saves clinicians time and the cost of healthcare. However, there is slow progress in implementing these digital advances in clinical practice and incorporation of AI in healthcare. More funding, infrastructure, and multidisciplinary personnel are needed to support the exponential growth of AI technology and take maximum advantage of its transformative capacity.

References

Abbasi, M., Santos, B. P., Pereira, T. C., Sofia, R., Monteiro, N. R. C., Simões, C. J. V., Brito, R. M. M., Ribeiro, B., Oliveira, J. L., & Arrais, J. P. (2022). Designing optimized drug candidates with generative adversarial network. *Journal of Cheminformatics, 14*, 40.

Ahmad, A. (2023). Pathways to breast cancer recurrence. *ISRN Oncology, 2013*, 290568.

Arnold, M., Morgan, E., Rumgay, H., Mafra, A., Singh, D., Laversanne, M., Vignat, J., Gralow, J. R., Cardoso, F., Siesling, S., & Soerjomataram, I. (2022). Current and future burden of breast cancer: Global statistics for 2020 and 2040. *The Breast: Official Journal of the European Society of Mastology, 66*, 15–23. https://doi.org/10.1016/j.breast.2022.08.010

Barretina, J., Caponigro, G., Stransky, N., Venkatesan, K., Margolin, A. A., Kim, S., et al. (2012). The cancer cell line encyclopedia enables predictive modelling of anticancer drug sensitivity. *Nature, 483*, 603–607.

Beck, J. T., Rammage, M., Jackson, G. P., Preininger, A. M., Dankwa-Mullan, I., Roebuck, M. C., Torres, A., Holtzen, H., Coverdill, S. E., Williamson, M. P., Chau, Q., Rhee, K., & Vinegra, M. (2020). Artificial intelligence tool for optimizing eligibility screening for clinical trials in a large community cancer center. *JCO Clinical Cancer Informatics, 4*, 50–59. https://doi.org/10.1200/CCI.19.00079

Bomane, A., Gonçalves, A., & Ballester, P. J. (2019). Paclitaxel response can be predicted with interpretable multi-variate classifiers exploiting DNA-methylation and miRNA data. *Frontiers in Genetics, 25*(10), 1041. https://doi.org/10.3389/fgene.2019.01041

Born, J., Manica, M., Oskooei, A., Cadow, J., Markert, G., & Rodríguez Martínez, M. (2021). PaccMann(RL): De novo generation of hit-like anticancer molecules from transcriptomic data via reinforcement learning. *IScience, 24*, 102269.

Bray, F., Ren, J. S., Masuyer, E., & Ferlay, J. (2013). Global estimates of cancer prevalence for 27 sites in the adult population in 2008. *International Journal of Cancer, 132*(5), 1133–1145. https://doi.org/10.1002/ijc.27711

Broeders, M., Moss, S., Nyström, L., Njor, S., Jonsson, H., Paap, E., Massat, N., Duffy, S., Lynge, E., Paci, E., & EUROSCREEN Working Group. (2012). The impact of mammographic screening on breast cancer mortality in Europe: A review of observational studies. *Journal of Medical Screening, 19*(1), 14–25. https://doi.org/10.1258/jms.2012.012078

Casparie, M., Tiebosch, A. T., Burger, G., Blauwgeers, H., Van De Pol, A., Van Krieken, J. H., & Meijer, G. A. (2007). Pathology databanking and biobanking in The Netherlands, a central role for PALGA, the nationwide histopathology and cytopathology data network and archive. *Cellular Oncology, 29*, 19–24.

Chakraborty, S., Hosen, M. I., Ahmed, M., & Shekhar, H. U. (2018). Onco-multi-OMICS approach: A new frontier in cancer research. *BioMed Research International, 2018*, 9836256.

Chica-Parrado, M. R., Godoy-Ortiz, A., Jiménez, B., Ribelles, N., Barragan, I., & Alba, E. (2020). Resistance to neoadjuvant treatment in breast cancer: Clinicopathological and molecular predictors. *Cancers, 12*, 2012.

Christensen, J. (2023). AI-supported mammogram screening increases breast cancer detection by 20%. Retrieved August 23, 2023, from https://edition.cnn.com/2023/08/01/health/ai-breast-cancer-detection/index.html#

Conner-Simons, A., & Gordon, R. (2019). Using AI to predict breast cancer and personalize care MIT/MGH's image-based deep learning model can predict breast cancer up to five years in advance, CSAIL. Retrieved August 23, 2023, from https://news.mit.edu/2019/using-ai-predict-breast-cancer-and-personalize-care-0507

Consortium GO. (2004). The gene ontology (GO) database and informatics resource. *Nucleic Acids Research, 32*, D258–D261.

Corti, C., Cobanaj, M., Marian, F., Dee, E. C., Lloyd, M. R., Marcu, S., Dombrovschi, A., Biondetti, G. P., Batalini, F., Celi, L. A., & Curigliano, G. (2022). Artificial intelligence for prediction of treatment outcomes in breast cancer: Systematic review of design, reporting standards, and bias. *Cancer Treatment Reviews, 108*, 102410.

Darby, S., Davies, C., & Paul McGale, P. (2005). The early breast cancer Trialists' collaborative group: A brief history of results to date. In Y. Dodge & N. Wermuth (Eds.), *Celebrating statistics'AC davison*. Oxford University Press.

DePolo, J. (2023). AI-supported mammogram reading detects 20% more cancers. Written. Retrieved August 23, 2023, from https://www.breastcancer.org/research-news/ai-mammogram-reading

Ding, Z., Zu, S., & Gu, J. (2016). Evaluating the molecule-based prediction of clinical drug responses in cancer. *Bioinformatics, 32*(19), 2891–2895. https://doi.org/10.1093/bioinformatics/btw344

Edgar, R., Domrachev, M., & Lash, A. E. (2002). Gene expression omnibus: NCBI gene expression and hybridization array data repository. *Nucleic Acids Research, 30*, 207–210.

Emran, T. B., Shahriar, A., Mahmud, A. R., Rahman, T., Abir, M. H., Faijanur-Rob Siddiquee, M., Ahmed, H., Rahman, N., Nainu, F., Wahyudin, E., Mitra, S., Dhama, K., Habiballah, M. M., Haque, S., Islam, A., & Hassan, M. M. (2022). Multidrug resistance in cancer: Understanding molecular mechanisms, immunoprevention and therapeutic approaches. *Frontiers in Oncology, 12*, 1–38. https://doi.org/10.3389/fonc.2022.891652

Evans, K. K., Birdwell, R. L., & Wolfe, J. M. (2013). If you don't find it often, you often don't find it: Why some cancers are missed in breast cancer screening. *PLoS One, 8*(5), e64366.

Fang, Y., Pan, X., & Shen, H.-B. (2023). De novo drug design by iterative multiobjective deep reinforcement learning with graph-based molecular quality assessment. *Bioinformatics, 39*, 1–10.

Feinberg, E. N., Sur, D., Wu, Z., Husic, B. E., Mai, H., Li, Y., Sun, S., Yang, J., Ramsundar, B., & Pande, V. S. (2018). PotentialNet for molecular property prediction. *ACS Central Science, 4*, 1520–1530.

Forbes, S. A., Bindal, N., Bamford, S., Cole, C., Kok, C. Y., Beare, D., Jia, M., Shepherd, R., Leung, K., Menzies, A., Teague, J. W., Campbell, P. J., Stratton, M. R., & Futreal, P. A. (2011). COSMIC: Mining complete cancer genomes in the catalogue of somatic mutations in cancer. *Nucleic Acids Research, 39*, D945–D950.

Fradkin, P., Young, A., Atanackovic, L., Frey, B., Lee, L. J., & Wang, B. (2022). A graph neural network approach for molecule carcinogenicity prediction. *Bioinformatics, 38*, i84–i91.

Gaulton, A., Bellis, L. J., Bento, A. P., Chambers, J., Davies, M., Hersey, A., Light, Y., Mcglinchey, S., Michalovich, D., Al-Lazikani, B., & Overington, J. P. (2012). ChEMBL: A large-scale bioactivity database for drug discovery. *Nucleic Acids Research, 40*, D1100–D1107.

Gehrmann, M., Schmidt, M., Brase, J. C., Roos, P., & Hengstler, J. G. (2008). Prediction of paclitaxel resistance in breast cancer: Is CYP1B1*3 a new factor of influence? *Pharmacogenomics, 9*, 969–974.

Goel, M., Raghunathan, S., Laghuvarapu, S., & Priyakumar, U. D. (2021). MoleGuLAR: Molecule generation using reinforcement learning with alternating rewards. *Journal of Chemical Information and Modeling, 61*, 5815–5826.

Goldenberg, S. L., Nir, G., & Salcudean, S. E. (2019). A new era: Artificial intelligence and machine learning in prostate cancer. *Nature Reviews Urology, 16*(7), 391–403.

Goodman, L. S., Wintrobe, M. M., Dameshek, W., Goodman, M. J., Gilman, A., & McLennan, M. T. (1946). Use of methyl-Bis (Beta-Chloroethyl)amine hydrochloride and Tris(Beta-Chloroethyl)amine hydrochloride for Hodgkin's disease, Lymphosarcoma, leukemia and certain allied and miscellaneous disorders. *Journal of the American Medical Association, 132*, 126–132.

Gore, J. C. (2020). Artificial intelligence in medical imaging. *Magnetic Resonance Imaging, 68*, A1–A4.

Grisoni, F., Moret, M., Lingwood, R., & Schneider, G. (2020). Bidirectional molecule generation with recurrent neural networks. *Journal of Chemical Information and Modeling, 60*, 1175–1183.

Gromski, P. S., Granda, J. M., & Cronin, L. (2020). Universal chemical synthesis and discovery with 'the Chemputer'. *Trends in Chemistry, 2*, 4–12.

Hamosh, A., Scott, A. F., Amberger, J. S., Bocchini, C. A., & Mckusick, V. A. (2005). Online Mendelian Inheritance in Man (OMIM), a knowledgebase of human genes and genetic disorders. *Nucleic Acids Research, 33*, D514–D517.

ICGC/TCGA Pan-Cancer Analysis of Whole Genomes Consortium. (2020). Pan-cancer analysis of whole genomes. *Nature, 578*(7793), 82–93.

Independent UK Panel on Breast Cancer Screening. (2012). The benefits and harms of breast cancer screening: An independent review. *Lancet, 380*(9855), 1778–1786.

Irwin, J. J., Tang, K. G., Young, J., Dandarchuluun, C., Wong, B. R., Khurelbaatar, M., Moroz, Y. S., Mayfield, J., & Sayle, R. A. (2020). ZINC20—A free ultralarge-scale chemical database for ligand discovery. *Journal of Chemical Information and Modeling, 60*, 6065–6073.

Kanehisa, M., & Goto, S. (2000). KEGG: Kyoto encyclopedia of genes and genomes. *Nucleic Acids Research, 28*, 27–30.

Khan, A., Ali, L., & Wei, D. Q. (2022). Editorial: Breast cancer resistance, biomarkers and therapeutics development in the era of artificial intelligence. *Frontiers in Molecular Biosciences, 9*, 1034990.

Koh, D. M., Papanikolaou, N., Bick, U., Illing, R., Kahn, C. E., Jr., Kalpathi-Cramer, J., Matos, C., Martí-Bonmatí, L., Miles, A., Mun, S. K., Napel, S., Rockall, A., Sala, E., Strickland, N., & Prior, F. (2022). Artificial intelligence and machine learning in cancer imaging. *Communications Medicine (Lond), 2*, 133.

Koscielny, S. (2010). Why most gene expression signatures of tumors have not been useful in the clinic. *Science Translational Medicine, 2*, 14ps2.

Lauritzen, A. D., Rodríguez-Ruiz, A., von Euler-Chelpin, M. C., Lynge, E., Vejborg, I., Nielsen, M., Karssemeijer, N., & Lillholm, M. (2022). An artificial intelligence-based mammography screening protocol for breast cancer: Outcome and radiologist workload. *Radiology, 304*(1), 41–49.

Leventakos, K., Helgeson, J., Mansfield, A. S., Deering, E., Schwecke, A., Adjei, A., Molina, J., Hocum, C., Halfdanarson, T., Marks, R., Parikh, K., Pomerleau, K., Coverdill, S., Rammage, M., & Haddad, T. (2019). Implementation of artificial intelligence (AI) for lung cancer clinical trial matching in a tertiary cancer center. *Annals of Oncology, 30*(Suppl 2), ii74.

Liang, G., Fan, W., Luo, H., & Zhu, X. (2020). The emerging roles of artificial intelligence in cancer drug development and precision therapy. *Biomedicine & Pharmacotherapy, 128*, 110255.

Liao, J., Li, X., Gan, Y., Han, S., Rong, P., Wang, W., Li, W., & Zhou, L. (2022). Artificial intelligence assists precision medicine in cancer treatment. *Frontiers in Oncology, 12*, 998222.

Lind, A. P., & Anderson, P. C. (2019). Predicting drug activity against cancer cells by random forest models based on minimal genomic information and chemical properties. *PLoS One, 14*(7), e0219774.

Ma, C. X., & Ellis, M. J. (2013). The cancer genome atlas: Clinical applications for breast cancer. *Oncology (Williston Park), 27*(1263–1269), 1274–1279.

MacEachern, S. J., & Forkert, N. D. (2021). Machine learning for precision medicine. *Genome, 64*(4), 416–425.

Mayr, A., Klambauer, G., Unterthiner, T., & Hochreiter, S. (2016). DeepTox: Toxicity prediction using deep learning. *Frontiers in Environmental Science, 3*, 80.

Maziarka, Ł., Pocha, A., Kaczmarczyk, J., Rataj, K., Danel, T., & Warchoł, M. (2020). Mol-CycleGAN: A generative model for molecular optimization. *Journal of Cheminformatics, 12*, 2.

Mazo, C., Aura, C., Rahman, A., Gallagher, W. M., & Mooney, C. (2022). Application of artificial intelligence techniques to predict risk of recurrence of breast cancer: A systematic review. *Journal of Personalized Medicine, 12*(9), 1496.

Nguyen, L. C., Naulaerts, S., Bruna, A., Ghislat, G., & Ballester, P. J. (2021). Predicting cancer drug response in vivo by learning an optimal feature selection of tumour molecular profiles. *Biomedicine, 9*(10), 1319.

Nordenskjöld, B., & Rutqvist, L. E. (2002). Long-term effects of mammography screening: Updated overview of the Swedish randomised trials. *Lancet, 359*(9310), 909–919.

Ogunleye, A. Z., Piyawajanusorn, C., Gonçalves, A., Ghislat, G., & Ballester, P. J. (2022). Interpretable machine learning models to predict the resistance of breast cancer patients to doxorubicin from their microRNA profiles. *Advanced Science (Weinh), 9*(24), e2201501.

Paul, D., Sanap, G., Shenoy, S., Kalyane, D., Kalia, K., & Tekade, R. K. (2021). Artificial intelligence in drug discovery and development. *Drug Discovery Today, 26*, 80–93.

Pinheiro, G. A., Mucelini, J., Soares, M. D., Prati, R. C., Da Silva, J. L. F., & Quiles, M. G. (2020). Machine learning prediction of nine molecular properties based on the SMILES representation of the QM9 quantum-chemistry dataset. *The Journal of Physical Chemistry A, 124*, 9854–9866.

Popova, M., Isayev, O., & Tropsha, A. (2018). Deep reinforcement learning for de novo drug design. Science. *Advances, 4*, eaap7885.

Prihantono, F. M. (2021). Breast cancer resistance to chemotherapy: When should we suspect it and how can we prevent it? *Annals of Medicine and Surgery (Lond), 70*, 102793.

Ramsundar, B. (2018). Molecular machine learning with DeepChem (Doctoral dissertation, Stanford University).

Ren, F., Ding, X., Zheng, M., Korzinkin, M., Cai, X., Zhu, W., Mantsyzov, A., Aliper, A., Aladinskiy, V., Cao, Z., Kong, S., Long, X., Man Liu, B. H., Liu, Y., Naumov, V., Shneyderman, A., Ozerov, I. V., Wang, J., Pun, F. W., Polykovskiy, D. A., Sun, C., Levitt, M., Aspuru-Guzik, A., & Zhavoronkov, A. (2023). Alpha fold accelerates artificial intelligence powered drug discovery: Efficient discovery of a novel CDK20 small molecule inhibitor. *Chemical Science, 14*, 1443–1452.

Samanta, B., De, A., Jana, G., Gómez, V., Chattaraj, P. K., Ganguly, N., & Gomez-Rodriguez, M. (2020). Nevae: A deep generative model for molecular graphs. *The Journal of Machine Learning Research, 21*, 4556–4588.

Stork, C., Wagner, J., Friedrich, N. O., De Bruyn, K. C., Šícho, M., & Kirchmair, J. (2018). Hit dexter: A machine-learning model for the prediction of frequent hitters. *ChemMedChem, 13*, 564–571.

Sung, H., Ferlay, J., Siegel, R. L., Laversanne, M., Soerjomataram, I., Jemal, A., et al. (2021). Global cancer statistics 2020: GLOBOCAN estimates of incidence and mortality worldwide for 36 cancers in 185 countries. *CA: A Cancer Journal for Clinicians, 71*(3), 209–249.

Szklarczyk, D., Gable, A. L., Nastou, K. C., Lyon, D., Kirsch, R., Pyysalo, S., Doncheva, N. T., Legeay, M., Fang, T., Bork, P., Jensen, L. J., & Von Mering, C. (2021). The STRING database in 2021: Customizable protein-protein networks, and functional characterization of user-uploaded gene/measurement sets. *Nucleic Acids Research, 49*, D605–D612.

Tai, C. A., Hodzic, N., Flanagan, N., Gunraj, H., & Wong, A. (2023). Cancer-net BCa: Breast cancer pathologic complete response prediction using volumetric deep radiomic features from synthetic correlated diffusion imaging. Submitted to arXiv.

The ENCODE Project Consortium. (2012). An integrated encyclopedia of DNA elements in the human genome. *Nature, 489*, 57–74.

The Institute of cancer Research. (2023). New AI drug discovery collaboration aims to design new precision cancer drugs. Retrieved August 24, 2023, from https://www.icr.ac.uk/news-archive/new-ai-drug-discovery-collaboration-aims-to-design-new-precision-cancer-drugs

Torre, L. A., Siegel, R. L., Ward, E. M., & Jemal, A. (2016). Global cancer incidence and mortality rates and trends–an update. *Cancer Epidemiology, Biomarkers & Prevention, 25*(1), 16–27.

Vamathevan, J., Clark, D., Czodrowski, P., Dunham, I., Ferran, E., Lee, G., Li, B., Madabhushi, A., Shah, P., Spitzer, M., & Zhao, S. (2019). Applications of machine learning in drug discovery and development. *Nature Reviews Drug Discovery, 18*, 463–477.

Verghese, G., Li, M., Liu, F., Lohan, A., Kurian, N. C., Meena, S., Gazinska, P., Shah, A., Oozeer, A., Chan, T., Opdam, M., Linn, S., Gillett, C., Alberts, E., Hardiman, T., Jones, S., Thavaraj, S., Jones, J. L., Salgado, R., Pinder, S. E., Rane, S., Sethi, A., & Grigoriadis, A. (2023). Multiscale deep learning framework captures systemic immune features in lymph nodes predictive of triple negative breast cancer outcome in large-scale studies. *The Journal of Pathology, 260*(4), 376–389.

Wang, C., & Zhang, Y. (2017). Improving scoring-docking-screening powers of protein-ligand scoring functions using random forest. *Journal of Computational Chemistry, 38*, 169–177.

Wang, L., McLeod, H. L., & Weinshilboum, R. M. (2011). Genomics and drug response. *New England Journal of Medicine, 364*(12), 1144–1153.

Wang, L., Song, Y., Wang, H., Zhang, X., Wang, M., He, J., Li, S., Zhang, L., Li, K., & Cao, L. (2023). Advances of artificial intelligence in anti-cancer drug design: A review of the past decade. *Pharmaceuticals, 16*, 253.

Wang, X., Zhang, H., & Chen, X. (2019). Drug resistance and combating drug resistance in cancer. *Cancer Drug Resistance, 2*(2), 141–160.

Wang, Y., Wang, Z., Xu, J., Li, J., Li, S., Zhang, M., & Yang, D. (2018). Systematic identification of non-coding pharmacogenomic landscape in cancer. *Nature Communications, 9*(1), 3192.

Wang, Y., Xiao, J., Suzek TO, Zhang, J., Wang, J., & Bryant, S. H. (2009). PubChem: A public information system for analyzing bioactivities of small molecules. *Nucleic Acids Research, 37*, W623–W633.

Wang, Y., Zhang, S., Li, F., Zhou, Y., Zhang, Y., Wang, Z., Zhang, R., Zhu, J., Ren, Y., Tan, Y., Qin, C., Li, Y., Li, X., Chen, Y., & Zhu, F. (2019). Therapeutic target database 2020: Enriched resource for facilitating research and early development of targeted therapeutics. *Nucleic Acids Research, 48*, D1031–D1041.

Wishart, D. S., Feunang, Y. D., Guo, A. C., Lo, E. J., Marcu, A., Grant, J. R., Sajed, T., Johnson, D., Li, C., Sayeeda, Z., Assempour, N., Iynkkaran, I., Liu, Y., Maciejewski, A., Gale, N., Wilson, A., Chin, L., Cummings, R., Le, D., Pon, A., Knox, C., & Wilson, M. (2018). DrugBank 5.0: A major update to the DrugBank database for 2018. *Nucleic Acids Research, 46*, D1074–D1082.

Xu, Y. (2022). Deep neural networks for QSAR. *Methods in Molecular Biology, 2390*, 233–260.

Yersal, O., & Barutca, S. (2014). Biological subtypes of breast cancer: Prognostic and therapeutic implications. *World Journal of Clinical Oncology, 5*, 412–424.

You, Y., Lai, X., Pan, Y., Zheng, H., Vera, J., Liu, S., Deng, S., & Zhang, L. (2022). Artificial intelligence in cancer target identification and drug discovery. *Signal Transduction and Targeted Therapy, 7*, 156.

Zeng, L., Liu, L., Chen, D., Lu, H., Xue, Y., Bi, H., & Yang, W. (2023). The innovative model based on artificial intelligence algorithms to predict recurrence risk of patients with postoperative breast cancer. *Frontiers in Oncology, 13*, 1117420.

Zhou, J., Sun, H., Wang, Z., Cong, W., Wang, J., Zeng, M., et al. (2020). Guidelines for the diagnosis and treatment of hepatocellular carcinoma (2019 edition). *Liver Cancer, 9*(6), 682–720.

Part IV
Future Directions and Advancements in Overcoming Drug Resistance

The Microbiome: A New Frontier in Overcoming Drug Resistance in Breast Cancer

Thifhelimbilu Emmanuel Luvhengo, Thabiso Victor Miya, Afra Basera, Olalekan Fadebi, Ravi Mehrotra, and Zodwa Dlamini

Abstract The gut microbiome comprises bacteria, fungi, viruses, archaea, and their genetic materials. The gut microbiome influences the physiological and immunological functions of the body. When there is a change in the composition of microbiota in the gut, this is called dysbiosis. Dysbiosis is linked with several gastrointestinal and extra-gastrointestinal diseases, including some cases of breast cancer (BC). Molecular Subtype and stage of diagnosis both affect the way patients with BC are managed. BC is a heterogeneous disease and, in some cases, the response to treatment may not be as predicted. Dysbiosis of the gut and breast

T. E. Luvhengo (✉)
SAMRC Precision Oncology Research Unit (PORU), Precision Oncology and Cancer Prevention (POCP), Pan African Cancer Research Institute (PACRI), University of Pretoria, Pretoria, South Africa

Department of Surgery, University of the Witwatersrand, Johannesburg, South Africa
e-mail: Thifhelimbilu.Luvhengo@wits.ac.za

T. V. Miya · Z. Dlamini
SAMRC Precision Oncology Research Unit (PORU), DSI/NRF SARChI Chair in Precision Oncology and Cancer Prevention (POCP), Pan African Cancer Research Institute (PACRI), University of Pretoria, Pretoria, South Africa
e-mail: thabiso.miya@up.ac.za; Zodwa.Dlamini@up.ac.za

A. Basera · O. Fadebi
SAMRC Precision Oncology Research Unit (PORU), Precision Oncology and Cancer Prevention (POCP), Pan African Cancer Research Institute (PACRI), University of Pretoria, Pretoria, South Africa
Department of Medical Oncology, Faculty of Health Sciences, Steve Biko Academic Hospital, University of Pretoria, Hatfield, South Africa
e-mail: u22800370@tuks.co.za; u22493591@tuks.co.za

R. Mehrotra
SAMRC Precision Oncology Research Unit (PORU), Precision Oncology and Cancer Prevention (POCP), Pan African Cancer Research Institute (PACRI), University of Pretoria, Pretoria, South Africa

Indian Cancer Genomic Atlas, Centre for Health, Innovation and Policy Foundation, Noida, India
e-mail: ravi.mehrotra@gov.in

Z. Dlamini (ed.), *Overcoming Breast Cancer Therapy Resistance*,
https://doi.org/10.1007/978-3-031-52860-6_11

microbiota may influence the progression of BC and its response to treatment. Furthermore, treatment of BC may also alter the microbiota, leading to dysbiosis. This chapter reviews the relationship between dysbiosis and BC. Furthermore, how dysbiosis can be manipulated to improve tumor response or reverse resistance to drug treatment is also elaborated on.

Keywords Breast cancer · Microbiome · Microbiota · Dysbiosis · Chemotherapy · Drug resistance · Innate immunity

Introduction

Close to 90% of breast cancers (BCs) are sporadic and related to modifiable factors such as lifestyle and overweight or obesity (Bowers et al., 2022; De Oliveira Andrade et al., 2022; Kang et al., 2018). Both obesity and BC are commonly associated with chronic systemic inflammation that is driven from the gut. Changes in either the total number of bacteria or the variety of the phyla of the microbiota in the gut, triggers dysbiosis (Khandekar et al., 2011; Kang et al., 2018; Untersmayr et al., 2022). Several factors may cause the dysbiosis of the gut microbiota, among them physical activity, dietary habits, smoking, alcohol intake, antimicrobial therapy, chemotherapy (CT), immunotherapy, targeted therapy, and radiotherapy (Rosean et al., 2019; Ruo et al., 2021; Sevcikova et al., 2022; Nandi et al., 2023).

The mainstay of curative treatment for BC is surgery, and whether hormone therapy, CT, targeted therapy, or immunotherapy is used also depends on the tumor's stage and molecular subtype (Yin et al., 2020). Although early detection and timeous treatment are the most effective weapons against BC, in some patients, the cancer is not curable despite the institution of appropriate treatment for less aggressive and non-metastatic tumors (Sevcikova et al., 2022). Some of the patients may respond transiently and then become resistant to hormonal therapy, CT, trastuzumab, and immune checkpoint inhibitors (Bruce et al., 2021; Sevcikova et al., 2022).

The divergent response of BC to treatment is partly explained by the heterogeneity of the patients, histological features, tumor microenvironment, and the genomic landscape (Bruce et al., 2021; Lu et al., 2022; Qiu et al., 2021). BC that was initially responsive to therapy may become resistant and de novo resistance to standard treatment is more likely in patients who have triple-negative BC (TNBC) (Bowers et al., 2022). TNBC is more common in women below the age of 40 years, premenopausal, and/or overweight or obese (Bowers et al., 2022; De Oliveira Andrade et al., 2022). Adiposity and adipokines elaborated from adipose tissue help to sustain chronic systemic inflammation, which may promote the progression of the tumor, metastatic spread, or recurrence following treatment (Kolb & Zhang, 2020). The response to BC may also be influenced by the dysbiosis of the microbiota within a tumor or in the gut (Kang et al., 2018; Kothari et al., 2020; Laborda-Illanes et al., 2020; Li et al., 2022).

Gut Microbiota in Innate Immunity and Normal Physiology

The gut in humans harbors more than 300 species of bacteria and the total bacterial count is higher in the colon, where the count is around 10^{14} (Zhao et al., 2023). The Firmicutes, Proteobacteria, and Bacteroidetes phyla account for more than 90% of the bacterial species that are in a healthy state (Arnone & Cook, 2022; German et al., 2023; Liu et al., 2021, 2021; Nandi et al., 2023; Sevcikova et al., 2022). Colonization starts in utero and is influenced by the nature of delivery and the weaning diet (Nakamura et al., 2016; Wilson et al., 2020). Once established, the gut microbiome, comprising the microbiota together with their genome, is critical for the defense and normal function of the body (Hills et al., 2019; Nakamura et al., 2016; Sampsell et al., 2020; Wilson et al., 2020).

There are 65–80% of the cells involved in innate and adaptive immunity within the tissues of the GI tract, which is the area of the body most exposed to external threats and harbors the largest number of bacteria (Hendel et al., 2022; Zhao et al., 2023). The microorganisms in various niches along the GIT compete among themselves for nutrients and some species of bacteria possess quorum sensors and secrete bacteriocins to also prevent dysbiosis; while others assist in the digestion of indigestible fibers (Zhao et al., 2022). The virome composed of viruses and bacteriophages in the gut also participates in innate defense and prevention of dysbiosis (Stern et al., 2019).

The innate immunity of the gut provides the first line of defense against pathogens as the gut microbiota and intestinal epithelial cells (IECs) along the GIT are key role players in innate immunity, especially in the colon and the small intestine (Uribe-Herranz et al., 2020). IECs are produced from intestinal stem cells (ISCs) found at the base of the Lieberkuhn crypt (intestinal crypt) (Kurokawa et al., 2021). The majority of IECs have pathogen recognition receptors (PRRs), which they utilize to monitor and regulate the microbiota in the gut lumen to prevent dysbiosis (Sevcikova et al., 2022).

The IECs that are among the major contributors to innate immunity in the gut are the Paneth cells (Wallaeys et al., 2023), goblet cells (Gierynska et al., 2022), tuft cells and M-cells (Hendel et al., 2022; Kanaya et al., 2020; Markandey et al., 2021). Paneth cells secrete antimicrobial peptides that shape the gut microbiota to prevent dysbiosis and ligands lipopolysaccharides from Gram-negative bacteria to prevent translocation and subsequent systemic inflammation (Jiang & Miao, 2023; Nakamura et al., 2016). Paneth cells also collaborate with cells in the lamina propria, among them fibroblasts, smooth muscle cells, and endothelial cells, to produce the niche factors that govern the proliferation and differentiation of the ISCs (Zhu et al., 2021). The MUC2 from goblet cells forms a protective layer of mucus on the luminal surface of the IECs (Lee et al., 2021; Zhao et al., 2022). Mucus is a preferred nutrient for some of the bacteria that reside in the lumen of the gut (Cheng et al., 2020). The gut microbiota interacts with the IECs and cells in the lamina propria for coordination of the local innate and adaptive immunity, and subsequently of the entire body (Rumbo et al., 2004) (Fig. 1).

Bile acids and metabolites of dietary products also assist in the maintenance of normal microbial flora (eubiosis) in the gut (Ruo et al., 2021). An extended state of eubiosis restricts the release of pro-inflammatory cytokines and local inflammation,

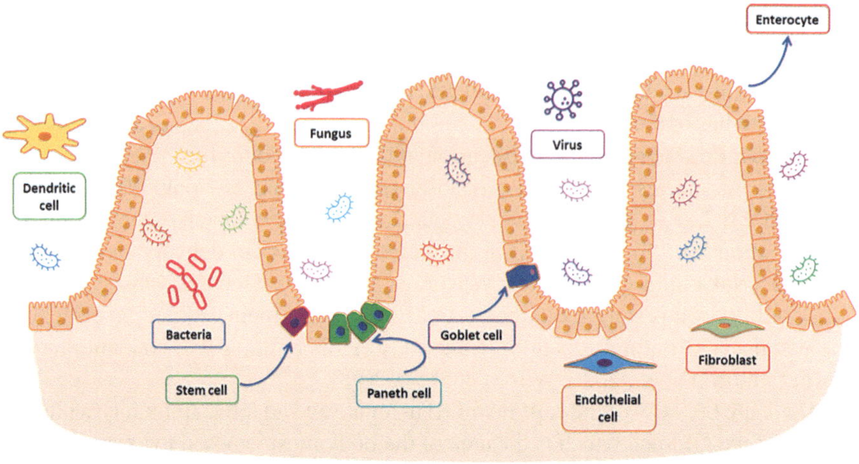

Fig. 1 Schematic diagram depicting the intestinal crypt of Lieberkühn, the gut microbiota, IECs, and cells found in the lamina propria which link innate immunity with adaptive immunity. The microbiome of the gut is made of viruses, bacteria, and fungi. Paneth cells and ISCs are found near each other. Also depicted are cells of the lamina propria that are critical for innate immunity and the production of niche factors for the ISCs, such as dendritic and endothelial cells

which could harm the intestinal epithelium, increase gut permeability, and allow endotoxins to move to other parts of the body (Untersmayr et al., 2022). Some of the pathogens may produce excessive amounts of reactive oxygen and nitrogen species and overwhelm the local antioxidant mechanisms, leading to damage to intestinal epithelium (Zhao et al., 2023). The beneficial effects of microbial species in the GIT are not limited to innate immunity as some species of bacteria help with digestion and absorption of nutrients like vitamins and short-chain fatty acids, among them butyrate (Wilson et al., 2020). Butyrate is critical in the maintenance of the integrity of the IECs, especially colonocytes and its deficiency may lead to an increase in epithelial permeability (Wilson et al., 2020). Regulation of the proliferation and differentiation of intestinal stem cells, as well as regulation of the entero-endocrine system, are additional advantages of the gut microbiota (Bruce et al., 2021; Ervin et al., 2019; Klement et al., 2020). Certain bacteria in the gut microbiota play a role in the metabolism of hormones that affect the onset, progression, and treatment response of several malignancies (Bruce et al., 2021; Ervin et al., 2019).

Dysbiosis of the Microbiota of the Gut Microbiome and Diseases

Dysbiosis may lead to an increase in the local production of reactive oxygen and nitrogen species, a reduction in the production of short-chain fatty acid, pro-inflammatory cytokines production, local inflammation, and upregulated gut permeability (Nagpal et al., 2018). The increase in gut permeability allows the translocation of bacteria and their products, including endotoxins and a spillover of pro-inflammatory cytokines into the systemic circulation (Liu et al., 2021, 2021; Nagpal et al., 2018; Sevcikova et al., 2022; Wilson et al., 2020). The systemic inflammatory state disrupts mitochondrial function and causes increased oxidative stress (Sevcikova et al., 2022). Dysbiosis, increased gut permeability, mitochondrial dysfunction, systemic inflammation, and increased oxidative stress all contribute to the creation of a favorable environment for carcinogenesis. (Arnone & Cook, 2022; German et al., 2023; Nandi et al., 2023; Ruo et al., 2021; Zou et al., 2018). Individuals who develop cancer that is preceded by dysbiosis of the gut microbiota are likely to be obese and the cancer is likely to be aggressive and linked with poorer outcomes, for instance, TNBC (Bowers et al., 2022).

Dysbiosis is a change in the number or composition of microbes in a niche. Common causes of microbiota dysbiosis include the use of antimicrobials or other drugs, change of diet or lifestyle, surgical intervention, radiation therapy, CT, and psychological stress (Ransohoff et al., 2023; Rosean et al., 2019; Zidi et al., 2021). Dysbiosis of the gut microbiota has been shown to be involved in the pathogenesis of most non-communicable illnesses including cardiovascular disease, diabetes mellitus, arthritis, obesity, and cancers (Kang et al., 2018; Liu et al., 2021, 2021; Wilson et al., 2020). The impact of dysbiosis is not limited to carcinogenesis but includes tumor progression, de-differentiation, the composition of the tumor microenvironment, response to treatment, and the likelihood of recurrence of cancer (Qiu et al., 2021). Figure 2 contains some of the factors that may predispose to dysbiosis of the breast and/or gut microbiota.

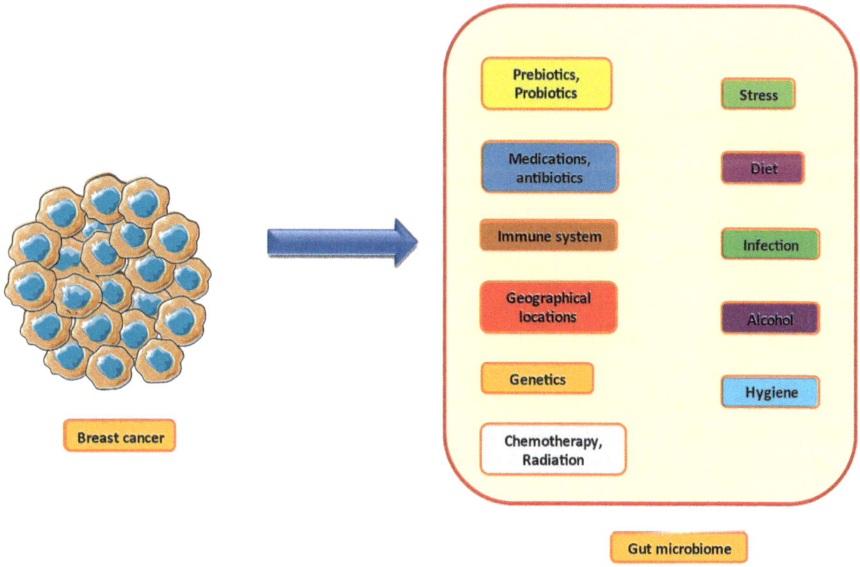

Fig. 2 Factors affecting the composition of the gut microbiota leading to dysbiosis. Multiple factors affect the composition of the gut microbiota that can lead to dysbiosis. These factors include stress, prebiotics, diet, and immune system to name a few

Dysbiosis of the Breast and Gut Microbiome and Pathogenesis of Breast Cancer

Dysbiosis of breast and gut microbiota is associated with some of the cases of BC and mechanisms include induction of inflammation, production of genotoxins, suppression of DNA repair mechanism, immunomodulation, or alteration of the levels of circulating estrogens (Viswanathan et al., 2023). Most of the unconjugated estrogen in a premenopausal woman is produced by the ovary, with less amount coming from the adrenal gland and adipose tissue (Bruce et al., 2021). The circulating estrogen is taken up, conjugated, and secreted into the bile by the liver. The conjugated bile is de-conjugated by β-glucuronidase produced by some of the species of bacteria in the gut (Arnone & Cook, 2022; Bruce et al., 2021; Rashed et al., 2022; Viswanathan et al., 2023). The de-conjugated estrogen is absorbed and recycled via the enterohepatic circulation (Bruce et al., 2021; Ervin et al., 2019) Dysbiosis of the gut microbiota may lead to an overgrowth of bacteria that increases the activities of β-glucuronidase and excessive production of estrogen which may induce cancer or alter the response to treatment of an already diagnosed BC (Fig. 3).

Elevated Estrogen Levels

While previous research has emphasized the importance of changes in the breast microbiome in BC tumorigenesis, the ramifications of changes in the gut microbiota have received less attention in the literature. It has been shown that altering the gut microbial ecology can have an impact on intestinal metabolite levels, which can both contribute to the development of cancer and result in carcinogenesis distal from the site of origin (Tsvetikova & Koshel, 2020). Research studies that compared the gut microbiota of healthy controls and BC patients using microbial profile methodologies found that the diversity of bacterial species was significantly lower in the BC patients compared to healthy controls (Flores et al., 2012; Fuhrman et al., 2014; Goedert et al., 2015). The gastrointestinal microbiota modulates systemic estrogen, and postmenopausal breast development is linked to abnormal (high) estrogen concentrations in the body (Iida et al., 2013). Estrogen is broken down in the liver, and there conjugation of the metabolites occurs and they are released into the gastrointestinal lumen (Rea et al., 2018). Bacterial β-glucuronidases can deconjugate excreted estrogens, allowing them to be reabsorbed and transported to the breast (Mikó et al., 2019). β-Glucuronidases secreting bacteria, *Clostridium coccoides* and *Clostridium leptum* subspecies levels are elevated in individuals with BC (Flores et al., 2012; Fuhrman et al., 2014; Goedert et al., 2015, 2018).

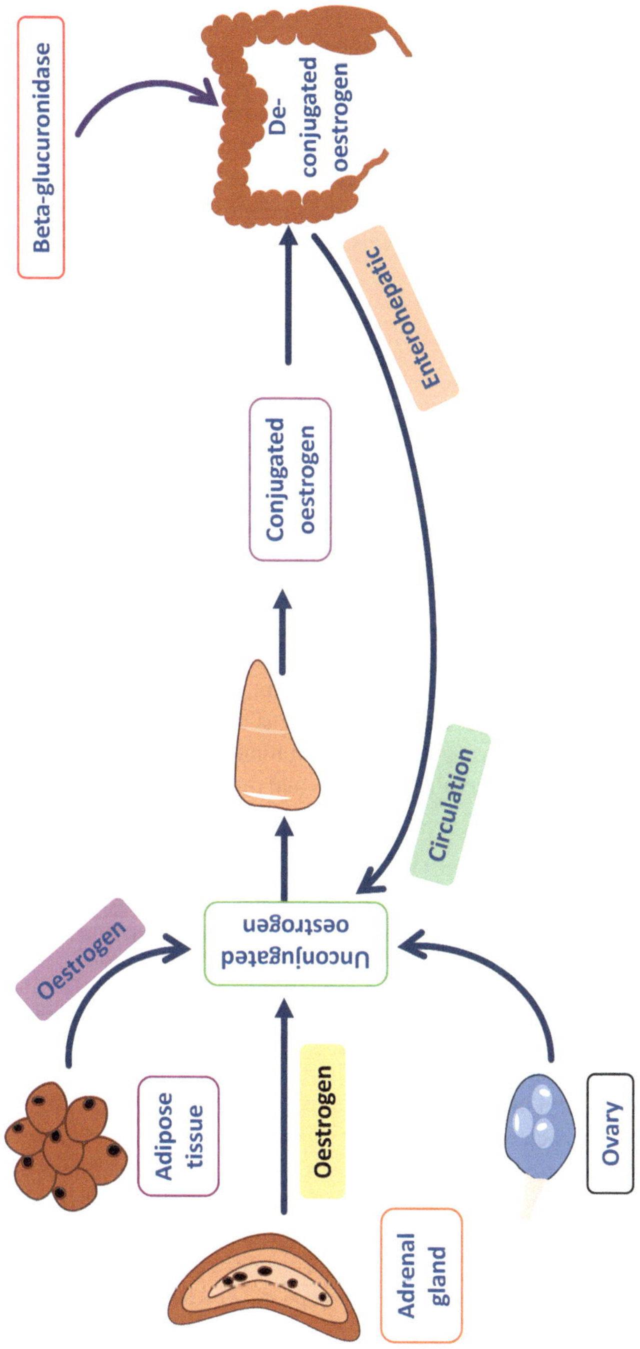

Fig. 3 Schematic diagram showing the metabolism of estrogens. Unconjugated estrogens are produced by the ovary, adrenal gland, and adipose tissue. The unconjugated estrogens are conjugated in the liver and secreted into the bile. Some of the conjugates that enter the gut are de-conjugated through an enzyme β-glucuronidase which is produced by some of the bacteria in the colon. The de-conjugated estrogens are reabsorbed and return to the circulation

Chronic Inflammation

The microbial community may elevate cancer risk by causing persistent inflammation, upsetting the body's delicate balance between cell growth and cell death, and promoting unchecked innate and adaptive immunity (Arumugam et al., 2011; Crusz & Balkwill, 2015). The overexpression of prostaglandin E2 (PGE) and cyclooxygenase 2 (COX2) is shown to be an inflammatory mechanism linked to BC, which would cause an upregulation of aromatase in adipose tissue, mediating the metabolism of androgen precursors to estrogens, and elevating the likelihood of breast malignancy (Bowers et al., 2015).

Obesity

A dysbiosis of the gut microbiota can lead to obesity. The idea of microbe-induced obesity was postulated as a state in which extra fat develops due to the primary alteration of the microbiome in childhood by numerous causes including antibiotics (Cox et al., 2014). Due to its impact on estrogen levels, obesity is a recognized risk factor for BCs. Obesity raises the risk of BC by proximal aromatization of androgens and reduction of liver hormone-binding protein synthesis, culminating in increased levels of estrogens (Newman et al., 2019). A link was discovered between the likelihood of malignancy and adult weight gain, with each 5-kg rise in weight related to a further 11% rise in the chance of postmenopausal breast malignancy (Cox et al., 2014). Thus, altering the gut microbiome to re-establish eubiosis may serve as a targeted strategy to combat adiposity and the elevated likelihood of malignancy (Xiong et al., 2018).

Short-Chain Fatty Acids and Breast Cancer Carcinogenesis

Bacterial metabolites can reach the blood system and disrupt the balance of the intestine and other proximal organs, serving as signaling mediators and influencing BC advancement (Zhang et al., 2022). Short-chain fatty acids (SCFAs) are an extremely frequent form of gut metabolite, generated from non-digestible carbohydrates, mostly by the bacterial species *Clostridium leptum*, *Faecalibacterium prausnitzii*, *Eubacterium rectale*, *Eubacterium hallii*, and *Anaerostipes*. The growth, cell death, invasion, gene expression, and metabolic activity, amongst other malignancy hallmarks, are all modulated by SCFAs in breast neoplasia (Bindels et al., 2012; Hopkins & Meier, 2017; Salimi et al., 2017; Thirunavukkarasan et al., 2017). The primary SCFA receptors are free fatty acid receptors (FFARs), which are only found on tumor cells and on stromal cells (such as adipocytes) (Hopkins & Meier, 2017; Huang et al., 2017; Iván et al., 2017). Depending on the situation, SCFA actions in breast neoplasia can be both beneficial and unfavorable (Huang et al., 2017; Thirunavukkarasan et al., 2017). The significance of SCFAs in regulating metabolic processes in breast carcinoma cells is poorly understood. BC cells can use even SCFAs, acetate, butyrate, or lactate as fuel molecules and sodium butyrate increases the intake of oxygen in cancer cell lines (Rodrigues et al., 2015) and the suppression of lactate metabolism decreases BC cell viability (Martinez-Outschoorn et al., 2014). Additionally, butyrate can cause apoptosis by increasing reactive oxygen species production in the mitochondria (Salimi et al., 2017). SCFAs can hinder tumor cell growth, epithelial-to-mesenchymal cell change, cancer metastasis, as well as stimulate anticancer immunity, remodel cell metabolism, trigger senescence, and decrease the quantity of cancer stem cells (Kovács et al., 2019; Luu et al., 2018; Yoshimoto et al., 2013).

BC pathogenesis is regulated by the gastrointestinal microbiome's estrogen and non-estrogen-dependent actions, which involve the synthesis of bioactive metabolites (Mikó et al., 2019; Rea et al., 2018). Some of the effects of dysbiosis include promotion of tumorigenesis, modification of immune response to tumor cells and alteration of metabolism of CT and other drugs used in the treatment of patients with BC (Untersmayr et al., 2022) (Fig. 4).

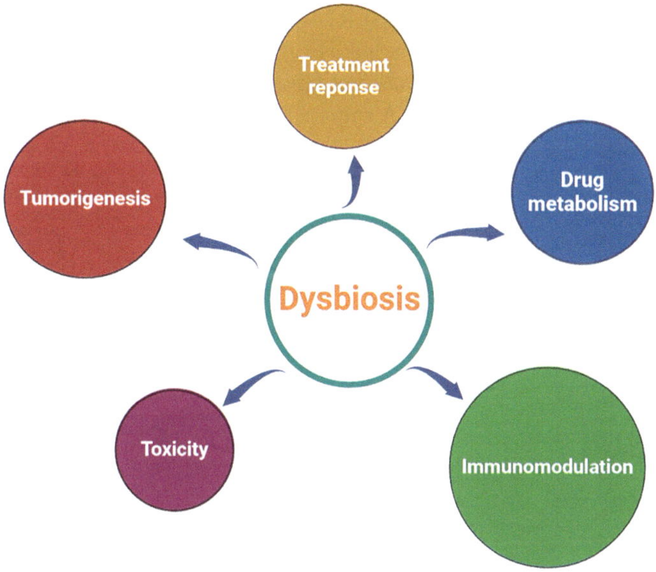

Fig. 4 Schematic diagram of the influence of dysbiosis on the development and treatment of breast cancer. Dysbiosis can lead to the promotion of tumorigenesis, modification of immune response to tumor cells, and alteration of metabolism

Management of Breast Cancer

BC treatment options include surgery, radiation (Viswanathan et al., 2023), CT (Li et al., 2022; Sun et al., 2018), hormonal therapy (Zhao et al., 2023), targeted therapy (Bonizzi et al., 2021; Bruce et al., 2021), and immunotherapy (Nandi et al., 2023). The overall aim in the management of patients with BC may be curative or palliative. Patients with early or locally advanced BC are amenable to treatment with curative intent. Surgery is the mainstay of treatment, and the surgical options are mastectomy or breast-conserving procedures. Surgery for BC may be instituted de novo or following a course of neoadjuvant therapy (Li et al., 2022). The choice of neoadjuvant or adjuvant therapy in BC depends on the molecular subtype of the tumor (Li et al., 2015; Yin et al., 2020). There are four main molecular subtypes of BC and the categorization of BC into subtypes is based on the expression of estrogen, progesterone, and human epidermal receptor 2 (HER 2), and the Ki67 index of the tumor (Li et al., 2015).

Luminal A BC is responsive to endocrine therapy and is treatable with estrogen receptor modulators, aromatase inhibitors, or ovarian ablation (Hanker et al., 2020; Korde et al., 2021). Although luminal A breast is supposed to be less aggressive but, in some patients, it may be aggressive and present with metastatic disease that is resistant to endocrine or CT and is associated with gut microbiota dysbiosis (Hanker et al., 2020). The use of hormonal therapy is also justifiable in patients with Lumina B cancer but not HER2-enriched tumors (Korde et al., 2021). Neoadjuvant or adjuvant chemotherapy is a requisite in all patients with BC except if the tumor is early and tumor does not have other markers of aggressive disease (Li et al., 2022; Zidi et al., 2021). A summary of the options available for the management of BC (Fig. 5).

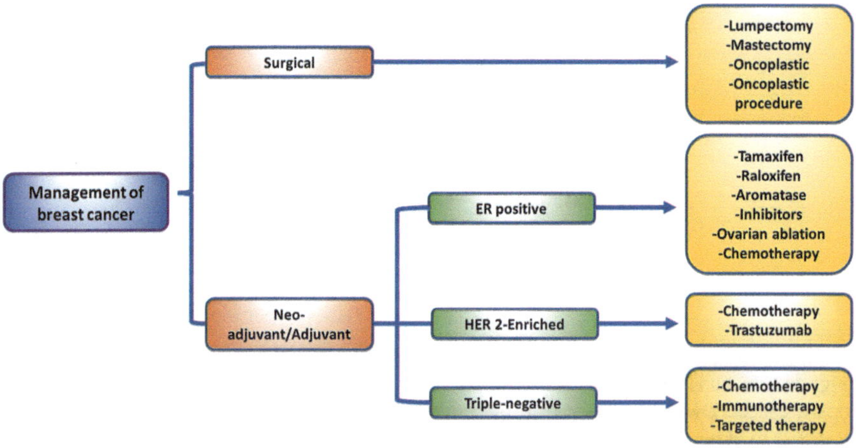

Fig. 5 Summary of the options available for the management of breast cancer. Breast cancer can be managed via surgical or neoadjuvant or adjuvant options. Depending on the type of breast cancer, numerous treatment options are available

Influence of Management Options for Breast Cancer on the Gut Microbiota

All the options used in the management of patients with BC can induce dysbiosis of the microbiota of the gut (Nandi et al., 2023). Radiotherapy, CT, hormonal therapy, targeted therapy, or immunotherapy may act directly on the gut microbiota or interfere with the protective function of the intestinal epithelial cells (Bruce et al., 2021). Patients for surgical treatment of BC may require antibiotics during the perioperative period for prophylaxis or treatment of postoperative complications, which may alter the composition of the microbiota of the gut (Di Modica et al., 2021; Rosean et al., 2019). Some of the chemotherapeutic agents such as cyclophosphamide have antimicrobial effects and may either kill or enhance the growth of some bacteria in the lumen of the gut (Zidi et al., 2021). Chemotherapeutic drugs and radiation may have an impact on the proliferation and differentiation of ISCs, as well as the synthesis of junctional proteins (Zhang et al., 2022). Reduced Paneth cell, goblet cell, and other IEC secretory functions decrease the gut's innate immunity, leading to dysbiosis (Luvhengo et al., 2023). Among the detrimental consequences of radiotherapy and CT on Paneth cells and goblet cells are impaired secretion of antimicrobial peptides and decreased synthesis of mucin, respectively (Luvhengo et al., 2023). Low levels of antimicrobial peptides and poor quality of mucin create an environment that is conducive to the overgrowth of pathogens (Cheng et al., 2020). Most significant complications of immunotherapy involve the gastrointestinal tract (GIT) and may include colitis or bloody diarrhea (Kennedy & Salama, 2020).

Microbiome, Dysbiosis, and Breast Cancer

The cause of over 70% of BC is not known, but alteration of the microbiota of the breast, gut, or both is seen in a significant number of cases (Arnone & Cook, 2022). Bacteria colonize the breast, most of which originate from the gut (Goto, 2022; Li et al., 2022). The species of bacteria may promote tumorigenesis through direct toxic effects, inducing inflammation, modification of chemicals, or changing the hormonal milieu (Viswanathan et al., 2023). Dysbiosis of the gut microbiota may lead to the dominance of organisms that potentiate the activity of beta-glucuronidase and increase deconjugation of estrogens and increase re-absorption and elevate circulating levels of estrogens, which increase the risk of BC especially in postmenopausal women (Arnone & Cook, 2022; Bruce et al., 2021; Ervin et al., 2019; Rashed et al., 2022; Viswanathan et al., 2023).

A high-fat diet stimulates the secretion of bile acids and subsequently increases the production of secondary bile acids, leading to dysbiosis (Jiang & Miao, 2023). Dysbiosis may reduce the number of bacteria that promote the generation of SCFA following the fermentation of indigestible fiber to form SCFA that are a significant source of energy for colonocytes (Wilson et al., 2020). Deficiency of SCFA weakens the intestinal epithelium, increases gut permeability, and predisposes to translocation of intact bacteria and/or lipopolysaccharides (De Oliveira Andrade et al., 2022; Jiang & Miao, 2023). The translocation of bacteria and LPS initiates systemic inflammation, mitochondrial dysfunction, and carcinogenesis (Arnone & Cook, 2022; Sevcikova et al., 2022; Viswanathan et al., 2023). The chronic systemic inflammatory state predisposes to obesity, which is a risk factor for BC and individuals who are obese are at an elevated risk of aggressive types of BC, including the TNBC (Bowers et al., 2022; Ransohoff et al., 2023; Yin et al., 2020). Furthermore, BC in individuals who are obese is likely to be resistant to treatment and prone to recurrence or distant metastasis (Klement et al., 2020). The dysbiosis in the breast also promotes inflammation in the tumor microenvironment, which together with the adiposity creates a fertile milieu for aggressive tumor behavior (Jaye et al., 2022; Marwaha et al., 2016; Nandi et al., 2023).

Dysbiosis and Drug Resistance in Breast Cancer

The stage and molecular subtype of the tumor can indicate treatment choices and the risk of drug resistance in patients with BC (Li et al., 2015; Turner et al., 2021; Viswanathan et al., 2023). Patients with luminal A BC are likely to benefit from hormonal therapy (Zhao et al., 2023). Similarly, HER 2-enriched tumors are responsive to trastuzumab (Di Modica et al., 2021). Hormonal therapy, standard CT, targeted therapy, and immunotherapy are not effective in the treatment of TBNC (Bowers et al., 2022; Ransohoff et al., 2023; Yin et al., 2020). Regrettably, luminal A, luminal B, and HER 2-enriched may not respond to treatment as expected (Bruce et al., 2021; Di Modica et al., 2021; Ruo et al., 2021).

Dysbiosis of the microbiota of the gut may alter the effectiveness of hormonal therapy, CT, immunotherapy, and targeted therapy (Bowers et al., 2022; Nandi et al., 2023; Viswanathan et al., 2023). Dysbiosis may alter the bioavailability of a drug, interfere with its receptors, reduce its potency or increase its toxic or side effects (Bonizzi et al., 2021; German et al., 2023; Nandi et al., 2023; Ruo et al., 2021; Sevcikova et al., 2022; Viswanathan et al., 2023; Zou et al., 2018). Dysbiosis may alter the level of circulating estrogens and affect the response to treatment (Ervin et al., 2019). Some of the chemotherapeutic agents, such as cyclophosphamide have an antimicrobial effect and may worsen dysbiosis, leading to among other toxic effects, mucositis that may cause suspension or reduction of the dose (Cheng et al., 2020; Zidi et al., 2021). Allochthonous species of bacteria may enhance metabolism of hormonal therapy, CT, or targeted therapy leading to a reduction in their bioavailability (Rosean et al., 2019).

Management of Dysbiosis in Drug-Resistant Breast Cancer

The gut microbiome may either potentiate or weaken the effect of CT, hormonal therapy, targeted therapy, or immunotherapy on cancer (Bonizzi et al., 2021; Jaye et al., 2022; Rosean et al., 2019; Zhao et al., 2022). Manipulation of the gut microbiota may alter the response of BC to treatment (Zhao et al., 2022). Obesity is a risk factor for BC, is linked with poor treatment response, and raises the risk of recurrence (Klement et al., 2020; Zhang et al., 2020). Chronic inflammation around the tumor and adipokines from adipose tissues within and outside the breast make BC aggressive and resistant to treatment (Klement et al., 2020). Obesity should therefore be prevented before, during, and after curative treatment of BC (Klement et al., 2020). Similar strategies that are used in the management of obesity are useful for the reversal of dysbiosis associated with BC and are broadly categorized into non-surgical and surgical (bariatric procedures) (Zhang et al., 2020). Non-surgical options to reverse dysbiosis and drug resistance in patients with BC are physical exercise, dietary manipulation, the use of probiotics (Zhao et al., 2023), prebiotics (Ruo et al., 2021), synbiotics (Wilson et al., 2020), postbiotics (Rashed et al., 2022), antimicrobial therapy (Ruo et al., 2021), fecal microbial transplantation (Chen et al., 2022; Wang et al., 2022, b), administration of exogenous LPS (Bawaneh et al., 2022), genetic engineering of commensal bacteria (Zhao et al., 2023), and bacteria spore-based technology (Zhao et al., 2023) are amongst the strategies that are available for use to alter the gut microbiota. Cessation of smoking may also restore eubiosis and reduce the incidence of BC or ameliorate resistance to drugs during treatment (Baron et al., 2021; Shapiro et al., 2022; Tyagi et al., 2021).

Physical Exercise

Cancer is distinguished by chronic low-grade systemic inflammation, mitochondrial dysfunction, and the production of large amounts of reactive oxygen species (ROS) and reactive nitrogen species (RNS) (Mittal et al., 2014; Villarreal-Garcia et al., 2022). Although physical exercise leads to an increase in the production of RNS and ROS, regular exercise teaches the body and programs it to expeditiously reduce the high level of toxic-free radicals (Powers et al., 2020). Another benefit of physical exercise is its ability to alter the gut microbiota and potentially reverse dysbiosis (Wegierska et al., 2022). Physical exercise also modulates the body's immunity and can prevent cancer of the breast, improve response to treatment, and prevent recurrence (Dilnaz et al., 2021).

Exercise can affect the GIT, lowering transient stool time and thus pathogen contact time with the GIT mucus layer (Monda et al., 2017). Exercise increases the diversity of gut microbiota in humans and correlates with protein consumption and creatinine levels (Clarke et al., 2014). Exercise causes an increase in gut microbiota by increasing a diverse bacteria population via internal and external factors. Athletes are exposed to their environmental biosphere and follow healthy lifestyles that promote richer microbiota. However, intrinsic causes such as decreased blood supply and tissue hypoxia could result in GIT alterations. Exercise-induced changes in the gut microbiota and bacterial translocation into the circulation may be an approach to enhance therapy response.

Dietary Management

The gut microbiota is significantly influenced by fiber from fruits, vegetables, and other plant foods, and dietary changes can have a major impact on this microbiome. The primary role of the gut microbiota is to assist in food digestion and to absorb vital nutrients that the host is unable to break down on its own (Gopalakrishnan et al., 2018). However, dietary interventions might encourage differences in the gut microbiota composition, as evidenced by research showing that substantial dietary modifications can alter the gut microbiota (David et al., 2014). Insights into how dietary modification could be utilized to improve the gut microbiome come from the susceptibility of some bacterial groups and their metabolites to a range of nutrients and immunological parameters (Ma et al., 2018; Shortt et al., 2018), with analogies that can be drawn to the treatment of cancer. Dietary interventions emphasize adding plant polysaccharides to the diet or cutting off animal fats, which shows a decrease in harmful Bacteroidetes bacteria (Turnbaugh et al., 2007). The significance of these bacteria in cancer treatment may offer a way to improve results by modifying the microbiome.

The composition of the diet can alter the microbiota and therefore the microbiome (Ruo et al., 2021; Sevcikova et al., 2022; Zhao et al., 2022). High calorie, low fat, or low diet predisposes to dysbiosis, which is sometimes seen in patients with BC that is resistant to treatment (Sevcikova et al., 2022). High-fat diet leads to dysbiosis, impairs the function of Paneth cells, promotes the overgrowth of bacteria that produce excessive amounts of ROS and pro-inflammatory cytokine, and increases epithelial permeability (Bawaneh et al., 2022). Low-fat and/high-fiber diet can restore eubiosis and improve response to treatment, reduce side effects of treatment, and prevent recurrence (Wilson et al., 2020). The dietary regimens that can reverse the dysbiosis seen in patients with BC include low-fat diet, low carbohydrate, high fiber, Mediterranean diet, and ketogenic diet (Klement et al., 2020).

Mediterranean Diet

One of the best dietary paradigms is the Mediterranean diet (MD). Many of its distinctive elements have practical qualities that improve health and wellness, such as lowering the prevalence of chronic diseases (like BC) (Biondi et al., 2012). Metabolic profiles show a strong correlation between MD and high quality of life. A reduction in cancer has been associated with improved diet (La Vecchia & Franceschi, 2000). BC, for example, has a complex etiology that includes genetics, behavior, and exposure to environmental agents including food. However, certain MD-related food nutrients may have an impact on BC (De Lima et al., 2008; Torres-Sanchez et al., 2009). The consumption of foods high in phytosterols, beta-carotene, vitamins C and E, and calcium can reduce cell growth by acting as an antioxidant on estrogen metabolic pathways (Albuquerque et al., 2014).

Ketogenic Diet

Ketogenic diet (KD) is rich in fat but low in carbohydrate and the source of 85–90% of calories in KD are from fat with only 10% from carbohydrates with restriction on protein intake (Jemal et al., 2021; Sevcikova et al., 2022; Zou et al., 2018). The intake of carbohydrates is limited to less than less than 50 g per day and consumption of dairy products and processed food is minimized (Klement et al., 2020). The classical KD contains medium-chain triglyceride-aldehyde, olive oil, virgin oil, legumes, and animal protein. Ketogenic diet leads to more weight loss than low-calorie diet, reverses dysbiosis, and enhances the proliferation of species of bacteria that produce SCFA (Klement et al., 2020). Additional benefits of KD are reduction of gut permeability, systemic inflammation, glucose, and insulin levels (Jemal et al., 2021). A ketogenic diet lowers the risk of BC and its recurrence following treatment (Jemal et al., 2021; Sevcikova et al., 2022; Zou et al., 2018).

Probiotics, Prebiotics, Synbiotics, and Postbiotics

Probiotics, prebiotics, postbiotics, and synbiotics are frequently used for the restoration of eubiosis in patients with diseases associated with dysbiosis such as diabetes mellitus, inflammatory bowel disease, radiation enteritis, and cancer including BC (Ruo et al., 2021; Thu et al., 2023; Viswanathan et al., 2023). Probiotics contain live bacteria that are found in healthy guts, for example, the *Lactobacillus* and *Bifidobacterium* species (Vallianou et al., 2020). Prebiotics are made of compounds that promote the growth of commensal bacteria and often include oligo- or polysaccharides whereas synbiotics are a combination of probiotics and prebiotics (Rashed et al., 2022; Thu et al., 2023). Synbiotics combine probiotics and prebiotics. Postbiotic therapy uses metabolites generated by the bacteria in the lumen of the gut, for example, SCFA. Probiotics, prebiotics, and postbiotics can modify the gut microbiome, reverse dysbiosis of the microbiota of gut improve response to treatment of all the molecular subtypes of BC (Bruce et al., 2021; Ruo et al., 2021; Thu et al., 2023; Viswanathan et al., 2023; Wilson et al., 2020).

Bariatric Surgery

Bariatric surgery is more effective than lifestyle change and medical treatment of obesity (Eisenberg et al., 2023; Lee et al., 2022). Indications of bariatric surgery include at least severe obesity or morbid with a medical condition that is resistant to treatment, such as diabetes mellitus (Eisenberg et al., 2023). The effects of bariatric surgery are also the most durable and may lead to the reversal of diabetes mellitus and cardiovascular disease (Courcoulas et al., 2020). The other positive consequences of bariatric surgery are the prevention of BC and the reduction of the likelihood of recurrence after curative treatment (Lee et al., 2021; Zhang et al., 2020). The positive effects of bariatric surgery result from the reversal of dysbiosis and systemic inflammation (Debedat et al., 2019).

Fecal Microbial Transplant

Fecal microbial transplantation is the most effective strategy to reverse dysbiosis of the gut microbiota and is approved for treatment of persistent or recurrent pseudomembranous colitis (Stripling & Rodriguez, 2018). Using FMT is effective for the correction of dysbiosis and improvement of response to hormonal therapy, CT, trastuzumab, and immunotherapy in patients with BC (Bawaneh et al., 2022). Feces for use during transplantation are procured from either healthy individuals or patients who responded favorably to treatment such as chemotherapy for cancer (Stripling & Rodriguez, 2018). The donated feces are either administered immediately via a tube or inserted during colonoscopy, or frozen for storage and transplantation later, or administered orally as a tablet (Stripling & Rodriguez, 2018).

Other Strategies

Smoking and alcohol intake should be discouraged as they have negative effects on the prognosis and risk of recurrence of BC (Baron et al., 2021; Ruo et al., 2021). Although nicotine is not a risk factor for BC, it is detrimental in patients in whom the cancer has developed as it promotes the development of pulmonary metastases. Cigarette smoking leads to dysbiosis throughout the aero-digestive tract, including the gut. The other detrimental of nicotine on the gut is reduction of the synthesis of mucin, which is a nutrient for some of the physiologically beneficial bacteria. Alcohol intake is similarly detrimental to the gut microbiome and (breast) and disrupts the integrity of gut epithelium leading to translocation of bacteria and LPS.

Oral metformin, engineered bacteria, synthetic metabolites, nanotechnology, spore technology, and bacteriophage technology have also been effective in the reversal of dysbiosis and improve treatment outcomes in patients with BC (Kiani et al., 2021; Sun et al., 2018; Zhao et al., 2023). Metformin is an oral hypoglycemic medication that is used as the first-line treatment for type 2 diabetes mellitus (Lee et al., 2021). The beneficial effects of metformin include among others reversal of dysbiosis, promotion of the growth of SCFA-producing bacteria, reduction of intestinal permeability, anti-inflammatory effects, and immunomodulation (Lee et al., 2021). The advent of synthetic biology opens the way for the use of genetic engineering technology to synthesize favorable bacteria for use to modify the gut microbiota (Chowdhury et al., 2019). In some cases, the bacteria are inoculated into the tumor to enhance the antitumor effects of the tumor microenvironment (Chowdhury et al., 2019). Application of nanonutraceuticals to manipulate the gut microbiota by using nanoprobiotics, nanoprebiotics, or nanosynbiotics (Rathod & Yadav, 2023). The other strategy to reverse dysbiosis is the use of bacteriophage technology to eliminate pathogenic bacteria (Kiani et al., 2021) and the administration of exogenously generated LPS (Bawaneh et al., 2022).

Limitations of Targeting the Microbiota for Breast Treatment

BCA is a complex disease and often the tumor microenvironment which significantly influences clinical behavior and outcome is not adequately assessed. Dysbiosis of the breast and/or gut microbiota may not be the primary driver of drug resistance. The detected organism(s) may be due to contamination and not be involved in the development of the resistance. The organisms in the gut, including bacteria, fungi, and viruses, influence each other and do not act in isolation, and interventions that target one species may not be effective. There is a significant difference in the composition of the microbiota among individuals and metagenomics does not always pick up all the organisms. Furthermore, change in the microbiota is not uniform with different phyla reported in patients with similar molecular subtype and stage of BC. Most of the options used for manipulation of the gut microbiota such as KD, fecal microbiota transplantation, and bariatric surgery are expensive and may not be accessible for patients in low- and middle-income countries.

Conclusion and Future Perspectives

Dysbiosis of the gut microbiota has an integral part in the development of sporadic BC and can affect response to therapy. BC in some patients may be resistant to standard treatment even when diagnosed early and is of the less aggressive molecular subtype. Dysbiosis is seen in some of the patients with BC and is resistant to treatment. Restoration of eubiosis in the gut microbiota through regular exercise, healthy dietary habits, intake of probiotics, fecal transplantation and bariatric surgery may reverse the resistance and prevent progression or recurrence of BC. Manipulation of the gut microbiota should be included as adjuvant therapy in patients with BC that is of the aggressive molecular subtype, resistant to standard treatment or is recurrent.

References

Albuquerque, R. C., Baltar, V. T., & Marchioni, D. M. (2014). Breast cancer and dietary patterns: A systematic review. *Nutrition Reviews, 72*(1), 1–17.

Arnone, A. A., & Cook, K. L. (2022). Gut and breast microbiota as endocrine regulators of hormone receptor-positive breast cancer risk and therapy response. *Endocrinology, 164*(1), bqac177. https://doi.org/10.1210/endocr/bqac177

Arumugam, M., Raes, J., Pelletier, E., Le Paslier, D., Yamada, T., Mende, D. R., Fernandes, G. R., Tap, J., Bruls, T., & Batto, J.-M. (2011). Enterotypes of the human gut microbiome. *Nature, 473*, 174–180.

Baron, J. A., Nichols, H. B., Anderson, C., & Safe, S. (2021). Cigarette smoking and estrogen-related cancer. *Cancer Epidemiology, Biomarkers & Prevention, 30*(8), 1462–1471. https://doi.org/10.1158/1055-9965.EPI-20-1803

Bawaneh, A., Wilson, A. S., Levi, N., Howard-Mcnatt, M. M., Chiba, A., Soto-Pantoja, D. R., & Cook, K. L. (2022). Intestinal microbiota influence doxorubicin responsiveness in triple-negative breast cancer. *Cancers, 14*, 4849. https://doi.org/10.3390/cancers14194849

Bindels, L. B., Porporato, P., Dewulf, E., Verrax, J., Neyrinck, A. M., Martin, J., Scott, K., Buc Calderon, P., Feron, O., & Muccioli, G. (2012). Gut microbiota-derived propionate reduces cancer cell proliferation in the liver. *British Journal of Cancer, 107*, 1337–1344.

Biondi, A., Fisichella, R., Fiorica, F., Malaguarnera, M., & Basile, F. (2012). Food mutagen and gastrointestinal cancer. *European Review for Medical and Pharmacological Sciences, 16*(9), 1280–1282.

Bonizzi, A., Ariolli, S., Bianchi, F., Corsi, F., Guglielmetti, S., & Balsari, A. (2021). Gut microbiota condition the therapeutic efficacy of trastuzumab in HER2-positive breast cancer. *Cancer Research, 81*(8), 2195–2206. https://doi.org/10.1158/0008-5472-Can-20-1659

Bowers, L. W., Brenner, A. J., Hursting, S. D., Tekmal, R. R., & Degraffenried, L. A. (2015). Obesity-associated systemic interleukin-6 promotes pre-adipocyte aromatase expression via increased breast cancer cell prostaglandin E2 production. *Breast Cancer Research and Treatment, 149*, 49–57.

Bowers, L. W., Doerstling, S. S., Shamsunder, M. G., Lineberger, C. G., Rossi, E. L., Montgomery, S. A., Coleman, M. F., Gong, W., Parker, J. S., Howell, A., Harvie, M., & Hursting, S. D. (2022). Reversing the genomic, epigenetic, and triple negative breast cancer-enhancing effects of obesity. *Cancer Prevention Research, 15*(9), 581–594. https://doi.org/10.1158/1940-6207.Capr-22-0113

Bruce, E., Makaranka, S., Urquhart, G., & Elsberger, B. (2021). Does the gut microbiome environment influence response to systemic breast cancer treatment? *Exploration of Targeted Anti-Tumor Therapy, 2*, 374–384. https://doi.org/10.37349/etat.2021.00051

Chen, D., Wu, J., Jin, D., Wang, B., & Cao, H. (2022). Fecal microbiota transplantation in cancer management: Current status and perspectives. *International Journal of Cancer, 145*, 2021–2031. https://doi.org/10.1002/ijc.32003

Cheng, W. Y., Wu, C. Y., & Yu, J. (2020). The role of gut microbiota in cancer treatment: Friend or foe? *Gut, 69*(10), 1867–1876. https://doi.org/10.1136/gutjnl-2020-321153

Chowdhury, S., Castro, S., Coker, C., Hinchliffe, T. E., Arpaia, N., & Danino, T. (2019). Programmable bacteria induce durable tumor regression and systemic antitumor immunity. *Nature Medicine, 25*, 1057–1063.

Clarke, S. F., Murphy, E. F., O'sullivan, O., Lucey, A. J., Humphreys, M., Hogan, A., Hayes, P., O'reilly, M., Jeffrey, I. B., Wood-Martin, R., Kerins, D. M., Quigley, E., Ross, R. P., O'toole, P., Molloy, M. G., Falvey, E., Shanahan, F., & Cotter, P. D. (2014). Exercise and associated dietary extremes impact on gut microbial diversity. *Gut, 63*(12), 1913–1920.

Courcoulas, A. P., Gallagher, J. W., Neiberg, R. H., Eagleton, E. B., DeLany, J. P., Lang, W., Punchai, S., Gourash, W., & Jakicic, J. M. (2020). Bariatric surgery vs lifestyle intervention for diabetes treatment: 5-year outcomes from a randomized trial. *The Journal of Clinical Endocrinology and Metabolism, 105*(3), 866–876. https://doi.org/10.1210/clinem/dgaa006

Cox, L. M., Yamanishi, S., Sohn, J., Alekseyenko, A. V., Leung, J. M., Cho, I., Kim, S. G., Li, H., Gao, Z., & Mahana, D. (2014). Altering the intestinal microbiota during a critical developmental window has lasting metabolic consequences. *Cell, 158*, 705–721.

Crusz, S. M., & Balkwill, F. R. (2015). Inflammation and cancer: Advances and new agents. *Nature Reviews Clinical Oncology, 12*, 584–596.

David, L. A., Maurice, C. F., Carmody, R. N., Gootenberg, D. B., Button, J. E., Wolfe, B. E., Ling, A. V., Devlin, A. S., Varma, Y., Fischbach, M. A., Biddinger, S. B., Dutton, R. J., & Turnbaugh, P. J. (2014). Diet rapidly and reproducibly alters the human gut microbiome. *Nature, 505*(7484), 559–563.

Debedat, J., Clement, K., & Aron-Wisnewsky, J. (2019). Gut microbiota dysbiosis in human obesity: Impact of bariatric surgery. *Current Obesity Reports, 8*(3), 229–242 https://doi.org/10.1007/s13679-019-00351-3

De Lima, F. E. L., Do Rosario Dias De Oliveira Latorre, M., Jose De Carvalho Costa, M., & Fisberg, R. M. (2008). Diet and cancer in Northeast Brazil: Evaluation of eating habits and food group consumption in relation to breast cancer. *Cadernos De Saude Publica, 24*, 820–828.

De Oliveira Andrade, F., Verma, V., & Hilakivi-Clarke, L. (2022). Maternal obesity, and resistance to breast cancer treatments among offspring: Link to gut dysbiosis. *Cancer Reports, 5*, e1752. https://doi.org/10.1002/cnr2.1752

Di Modica, M., Gargan, G., Regondi, V., Bonizzi, A., Arioli, S., Belmonte, B., De Cecco, L., Fasano, E., Bianchi, F., Bertolotti, A., Tripodo, C., Villani, L., Corsi, F., Guglielmetti, S., Balsari, A., Triulzi, T., & Tagliabue, E. (2021). Gut microbiota condition the therapeutic efficacy of trastuzumab in Her2-positive breast cancer. *Cancer Research, 81*(8), 2195–2206. https://doi.org/10.1158/0008-5472.Can-20-1659

Dilnaz, F., Zafar, F., Afroze, T., Zakia, U. B., Chowdhury, T., Swarna, S. S., Fathma, S., Tasmin, R., Sakibuzzaman, M., Fariza, T. T., & Eshan, S. H. (2021). Mediterranean diet and physical activity: Two imperative components in breast cancer prevention. *Cureus, 13*(8), e17306. https://doi.org/10.7759/cureus.17306

Eisenberg, D., Shikora, S. A., Aarts, E., Aminian, A., Angrisani, L., Cohen, R. V., De Luca, M., Faria, S. L., Goodpaster, K. P. S., Haddad, A., Himpens, J. M., Kow, L., Kurian, M., Loi, K., Mahawar, K., Nimeri, A., O'kane, M., Papasavas, P. K., Ponce, J., Pratt, J. S. A., Rogers, A. M., Steele, K. E., Suter, M., & Kothari, S. N. (2023). 2022 American Society of Metabolic and Bariatric Surgery (ASMBS) and International Federation for the Surgery of Obesity and Metabolic Disorders (IFSO) indications for metabolic and bariatric surgery. *Obesity Surgery, 33*(1), 3–14. https://doi.org/10.1007/s11695-022-06332-1

Ervin, S. M., Li, H., Lim, L., Roberts, L. R., Liang, X., Mani, S., & Redinbo, M. R. (2019). Gut microbial β-glucuronidases reactivate estrogens as components of the estrobolome that reactivate estrogens. *The Journal of Biological Chemistry, 294*(49), 18586–18599.

Flores, R., Shi, J., Fuhrman, B., Xu, X., Veenstra, T. D., Gail, M. H., Gajer, P., Ravel, J., & Goedert, J. J. (2012). Fecal microbial determinants of fecal and systemic estrogens and estrogen metabolites: A cross-sectional study. *Journal of Translational Medicine, 2012*(10), 1–11.

Fuhrman, B. J., Feigelson, H. S., Flores, R., Gail, M. H., Xu, X., Ravel, J., & Goedert, J. J. (2014). Associations of the fecal microbiome with urinary estrogens and estrogen metabolites in postmenopausal women. *The Journal of Clinical Endocrinology & Metabolism, 99*, 4632–4640.

German, R., Marino, N., Hemmerich, C., Podicheti, R., Rusch, D. B., Stiemsma, L. T., Gao, H., Xuei, X., Rockey, P., & Storniolo, A. M. (2023). Exploring breast tissue microbial composition and the association with breast cancer risk factors. *Breast Cancer Research, 25*, 82. https://doi.org/10.1186/s13058-023-01677-6

Gierynska, M., Szulc-Dabrowska, L., Struzik, J., Mielcarska, M. B., & Gregorczyk-Zboroch, K. P. (2022). Integrity of the intestinal barrier: The involvement of epithelial cells and microbiota-a mutual relationship. *Animals, 12*, 145. https://doi.org/10.3390/ani12020145

Goedert, J. J., Hua, X., Bielecka, A., Okayasu, I., Milne, G. L., Jones, G. S., Fujiwara, M., Sinha, R., Wan, Y., & Xu, X. (2018). Postmenopausal breast cancer and oestrogen associations with the IgA-coated and IgA-noncoated faecal microbiota. *British Journal of Cancer, 118*, 471–479.

Goedert, J. J., Jones, G., Hua, X., Xu, X., Yu, G., Flores, R., Falk, R. T., Gail, M. H., Shi, J., & Ravel, J. (2015). Investigation of the association between the fecal microbiota and breast cancer in postmenopausal women: A population-based case-control pilot study. *Journal of the National Cancer Institute, 107*, djv147.

Gopalakrishnan, V., Helmink, B. A., Spencer, C. N., Reuben, A., & Wargo, J. A. (2018). The influence of the gut microbiome on cancer, immunity, and cancer immunotherapy. *Cancer Cell, 33*(4), 570–580.

Goto, T. (2022). Microbiota and lung cancer. *Seminars in Cancer Biology, 86*, 1–10. https://doi.org/10.1016/j.semcancer.2022.07.006

Hanker, A. B., Sudhan, D. R., & Arteaga, C. L. (2020). Overcoming endocrine resistance in breast cancer. *Cancer, 37*(4), 496–513. https://doi.org/10.1016/j.ccell.2020.03.009

Hendel, S. K., Kellermann, L., Hausmann, A., Bindslev, N., Jensen, K. B., & Nielsen, O. (2022). Tuft cells and their role in intestinal diseases. *Frontiers in Immunology, 2022*, 822867. https://doi.org/10.3389/fimmu.2022.822867

Hills, R. D., Pontefract, B. A., Mishcon, H. R., Black, C. A., Sutton, S. C., & Theberge, C. R. (2019). Gut microbiome: Profound implications for diet and disease. *Nutrients, 11*, 1613. https://doi.org/10.3390/nu11071613

Hopkins, M. M., & Meier, K. E. (2017). Free fatty acid receptors and cancer: From nutrition to pharmacology. In *Free Fatty Acid Receptors* (pp. 233–251).

Huang, C.-K., Chang, P.-H., Kuo, W.-H., Chen, C.-L., Jeng, Y.-M., Chang, K.-J., Shew, J.-Y., Hu, C.-M., & Lee, W.-H. (2017). Adipocytes promote malignant growth of breast tumours with monocarboxylate transporter 2 expression via β-hydroxybutyrate. *Nature Communications, 8*, 1–13.

Iida, N., Dzutsev, A., Stewart, C. A., Smith, L., Bouladoux, N., Weingarten, R. A., Molina, D. A., Salcedo, R., Back, T., & Cramer, S. (2013). Commensal bacteria control cancer response to therapy by modulating the tumor microenvironment. *Science, 342*, 967–970.

Iván, J., Major, E., Sipos, A., Kovács, K., Horváth, D., Tamás, I., Bay, P., Dombrádi, V., & Lontay, B. (2017). The short-chain fatty acid propionate inhibits adipogenic differentiation of human chorion-derived mesenchymal stem cells through the free fatty acid receptor 2. *Stem Cells and Development, 2017*(26), 1724–1733.

Jaye, K., Chang, D., Li, C. G., & Bhuyan, D. J. (2022). Gut metabolites and breast cancer: The continuum of dysbiosis, breast cancer risk, and potential breast cancer therapy. *International Journal of Molecular Sciences, 23*(16), 9490. https://doi.org/10.3390/ijms23169490

Jemal, M., Molla, T. S., & Dejenie, T. A. (2021). Ketogenic diets and their therapeutic potential on breast cancer: A systemic review. *Cancer Management and Research, 13*, 9147–9155.

Jiang, S., & Miao, Z. (2023). High-fat diet induces intestinal mucosal barrier dysfunction in ulcerative colitis: Emerging mechanisms and dietary intervention perspective. *American Journal of Translational Research, 15*(2), 653–677.

Kanaya, T., Williams, I. R., & Ohno, H. (2020). Intestinal M cells: Tireless samplers of enteric microbiota. *Traffic, 21*, 34–44. https://doi.org/10.1111/tra.12707

Kang, C., Leroith, D., & Gallagher, E. J. (2018). Diabetes, obesity, and breast cancer. *Endocrinology, 159*(11), 3801–3812. https://doi.org/10.1210/en.2018-00574

Kennedy, L. B., & Salama, A. K. S. (2020). A review of cancer immunotherapy toxicity. *CA: a Cancer Journal for Clinicians, 70*, 86–104. https://doi.org/10.3322/caac.2i596

Khandekar, M. J., Cohen, P., & Spiegelman, B. M. (2011). Molecular mechanisms of cancer development in obesity. *Nature Reviews. Cancer, 11*(12), 886–895. https://doi.org/10.1038/nrc3174

Kiani, A. K., Dhuli, K. A. K., Paolacci, S., Manara, B. E., Guerri, G., Dautaj, A., Beccari, T., Dundar, M., & Bertelli, M. (2021). Naturally-occurring and cultured bacteriophages in human therapy. *European Review for Medical and Pharmacological Sciences, 25*(1 Suppl), 101–107. https://doi.org/10.26355/eurrev_202112_27339

Klement, R. J., Champ, C. E., Kammerer, U., Koebrunner, P. S., Krage, K., Schafer, G., Weigel, M., & Sweeney, R. A. (2020). Impact of a ketogenic diet intervention during radiotherapy on body composition: Iii-final results of the Ketocomp study for breast cancer patients. *Breast Cancer Research, 22*(1), 94. https://doi.org/10.1186/s13058-020-01331-5

Kolb, R., & Zhang, W. (2020). Obesity and breast cancer: A case of inflamed adipose tissue. *Cancers, 12*(6), 1686. https://doi.org/10.3390/cancers12061686

Korde, L. A., Somerfield, M. R., Carey, L. A., Crews, J. R., Denduluri, N., Hwang, E. S., Khan, S. A., Loibl, S., Morris, E. A., Perez, A., Regan, M. M., Spears, P. A., Sudheendra, P. K., Symmans, F., Yung, R. L., Harvey, B. E., & Hershman, D. L. (2021). Neoadjuvant chemotherapy, endocrine therapy, and targeted therapy for breast cancer: Asco guideline. *Journal of Clinical Oncology, 39*(13), 1385–1505. https://doi.org/10.1200/Jco.20.03399

Kothari, C., Diorio, C., & Durocher, F. (2020). The importance of breast adipose tissue in breast cancer. *International Journal of Molecular Sciences, 21*(16), 5760. https://doi.org/10.3390/ijms21165760

Kovács, T., Mikó, E., Vida, A., Sebő, É., Toth, J., Csonka, T., Boratkó, A., Ujlaki, G., Lente, G., & Kovács, P. (2019). Cadaverine, a metabolite of the microbiome, reduces breast cancer aggressiveness through trace amino acid receptors. *Scientific Reports, 9*, 1300.

Kurokawa, K., Hayakawa, Y., & Koike, K. (2021). Plasticity of intestinal epithelium: Stem cell niches and regulatory signals. *International Journal of Molecular Sciences, 2021*(22), 357. https://doi.org/10.3390/ijms22010357

La Vecchia, C., & Franceschi, S. (2000). Nutrition and gastric cancer. *Canadian Journal of Gastroenterology, 14*(Suppl D), 51D–54D.

Laborda-Illanes, A., Sanchez-Alcoholado, L., Dominguez-Recio, M. E., Jimenez-Rodriguez, B., Lavado, R., Comino-Mendez, I., Alba, E., & Queipo-Ortuno, M. I. (2020). Breast and gut microbiota action mechanisms in breast cancer pathogenesis and treatment. *Cancers, 12*(9), 2465. https://doi.org/10.3390/cancers12092465

Lee, C. B., Chae, S. U., Jo, S. J., Jerng, U. M., & Bae, S. K. (2021). The relationship between the gut microbiome and metformin as a key for treating type 2 diabetes mellitus. *International Journal of Molecular Sciences, 22*(7), 3566. https://doi.org/10.3390/ijms22073566

Lee, E., Kawaguchi, E. S., Zhang, J., Kim, S. E., Deapen, D., Liu, L., Sheidaee, N., Hwang, A. E., Kang, I., Sandhu, K., Ursin, G., Wu, A. H., & Garcia, A. A. (2022). Bariatric surgery in patients with breast and endometrial cancer in California: Population-based prevalence and survival. *Surgery for Obesity and Related Diseases, 18*(1), 42–52. https://doi.org/10.1016/j.soard.2021.09.017

Li, J., Chen, Z., Su, K., & Zeng, J. (2015). Clinicopathological classification and traditional prognostic indicators of breast cancer. *International Journal of Clinical and Experimental Pathology, 8*(7), 8500–8505.

Li, X., Sun, X., Zhang, A., Pang, J., Li, Y., Yan, M., Xu, Z., Yu, Y., Yang, Z., Chen, X., Wang, X., Cao, X. C., & Tang, N. J. (2022). Breast microbiome associations with breast tumor characteristics and neoadjuvant chemotherapy: A case-control study. *Frontiers in Oncology, 12*, 926920. https://doi.org/10.3389/fonc.2022.926920

Liu, X., Cheng, Y., Zang, D., Zhang, M., Li, X., Liu, D., Gao, B., Zhou, H., Sun, J., Han, X., Lin, M., & Chen, J. (2021). The role of gut microbiota in lung cancer: From carcinogenesis to immunotherapy. *Frontiers in Oncology, 11*, 720842. https://doi.org/10.3389/fonc.2021.720842

Liu, B. N., Liu, X. T., Liang, Z. H., & Wang, J. H. (2021). Gut microbiota in obesity. *World Journal of Gastroenterology, 27*(25), 3837–3850. https://doi.org/10.3748/wjg.v27.i25.3837

Lu, Y., Yuan, X., Wang, M., He, Z., Li, H., Wang, J., & Li, Q. (2022). Gut microbiota influence immunotherapy responses: Mechanisms and therapeutic strategies. *Journal of Hematology & Oncology, 15*(1), 47. https://doi.org/10.1186/s13045-022-01273-9

Luu, T. H., Bard, J.-M., Carbonnelle, D., Chaillou, C., Huvelin, J.-M., Bobin-Dubigeon, C., & Nazih, H. (2018). Lithocholic bile acid inhibits lipogenesis and induces apoptosis in breast cancer cells. *Cellular Oncology, 41*, 13–24.

Luvhengo, T. E., Khan, U., & Marumo, T. K. (2023). Paneth cells and Lgr5+ intestinal stem cells in radiation enteritis. *Applied Science, 13*(5), 2758. https://doi.org/10.3390/app13052758

Ma, N., Guo, P., Zhang, J., He, T., Kim, S. W., Zhang, G., & Ma, X. (2018). Nutrients mediate intestinal bacteria-mucosal immune crosstalk. *Frontiers in Immunology, 9*, 5.

Markandey, M., Bajaj, A., Ilott, N. E., Kedia, S., Travis, S., Powrie, F., & Ahuja, V. (2021). Gut microbiota: Sculptors of the intestinal stem cell niche in health and inflammatory bowel disease. *Gut Microbes, 13*(1), 1990827. https://doi.org/10.1080/19490976.2021.1990827

Martinez-Outschoorn, U. E., Lisanti, M. P., & Sotgia, F. (2014). Catabolic cancer-associated fibroblasts transfer energy and biomass to anabolic cancer cells, fueling tumor growth. In *Seminars in cancer biology* (pp. 47–60). Elsevier.

Marwaha, A. K., Morris, J. A., & Rigby, R. J. (2016). Hypothesis: Bacterial induced inflammation disrupts the orderly progression of the stem cell hierarchy and has a role in the pathogenesis of breast cancer. *Medical Hypotheses, 136*, 109530. https://doi.org/10.1016/j.mehy.2019.109530

Mikó, E., Kovács, T., Sebő, É., Tóth, J., Csonka, T., Ujlaki, G., Sipos, A., Szabó, J., Méhes, G., & Bai, P. (2019). Microbiome—microbial metabolome—cancer cell interactions in breast cancer—familiar, but unexplored. *Cells, 8*, 293.

Mittal, M., Siddiqui, M. R., Tran, K., Reddy, S. P., & Malik, A. B. (2014). Reactive oxygen species in inflammation and tissue injury. *Antioxidants & Redox Signaling, 20*(7), 1126–1167. https://doi.org/10.1089/ars.2012.5149

Monda, V., Villano, I., Messina, A., Valenzano, A., Esposito, T., Moscatelli, F., Viggiano, A., Cibelli, G., Chieffi, S., Monda, M., & Messina, G. (2017). Exercise modifies the gut microbiota with positive health effects. *Oxidative Medicine and Cellular Longevity, 2017*, 3831972. https://doi.org/10.1155/2017/3831972

Nagpal, R., Newman, T. M., Wang, S., Jain, S., Lovato, J. F., & Yadav, H. (2018). Obesity-linked gut microbiome dysbiosis associated with derangements in gut permeability and intestinal cellular homeostasis independent of diet. *Journal of Diabetes Research, 2018*, 3462092. https://doi.org/10.1155/2018/3462092

Nakamura, K., Sakuragi, N., Takakuwa, A., & Ayabe, T. (2016). Paneth cell α-defensins and enteric microbiota in health and disease. *Bioscience of Microbiota, Food and Health, 35*(2), 57–67.

Nandi, D., Parida, S., & Sharma, D. (2023). The gut microbiota in breast cancer development and treatment: The good, the bad, and the useful. *Gut Microbes, 15*(1), 2221452. https://doi.org/10.1080/19490976.2023.2221452

Newman, T. M., Vitolins, M. Z., & Cook, K. L. (2019). From the table to the tumor: The role of mediterranean and western dietary patterns in shifting microbial-mediated signaling to impact breast cancer risk. *Nutrients, 11*, 2565.

Powers, S. K., Deminice, R., Ozdemir, M., Yoshihara, T., Bomkamp, M. P., & Hyatt, H. (2020). Exercise-induced oxidative stress: Friend or foe? *Journal of Sport and Health Science, 9*(5), 415–425. https://doi.org/10.1016/j.jshs.2020.04.001

Qiu, Q., Lin, Y., Ma, Y., Li, X., Liang, J., Chen, Z., Liu, K., Huang, Y., Luo, H., Huang, R., & Luo, L. (2021). Exploring the emerging role of the gut microbiota and tumor microenvironment in cancer immunotherapy. *Frontiers in Immunology, 11*, 612202.

Ransohoff, J. D., Ritter, V., & Kurian, A. W. (2023). Antimicrobial exposure is associated with decreased survival in triple-negative breast cancer. *Nature Communications, 14*, 2053. https://doi.org/10.1038/s41467-023-37636-0

Rashed, R., Valcheva, R., & Dieleman, L. A. (2022). Manipulation of gut microbiota as a key target for Crohn's disease. *Frontiers in Medicine, 9*, 887044. https://doi.org/10.3389/fmed.2022.887044

Rathod, P., & Yadav, R. P. (2023). Gut microbiome as therapeutic target for diabesity management: Opportunity for nanonutraceuticals and associated challenges. *Drug Delivery and Translational Research, 14*, 17–29. https://doi.org/10.1007/s13346-023-01404-w

Rea, D., Coppola, G., Palma, G., Barbieri, A., Luciano, A., Del Prete, P., Rossetti, S., Berretta, M., Facchini, G., & Perdonà, S. (2018). Microbiota effects on cancer: From risks to therapies. *Oncotarget, 9*, 17915.

Rodrigues, M. F., Carvalho, É., Pezzuto, P., Rumjanek, F. D., & Amoêdo, N. D. (2015). Reciprocal modulation of histone deacetylase inhibitors sodium butyrate and trichostatin A on the energy metabolism of breast cancer cells. *Journal of Cellular Biochemistry, 116*, 797–808.

Rosean, C. B., Bostic, R. R., Ferey, J. C. M., Feng, T.-Y., Azar, F. N., Tung, K. S., Dozmorov, M. G., Smirnova, E., Bos, P. D., & Rutkowski, M. R. (2019). Pre-existing commensal dysbiosis is a host-intrinsic regulator of tissue inflammation and tumor cell dissemination in hormone receptor-positive breast cancer. *Cancer Research, 79*(14), 3662–3675. https://doi.org/10.1158/0008-5472.Can-18-3464

Rumbo, M., Anderle, P., Didierlaurent, A., Sierro, F., Debard, N., Sirard, J. C., Finke, D., & Kraehenbuhl, L. P. (2004). How the gut links innate and adaptive immunity. *Annals of the New York Academy of Sciences, 1029*, 16–21. https://doi.org/10.1196/annals.1309.003

Ruo, S. W., Alkayyali, T., Win, M., Tara, A., Joseph, C., Kannan, A., Srivastava, K., Ochuba, O., Sandhu, J. K., Went, T. R., Sultan, W., Kantamaneni, K., & Poudel, S. (2021). Role of gut microbiota dysbiosis in breast cancer and novel approaches in prevention, diagnosis, and treatment. *Cureus, 13*(8), e17472. https://doi.org/10.7759/cureus.17472

Salimi, V., Shahsavari, Z., Safizadeh, B., Hosseini, A., Khademian, N., & Tavakoli-Yaraki, M. (2017). Sodium butyrate promotes apoptosis in breast cancer cells through reactive oxygen species (Ros) formation and mitochondrial impairment. *Lipids in Health and Disease, 16*, 1–11.

Sampsell, K., Hao, D., & Reimer, R. A. (2020). The gut microbiota: A potential gateway to improved health outcomes in breast cancer treatment and survivorship. *International Journal of Molecular Sciences, 21*(23), 9239. https://doi.org/10.3390/ijms21239239

Sevcikova, A., Izoldova, V., Stevurkova, V., Kasperova, B., Chovanec, M., Ciernikova, S., & Mego, M. (2022). The impact of the microbiome on resistance to cancer treatment with chemotherapeutic agents and immunotherapy. *International Journal of Molecular Sciences, 23*(1), 488. https://doi.org/10.3390/ijms23010488

Shapiro, H., Goldenberg, K., Ratiner, K., & Elinav, E. (2022). Smoking-induced microbial dysbiosis in health and disease. *Clinical Science, 136*(18), 1371–1387. https://doi.org/10.1042/Cs20220175

Shortt, C., Hasselwander, O., Meynier, A., Nauta, A., Fernandez, E. N., Putz, P., Rowland, I., Swann, J., Turk, J., Vermeiren, J., & Antoine, J.-M. (2018). Systematic review of the effects of the intestinal microbiota on selected nutrients and non-nutrients. *European Journal of Nutrition, 57*(1), 25–49.

Stern, J., Millr, G., Li, X., & Saxena, D. (2019). Virome and bacteriome: Two sides of the same coin. *Current Opinion in Virology, 37*, 37–43. https://doi.org/10.1016/j.coviro.2019.05.007

Stripling, J., & Rodriguez, M. (2018). Current evidence in delivery and therapeutic uses of fecal microbiota transplantation in human diseases-clostridium difficile disease and beyond. *The American Journal of the Medical Sciences, 356*(5), 424–432. https://doi.org/10.1016/j.amjms.2018.08.010

Sun, J., Li, D., Chen, Q., Li, M., Su, L., Luo, T., Liang, D., Lai, G., Shuai, O., Jiao, C., Wu, Q., Xie, Y., & Zhou, X. (2018). Anti-breast cancer enhancement of polysaccharide from spore of ganoderma lucidum with paclitaxel: Suppression of tumor metabolism with gut microbiota reshaping. *Frontiers in Microbiology, 9*, 3099. https://doi.org/10.3389/fmicb.2018.03099

Thirunavukkarasan, M., Wang, C., Rao, A., Hind, T., Teo, Y. R., Siddiquee, A. A.-M., Goghari, M. A. I., Kumar, A. P., & Herr, D. R. (2017). Short-chain fatty acid receptors inhibit invasive phenotypes in breast cancer cells. *PLoS One, 12*, e0186334.

Thu, M. S., Ondee, T., Nopsopon, T., Karzana, I. A. K., Fothergill, J. L., Hirankarn, N., Campbell, B. J., & Pongpirul, K. (2023). Effect of probiotics in breast cancer: A systematic review and meta-analysis. *Biology, 12*, 280. https://doi.org/10.3390/biology12020280

Torres-Sanchez, L., Galvan-Portillo, M., Wolff, M. S., & Lopez-Carillo, L. L. (2009). Dietary consumption of phytochemicals and breast cancer risk in Mexican women. *Public Health Nutrition, 12*(6), 825–831.

Tsvetikova, S. A., & Koshel, E. I. (2020). Microbiota and cancer: Host cellular mechanisms activated by gut microbial metabolites. *International Journal of Medical Microbiology, 310*, 151425.

Turnbaugh, P. J., Ley, R. E., Hamady, M., Fraser-Liggett, C. M., Knight, R., & Gordon, J. I. (2007). The human microbiome project. *Nature, 449*(7164), 804–810.

Turner, K. M., Yeo, S. K., Holm, T. M., Shaughnessy, E., & Guan, J. L. (2021). Heterogeneity within molecular subtypes of breast cancer. *American Journal of Physiology. Cell Physiology, 321*(2), C343–C354. https://doi.org/10.1152/ajpcell.00109.2021

Tyagi, A., Sharma, S., Wu, K., Wu, S. Y., Xing, F., Liu, Y., Zhao, D., Deshpande, R. P., D'agostino, R. B., Jr., & Watabe, K. (2021). Nicotine promotes breast cancer metastasis by stimulating N2 neutrophils and generating pre-metastatic niche in lung. *Nature Communications, 12*(1), 474. https://doi.org/10.1038/s1467-020-20733-9

Untersmayr, E., Brandt, A., Koidl, L., & Bergheim, I. (2022). The intestinal barrier dysfunction as driving factor of inflammation. *Nutrients, 14*(5), 949. https://doi.org/10.3390/nu14050949

Uribe-Herranz, M., Rafali, S., Beghi, S., Gil-De-Gomez, L., Verginadis, I., Bittinger, K., Pustylnikov, S., Pierini, S., Perales-Linares, R., Blair, I. A., Mesaros, C. A., Snyder, N. W., Bushman, F., Koumenis, C., & Facciabene, A. (2020). Gut microbiota modulate dendritic cell antigen presentation and radiotherapy-induced antitumor immune response. *The Journal of Clinical Investigation, 130*(1), 466–479.

Vallianou, N., Stratigou, T., Christodoulatos, G. S., Tsigalou, C., & Dalamaga, M. (2020). Probiotics, prebiotics, synbiotics, postbiotics and obesity: Current evidence, controversies, and perspectives. *Current Obesity Reports, 9*(3), 179–192. https://doi.org/10.1007/s13679-020-00379-w

Villarreal-Garcia, V., Estupinan-Jiminez, J. R., Vivas-Mejia, P. E., Gonzalez-Villasana, V., Vazquez-Guillen, J. M., & Resendez-Perez, D. (2022). A vicious circle in breast cancer: The interplay between inflammation, reactive oxygen species, and micrornas. *Frontiers in Oncology, 12*, 980694. https://doi.org/10.3389/fonc.2022.980694

Viswanathan, S., Parida, S., Lingipilli, B. T., Krishnan, R., Podipireddy, D. R., & Muniraj, N. (2023). Role of gut microbiota in breast cancer and drug resistance. *Pathogens, 12*(3), 468. https://doi.org/10.3390/pathogens12030468

Wallaeys, C., Garcia-Gonzalez, N., & Libert, C. (2023). Paneth cells as the cornerstones of intestinal and organismal health: A primer. *EMBO Molecular Medicine, 15*, e16427. https://doi.org/10.15252/emmm.202216427

Wang, N., Yang, J., Han, W., Han, M., Liu, X., Jiang, L., Cao, H., Jing, M., Sun, T., & Xu, J. (2022). Identifying distinctive tissue and fecal microbial signatures and the tumor-promoting effects of deoxycholic acid on breast cancer. *Frontiers in Cellular and Infection Microbiology, 12*, 1029905. https://doi.org/10.3389/fcimb.2022.1029905

Wang, Y., Zhang, S., Borody, T. J., & Zhang, F. (2022). Encyclopedia of fecal microbiota transplantation: A review of effectiveness in the treatment of 85 disease. *Chinese Medical Journal, 135*(16), 1927–1939. https://doi.org/10.1097/Cm9.0000000000002339

Wegierska, A. E., Charitos, I. A., Topi, S., Potenza, M. A., Montagnani, M., & Santacroce, L. (2022). The connection between physical exercise and gut microbiota: Implications for competitive sports athletes. *Sports Medicine, 52*(10), 2355–2369. https://doi.org/10.1007/s40279-022-01696-x

Wilson, A. S., Koller, K. R., Ramaboli, M. C., Nesengani, L. T., Ocvirk, S., Chen, C., Flanagan, C. A., Sapp, F. R., Merritt, Z. T., Bhatti, F., Thomas, T. K., & O'keefe JD. (2020). Diet and the human gut microbiome: An international review. *Digestive Diseases and Sciences, 65*(3), 723–740. https://doi.org/10.1007/s10620-020-06112-w

Xiong, Z., Deng, G., Huang, X., Li, X., Xie, X., Wang, J., Shuang, Z., & Wang, X. (2018). Bone metastasis pattern in initial metastatic breast cancer: A population-based study. *Cancer Management and Research, 10*, 287–295.

Yin, L., Duan, J. J., Bian, X. W., & Yu, S. (2020). Triple-negative breast cancer molecular subtyping and treatment progress. *Breast Cancer Research, 22*, 61. https://doi.org/10.1186/s13058-020-01296-5

Yoshimoto, S., Loo, T. M., Atarashi, K., Kanda, H., Sato, S., Oyadomari, S., Iwakura, Y., Oshima, K., Morita, H., & Hattori, M. (2013). Obesity-induced gut microbial metabolite promotes liver cancer through senescence secretome. *Nature, 499*, 97–101.

Zhang, S., Ikramuddin, S., Beckwith, H. C., Sheka, A. C., With, K. M., & Blaes, A. H. (2020). The impact of bariatric surgery on breast cancer recurrence: Case series and review of literature. *Obesity Surgery, 30*(2), 780–785. https://doi.org/10.1007/s11695-019-04099-6

Zhang, J., Xie, Q., Huo, X., Liu, Z., Da, M., Yuan, M., Zhao, Y., & Shen, G. (2022). Impact of intestinal dysbiosis on breast cancer metastasis and progression. *Frontiers in Oncology, 12*, 1037831.

Zhao, L. Y., Mei, J. X., Yu, G., Lei, L., Zhang, W. H., Liu, K., Chen, X. L., Kolat, D., Yang, K., & Hu, J. K. (2023). Role of the gut microbiota in anticancer therapy: From molecular mechanisms to clinical applications. *Signal Transduction and Targeted Therapy, 8*(1), 201. https://doi.org/10.1038/s41392-023-01406-7

Zhao, H., Wang, D., Zhang, Z., Xian, J., & Bai, X. (2022). Effect of gut microbiota-derived metabolites on immune checkpoint inhibitor therapy: Enemy or friend? *Molecules, 27*(15), 4799. https://doi.org/10.3390/molecules27154799

Zhu, G., Hu, J., & Xi, R. (2021). The cellular niche for intestinal stem cells: A team effort. *Cell Regeneration, 10*, 1. https://doi.org/10.1186/s13619-020-00061-5

Zidi, O., Souai, N., Raies, H., Ayed, F. B., Mezlini, A., Mezrioui, S., Tranchida, F., Sabatier, J. M., Mosbah, A., Cherif, A., Shintu, L., & Kouidhi, S. (2021). Fecal metabolic profiling of breast cancer patients during neoadjuvant chemotherapy reveals potential biomarkers. *Molecules, 26*(8), 2266. https://doi.org/10.3390/molecules26082266

Zou, S., Fang, L., & Lee, M. H. (2018). Dysbiosis of gut microbiota in promoting the development of colorectal cancer. *Gastroenterology Report, 6*(1), 1–12. https://doi.org/10.1093/gastro/gox031

Molecular Profiling and Personalized Medicine in Drug-Resistant Breast Cancer

Lloyd Mabonga, Aristotelis Chatziioannou, and Zodwa Dlamini

Abstract The utilization of molecular profiling techniques and personalized medicine approaches in the management of breast cancer is driven by molecular targets that can selectively target drug-resistant molecular pathways. The peremptory need for molecular profiling and personalized medicine in the management of drug resistance in breast cancer has revolutionized the concept of precision oncology. Molecular profiling and personalized medicines have drawn increased interest and funding in integrating diagnostics and therapeutics in breast cancer management. Drug resistance in breast cancer accounts for more than forty percent of breast cancer deaths leading to chemoresistance, metastases, relapses, and the subsequent decrease in the effectiveness of chemotherapy medications. The drug resistance mechanisms include the epithelial-to-mesenchymal transition (EMT), epigenetic alterations, increased drug efflux, tumor microenvironment (TME), senescence escape, enhanced DNA repair, and tumor heterogeneity. Deciphering the molecular pathways linked to drug resistance in breast cancer is an indispensable tool in cancer management. The rapidly evolving landscape in the management of breast cancer makes it imperative that the oncologists' knowledge of the biological disease spectrum aligns with contemporary practice. And precision oncology is no longer a distant promise but a growing reality, and the demand for molecular profiling and personalized medicine is continuously increasing. Various attempts have been made to curb chemoresistance and to overcome drug resistance in drug-resistant breast cancer. However, the effects are still unsatisfactory, which makes it challenging to overcome. The chapter focuses on the utilization of molecular profiling techniques and personalized medicine approaches in the management of drug-resistant breast

L. Mabonga (✉) · Z. Dlamini
SAMRC Precision Oncology Research Unit (PORU), DSI/NRF SARChI Chair in Precision Oncology and Cancer Prevention (POCP), Pan African Cancer Research Institute (PACRI), University of Pretoria, Pretoria, South Africa
e-mail: Lloyd.Mabonga@up.ac.za; zodwa.dlamini@up.ac.za

A. Chatziioannou
Centre of Systems Biology, Biomedical Research Foundation of the Academy of Athens, Athens, Greece
e-mail: achatzi@bioacademy.gr

Z. Dlamini (ed.), *Overcoming Breast Cancer Therapy Resistance*,
https://doi.org/10.1007/978-3-031-52860-6_12

cancer. It emphasizes the potential use of molecular profiling and personalized medicine in guiding treatment decisions and improving outcomes for patients with drug-resistant breast cancer.

Keywords Breast cancer · Drug resistance · Biomarkers · Molecular profiling · Personalized medicine

Introduction

The realization that most orthodox clinical-pathological approaches are poorly suited in the management of breast cancer has provided a powerful impetus for research endeavors aimed at discovering entirely new disruptive innovations that could fill the existing gaps in the management of drug-resistant breast cancer (Kinnel et al., 2023; Tendl & Bago-Horvath, 2020). The peremptory need to find solutions in the management of drug-resistant breast cancer has ushered an important juncture, transitioning from the dominant clinicopathological approach to the emerging molecular profiling paradigm (Davey & Kerin, 2023; Kinnel et al., 2023; Mehmood et al., 2022). Over the years, drug resistance has been a large hurdle in the management of breast cancer and in reducing breast cancer deaths. Drug resistance in breast cancer accounts for a significant proportion of cancer deaths globally (Kinnel et al., 2023; Siegel et al., 2023), and drug resistance leading to metastasis and relapses hinders the efficacy of chemotherapeutic drugs (Davey & Kerin, 2023; Kinnel et al., 2023; Mehmood et al., 2022; Kittaneh et al., 2013).

Breast cancer is difficult to treat due to several drug resistance mechanisms, such as altered tumor microenvironment, improved DNA repair, epigenetic modifications, epithelial-to-mesenchymal transition (EMT), and increased drug efflux (Kinnel et al., 2023; Tufail et al., 2022; Ahmed, 2020). The roles of genes involved in drug-resistant breast cancer remain elusive and yet to be fully characterized (Mehmood et al., 2022). Thus, deciphering the underlying mechanisms is critical to overcome drug-resistant breast cancer (Kinnel et al., 2023; Tufail et al., 2022; Ahmed, 2020).

The herald of molecular profiling approaches has opened novel diagnostic and therapeutic possibilities to deal with drug resistance in breast cancer management. Molecular profiling involves analyzing the genetic and molecular characteristics of tumors to gain insights into their biology and drug response patterns (Kinnel et al., 2023; Siegel et al., 2023). It analyzes the genomic and gene expression profiles of tumors to identify potentially actionable genetic alterations (Tufail et al., 2022; Ahmed, 2020), which can then be used to develop precision cancer therapies. Molecular profiling is used to characterize and identify different subtypes of breast cancer in patients (Kinnel et al., 2023; Siegel et al., 2023). The treatment of drug resistance in breast cancer has changed from a one-size-fits-all strategy to finding more focused therapeutic choices because of the heterogeneity of breast cancer. Hence, drug resistance in breast cancer is treated based on the identified subtypes

(Kinnel et al., 2023), and molecular profiling is a useful tool in the management of drug-resistant breast cancer as it allows for more personalized treatment approaches based on the specific molecular changes present in a patient's tumor (Kinnel et al., 2023; Herzog & Fuqua, 2022; Garcia-Martinez et al., 2021).

Molecular profiling techniques are used to investigate the genomic alterations in drug-resistant breast cancer tumors (Herzog & Fuqua, 2022; Garcia-Martinez et al., 2021). They allow for the identification of hereditary cancer syndromes in patients with a family history of malignancies, help match patients in clinical trials to establishing personalized treatments or medicines for one or more alterations associated with drug resistance in breast cancer, and contribute to the successful prevention of drug-resistant breast cancers (Mehmood et al., 2022; Sabatier et al., 2014). The chapter focuses on the utilization of molecular profiling techniques and personalized medicine approaches in the management of drug resistance in breast cancer. It emphasizes the potential use of molecular profiling and personalized medicine in guiding treatment decisions and improving outcomes for patients with drug-resistant breast cancer.

Molecular Profiling Techniques for Breast Cancer Patients

Molecular profiling is an emerging panomics technology that has ushered in a new dawn in the management of drug-resistant breast cancer. It muzzles an integrative multi-analytical omics approach that combines panomics techniques to answer the elusive biological question of heterogeneity and drug resistance in breast cancer (Mehmood et al., 2022; Woodhouse et al., 2020). The aim of the approach is to move from a single gene single therapy approach toward personalized decisions and treatment options as shown in Fig. 1 (Falcone et al., 2023; Kinnel et al., 2023; Mehmood et al., 2022; Woodhouse et al., 2020). Molecular profiling assays target multiple genes that provide predictive or prognostic information that aids clinicians in choosing whether to use adjuvant therapy, particularly when such decisions are elusive from the perspective of traditional clinicopathologic approaches. Multigene assays are used for initial diagnosis and surgical resection. And for the molecular

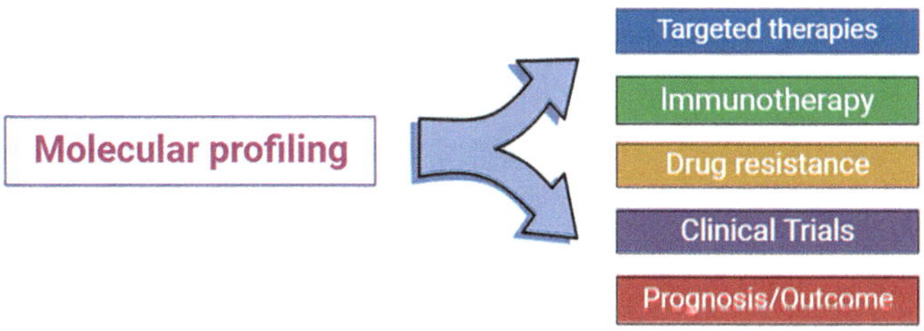

Fig. 1 Molecular profiling unlocks the full potential of personalized medicine. The approach aims to move from a single gene single therapy approach toward personalized decisions and treatment options

profiling of breast cancer patients, several commercially available multigene assays (MGAs) have been created and validated (Falcone et al., 2023; Kinnel et al., 2023).

Molecular profiling techniques aid in identifying diagnostic, prognostic, and predictive biomarkers that are linked to response, lack of response, or resistance to treatment plans by collective characterization and quantification of high-value biological data (Kinnel et al., 2023; Mehmood et al., 2022). The diagnosis, prediction of treatment responses, and prognostics in breast cancer have been a success over the years using biomarkers designed from oncogenic driver mutations (Falcone et al., 2023; Kinnel et al., 2023; Woodhouse et al., 2020). A new era of precision medicine and focused therapeutic oncology medication development has emerged because of the characterization of such biomarkers and molecular profiles. Precision medicine involves different steps as shown in Fig. 2. High-throughput sequencing or molecular profiling is performed on the patient samples. The gathered information is examined for cancer-related mutations and target genes. To treat cancer, a precise medicine is chosen based on the determined target (Falcone et al., 2023; Kinnel et al., 2023). Today, combinations of tumor-specific biomarkers can be found, and these combinations can aid in the detection, prognosis, and therapy of breast cancer. Using this knowledge, targeted medicines that are created to be more efficient for a certain tumor profile can be created. A "profile" is data on the genes present in cancer cells (Falcone et al., 2023; Kinnel et al., 2023; Mehmood et al., 2022; Woodhouse et al., 2020).

The specific protein, ribonucleic acid (RNA) or deoxyribonucleic acid (DNA) molecule linked to an illness is identified through molecular profiling (Falcone et al., 2023; Woodhouse et al., 2020). The patient's sample is first taken through a

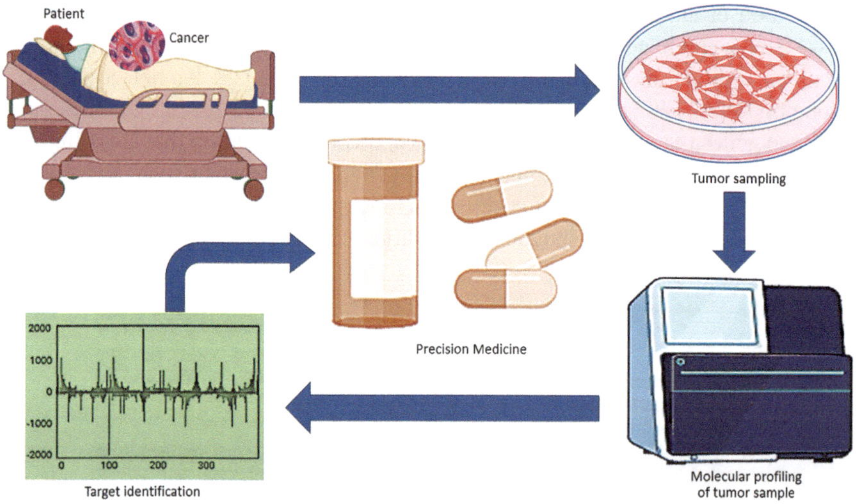

Fig. 2 There are various steps in precision medicine. Patients who undergo molecular profiling or high-throughput sequencing provide the sample. The gathered information is examined for mutations and target genes related to malignancy. To treat cancer, a precise medicine is chosen based on the determined target

biopsy technique from the lymph node (for some blood cancers), bone marrow, tumor tissue, or peripheral blood in cases where there are circulating tumor cells. The sample goes through several molecular profiling tests to observe the specific biomarkers that are linked with the patient's cancer (Kinnel et al., 2023; Mehmood et al., 2022). The creation of specialized, extremely targeted, and efficient treatments that can enhance patient outcomes is the aim of molecular profiling. The kind and quantity of mutations can be used to forecast how a patient will react to a given medication (Falcone et al., 2023; Kinnel et al., 2023; Mehmood et al., 2022; Woodhouse et al., 2020). The molecular profiling techniques used for tumor profiling for breast cancer are highlighted below.

Next-Generation Sequencing (NGS) Techniques

The potential use of genomics-based molecular profiling techniques as standard of care of management in breast cancer has allowed the rapid sequencing of DNA or RNA covering the whole genome (Falcone et al., 2023; Kinnel et al., 2023; Mehmood et al., 2022; Woodhouse et al., 2020). Next-generation sequencing (NGS) has helped detect copy number variations, gene fusions, and DNA mutations across the genome and provides information about prognosis and treatment as shown in Fig. 3. It has redefined subtypes of breast cancer and assists in pinpointing single nucleotide polymorphisms (SNPs) and mutations as biomarkers in breast cancer (Mehmood et al., 2022; Parsons & Francavilla, 2020). In this context, stem cells from breast cancer have also been used as novel therapeutic tools and with other

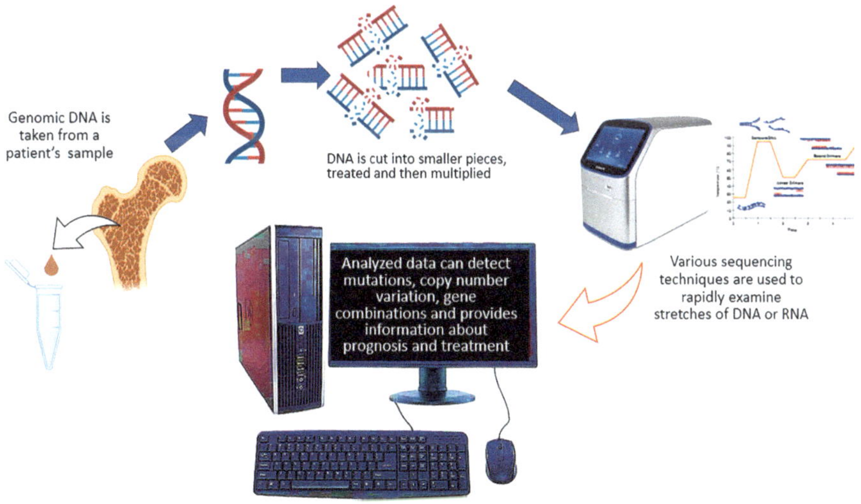

Fig. 3 Next-Generation Sequencing (NGS). A molecular profiling tool that can identify gene fusions, copy number variations, and DNA mutations throughout the genome and offer data on the prognosis and management of breast cancer

molecular signatures have intensified personalized treatments for breast cancer patients (Mehmood et al., 2022). Next-generation sequencing (NGS) technologies targeting molecular profiling signatures such as estrogen receptor (ER), human epidermal growth factor receptor 2 (HER2) and progesterone receptor (PR) are vital in the prediction of therapeutic targets for breast cancer patients (Rakha et al., 2010). One example of an assay derived from Next-Generation Sequencing (NGS) techniques is the FoundationOne®CDx (F1CDx).

FoundationOne®CDx (F1CDx) is a pan-cancer circulating a novel 324-Gene cell-free DNA (cfDNA)-based molecular profiling technique that utilizes next-generation sequencing (NGS)-based comprehensive genomic profiling (CGP) technology to evaluate the presence of cancer genes in solid tumors (Milbury et al., 2022; Woodhouse et al., 2020). According to the approved therapeutic product labelling for various drug therapies, it is used to identify individuals who might benefit from treatment (Sabari et al., 2019; Rolfo et al., 2018). The use of procedures based on circulating cell-free DNA (cfDNA)—often referred to as liquid biopsy assays—is increasing to deliver genomic profile data to patients. They are created for patients who cannot donate tissue that can be evaluated or when tissue quality or quantity is poor in several malignancies (Sabari et al., 2019; Rolfo et al., 2018). Due to the longer turnaround time for providing a tumor sample for testing than tumor tissue tests, circulating cell-free DNA (cfDNA)-based approaches give a shorter time to obtain results. A tumor biopsy may only contain a tiny portion of the total tumor cell population because of intratumor heterogeneity. CfDNA may be able to help overcome this limitation (Sabari et al., 2019; Rolfo et al., 2018).

FoundationOne®CDx (F1CDx), a cfDNA-based method, may be therapeutically useful (Bronkhorst et al., 2019; Merker et al., 2018), although it can be technically difficult. Liquid biopsies are used more frequently in clinical practice; however, more clinical validity and usefulness evidence are still required (Merker et al., 2018). The degree to which an NGS assay successfully detects a certain genetic trait, such as a genomic change or genomic signature, is referred to as its analytical validity (Bronkhorst et al., 2019; Merker et al., 2018). To show that a test reliably and accurately detects genetic changes in a sample, analytical validation is crucial. Clinical utility, on the other hand, refers to the link between a genetic mutation and the presence or absence of a certain disease (Woodhouse et al., 2020; Bronkhorst et al., 2019; Merker et al., 2018). The evaluation of the relationship between test results and health outcomes requires clinical validation. Numerous studies that evaluate the concordance between tumor tissue and plasma samples when evaluating the analytical validity of cfDNA assays introduce confounding factors like tumor heterogeneity and run the risk of confusing clinical validity with analytical validity (Woodhouse et al., 2020; Merker et al., 2018). These issues can be resolved by evaluating the analytical authenticity of samples with known variants at variant allele fractions, such as cell line DNA diluted in the appropriate matrix. The potential effects of preanalytical and analytical variables must also be assessed according to several researchers (Woodhouse et al., 2020; Bronkhorst et al., 2019; Merker et al., 2018).

To identify the 4 main classes of genomic alterations, namely base substitutions (subs), insertions or deletions (indels), copy number alterations (CNAs), and gene rearrangements, FoundationOne®CDx (F1CDx) uses NGS technology to assess entire exonic regions of cancer-vulnerable genes for all types of tumors (Milbury et al., 2022; Woodhouse et al., 2020). Precision medicine can only enhance treatment choices and outcomes for cancer patients if test results are exact, precise, and confirmed clinically and analytically to the highest degree feasible. Comprehensive genomic profiling (CGP) services can decrease the complexity of biomarker testing (Woodhouse et al., 2020). To present complex indicators like microsatellite instability (MSI) and blood tumor mutational burden (bTMB) and to guide cancer therapy decisions utilizing a single test, the CGP assays may evaluate genomic aberration patterns across linked genes in orthodox cancer pathways (Milbury et al., 2022).

The therapeutic value of tissue based CGP has been demonstrated to be higher than that of non-CGP testing, and liquid testing will probably be more valuable because it can locate supplementary data and furnish biomarker results for patients who cannot undergo tissue testing (Woodhouse et al., 2020). Collectively, F1CDx reports copy number alterations (CNAs), short variants (SVs), and specific rearrangements that are known or highly likely to be pathogenic, as well as compounded biomarkers like tumor mutational burden (TMB), microsatellite instability (MSI), and genomic losses of heterozygosity (gLOH). By providing guideline-based biomarker testing, F1CDx satisfies the clinical needs of healthcare professionals and patients, enabling them to stay up with the fast-developing field of medicine (Milbury et al., 2022; Woodhouse et al., 2020).

Quantitative Polymerase Chain Reaction (qPCR)

To evaluate copy number variation (CNV), quantitative real-time polymerase chain reaction (qPCR) is frequently utilized. In formalin-fixed paraffin-embedded (FFPE) tissues, it has been suggested that qPCR may be a very sensitive, accurate, and reliable approach for the assessment of CNV in breast cancer cells (Angius et al., 2023; Pu et al., 2015). Because FFPE samples' genomic DNA is usually fragmented, measuring the HER-2 gene CNV using qPCR, which concentrates on short sequences, may yield more sensitive and precise results (Angius et al., 2023). To study a particular DNA segment, the molecular profiling technique known as quantitative real-time polymerase chain reaction (qPCR) increases tiny amounts of DNA. This technique now allows the detection of a very low concentration of blood cancer cells, too little to be seen under a microscope. A qPCR test can detect one blood cancer cell in 100,000 to 1,000,000 blood cells that are normal (Angius et al., 2023; Pu et al., 2015).

As shown in Fig. 4, qPCR utilizes a patient's blood or bone marrow. The strands are split once a single section has been retrieved. Artificial DNA fragments that bind at the correct position are added. A specific gene signal can be amplified so that even minute amounts can be used to determine if the cancer gene is present or absent.

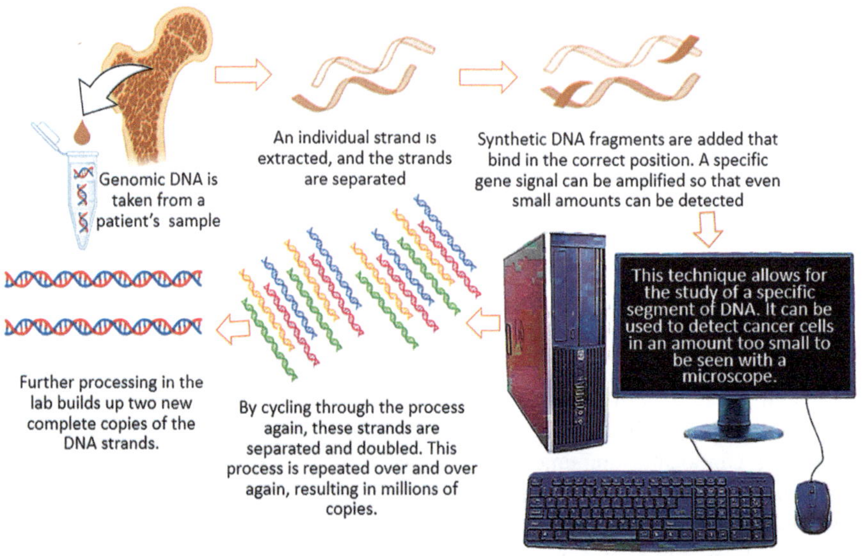

Fig. 4 Quantitative Polymerase Chain Reaction (qPCR). A method of molecular profiling that enlarges tiny bits of DNA so that a particular DNA section may be examined. The method has proven effective in identifying blood cancer cells in extremely low concentrations that are too small to be detected under a microscope. One blood cancer cell among 100,000 to 1,000,000 healthy blood cells can be found using a qPCR test. This test utilizes a patient's blood or bone marrow

These strands are split apart, then doubled by repeating the process. Millions of copies are produced because of this process being done over and over. Two fresh, full copies of the DNA strands are created in the lab by additional processing. This method enables the examination of a particular DNA section. Cancer cells that are too small to be detected under a microscope can be found using this method (Angius et al., 2023; Pu et al., 2015).

Quantitative real-time polymerase chain reaction (qPCR) has several advantages. It is a quick and simple, effective, credible, and accurate molecular profiling technique, which allows for the quick screening of several samples in a short period of time (Angius et al., 2023; Pu et al., 2015). Furthermore, qPCR amplification and quantification are performed in the same reaction tube, which reduces the systematic errors to some extent (Angius et al., 2023). Quantitative real-time polymerase chain reaction (qPCR) is a viable option because of its superior performance and considerable potential for extensive applications. It can serve as a useful and complementary screening tool for the detection of the HER-2 gene level in FFPE tissue samples (Pu et al., 2015). Quantitative real-time polymerase chain reaction (qPCR) can compensate for the inadequacy of IHC and FISH and produce specific quantitative results. HER-2 detection with qPCR provides decisive information for the assessment of the effects of trastuzumab therapy in breast cancer patients (Pu et al., 2015).

Key clinical screening and prevention tests for 19 hereditary predisposition genes have been successfully identified (Mehmood et al., 2022; Hamdan et al., 2019; Rakha et al., 2010). Genetic modifications based on GATA3, PIK3CA, TP53, BRCA1, BRCA2, and RB1 genes identified in more than 9% of breast cancer patients have been isolated (Koboldt et al., 2012; Ellsworth et al., 2010). Breast cancer screening for the detection of mutations in BRCA2 and BRCA1 using BRACAnalysis® has been successfully recommended for early age diagnosis in women with a cancer family history (Ellsworth et al., 2010).

Transcriptomics Profiling Techniques

Transcriptomics-based molecular profiling techniques such as microarrays and RNA-Seq have been widely used to investigate prognostic or predictive biomarkers that could be used in breast cancer subtype identification, risk assessment, disease progression, invasion, survival, and assessment of treatment success and clinical trials. The biomarkers have been used to plan hormonal therapy, molecular targeted therapy, and chemotherapy for breast cancer patients. Transcriptome-wide association studies (TWAS) revealed 1196 genes related to 30 complex biological pathways from whole genome sequencing and RNA-Seq data to gain insights into the management of breast cancer (Wainberg et al., 2019). ANKLE1 (Ankyrin Repeat and LEM Domain Containing 1) and U4C, RCCD1 (RCC1 domain containing 1) and DHODH, and TP53INP2 (tumor protein p53-inducible nuclear protein 2) and ER-negative have been linked to the therapy of breast cancer (You et al., 2019). Expression quantitative trait loci (eQTL) have been used to investigate how genes affect cell proliferation and colony-forming effectiveness to shed light on breast cancer (Feng et al., 2018). Six molecular profiling methods, including Oncotype DX, Prosigna, Breast Cancer Index, EndoPredict, MammaPrint, and genomic grade index, have been developed in this context based on transcriptome signatures for the early identification of breast cancer (You et al., 2019).

The breast cancer index evaluates the expression of the genomic grade index genes RRM2, RACGAP1, NEK2, CENPA, and BUB1B, as well as the ratio of the IL17BR and HOXB13 genes. It was created using 60 ER+ tumor samples from patients who had taken tamoxifen. The ratio of the genes IL17BR and HOXB13, as well as the genomic grade index genes RRM2, RACGAP1, NEK2, CENPA, and BUB1B, is all measured. According to Lal et al. (2017), the breast cancer index is used to assess the prognosis of women with lymph node-negative and estrogen receptor-positive illness. The EndoPredict is designed for patients with LN ± disease treated with tamoxifen on 964 ER+ tumor samples. This assay encompasses the expression of tumor-associated genes (MGP, DHCR7, RBBP8, IL6ST, BIRC5, UBE2C, STC2, and AZGP1) and control genes (OAZ1, RPL37A, and CALM2). The EndoPredict is utilized in examining the prognosis of women with lymph node ± and estrogen receptor-positive disease (Dinh et al., 2022). Angiogenesis resistance (12 genes), growth factor signal transduction (6 genes), apoptosis (2 genes), cell-cycle dysregulation (15 genes), invasion and metastasis (8 genes), proliferation and oncogenic transformation (11 genes), and other/unknown function (16 genes) are all quantified in MammaPrint, a microarray technology test. The assay was authorized by the FDA in 2007 to assess a patient's risk of developing metastases. The MammaPrint test is a 70-gene assay created using 78 samples of ER tumors. It affects whether women with LN and ER disease in stages 1 or 2 have a favorable prognosis (Mehmood et al., 2022; Dinh et al., 2022).

Oncotype DX is used to forecast 10-year recurrence risk in patients with LN− and ER+ disease. The test measures genes for estrogen (4), invasion (2), proliferation (5), HER2 (2), BAG1, GSTM1, CD68 as well as other five genes for reference. Oncotype DX has been evaluated on 447 ER ± tumor samples from patients with LN ± disease including tamoxifen treated patients. It is used to predict 10-year recurrence risk in patients with ER+ and LN− disease (Chen et al., 2023). To categorize breast cancer into one of four intrinsic subtypes, the Prosigna test examines the expression levels of 50 genes together with five reference genes. It is built using 29 non-malignant breast tissue biopsy samples and 189 ER tumor samples from individuals with LN illness. In clinical settings, the test has been used to assess the prognosis of postmenopausal women with ER+ and stage 1 or 2 LN illness. It is inevitable that more research will be done to find the biomarkers for various types of breast cancer, despite the identification of biomarkers for breast cancer therapy end point, progression, and diagnosis (Chen et al., 2023).

Fluorescence In Situ Hybridization (FISH)

To assess genes and DNA sequences on chromosomes and identify tumor-specific abnormalities, fluorescence in situ hybridization (FISH), a common cytogenetic-molecular profiling technique, is used in routine diagnostics of genetic aberrations (Bogdanovska-Todorovska et al., 2018; Hastings et al., 2016; Broholm et al., 2008). Targets in customized oncology include gene rearrangements, deletions of crucial areas, gene fusions, genomic imbalances, and amplifications. A final diagnosis or the beginning of a specific, targeted treatment is frequently directly indicated by the confirmation of a genetic marker (Huber et al., 2018). FISH can be used to examine the genomic status of cells derived from a primary tumor or metastasis in formalin-fixed paraffin-embedded tissue samples (FFPE) (Hastings et al., 2016; Broholm et al., 2008).

In a FISH protocol (Fig. 5), segments of DNA are transformed by the addition of a fluorescent dye, and then the modified DNA is put to cells or tissues on a glass slide. When seen through a microscope with a special light, these DNA fragments "glow" when they bind to genes or regions of chromosomes on the slide (Chrzanowska et al., 2020). This makes it possible to pinpoint chromosomal regions that have changed in size, quantity, or arrangement. FISH can be useful for diagnosis, risk assessment, determining the necessity for treatment, and evaluating the efficacy of that treatment (Chrzanowska et al., 2020; Huber et al., 2018). The tissue

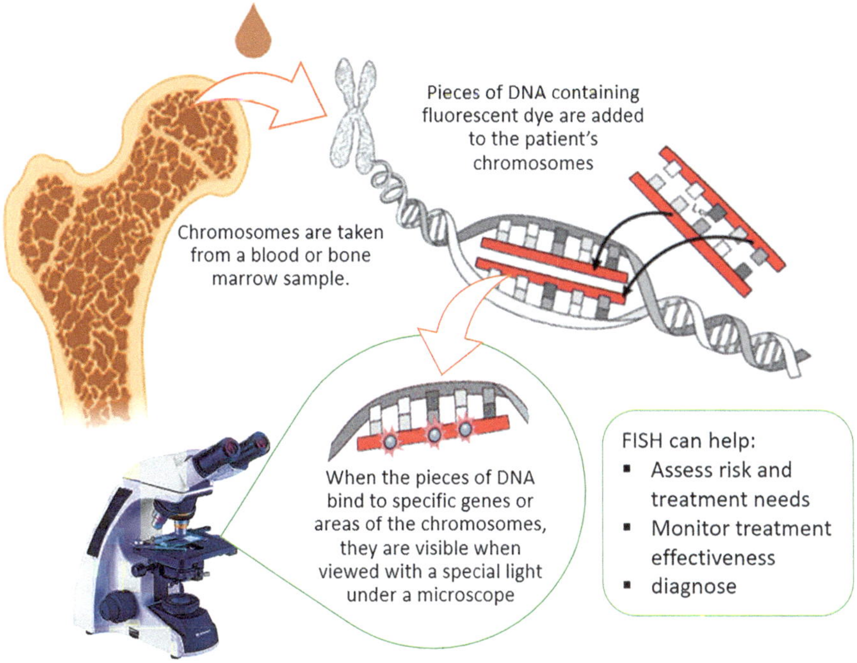

Fig. 5 Fluorescence in situ hybridization (FISH). A molecular profiling technique that assesses chromosomal genes and/or DNA sequences. Tests on the blood or marrow are used to remove cells and tissue. Segments of DNA are transformed in the lab by the addition of a fluorescent dye, and then the modified DNA is put to cells or tissues on a glass plate. When seen through a microscope that has a special light, these DNA fragments "glow" when they link to genes or regions of chromosomes on the slide. This makes it possible to pinpoint chromosomal regions that have changed in size, quantity, or arrangement. FISH can be useful for diagnosis, risk assessment, determining the need for treatment, and gauging the efficacy of that treatment

and cells are removed using either blood or marrow assays. However, the technique is limited to designed probe types (Bogdanovska-Todorovska et al., 2018).

Microfluidic platforms are now available for the study of circulating tumor cells (CTCs) using the modern FISH technique. A patient's blood sample can be utilized to collect the cells, which can then be employed as a tumor biomarker for diagnosis and metastasis prognosis (Chrzanowska et al., 2020). Cellular DNA applied to a microarray is placed in a microchannel, allowing for flow-based chemical incubation. This improves the kinetics of the hybridization procedure between the probe and the target sequence. Signal strength is greatly improved by this. The approach also lowered labor time and increased reproducibility. The technique has been examined for the lysine methyl transferase 2A (KMT2A), HER2, and other genes. According to several studies (Chrzanowska et al., 2020; Huber et al., 2018; Bogdanovska-Todorovska et al., 2018; Hastings et al., 2016; Broholm et al., 2008), the microfluidic platform's method of accepting CTCs appears to be its major hurdle.

By using labelled nucleic acid probes, fluorescence in situ hybridization (FISH) can identify specific DNA or RNA sequences in tissue samples. Gene amplifications, deletions, fusions, and translocations can all be found using fluorescence in situ hybridization (Chrzanowska et al., 2020). FISH testing is dependable and simple to use; however, it only detects DNA rearrangements and does not catch sequence alterations. Since FISH can discriminate between HER2-amplified vs. HER2-low status, it is frequently utilized when HER2 amplification on initial testing in breast cancer is ambiguous (Huber et al., 2018; Bogdanovska-Todorovska et al., 2018).

Immunohistochemistry (IHC)

A molecular profiling method that aids in directing patient care is immunohistochemistry. According to Sun et al., 2021, the technique is used to classify metastases, pinpoint genetic alterations in special-type breast cancer, and determine the status of PD-L1 as a newly emerging biomarker in triple-negative (estrogen receptor [ER]/progesterone receptor [PR]/human epidermal growth factor receptor-2 [HER-2]) breast cancer. As seen in Fig. 6, immunohistochemistry is a crucial part in diagnosing breast disease. New interpretation standards and associated problems

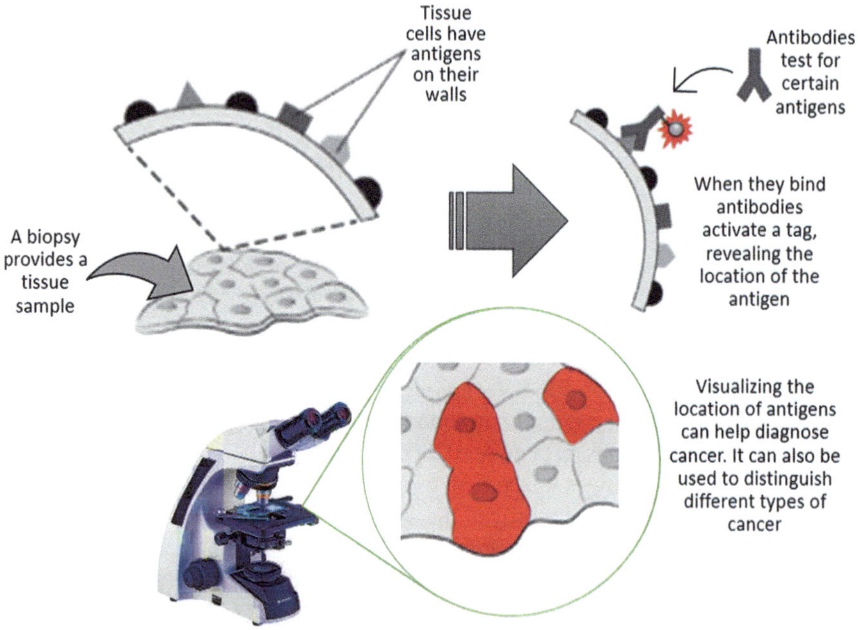

Fig. 6 Immunohistochemistry (IHC). A molecular profiling technique evaluates alterations in the expression or quantity of proteins in tissue samples. Antibodies are used in immunohistochemistry to identify proteins that are linked to cancer, such as tumor-specific antigens, oncogenic proteins that promote cell development, or indicators of cellular proliferation. It employs antibodies to find certain antigens (markers) in a biopsy-derived tissue sample

arise along with fresh tests and applications. No single immunostain is entirely sensitive or specific, although immunohistochemistry aids in demonstrating breast cancer origin for primary or metastatic malignancies and pinpointing non-mammary metastases to the breast (Sun et al., 2021).

Using antibodies, the IHC technique can identify specific antigens (markers) in a tissue sample taken from a biopsy. Fluorescent dyes or enzymes connected to the antibodies are triggered when they attach to the antigen in the tissue sample, making the antigen easily viewed under a microscope. The information provided by immunohistochemistry aids in the diagnosis of disorders like cancer. It can also be utilized to differentiate between various cancer kinds. The same concepts apply to flow cytometry, with the exception that it is performed on cells that are embedded in liquid as opposed to cells that have been implanted in a tissue sample (Zhang, 2023). Immunohistochemistry (IHC) measures alterations in the presence or expression of proteins in tissue samples. Antibodies are used in immunohistochemistry to identify proteins that are linked to cancer, such as tumor-specific antigens, oncogenic proteins that promote cell development, or indicators of cellular proliferation. The benefit of immunohistochemistry is that it can show where a protein is expressed within the context of a tumor tissue sample. However, because each of the target proteins in this test requires a different antibody, not all targeted targets or antigens may be detectable. The presence or absence of distinctive markers can assist in determining the primary tumor site when using immunohistochemistry for the diagnosis of cancer with an unknown primary (Sun et al., 2021).

According to Cimino-Mathews, 2021, when identifying triple-negative breast cancer, which frequently tests negative for markers of mammary differentiation, GATA3 and Sox10 are very helpful immunostains. A pan-cytokeratin immunostain ought to be perpetually used for this differential diagnosis because S-100 and Sox10 label both triple-negative breast cancer and metastatic melanoma. Sox10 labelling is a significant potential diagnostic trap. The genetic abnormalities specific to several special-type breast cancers are represented by novel immunohistochemistry, such as the usage of pan-TRK in secretory carcinoma, MYB in adenoid cystic carcinoma, and mutant IDH2 in tall cell carcinoma with reversed polarity (TCCRP). Furthermore, PD-L1 immunohistochemistry is a developing, albeit unreliable, biomarker for immunotherapy for breast cancer, with distinct test settings and scoring standards in breast carcinoma in comparison with other tumor types. Additional diagnostic tools and biomarkers are made available by the growing library of innovative immunohistochemical techniques, which enhances patient care and diagnostic breast pathology (Cimino-Mathews, 2021).

Proteomics Profiling Techniques

The development of predictive biomarkers for breast cancer diagnosis is crucial to the success of proteomics-based molecular profiling approaches. Protein biomarkers that can distinguish biologically between distinct subgroups of breast cancer have already been found, and they are clinically more accurate than prognostic indicators (Kalocsay et al., 2023). Nine tryptic peptides with differential expression that were connected to stromal and tumor analyses were found using laser capture microdissection. Protein-specific patterns may be to blame for early diagnosis in breast cancer patients, according to mass spectrometry examination of the breast cancer proteome. According to Johansson et al. (2019), numerous peptide biomarkers have been discovered recently, including fragments of C3, bradykinin, C3adesArg, apoA-IV, fibrinogen, factor XIIIa, FPA, transthyretin, and ITIH4.

According to Kalocsay et al. (2023), there are more than 37 protein biomarkers that can be categorized using proteomics. Among them, it has been discovered that D3 cyclins are linked to CDK4, and BRCA2-mediated malignancies are linked to D1. In 28 ER-positive patients, the possible biosignature function of retinoic acid receptor alpha has also been detected. Using MS and ELISA, it has been revealed that HSP27, CD14, and ANXV may serve as breast cancer biomarkers. Using MALDI-TOF/MS, 2D-DIGE, LC-MS/MS, and IHC, biosignatures for breast cancer have been identified. These methods allowed the identification of the proteins peroxiredoxin, fibronectin, glycolytic enzymes, vimetin, annexin-1, cytokeratin, L-plastin, and annexin-2 (Kuburich et al., 2022). Several proteins that are differentially expressed during cancer invasion include tumor-suppressor genes, structural proteins, cytokines, signal-transducers, and cell-cycle regulators, indicating that they actively participate in tumor suppression. These include Maspin, DSG3, and DCC. Contrarily, during cancer invasion, CGG3, HER-3, CATH, and HSP-27 are overexpressed and play a big part in breast cancer's malignant transformation (Caporossi et al., 2021).

From a meta-analysis of genomic assays, protein-based "signatures" such as trinucleotide repeat containing 9 (TNRC9/LOC643714), lymphocyte-specific protein (LSP1), mitogen-activated kinase-1 (MAP 3K1), FGFR2 oncogene protein, ER, fibroblast growth factor receptor-2 (FGFR2), Ki67, PR, and HER2 were discovered. Different prediction algorithms have been created and validated for the diagnosis of breast cancer recurrence risks in breast cancer management using protein-based "signatures" along with clinicopathological biosignature data. To assist clinicians in choosing whether to proceed with surgery or adjuvant therapy, several molecular profiling systems have been developed, including Predict, Online, Adjuvant! and the Nottingham Prognostic Index. These instruments combine molecular markers of tumor expression (ER, Ki67, PR, and HER2) that aid in predicting whether breast cancer patients will survive with or without adjuvant therapy. Nevertheless, despite all these developments, it is still unclear how DNA variations in intronic or intergenic areas cause breast cancer (Qing et al., 2023).

Proteomics and pathological assays have identified more than 97 breast cancer biomarkers, including E-cadherin, ER, CK8/18, cyclin E, p53, Ki-67, cyclin D1, HER-2, cyclin E, BCL2, PR, and CK5/6. Although advances in this area are essential for the quick management of breast cancer, molecular tests for preclinical decision-making and breast cancer diagnosis still need to be developed and validated. According to Kuburich et al., 2022, these biosignatures can serve as a backdrop for the early detection of breast cancer.

Metabolomic Profiling Techniques

Arguably the most intriguing field of research for breast cancer treatment is metabolomics. It takes a very different approach from the typical cell pathways in that it focuses on metabolites and metabolic pathways (Cheung et al., 2019). The field of precision medicine, where individualized treatments are created for patients based on their distinct molecular anomalies indicated by their metabolomics profile and fingerprints, is rapidly embracing metabolomics. There are two types of metabolomics profiling techniques: targeted and untargeted. Metabolomics data has been employed over time to produce novel molecular biomarkers for breast cancer prognosis, treatment response, monitoring their metastatic condition, and therapeutic decision-making (Schmidt et al., 2021).

Pharmacometabolomics can be utilized to assess treatment response in breast cancer patients by monitoring the patients' metabolic profiles. According to the risk of breast cancer development and susceptibility, diet-related metabolites are thoroughly investigated (Playdon et al., 2017). Circulating metabolites such as tocopherols (vitamin E), caprate, SFA, 2-hydroxyoctanoate, MUFA, hydroxy fatty acids, fat metabolites, and g-CEHC, which are reliable and informative, can be used to provide a suggestion as to the likelihood that breast cancer would develop in ER+ individuals. The alteration of numerous physiological processes, including immune function, tumor suppression, and breast cells' response to growth factors, as well as inflammation and an increase in estrogen synthesis in adipose tissues, are among the mechanisms by which diet-related metabolites can cause breast cancer (Schmidt et al., 2021). Dietary biomarkers that promote androgen-dependent and androgen-independent pathways, which may cause alcohol-related breast cancer, notably in postmenopausal ER+ patients, can be seen to have the same effects. Breast cancer patients' metabolic profiles and diet-related metabolites can be studied to learn a lot about how to manage the disease. However, there are still difficulties when combining metabolomics data with other omics datasets. Nevertheless, metabolomics is unavoidably important for the detection and treatment of breast cancer (Mehmood et al., 2022; Playdon et al., 2017).

The management of drug-resistant breast cancer makes use of several molecular profiling techniques, such as FoundationOne®CDx (F1CDx), IntelliGEN Oncology Therapeutic Panel, Molecular Intelligence, and numerous other internal broad molecular profiling tests developed by major academic institutions (Schmidt et al., 2021). To manage drug-resistant breast cancer, molecular profiling techniques use samples of tumor tissue and blood, depending on the type of breast cancer a person has been diagnosed with. To match advanced-stage drug-resistant breast cancer tumors with targeted and individualized treatments, molecular profiling approaches are used in this context (Schmidt et al., 2021; Mehmood et al., 2022). The use of molecular profiling methods differs from tests like the Breast Cancer Index, Oncotype DX, Prosigna Breast Cancer Prognostic Gene Signature Assay, MammaPrint, and EndoPredict, which only examine a subset of the genome and are focused on a single type of cancer. Techniques for molecular profiling are used to manage diseases in their early stages. Although it is still not fully understood, there is encouraging progress in the direction of using molecular profiling tools as the pinnacle of care in the management of drug-resistant breast cancer (Schmidt et al., 2021).

An assessment of attainable mutations within a panel consisting of 50 cancer genes believed to be involved in the initiation, progression, and therapy of tumors is provided by the IntelliGEN oncology therapeutic panel. The panel contains well-known biomarkers that could guide therapy choices (Bitterman et al., 2023). IntelliGEN may be useful as a tool when there is insufficient tissue for guideline-recommended biomarker evaluation, disease progression or relapse has happened after prior therapies, the tumor is poorly differentiated and of uncertain origin, the cancer lacks an effective standard-of-care therapy at the time of diagnosis, there is insufficient tissue for guideline-recommended biomarker assessment, and in many other clinical situations. The IntelliGEN assay from Integrated Oncology evaluates an array profile of 50 cancer genes dubbed to relate to the initiation, progression, and treatment of cancers for targetable mutations, providing medical professionals with the knowledge they need to diagnose and treat cancers effectively (Bitterman et al., 2023).

Role of Biomarkers in Treatment Decision-making

Biomarkers are "biological molecules in the blood, other body fluids, or tissues that indicate a normal or abnormal process" or "an assessable index of biologic procedures, whether gained from tissue, imaging, or other sources" (Tarighati et al., 2023). Biomarkers can be diagnostic, pharmacodynamic/response, monitoring, prognostic, or predictive depending on the intended purpose (Provenzano et al., 2020). The three biomarkers that oncologists most frequently utilize in clinical practice to determine treatment options for breast cancer patients are the estrogen receptor (ER), human epidermal growth factor receptor 2 (HER2), and progesterone receptor (PR). Both germline and somatic genetic changes can be thought of as cancer biomarkers in a broader sense and offer helpful information on therapy options. There have also been reports of other indicators, including tumor HGF levels and circulating tumor DNA (ctDNA). Diagnostic, prognostic, and predictive biomarkers together provide valuable information; however, prognostic and predictive biomarkers represent the most developed biomarkers used in treatment decision-making (Sarhadi & Armengol, 2022). As shown in Fig. 7, the roles of biomarkers include selection of patients in MASTER trial protocols, risk-based enrichment, and adaptive enrichment.

To predict the likelihood of a clinical outcome in individuals who are already afflicted with the target disease, prognostic biomarkers are used. They enable the selection of patients who require adjuvant therapy or more intense surveillance. They evaluate the connection between the disease and the clinical outcome in the absence of therapy or with the typical therapy that most patients are likely to get

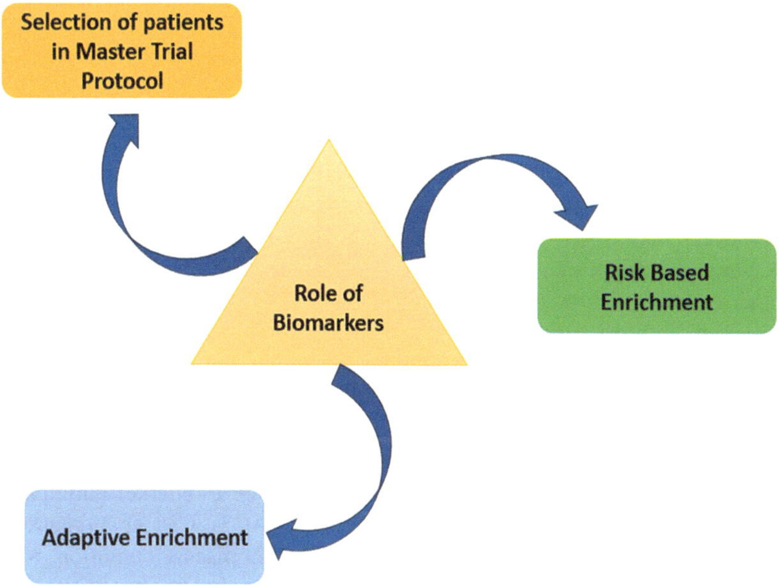

Fig. 7 Clinical trial patient selection methods based on biomarkers. By identifying patients who are more likely to experience risk-based enrichment, choosing a population based on how they respond to predictive response enrichment or adaptive enrichment, and identifying subgroups of similar patients within a pinnacle protocol, biomarkers play a key role in enriching clinical trial populations

(Tarighati et al., 2023). A prognostic marker evaluates tumor-specific molecular and histological traits that are related to long-term outcome or progression of a disease, such as somatic or germline mutations, micro-RNA levels, alterations in DNA methylation, or circulating tumor cells in blood. These characteristics are identified before treatment. A prognostic biomarker's likelihood of surviving depends on whether it is expressed. Survival is comparable between treated and untreated patients in patients who express the relevant biomarker (Tarighati et al., 2023). Prognostic indicators for patients with breast cancer include increased expression of the estrogen receptor (ER) and/or the progesterone receptor (PR), both of which are linked to improved overall survival. Another biomarker that predicts a patient's likelihood of responding to trastuzumab therapy is HER2/neu gene amplification (Provenzano et al., 2020).

To assess a patient's likelihood of benefiting from a certain medication, predictive biomarkers are used. A positive biomarker could indicate a successful response to a medicine, or it could indicate a lack of gain from the same medication, which could spare a patient from drug toxicity or unintended side effects (Provenzano et al., 2020). A predictive biomarker is typically evaluated prior to treatment and offers data on the likelihood of responding to a specific medication. While both prognostic and predictive cancer biomarkers are used to predict clinical results, predictive biomarkers are only used to link a particular medication to a certain clinical outcome. The likelihood of survival in patients who show the biomarker linked to responsiveness to a specific medication depends on the course of treatment (Sarhadi & Armengol, 2022). There is no disparity in longevity between treated and untreated patients for those who test negative for biomarkers. The expression of the HER2/neu protein is one instance of a breast cancer prognostic biomarker. In 15% to 20% of patients with intrusive breast cancer, the HER2/neu protein, a member of the EGFR family of transmembrane receptors, is expressed more frequently. This higher level of expression is associated with how well these patients respond to anti-HER2-targeted drugs like trastuzumab, pertuzumab, and trastuzumab-emtansine. Another example is how the expression of the estrogen receptor in breast cancer corresponds with the responsiveness to hormonal therapies used as adjuvant and metastatic therapy (Tarighati et al., 2023).

The effectiveness of drug development milestones is evaluated using cancer biomarkers (Provenzano et al., 2020). They are used to answer critical questions like "Does this novel drug impact the organized target?"; "Is this drug assured?"; "Is the remedy more effectual in one population?"; "Does the biomarker anticipate survival?"; and other such questions (Tarighati et al., 2023). Cancer biomarkers are employed to determine whether a patient has a certain disease condition, relate to remedial choices, lead to specific therapeutic objectives, and forecast responses to therapeutic procedures (Tarighati et al., 2023; Moorcraft et al., 2015). They can be used to evaluate patients in a variety of clinical settings, including risk assessment, screening for latent primitive cancers, identifying benign from malignant detections or one type of malignancy from another, describing prognosis and prediction for patients who have been diagnosed with cancer, and monitoring disease conditions to ascertain whether the disease is progressing or relapsing as well as how well it is responding to treatment (Moore & Guinigundo, 2023). As shown in Fig. 8, biomarkers play a crucial role in enlarging clinical trial populations by identifying patients who are more likely to experience an event (risk-based enrichment), selecting a population based on how they respond to a drug of interest (predictive response enrichment or adaptive enrichment), and identifying subgroups of related patients within a master trial protocol (Li et al., 2020).

Biomarkers can be used to assess the prognosis of certain malignancies in cancer patients and assist gauge the risk of treatment-independent illness. For instance, several gene expression signatures have been discovered that can be used to evaluate the tumor prognosis for breast cancer patients (Tarighati et al., 2023; Li et al., 2020) and that can be assessed at all stages of cancer management, including metastasis, diagnosis, treatment, and screening (Moore & Guinigundo, 2023). Using high-throughput sequencing, gene expression arrays, and mass spectroscopy, biomarkers reconnaissance can be used to uncover specific biomarkers or groupings of biomarkers that differ between cohorts. The likelihood of false positives can be reduced by using the gathered data. In phase II or III evaluation, numerous prognostic biomarkers based on specific genes or proteins work in concert with treatment drugs (Tarighati et al., 2023).

Predictive biomarkers are becoming increasingly significant (Provenzano et al., 2020). The rapid advancements in the field are also benefiting reliabilities in

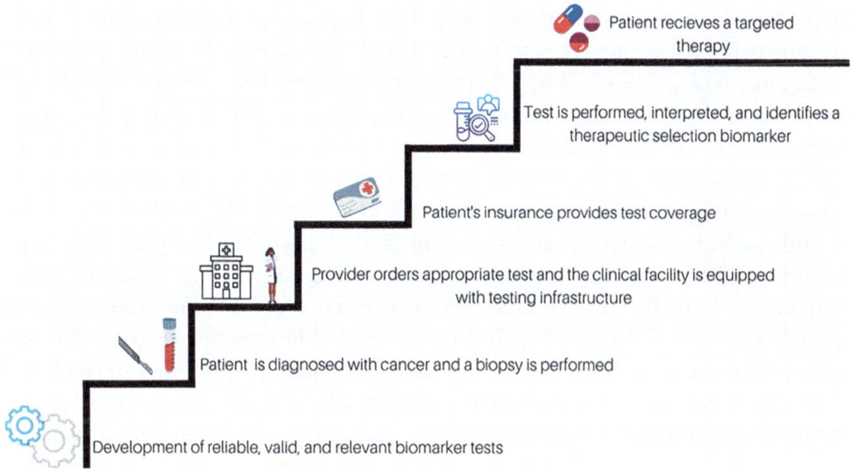

Fig. 8 Actions to improve patient outcomes through biomarker-driven personalized cancer therapy. Precision medicine's understanding and use in the treatment of cancer has advanced quickly, and these developments have produced targeted cancer medicines that can increase patient survival and quality of life. Targeted therapy frequently calls for diagnostic tests to examine biological samples from patients to find and assess cancer biomarkers. Precision medicine in the treatment of cancer relies heavily on testing patients for specific biomarkers

alternative malignancies underlying certain similar oncogenic drivers and less common cancers (Tarighati et al., 2023). The search is on for biomarkers recognized in a specific type of cancer. In a significant prospective trial involving more than 6600 participants in 9 countries (MINDACT study), the 70-gene breast cancer signature is currently being tested for its capacity to predict the likelihood of recurrence in comparison with a clinicopathological evaluation. The primary outcomes suggest that the 70-gene signature added information to common valuation (Moorcraft et al., 2015). In current conventional clinical practice, only HER2 status and hormone receptor status are considered when treating patients with breast cancer. The identification of biomarkers—typically testing for mutations or monitoring gene expression—has been included or will be included in the future, according to the designs of various clinical studies (Tarighati et al., 2023; Moorcraft et al., 2015). Some studies demand certain test results as a prerequisite for inclusion. Other studies employ the test results for stratification and/or prospectively planned subgroup analysis (Tarighati et al., 2023).

One study that demands a specific test result is the ongoing PARP inhibitor research. For inclusion in most of these trials, BRCA mutation proof is required. In other studies, patients with triple-negative breast cancer are the only ones who are included. Other research (Tarighati et al., 2023; Moorcraft et al., 2015) has prospectively included test data into the treatment options and randomization algorithms. Which patients should get adjuvant chemotherapy was determined by the NNBC3 research using the invasion variables uPA/PAI1. Multigene assays have been employed in more recent investigations. The ADAPT research concept identified individuals with a great prognosis who were hypothesized to not require chemotherapy using a 21-gene assay and serial analysis of tumors (Tarighati et al., 2023).

Studies where investigation of anticipated subgroups is planned include PI3K mutation testing. Although the biological importance of PI3K mutations, particularly in HER2-positive and hormone receptor-positive breast cancer, has been well documented and there are indications that tumor response to anti-HER2 treatment is contingent upon mutation status (Tarighati et al., 2023; Moorcraft et al., 2015), it is still unclear whether the mutation can predict effectiveness when the enzyme itself is inhibited. In fact, preliminary research suggests that the mutation status of patients receiving the PI3K inhibitor pictilisib did not foresee effectiveness as determined by progression-free survival (Li et al., 2020; Moorcraft et al., 2015). In recent years, the variety of molecular assays used in clinical research has expanded. To assess the efficacy of anti-estrogen medications, clinicians have been employing the estrogen receptor (ER) status. Tamoxifen, anastrozole, letrozole, exemestane, fulvestrant, and other endocrine medications are used in a variety of circumstances. Genetic risk assessment, which has treatment and hereditary consequences, is also a part of the workup for DCIS through stage IV illness (Li et al., 2020).

Another long-used breast cancer biomarker is HER2 (human epidermal growth factor receptor 2). All invasive breast tumors should be screened, even if we do not currently test for HER2 (Li et al., 2020). Prior to recently, only patients with an IHC (immunohistochemistry) 3+ score and/or FISH positive status were eligible for HER2-directed therapy. In adult patients with metastatic or unresectable "HER2-low" cancers, denoted as IHC 1+ or 2+/ISH negative, recent studies suggest the use of fam-trastuzumab deruxtecan-nxki (Narayan et al., 2021). Chemotherapy and HER2 therapy are options for patients with tumors smaller than 1 cm in size in the adjuvant context. Chemotherapy and trastuzumab (Herceptin) are advised for patients with tumors greater than 1 cm. The additional HER2-directed drug pertuzumab (Perjeta) may be introduced to the same 1 cm tumor in combination with a pN1 or higher. If the condition is operable and HER2-positive at the cT1c or cN1 stage or higher, or if the condition is inoperable, neoadjuvant chemotherapy combined with HER2-directed therapy may be an option. Trastuzumab, with or without pertuzumab, should be continued for a total of one year of HER2 therapy if a pathologic complete response (CR) is attained. Ado-trastuzumab emtansine may be substituted for trastuzumab with or without pertuzumab for the remainder of the prescribed one-year course of treatment if residual disease is found (Moore & Guinigundo, 2023; Narayan et al., 2021).

Lapatinib is one more HER2 agent that is approved for use in conjunction with capecitabine in patients with metastatic illness who have already taken anthracycline, taxane, or trastuzumab. In postmenopausal, HER2-positive, and ER-positive metastatic illness, it can also be used with letrozole (Moore & Guinigundo, 2023). Neratinib, an oral HER2 drug, has been utilized in conjunction with capecitabine in patients with advanced illnesses who have previously taken two or more HER2-directed drugs (Moore & Guinigundo, 2023; Narayan et al., 2021). In the ExteNET trial, HER2-positive patients who had finished trastuzumab in the adjuvant context were given neratinib within 2 years after finishing trastuzumab, which was a unique application for neratinib (Chan et al., 2021). According to the research, neratinib had a 0.66 hazard ratio for invasive disease-free survival in comparison with placebo (Narayan et al., 2021). A kinase inhibitor called tucatinib is given to patients with advanced or metastatic HER2-positive breast cancer who have already received one or more HER2-directed treatments in conjunction with trastuzumab and capecitabine (Casak et al., 2023). For patients who have had at least two anti-HER2 therapies, at least one of which was administered in a metastatic context, margetuximab-cmkb is another HER2-directed therapy that can be used in conjunction with chemotherapy (Markham, 2021).

Drugs targeting MSI-H, TMB-high, NTRK or RET fusions, among others, should be investigated as biomarker-directed therapy for triple-negative breast cancer (TNBC) in the third-line setting and beyond. Pathogenic biomarkers, such as germline (hereditary) BRCA1 and BRCA2 mutations (gBRCAm) are some additional biomarkers to consider (Tarighati et al., 2023). This calls for germline genetic testing to be considered for all breast cancer patients. Only olaparib is authorized in this situation for HER2-negative illness, and gBRCAm are the only recognized biomarkers for breast cancer (Robson et al., 2017). Along with Ki-67, TMB, and homologous recombination deficit (HRD), somatic BRCA is referred to as an "emerging biomarker" (Mohyuddin et al., 2020). Olaparib can be given in the adjuvant situation, following chemotherapy, for up to a year. When olaparib was compared to a placebo, this treatment was related to a hazard ratio of 0.68 for overall survival. Olaparib can be utilized in the metastatic situation in patients with *gBRCAm* who have undergone prior chemotherapy and endocrine therapy (or were ruled ineligible for endocrine therapy) (Robson et al., 2017).

The roles of biomarkers in treatment decision-making include assessing an individual's risk of contracting cancer, determining an individual's risk of cancer recurrence, predicting the possibility that a particular therapy will be beneficial for a specific patient, monitoring a disease's progression to assess whether a therapy is effective, identifying the mechanisms underlying a disease to find potential new therapeutic crucial targets, and screening healthy patients for malignancies.

Implementation of Personalized Medicine Approaches

Personalized medicine (PM), also known as precision medicine in oncology, is a new approach to avoiding the development as well as treatment of tumors that takes into consideration the inter- and intra-tumor genetic variability, as well as the lifestyle and pathologies of each person suffering from cancer. According to Hoeben et al. (2021), it has the capacity to alter the tumor immune environment and direct therapy toward the oncogenic tumor drivers. Personalized medicine (PM) aims to maximize tumor response while accounting for each patient's unique adverse reactions of the medication. In this way, the quality of life and organ function are maintained while the tumor response is maximized. Furthermore, this ensures enhanced patient care in the end, which is undoubtedly its objective (Hoeben et al., 2021). It has become easier to diagnose cancer, forecast how it will respond to treatment, and determine the prognosis thanks to the discovery of biomarkers based on oncogenic driver mutations. Precision medicine and targeted therapeutic oncology medication development have entered a new age because of the characterization of such biomarkers and molecular profiles (Moore & Guinigundo, 2023).

The molecular subtyping has enabled the development of individualized therapeutic approaches for breast cancer patients; however, primary or acquired resistances to these therapies present a significant clinical challenge, with a substantial percentage of patients experiencing progression of the disease and death while taking these drugs (Nabi, 2022). It is unclear why some people do not respond to endocrine or targeted therapy, and the fundamental mechanisms of resistance remain poorly understood. For individuals with cancers that are resistant to these medicines, choosing other treatment modalities would be encouraged by finding indicators of receptivity to various treatments (Moore & Guinigundo, 2023). The application of tailored techniques to the early identification and prevention of breast cancer has been made possible by technological advances. Using genetic and/or environmental risk variables, it is now possible to categorize healthy persons according to their individual risk of breast cancer and, therefore, customize preventative recommendations (Clift et al., 2022), changing from a prevention approach that is "one size fits all" to one that is "personalized or stratified." Patients are taking greater ownership of their health decisions and taking charge of it in accordance with their values, requirements, and preferences. It is intuitively believed that all—encompassing breast cancer prevention, treatment, and follow-up methods will probably prove futile in the long run (Clift et al., 2022; Nabi, 2022).

The most important groups of stakeholders, particularly the patients themselves, must be on board for the project to be successful adoption of a tailored breast cancer screening approach inside healthcare systems. Precision medicine's understanding and use in the treatment of cancer has advanced quickly, and these developments have produced targeted cancer medicines that can increase patient survival and quality of life (Goetz & Schork, 2018). Figure 8 below illustrates the steps to biomarker-driven tailored cancer therapy that aims to enhance patient outcomes. Targeted therapy frequently calls for diagnostic tests to examine biological samples from patients to find and assess cancer biomarkers. Precision medicine in the treatment of cancer relies heavily on testing patients for specific biomarkers (Goetz & Schork, 2018).

According to Goetz and Schork (2018), the foundation of personalized medicine (PM) is the notion that because each person has unique biological, physiological, environmental, and behavioral traits, they may need disease interventions that are tailored to these qualities. Because it is increasingly clear that individual features can affect how a disease develops and how well a treatment works, personalized medicine is rapidly evolving. Some people are more likely to experience serious side effects when taking medications due to their genetic makeup. Some people need a different dose of medication because they are more sensitive to what is typically advised. Additionally, the genetic makeup of a patient's tumor may vary from one patient to the next, offering chances to tailor the therapy based on tumor features. The use of PM necessitates both individualized therapies and patient stratification tools (Botham et al., 2021).

The adoption of PM in clinical practice demands careful planning and a disciplined approach to assure quality and sustainability over the long term. Only if the public is aware of and supportive of this transformation will the integration of PM into standard healthcare be successful (Holden et al., 2019). Major healthcare organizations and government leaders are striving for a quick conversion of these discoveries into advantages for patients. However, moving away from the current "one-size-fits-all" strategy to healthcare and toward "an innovative approach that takes into account individual differences in people's genes, environments, and lifestyles" necessitates that the public and other stakeholders have a better understanding of this new approach (Botham et al., 2021). Even though personalized medicine is becoming a novel approach for the management of some diseases, the financial implications of personalized medicine have only focused on assessing the efficacy of specific treatments and lack a theoretical framework analyzing the relationships between pharmaceutical firms and healthcare systems that led to the implementation of personalized treatments (Moore & Guinigundo, 2023).

Challenges and Limitations

Personalized medicines present several difficulties, particularly when it comes to getting regulatory agency approval for normal usage. The widespread acceptance of personalized pharmaceuticals by various stakeholders in the healthcare industry, including doctors, executives in the industry, insurance companies, and eventually patients, has also raised several problems. The necessity to demonstrate that customized medicine techniques simply outperform conventional medical strategies underlies nearly all these problems (Sadee et al., 2023). And before fulfilling the promise of customized cancer therapy, these difficulties must be overcome. The lack of effective treatments for most genetic disorders, tumor heterogeneity and molecular development, biopsy costs and corresponding morbidity, technical limitations on molecular diagnoses, reimbursement concerns, and regulatory impediments are a few of them. Realistic expectations that only include longer life durations for a portion of patients must be used to temper the "hype" around customized cancer therapy (Cecchin & Stocco, 2020).

Most of these potential drugs have had unsatisfactory results when tested in clinical trials, even though there are increasingly more focused therapeutic compounds available for clinical usage. This shows that there are still many problems that need to be handled to advance this discipline. New generations of clinical trials requiring biopsies to acquire relevant tumor material and cutting-edge statistical techniques are required to improve treatment outcomes. Clinical trials can only be successful if the appropriate biomarkers are discovered to help identify which therapies will be most beneficial for the participants (Sadee et al., 2023; Holden et al., 2019).

Gene-expression or protein-expression "signatures" and innovative imaging technologies have an opportunity to play key roles in the future despite being underutilized as biomarkers today. Any problems that could impede the rapid identification and translation of validated biomarkers with sufficient sensitivity and specificity from the laboratory to the clinic must be identified and resolved right away. Some of these challenges include regulatory and reimbursement norms, as well as the limitations of present biomarker research methodologies (Sadee et al., 2023).

The requirement for significant data gathering to identify criteria that distinguish between categories of people who are likely to benefit several from one or more interventions may give rise to privacy concerns and the danger that the information about those persons may be used for illicit reasons. The advent of increasingly effective methods for creating individualized medicines should satisfy all patients' needs, which could be challenging depending on each person's specific disease state (Cecchin & Stocco, 2020). Additionally, because personalized medicine procedures may cost more up front, paying for them down the road may be difficult. If multiple stakeholders are to embrace it, better ways for teaching and training healthcare professionals about customized medicine need to be developed and implemented (Jeibouei et al., 2019).

Conclusion

To improve diagnosis, prognosis, and clinical outcome prediction, genetic profiling tools in precision medicine are increasingly being combined with conventional clinicopathological examinations. Although the era of molecular characterization has seen some unmistakable achievements, panomics' promise is still largely untapped (Kingston et al., 2021). The future of precision medicine includes comprehensive multi-omics tumor characterization, dynamic liquid biopsy sample monitoring, automated inscription guided by clinical experts' input, patient enrolment in state-of-the-art clinical trials that not only examine molecular profile-drug matching but also examine the usefulness of various drug-assignment algorithms, and the addition of ionizing radiation in real-time (Gambardella et al., 2020). From a technical standpoint, the future of precision medicine will look beyond genomics and consider issues like the education and participation of end users like doctors and patients, the broadening of utilization of genotype-drug matching by means of versatile and other innovative clinical trial concepts, and the promotion of exchange of information to maximize knowledge acquisition.

The amount of druggable tumor-specific molecular abnormalities has increased significantly over the past ten years, and biomarker-matched medicines have significantly improved survival in several different cancers. Therefore, molecular pathology has become crucial for informing both treatment decisions in daily practice and tumor diagnosis and prognosis. Precision oncology has undergone a revolution thanks to the development of next-generation sequencing technology and the rise of large-scale tumor genetic profiling initiatives across institutions globally. Healthcare personnel are faced with the challenging responsibilities of result interpretation and translation as comprehensive genetic studies become more widely available in clinical and research settings. Identifying which individuals should have chemotherapy, which patients ought to receive adjuvant therapy, and which patients should not be the most important duty following an invasive breast cancer diagnosis. If adjuvant therapy is decided, the next challenge is determining which treatment or combination of treatments is best for a given patient. The first and second problems can both be solved using predictive and prognostic biomarkers, respectively (Kawaji et al., 2021).

The possibility to offer cancer patients a molecularly based customized approach is a desirable alternative in oncology. To accomplish a real and genuine transformation that could enhance every clinical result, a greater grasp of molecular biology is necessary. To advance, a multi-omics strategy will be necessary. Finding resistance mechanisms and the potential for novel combinations would be aided by the implementation of translational studies using liquid biopsies, organoids, or xenografts to examine molecular alterations triggered on by clonal pressure caused using target agents or tumor heterogeneity. To improve precision, more research is necessary.

References

Ahmed, Z. (2020). Practicing precision medicine with intelligently integrative clinical and multi-omics data analysis. *Human Genomics, 14*, 35–35.

Angius, A., Pira, G., Cossu-Rocca, P., Sotgiu, G., Saderi, L., Muroni, M. R., Virdis, P., Piras, D., Vincenzo, R., Carru, C., Coradduzza, D., Uras, M. G., Cottu, P., Fancellu, A., Orrù, S., Uva, P., & De Miglio, M. R. (2023). Deciphering clinical significance of BCL11A isoforms and protein expression roles in triple-negative breast cancer subtype. *Journal of Cancer Research and Clinical Oncology, 149*, 3951–3963.

Bitterman, D. S., Kamal, A., & Mak, R. H. (2023). An oncology artificial intelligence fact sheet for cancer clinicians. *JAMA Oncology, 9*(5), 612–614.

Bogdanovska-Todorovska, M., Petrushevska, G., Janevska, V., Spasevska, L., & Kostadinova-Kunovska, S. (2018). Standardization and optimization of fluorescence in situ hybridization (FISH) for HER-2 assessment in breast cancer: A single center experience. *Bosnian Journal of Basic Medical Sciences, 18*, 132–140.

Botham, J., Shilling, V., & Jones, J. (2021). Patient and public understanding of the concept of 'personalized medicine' in relation to cancer treatment: A systematic review. *Future Healthcare Journal, 8*, e703–e708.

Broholm, H., Born, P. W., Guterbaum, D., Dyrbye, H., & Laursμen, H. (2008). Detecting chromosomal alterations at 1p and 19q by FISH and DNA fragment analysis--a comparative study in human gliomas. *Clinical Neuropathology, 27*, 378–387.

Bronkhorst, A. J., Ungerer, V., & Holdenrieder, S. (2019). The emerging role of cell-free DNA as a molecular marker for cancer management. *Biomolecular Detection and Quantification, 17*, 100087.

Caporossi, D., Parisi, A., Fantini, C., Grazioli, E., Cerulli, C., & Dimauro, I. (2021). AlphaB-crystallin and breast cancer: Role and possible therapeutic strategies. *Cell Stress & Chaperones, 26*(1), 19–28.

Casak, S. J., Horiba, M. N., Yuan, M., Cheng, J., Lemery, S. J., Shen, Y. L., Fu, W., Moore, J. N., Li, Y., Bi, Y., Auth, D., Fesenko, N., Kluetz, P. G., Pazdur, R., & Fashoyin-Aje, L. A. (2023).

FDA approval summary: Tucatinib with trastuzumab for advanced unresectable or metastatic, chemotherapy refractory, HER2 positive RAS wild type colorectal cancer. *Clinical Cancer Research: An Official Journal of the American Association for Cancer Research*. CCR-23-1041.

Cecchin, E., & Stocco, G. (2020). Pharmacogenomics and personalized medicine. *Genes (Basel), 11*(6), 679.

Chan, A., Moy, B., Mansi, J., Ejlertsen, B., Holmes, F. A., & Chia, S. (2021). Final efficacy results of neratinib in HER2-positive hormone receptor-positive early-stage breast cancer from the phase III ExteNET trial. *Clinical Breast Cancer, 21*(1), 80–91.

Chen, S., Thacker, C., Wang, S., Young, K. A., Hoffman, R. L., & Blansfield, J. A. (2023). Adherence disparities and utilization trends of oncotype Dx assay: A national cancer database study. *The Journal of Surgical Research, 286*, 65–73.

Cheung, P. K., Ma, M. H., Tse, H. F., Yeung, K. F., Tsang, H. F., Chu, M. K. M., Kan, C. M., Cho, W. C. S., Ng, L. B. W., Chan, L. W. C., & Wong, S. C. C. (2019). The applications of metabolomics in the molecular diagnostics of cancer. *Expert Review of Molecular Diagnostics, 19*(9), 785–793.

Chrzanowska, N. M., Kowalewski, J., & Lewandowska, M. A. (2020). Use of fluorescence in situ hybridization (FISH) in diagnosis and tailored therapies in solid tumors. *Molecules, 25*(8), 1864.

Cimino-Mathews, A. (2021). Novel uses of immunohistochemistry in breast pathology: Interpretation and pitfalls. *Modern Pathology: An Official Journal of the United States and Canadian Academy of Pathology, Inc, 34*(Suppl 1), 62–77.

Clift, A. K., Dodwell, D., Lord, S., Petrou, S., Brady, S. M., Collins, G. S., & Hippisley-Cox, J. (2022). The current status of risk-stratified breast screening. *British Journal of Cancer, 126*, 533–550.

Davey, M. G., & Kerin, M. J. (2023). Molecular profiling in contemporary breast cancer management. *British Journal of Surgery, 110*, 743–745.

Dinh, P., Graham, J. D., Elder, E. N., Kabir, M., Doan, T. B., French, J., Meybodi, F., Hui, R., Wilcken, N. R., Harnett, P. R., Hsu, J., Stuart, K. E., Wang, T., Ahern, V., Brennan, M., Fox, S. B., Dear, R. F., Lim, E., White, M., Mann, G. B., et al. (2022). Impact of the EndoPredict genomic assay on treatment decisions for estrogen receptor-positive early breast cancer patients: Benefits of physician selective testing. *Breast Cancer Research and Treatment, 191*(3), 501–511.

Ellsworth, R. E., Decewicz, D. J., Shriver, C. D., & Ellsworth, D. L. (2010). Breast cancer in the personal genomics era. *Current Genomics, 11*(3), 146–161.

Falcone, R., Lombardi, P., Filetti, M., Fabi, A., Altamura, V., Scambia, G., & Daniele, G. (2023). Molecular profile and matched targeted therapy for advanced breast cancer patients. *Current Oncology (Toronto, Ont.), 30*(2), 2501–2509.

Feng, Y., Spezia, M., Huang, S., Yuan, C., Zeng, Z., Zhang, L., Ji, X., Liu, W., Huang, B., Luo, W., Liu, B., Lei, Y., Du, S., Vuppalapati, A., Luu, H. H., Haydon, R. C., He, T. C., & Ren, G. (2018). Breast cancer development and progression: Risk factors, cancer stem cells, signaling pathways, genomics, and molecular pathogenesis. *Genes & Diseases, 5*(2), 77–106.

Gambardella, V., Tarazona, N., Cejalvo, J. M., Lombardi, P., Huerta, M., Roselló, S., Fleitas, T., Roda, D., & Cervantes, A. (2020). Personalized medicine: Recent progress in cancer therapy. *Cancers, 12*(4), 1009.

Garcia-Martinez, L., Zhang, Y., Nakata, Y., Chan, H. L., & Morey, L. (2021). Epigenetic mechanisms in breast cancer therapy and resistance. *Nature Communications, 12*, 1786.

Goetz, L. H., & Schork, N. J. (2018). Personalized medicine: Motivation, challenges, and progress. *Fertility and Sterility, 109*, 952–963.

Hamdan, D., Nguyen, T. T., Leboeuf, C., Meles, S., Janin, A., & Bousquet, G. (2019). Genomics applied to the treatment of breast cancer. *Oncotarget, 10*(46), 4786–4801.

Hastings, R. J., Bown, N., Tibiletti, M. G., Debiec-Rychter, M., Vanni, R., & Espinet, B. (2016). Guidelines for cytogenetic investigations in tumors. *European Journal of Human Genetics, 24*, 6–13.

Herzog, S. K., & Fuqua, S. A. W. (2022). *ESR1* mutations and therapeutic resistance in metastatic breast cancer: Progress and remaining challenges. *British Journal of Cancer, 126*, 174–186.

Hoeben, A., Joosten, E. A., & van den Beuken-van Everdingen, M. H. (2021). Personalized medicine: Recent progress in cancer therapy. *Cancers, 13*(2), 242.

Holden, C., Bignell, L., Mukhopadhyay, S., & Jones, C. (2019). The public perception of the facilitators and barriers to implementing personalized medicine: A systematic review. *Personalized Medicine, 2019*(16), 151.

Huber, D., Voith von Voithenberg, L., & Kaigala, G. V. (2018). Fluorescence in situ hybridization (FISH): History, limitations and what to expect from micro-scale FISH? *Micro and Nano Engineering, 1*, 15–24.

Jeibouei, S., Akbari, M. E., Kalbasi, A., Aref, A. R., Ajoudanian, M., Rezvani, A., & Zali, H. (2019). Personalized medicine in breast cancer: Pharmacogenomics approaches. *Pharmacogenomics and Personalized Medicine, 12*, 59–73.

Johansson, H. J., Socciarelli, F., Vacanti, N. M., Haugen, M. H., Zhu, Y., Siavelis, I., Fernandez-Woodbridge, A., Aure, M. R., Sennblad, B., Vesterlund, M., Branca, R. M., Orre, L. M., Huss, M., Fredlund, E., Beraki, E., Garred, Ø., Boekel, J., Sauer, T., Zhao, W., Nord, S., et al. (2019). Breast cancer quantitative proteome and proteogenomic landscape. *Nature Communications, 10*(1), 1600.

Kalocsay, M., Berberich, M. J., Everley, R. A., Nariya, M. K., Chung, M., Gaudio, B., Victor, C., Bradshaw, G. A., Eisert, R. J., Hafner, M., Sorger, P. K., Mills, C. E., & Subramanian, K. (2023). Proteomic profiling across breast cancer cell lines and models. *Scientific Data, 10*(1), 514.

Kawaji, H., Kubo, M., Yamashita, N., Yamamoto, H., Kai, M., Kajihara, A., Yamada, M., Kurata, K., Kaneshiro, K., Harada, Y., Hayashi, S., Shimazaki, A., Mori, H., Akiyoshi, S., Oki, E., Oda, Y., Baba, E., Mori, M., & Nakamura, M. (2021). Comprehensive molecular profiling broadens treatment options for breast cancer patients. *Cancer Medicine, 10*, 529–539.

Kingston, B., Cutts, R. J., Bye, H., Beaney, M., Walsh-Crestani, G., Hrebien, S., Swift, C., Kilburn, L. S., Kernaghan, S., Moretti, L., Wilkinson, K., Wardley, A. M., Macpherson, I. R., Baird, R. D., Roylance, R., Reis-Filho, J. S., Hubank, M., Faull, I., Banks, K. C., Lanman, R. B., Garcia-Murillas, I., Bliss, J. M., Ring, A., & Turner, N. C. (2021). Genomic profile of advanced breast cancer in circulating tumor DNA. *Nature Communications, 12*, 2423.

Kinnel, B., Singh, S. K., Oprea-Ilies, G., & Singh, R. (2023). Targeted therapy and mechanisms of drug resistance in breast cancer. *Cancers, 15*(4), 1320.

Kittaneh, M., Montero, A. J., & Glück, S. (2013). Molecular profiling for breast cancer: A comprehensive review. *Biomark Cancer, 5*, 61–70.

Koboldt, D., Fulton, R., McLellan, M., Schmidt, H., Kalicki-Veizer, J., McMichael, J., Fulton, J. F., Dooling, L. L., Ding, D. J., Mardis, L., Wilson, E. R., Ally, R. K., Balasundaram, A., Butterfield, M., Carlsen, Y. S. N., Carter, R., Chu, C., Chuah, A., Chun, E., Coope, H. E., Dhalla, R. J. N., Guin, N., Hirst, R., Hirst, C., Holt, M., Lee, R. A., Li, D., Mayo, H. I., Moore, M., Mungall, R. A., Pleasance, A. J., & Gordon Robertson, E. A. (2012). Comprehensive molecular portraits of human breast Tumors. *Nature, 490*, 61–70.

Kuburich, N. A., den Hollander, P., Pietz, J. T., & Mani, S. A. (2022). Vimentin and cytokeratin: Good alone, bad together. *Seminars in Cancer Biology, 86*(Pt 3), 816–826.

Lal, S., McCart Reed, A. E., de Luca, X. M., & Simpson, P. T. (2017). Molecular signatures in breast cancer. *Methods, 131*, 135–146.

Li, C. J., Chen, H. M., & Lai, J. C. (2020). Diagnostic, prognostic, and predictive biomarkers in breast cancer. *Journal of Oncology, 2020*, 1835691.

Markham, A. (2021). Margetuximab: First approval. *Drugs, 81*(5), 599–604.

Mehmood, S., Faheem, M., Ismail, H., Farhat, S. M., Ali, M., Younis, S., & Asghar, M. N. (2022). Breast cancer resistance likelihood and personalized treatment through integrated multiomics. *Frontiers in Molecular Biosciences, 9*, 783494.

Merker, J. D., Oxnard, G. R., Compton, C., Diehn, M., Hurley, P., Lazar, A. J., Lindeman, N., Lockwood, C. M., Rai, A. J., Schilsky, R. L., Tsimberidou, A. M., Vasalos, P., Billman, B. L.,

Oliver, T. K., Bruinooge, S. S., Hayes, D. F., & Turner, N. C. (2018). Circulating tumor DNA analysis in patients with cancer: American Society of Clinical Oncology and College of American Pathologists joint review. *Archives of Pathology & Laboratory Medicine, 142*, 1242–1253.

Milbury, C. A., Creeden, J., Yip, W. K., Smith, D. L., Pattani, V., Maxwell, K., Sawchyn, B., Gjoerup, O., Meng, W., Skoletsky, J., Concepcion, A. D., Tang, Y., Bai, X., Dewal, N., Ma, P., Bailey, S. T., Thornton, J., Pavlick, D. C., Frampton, G. M., Lieber, D., & Vietz, C. (2022). Clinical and analytical validation of FoundationOne®CDx, a comprehensive genomic profiling assay for solid tumors. *PLoS One, 17*(3), e0264138.

Mohyuddin, G. R., Aziz, M., Britt, A., Wade, L., Sun, W., Baranda, J., Al-Rajabi, R., Saeed, A., & Kasi, A. (2020). Similar response rates and survival with PARP inhibitors for patients with solid tumors harboring somatic versus germline BRCA mutations: A meta-analysis and systematic review. *BMC Cancer, 20*, 507.

Moorcraft, S. Y., Gonzalez, D., & Walker, B. A. (2015). Understanding next generation sequencing in oncology: A guide for oncologists. *Critical Reviews in Oncology/Hematology, 96*, 463–474.

Moore, D. C., & Guinigundo, A. S. (2023). The role of biomarkers in guiding clinical decision-making in oncology. *Journal of the Advanced Practitioner in Oncology, 14*(1), 15–37.

Nabi, H. (2022). Personalized approaches for the prevention and treatment of breast cancer. *Journal of Personalized Medicine, 12*(8), 1201.

Narayan, P., Osgood, C. L., Singh, H., Chiu, H. J., Ricks, T. K., Chiu Yuen Chow, E., Qiu, J., Song, P., Yu, J., Namuswe, F., Guiterrez-Lugo, M., Hou, S., Pierce, W. F., Goldberg, K. B., Tang, S., Amiri-Kordestani, L., Theoret, M. R., Pazdur, R., & Beaver, J. A. (2021). FDA approval summary: Fam-trastuzumab Deruxtecan-Nxki for the treatment of unresectable or metastatic HER2-positive breast cancer. *Clinical Cancer Research: An Official Journal of the American Association for Cancer Research, 27*(16), 4478–4485.

Parsons, J., & Francavilla, C. (2020). Omics approaches to explore the breast cancer landscape. *Frontiers in Cell and Developmental Biology, 7*, 395.

Playdon, M. C., Moore, S. C., Derkach, A., Reedy, J., Subar, A. F., Sampson, J. N., Albanes, D., Gu, F., Kontto, J., Lassale, C., Liao, L. M., Männistö, S., Mondul, A. M., Weinstein, S. J., Irwin, M. L., Mayne, S. T., & Stolzenberg-Solomon, R. (2017). Identifying biomarkers of dietary patterns by using metabolomics. *The American Journal of Clinical Nutrition, 105*(2), 450–465.

Provenzano, M., Rotundo, S., Chiodini, P., Gagliardi, I., Michael, A., Angotti, E., Borrelli, S., Serra, R., Foti, D., De Sarro, G., & Andreucci, M. (2020). Contribution of predictive and prognostic biomarkers to clinical research on chronic kidney disease. *International Journal of Molecular Sciences, 21*(16), 5846.

Pu, T., Guo, P., Qiu, Y., Chen, S., Yang, L., Sun, L., Ye, F., & Bu, H. (2015). Quantitative real-time polymerase chain reaction is an alternative method for the detection of HER-2 amplification in formalin-fixed paraffin-embedded breast cancer samples. *International Journal of Clinical and Experimental Pathology, 8*(9), 10565–10574.

Qing, X., Yuan, C., & Wang, K. (2023). Characterization of protein-based risk signature to predict prognosis and evaluate the tumor immune environment in breast cancer. *Breast Cancer (Tokyo, Japan), 30*(3), 424–435.

Rakha, E. A., Reis-Filho, J. S., & Ellis, I. O. (2010). Combinatorial biomarker expression in breast cancer. *Breast Cancer Research and Treatment, 120*(2), 293–308.

Robson, M., Im, S. A., Senkus, E., Xu, B., Domchek, S. M., Masuda, N., Delaloge, S., Li, W., Tung, N., Armstrong, A., Wu, W., Goessl, C., Runswick, S., & Conte, P. (2017). Olaparib for metastatic breast cancer in patients with a germline BRCA mutation. *The New England Journal of Medicine, 377*(6), 523–533.

Rolfo, C., Mack, P. C., Scagliotti, G. V., Baas, P., Barlesi, F., Bivona, T. G., Herbst, R. S., Mok, T. S., Peled, N., Pirker, R., Raez, L. E., Reck, M., Riess, J. W., Sequist, L. V., Shepherd, F. A., Sholl, L. M., Tan, D. S. W., Wakelee, H. A., Wistuba, I. I., Wynes, M. W., et al. (2018). Liquid biopsy for advanced non-small cell lung cancer (NSCLC): A statement paper from the IASLC. *Journal of Thoracic Oncology, 13*(9), 1248–1268.

Sabari, J. K., Offin, M., Stephens, D., Ni, A., Lee, A., Pavlakis, N., et al. (2019). A prospective study of circulating tumor DNA to guide matched targeted therapy in lung cancers. *Journal of the National Cancer Institute, 111*(6), 575–583.

Sabatier, R., Gonçalves, A., & Bertucci, F. (2014). Personalized medicine: Present and future of breast cancer management. *Critical Reviews in Oncology/Hematology, 91*(3), 223–233.

Sadee, W., Wang, D., Hartmann, K., & Toland, A. E. (2023). Pharmacogenomics: Driving personalized medicine. *Pharmacological Reviews, 75*(4), 789–814.

Sarhadi, V. K., & Armengol, G. (2022). Molecular biomarkers in cancer. *Biomolecules, 12*(8), 1021.

Schmidt, D. R., Patel, R., Kirsch, D. G., Lewis, C. A., Vander Heiden, M. G., & Locasale, J. W. (2021). Metabolomics in cancer research and emerging applications in clinical oncology. *CA: A Cancer Journal for Clinicians, 71*(4), 333–358.

Siegel, R. L., Miller, K. D., Wagle, N. S., & Jemal, A. (2023). Cancer statistics, 2023. *CA: A Cancer Journal for Clinicians, 73*(1), 17–48.

Sun, L., Wu, A., Bean, G. R., Hagemann, I. S., & Lin, C. Y. (2021). Molecular testing in breast cancer: Current status and future directions. *The Journal of Molecular Diagnostics: JMD, 23*(11), 1422–1432.

Tarighati, E., Keivan, H., & Mahani, H. (2023). A review of prognostic and predictive biomarkers in breast cancer. *Clinical and Experimental Medicine, 23*(1), 1–16.

Tendl, K. A., & Bago-Horvath, Z. (2020). Molecular profiling in breast cancer - ready for clinical routine? *Memo, 13*, 445–449.

Tufail, M., Cui, J., & Wu, C. (2022). Breast cancer: Molecular mechanisms of underlying resistance and therapeutic approaches. *American Journal of Cancer Research, 12*(7), 2920–2949.

Wainberg, M., Sinnott-Armstrong, N., Mancuso, N., Barbeira, A. N., Knowles, D. A., Golan, D., Ermel, R., Ruusalepp, A., Quertermous, T., Hao, K., Björkegren, J. L. M., Im, H. K., Pasaniuc, B., Rivas, M. A., & Kundaje, A. (2019). Opportunities and challenges for transcriptome-wide association studies. *Nature Genetics, 51*(4), 592–599.

Woodhouse, R., Li, M., Hughes, J., Delfosse, D., Skoletsky, J., Ma, P., Meng, W., Dewal, N., Milbury, C., Clark, T., Donahue, A., Stover, D., Kennedy, M., Dacpano-Komansky, J., Burns, C., Vietz, C., Alexander, B., Hegde, P., & Dennis, L. (2020). Clinical and analytical validation of FoundationOne liquid CDx, a novel 324-gene cfDNA-based comprehensive genomic profiling assay for cancers of solid tumor origin. *PLoS One, 15*(9), e0237802.

You, Z., Xu, Y., Wan, W., Zhou, L., Li, J., Zhou, T., Shi, Y., & Liu, W. (2019). TP53INP2 contributes to autophagosome formation by promoting LC3-ATG7 interaction. *Autophagy, 15*(8), 1309–1321.

Zhang, X. (2023). Molecular classification of breast cancer: Relevance and challenges. *Archives of Pathology & Laboratory Medicine, 147*(1), 46–51.

Emerging Therapeutic Approaches in Drug-Resistant Breast Cancer

Thulo Molefi, Talent Chipiti, Victoria P. Belancio, and Zodwa Dlamini

Abstract Breast cancer, a heterogeneous and complex disease, remains a significant healthcare challenge around the world, with drug resistance being a major impediment to successful treatment. Traditional treatment regimens are frequently met with resistance mechanisms, resulting in treatment failure and disease progression. In the past few years, there has been a paradigm shift in the approach to battling drug-resistant breast cancer, with the introduction of innovative treatment techniques including immunotherapy, gene therapy, and epigenetic modelling. Immunotherapy has shown great promise in terms of boosting the host immunity to detect and eradicate cancer cells, as well as efficiently overcoming resistance mechanisms. New treatments for drug-resistant breast cancer show promise in clinical trials, including immune checkpoint inhibitors and CAR-T cell therapy. Another novel approach is gene therapy, which addresses drug resistance through targeted genetic modifications. Scientists are researching ways to combat drug-resistant breast cancer cells, including gene editing, gene silencing, and oncolytic viruses. The aim is to increase sensitivity in these cells and improve treatment outcomes for patients. Gene therapy can modulate drug metabolism and improve drug delivery

T. Molefi (✉)
SAMRC Precision Oncology Research Unit (PORU), SARChI Chair in Precision Oncology and Cancer Prevention (POCP), Pan African Cancer Research Institute (PACRI), University of Pretoria, Pretoria, South Africa

Department of Medical Oncology, Faculty of Health Sciences, Steve Biko Academic Hospital, University of Pretoria, Hatfield, South Africa
e-mail: thulo.molefi@up.ac.za

T. Chipiti · Z. Dlamini
SAMRC Precision Oncology Research Unit (PORU), DSI/NRF SARChI Chair in Precision Oncology and Cancer Prevention (POCP), Pan African Cancer Research Institute (PACRI), University of Pretoria, Pretoria, South Africa
e-mail: talent.chipiti@up.ac.za; Zodwa.Dlamini@up.ac.za

V. P. Belancio
Department of Structural and Cellular Biology, Tulane Cancer Center, Tulane School of Medicine, New Orleans, LA, USA
e-mail: vperepe@tulane.edu

Z. Dlamini (ed.), *Overcoming Breast Cancer Therapy Resistance*,
https://doi.org/10.1007/978-3-031-52860-6_13

which holds promise for circumventing resistance mechanisms. Epigenetic modelling is a powerful tool to reprogram cancer cells by manipulating epigenetic marks and overcoming drug resistance. Epigenetic modifiers hold the potential to revive the sensitivity of drugs in breast cancer cells that have lost their initial responsiveness. This valuable information suggests a promising avenue for the development of effective treatment options for patients with drug-resistant breast cancer. Combination therapy can be a valuable tool in attacking various oncogenic signaling pathways at the same time, which will aid in overcoming resistance to medication and achieving improved clinical results for patients with breast cancer.

Keywords Breast cancer · Drug resistance · Epigenetic modelling · Drug resistance · Immunotherapy · Gene therapy

Introduction

Cancer is the second-most common cause of mortality globally. As a result, there is an urgent need for novel approaches to treating tumors, particularly solid tumors. Solid tumors, including breast cancer, are the primary cause of cancer-related deaths among women. Breast cancer is a significant public health concern for women due to its wide variety of manifestations (Salvioni et al., 2020). Chemotherapy, radiation, surgery, and hormone therapy are effective in early breast cancer. However, they only provide palliative care in advanced stages and have various side effects. Moreover, individuals using present systemic medications are known to experience an array of adverse effects (Ramírez et al., 2018). Effective treatment of breast cancer requires innovative therapeutic techniques like immunotherapy, gene therapy, and epigenetic modelling (Jazieh et al., 2020; Li et al., 2023).

In recent years, there has been exploration of novel medicines for treating BC, from preclinical to clinical trial phases. This chapter will go through the unique therapy options available for each form of BC, as well as those that are currently being investigated. The motivation for the use of each treatment modality will be explored, also highlighting the limitations and prospects. Alternative therapies for breast cancer have been used recently due to the poor effectiveness of traditional treatments. Recent progress in comprehending the molecular foundation of breast cancer enables the use of genetic resources for therapeutic interventions. In this context, gene therapy has become a popular treatment for breast cancer and other tumors due to its potential efficacy. Due to this, there are multiple targets available for gene therapy to treat breast cancer (Sheikh-Hosseini et al., 2020). Immune checkpoint inhibitors in immunotherapy are a game-changing treatment that enables the immune system to recognize and attack cancer cells, revolutionizing cancer treatment. Immunological checkpoint inhibitors, such as programmed cell death protein 1 (PD-1), programmed death-ligand 1 (PD-L1), and cytotoxic T-lymphocyte-associated protein 4 (CTLA-4) agents, have demonstrated encouraging outcomes in the treatment of diverse types of cancers. These agents work by inhibiting the immune checkpoints, which are mechanisms that cancer cells use to evade detection and destruction by the immune system. By blocking these checkpoints, these inhibitors enable the immune system to recognize and attack cancer cells more effectively, thereby improving treatment outcomes (Abdou et al., 2022). Immunotherapy can target resistant cells in drug-resistant breast cancer and make them more receptive to standard treatments. Ongoing clinical trials are exploring the effectiveness of immune checkpoint inhibitors in this regard and shedding light on potential synergies between immunotherapy and standard therapies.

Gene-based techniques to combat resistance to medications in breast cancer have increased momentum. Gene therapy approaches, such as CRISPR-Cas9 gene editing, hold the potential to modify drug-resistant cells at the genetic level (Sheikh-Hosseini et al., 2020). Researchers hope to restore medication sensitivity by targeting critical genes implicated in resistance mechanisms, such as those involved in drug efflux pumps or altered drug metabolism. Epigenetic changes strongly impact breast cancer treatment resistance. Another alternative approach to explore is using epigenetic modifiers, such as DNA methyltransferase inhibitors and histone deacetylase inhibitors, to reverse drug-resistant epigenetic alterations (Terranova-Barberio et al., 2017; Vernier et al., 2020). Epigenetic therapies have the ability not only to sensitize drug-resistant cells to treatment but also to prevent resistance from developing in the first place. Also, directly delivering therapeutic genes encoding anticancer drugs into drug-resistant cells is a novel technique for selectively eliminating these cells while sparing normal tissues (Zhang et al., 2023). This chapter explores the most recent discoveries, problems, and possibilities afforded by these novel techniques, emphasizing their potential to influence the future of breast cancer treatment.

Immunotherapy

The field of oncology has seen significant advancements in recent times, particularly in the area of cancer immunotherapy. This form of treatment has shown promising results in terms of its antitumor capabilities and long-term therapeutic benefits for a range of cancer types, including triple-negative breast cancer (TNBC) (Debien et al., 2023). Currently, immune checkpoint inhibitors are the only immunotherapy approach for breast cancer (BC) that has approval from the FDA. Various novel immune-modulatory strategies are being investigated with promising results at different stages of preclinical and clinical trials (Savas et al., 2016). Breast cancer (BC) is a serious disease that often does not respond well to traditional treatments. Because of this, researchers are searching for new immunotherapeutic strategies to treat BC. The TNBC subtype of BC appears to be more responsive to immunotherapy, as it has higher levels of tumor-infiltrating lymphocytes, PD-L1 expression, and tumor mutation burden. As a result, immuno-oncology is a promising field for advancing TNBC research (Abdou et al., 2022; Li et al., 2023; Mohamed et al., 2013). Immunotherapies have become increasingly important in treating certain tumors due to the crucial role of the immune system in causing cancer (Guha et al., 2022). The roots of cancer immunotherapy date back to 1891 when Dr. William Coley set out on a quest to find a more effective way to treat sarcoma beyond surgery. During his research, he discovered that some patients' response to infection was connected to tumor regression. The journal *Science* praised cancer immunotherapy as a breakthrough of the year in 2013 (Li et al., 2023). Drs. James P. Alison and Tasuku Honjo won the 2018 Nobel Prize in Physiology and Medicine for discovering cancer therapy through immune regulation inhibition.

Cancer immunotherapy is a treatment that aggressively fights cancer cells using either drugs or the immune system. Immunotherapy could cure a wide range of cancers. It can be used on its own or in conjunction with chemotherapy and/or other cancer treatments. Our body's immune system is commonly breached by cancer, allowing cancer cells to thrive (Li et al., 2023). One of cancer hallmarks is the use of the process of immunoediting to its advantage to avoid immune destruction. Immunoediting occurs in three stages; ideally, cancer is discovered via cancer-specific antigens during the first phase of elimination and killed by immunosurveillance by the body's immune systems (Abbott & Ustoyev, 2019). Some tumors, however, survive this phase and proceed to the following equilibrium phase. In this stage, cancerous cells reside alongside the immune system for an extended period until they become resistant to the body's antitumor response and advance to the next phase. During the third evasion phase, cancer cells adopt adaptive and evasive tactics, including the loss of antigens, manipulation of cytokine expression, and an increase in immune checkpoint proteins (Abbott & Ustoyev, 2019; Kennedy & Salama, 2020; Li et al., 2023).

The current arsenal of cancer immunotherapies includes the use of monoclonal antibodies (mAbs), immune checkpoint inhibitors (ICIs), toxins, tumor necrosis factors, oncolytic viral platforms (OVPs), cancer vaccines, adoptive cell therapy (ACT), chimeric antigen receptor (CAR)-T cells, and a variety of combinatorial approaches (Guha et al., 2022; Li et al., 2023). Cutting-edge immunotherapies, such as immune checkpoint inhibitors (ICIs) and CAR-T cell therapies, show great promise in the field of cancer treatment. While CAR-T cell technologies have demonstrated remarkable efficacy in treating hematological tumors, they may not be as effective when it comes to solid tumors like breast cancer (BC). This is because CAR T-cells are delivered via the bloodstream and lymphatic system, providing a wider area of tumor contact in the bloodstream (Filin et al., 2020). Treating solid tumors has been difficult since the basic therapeutic methods for solid tumors, such as surgical resection, chemotherapy, and radiation, do not offer long-term disease control. If the hurdles provided by solid tumor treatment can be overcome, immunotherapy may be a promising treatment option (Lee Ventola, 2017). The ultimate aim of cancer immunotherapy is to stimulate the patient's immune system and redirect immune cells to attack and eliminate cancerous cells, thereby achieving sustainable disease control. Nonetheless, the weakened anticancer immunity of patients can lead to reduced effectiveness of immunotherapy. Cancer burden usually leads to an imbalance between immune stimulatory and inhibitory pathways in the tumor microenvironment (TME), in which immunosuppression outweighs effective immunotherapy responsiveness. Various mechanisms can either promote or inhibit tumor progression through changes in chemokines and cytokine profiles. This can activate transcription factors like STAT, SMAD, AP-1, NFκB, and caspases. Cytokines also can control the pro- or anti-tumorigenic activities. Pro-tumorigenic cytokines include TNFα, IL-6, IL-7, and IL-23, while antitumorigenic cytokines include IL-12, IFNγ, and TRAIL (Filin et al., 2020; Guha et al., 2022). The immune system relies on lymphocytes, M1, and DCs macrophages to mount an antitumor response, while MDSCs and Tregs impede tumor immunity (Guha et al., 2022). To achieve better outcomes in shrinking solid tumors, it is essential to create a tumor microenvironment (TME) that promotes normal cellular immune function and avoids immunosuppressive pathways (Lee Ventola, 2017).

Immune Checkpoint Inhibitors

Immune checkpoint inhibitors (ICIs), also known as monoclonal antibodies, are a vital component of cancer immunotherapy as they help boost the immune system. They work by stopping factors that prevent T-cells from being active, which helps to block targets that hinder the growth of T-lymphocytes. As a result, ICIs are an important weapon in the battle against cancer. The immune response is activated by regulators like CTLA-4, PD-1, and PD-L1, which protect the body from pathogens (Filin et al., 2020). The immune system in the human body has a built-in mechanism to prevent it from attacking healthy cells too harshly. Whenever certain molecules attach to either cancerous or suppressor immune cells, they trigger a signaling process in T-cells. This signal causes the immune system to become less effective in fighting threats, leading to reduced functionality and less favorable cytokine profiles. Fortunately, ICIs can help prevent the binding of these checkpoint proteins to their ligands, which stops the "off" signal and allows the immune system to continue fighting (Filin et al., 2020; Guha et al., 2022).

Back in 2011, the FDA approved ipilimumab as the initial checkpoint inhibitor of CTLA-4. In subsequent years, monoclonal antibodies like pembrolizumab, nivolumab, atezolizumab, and durvalumab, which target PD1 and PD-L1, have also gained approval. These antibodies effectively block the PD-L1/PD-1 signaling pathway and are widely recognized as valuable anticancer treatments (Filin et al., 2020; Robert, 2020). The combination of PD-1 and PD-L1, either alone or in conjunction with chemotherapy, has demonstrated efficacy in the treatment of over 50 different types of cancers (Robert, 2020). Approximately 3000 clinical trials to evaluate T-cell modulators are ongoing as recorded in 2020. Numerous clinical trials are currently investigating the PD-1/PD-L1 axis or CTLA-4 signaling. Some of the commonly used T-cell PD-1 inhibitors include Pembrolizumab (Keytruda), Nivolumab (Opdivo), and Cemiplimab (Libtayo). Additionally, PD-L1 inhibitors such as Atezolizumab (Tecentriq), Avelumab (Bavencio), and Durvalumab (Imfinzi) are available, while a CTLA-4 inhibitor called Ipilimumab (Yervoy) is also utilized. Both anti-CTLA-4 (ipilimumab) and anti-PD-1 (nivolumab and pembrolizumab) have shown effectiveness in immunotherapy (Guha et al., 2022; Lisi et al., 2022).

A clinical trial was conducted to study the effects of combining nivolumab and ipilimumab, which are PD-L1 and CTLA-4 inhibitors, respectively. The results showed that patients with various types of cancer, including breast cancer, had a higher objective response rate, longer progression-free survival, and a lower risk of disease progression or mortality (Larkin et al., 2015). An effective approach for enhancing the efficacy of PD-1/PDL-1 ICIs is to focus on additional immune checkpoint molecules present in the TME, like TIM-3 and LAG-3. Given the substantial redundancy and physiological intricacy of solid organ TMEs, a combination immunotherapy tactic employing multiple checkpoint inhibitors appears to be a viable solution.

Recent studies have shown that immunotherapy can be an effective treatment for certain types of tumors such as melanoma, renal cell carcinoma, lung cancer, and bladder cancer. However, early research suggests that using immunotherapy as the sole form of treatment for breast cancer may have limited success (Guha et al., 2022). This is because breast cancer has lower immunogenicity compared to other types of cancer, which may impact the effectiveness of immunotherapy (Savas et al., 2016).

Toxins and Tumor Necrosis Factor

Between the 1930s and 1960s, bacteria were used to treat tumors by causing necrosis (O'Malley et al., 2009; Abbott & Ustoyev, 2019). However, this approach was not very effective and was not widely adopted. In the 1970s, tumor necrosis factor (TNF) was identified as a significant development in cancer immunotherapy (Abbott & Ustoyev, 2019). Unfortunately, TNF had severe side effects such as fever, rigors, and pulmonary edema when delivered through systemic infusion (Balkwill, 2009). Due to these harmful effects, TNF's usage was limited, and it has since been replaced by other superior medications (Abbott & Ustoyev, 2019).

Vaccination by DNA and RNA

Cancer vaccines come in three types: cellular, viral vector, and molecular (DNA, peptide, or RNA). Cellular vaccines can be made with either an autologous or allogeneic tumor cell line. Dendritic cells are used in the development of cellular cancer vaccines because they can produce antigens (Jou et al., 2021). Since breast cancer can spread throughout the body, vaccination techniques that activate the immune system may potentially reduce cancer in patients (Dastjerd et al., 2022). Recombinant vaccines, which typically contain bare DNA expressing tumor-associated antigens (TAA), are administered locally (intramuscular or intradermal) or systemically to stimulate an anticancer immune response. In addition to DNA-based vaccinations,

RNA-based vaccines, primarily mRNA vaccines, have been created in the last decade (Shanmugaraj et al., 2020).

Research conducted by Debien et al. in 2023 suggests that viral vector vaccines can activate immune responses that target tumors by introducing antigens through T-cell priming. Similarly, mRNA vaccines can encode antigens that lead to the production of proteins upon internalization, which can trigger an immunological response. However, developing vaccines for solid tumor types can be challenging due to pre-existing immunosuppressive TMEs that can limit patients' ability to mount significant antitumor responses to tumor antigens, as noted by Jou et al. in 2021. Cancer vaccines can be divided into two categories: prophylactic or preventative vaccines that aim to reduce cancer incidence, morbidity, and mortality, and therapeutic cancer vaccines that are used to treat an existing disease or prevent relapse or metastases (Lollini et al., 2006; Morse et al., 2021).

When DNA and RNA vaccines are administered, they present antigens via major histocompatibility complex class I (MHC-I), which stimulates cell-mediated immune responses that are comparable to those seen in viral infections. This is a desirable characteristic of vaccines (Arabi et al., 2022). Cancer vaccines that use DNA or RNA offer a potential way to elicit a targeted and long-lasting immune response against tumor antigens (TAs). TAs are mostly proteins that are overexpressed in tumor tissue and play a significant role in tumor development, progression, and metastasis (Lopes et al., 2019). However, compared to protein-based or whole viral immunizations, a significant drawback of DNA and RNA vaccines is their lack of immunogenicity. Cancer vaccines can be categorized as either prophylactic or therapeutic immunizations.

DNA vaccines containing genes that encode TAs are called plasmids. These vaccines can activate or boost the adaptive immune response against tumor cells that carry TAs. Additionally, they serve as potent "danger signals" that stimulate DNA-sensing pathways within cells, leading to an innate immune response. The presence of CpG motifs and the double-stranded structure of cancer DNA vaccines are responsible for this effect (Lopes et al., 2019). The targets for mRNA-based vaccines are more diverse, ranging from tumor-associated antigens (TAAs) to tumor-specific antigens (TSAs) and tumor microenvironment (TME) antigens (Jiang & Liu, 2023). For cancer vaccines to be effective, they should ideally elicit type 1 CD4+ and CD8+ T-cell responses against tumor-associated antigens (TAAs) and/or tumor-specific antigens (TSAs). The most commonly targeted breast cancer antigens in DNA and RNA vaccine technology include MUC-1, HER2/neu, hTERT, CD105, Yb-1, SOX2, CDH3, and MDM2 antigens (Solinas et al., 2020). Currently, phase III clinical trials on BC vaccines performed in metastatic settings using MUC-1 and adjuvant settings utilizing the HER2-peptide vaccine (NeuVax) have not yielded favorable outcomes (Jiang & Liu, 2023; Solinas et al., 2020). This failure might be attributed to patient selection considerations (disease burden, degree of past treatment, tumor immune contexture, and TAAs to target). According to Ayers et al. (2017), poor immunogenicity of the vaccine can be due to the antigen used or the delivery platform used, such as a peptide, dendritic cell, DNA, RNA, or tumor cell lysate.

Breast cancer is a type of cancer that is extensively studied for the development of vaccines. It ranks third in frequency. The most common antigens associated with the tumor that is targeted for treatment are HER2, MUC-1, carcinoembryonic antigen (CEA), and hTERT. However, standard cancer vaccines are currently not available for treating breast cancer. Instead, researchers are exploring alternative platforms for vaccine development and combination immunotherapy techniques, such as the use of ICB (Solinas et al., 2020). Unfortunately, none of the cancer vaccines developed so far have shown significant therapeutic benefits in phase III studies, whether in the metastatic or adjuvant context. The lack of success is due to ineffective vaccination formulations (tumor antigens and adjuvants) that do not efficiently activate tumor-specific T-cells and immune suppression pathways that dominate the tumor site, as well as a lack of relevant response indicators (Jiang & Liu, 2023).

Combinational Therapy of Breast Cancer Vaccines (BCVs)

Recent studies have revealed that Immune Checkpoint Blockers (ICB) show promise as an effective treatment for metastatic TNBC. However, when combined with Trastuzumab, ICB has been associated with increased side effects and does not significantly improve progression-free survival for HER2-positive metastatic BC, as noted by Antonarelli et al. (2021) and Emens et al. (2020). Fortunately, there is a promising and innovative approach that combines immunization with ICB to combat cancer tolerance. ICB can block inhibitory receptors like PD-1/PD-L1 and CTLA-4, enabling effector immune cells to attack cancer cells. Studies have also shown that cancer vaccines can stimulate T-cells, resulting in increased inhibitory receptor expression on the cell surface (Lai et al., 2021). Increased IFN production by tumor-specific T-cells may be the cause of this. IFN triggers the expression of PD-L1 on cancer cells and APCs. Initially, PD-L1 helps to keep the body's immune reactions from becoming too intense (Fares et al., 2020; Fujiwara et al., 2018; Lai et al., 2021). Consequently, administering ICB may potentially decrease the immunosuppressive effects of vaccines, which weaken antitumor immunity. Combining BC vaccination with ICB is a promising technique that has the potential to boost and prolong the immune response, resulting in significant therapeutic benefits. Combining cancer vaccines with approved drugs may also enhance their effectiveness. An increase in IFN production by T-cells specific to the tumor may be the culprit. This results in the expression of PD-L1 on cancer cells and APCs. At first, PD-L1 helps to prevent the body's immune responses from becoming too intense (Fares et al., 2020; Fujiwara et al., 2018; Lai et al., 2021). As a result, administering ICB may reduce the immunosuppressive effects of vaccines that weaken antitumor immunity. Combining BC vaccination with ICB is a promising technique that has the potential to enhance and prolong the immune response, leading to significant therapeutic benefits. The combination of cancer vaccines with approved drugs may also increase their efficacy.

Clinical Trials

Although there have been efforts to create cancer vaccines through clinical trials, the success rate has been low, with only a few vaccines licensed in the USA and EU. Unfortunately, some phase 3 trials have been stopped due to unsatisfactory results. However, there have been some notable breakthroughs with BCG (TheraCys & TICE), Sipuleucel-T (PROVENGE), and T-Vec (IMLYGIC) (DeMaria & Bilusic, 2019). BCG, which was approved by the FDA as TheraCys in 1990, showed a 5-year disease-free survival rate in a phase 3 trial conducted by Debien et al. in 2023. In 2010, Sipuleucel-T gained approval for use as an immunotherapy that utilizes a patient's cells. While GVAX vaccines have been genetically modified to release immune stimulatory GM-CSF, clinical trials have shown they are insufficiently effective for various types of cancer (DeMaria & Bilusic, 2019). Unfortunately, vaccines like Theratope® and Enhanzyn™ were removed from clinical trial enrollment (Antonarelli et al., 2021). However, early tests of some breast cancer vaccines (BCVs) have revealed promising results, with noticeable immune responses and good tolerance (Debien et al., 2023). Phase 3 studies have demonstrated significant therapeutic benefits for many of these BCVs. Recently, Galena Biopharma, a US-based biotech company, received a Special Protocol Assessment for its Phase 3 trial of the NeuVax™ vaccine. Administered with Leukine®, the vaccine is designed to prevent recurrence in early-stage, node-positive breast cancer patients with intermediate to low HER2 expression (Antonarelli et al., 2021).

Ongoing Challenges for Cancer Immunotherapy and Therapeutic Cancer Vaccines

Cancer immunotherapy using T-cells faces several challenges such as low immune response due to ageing or exhaustion of immune cells after previous treatments, a high amount of cancer cells, and a suppressive tumor microenvironment. This environment allows cancer cells to evade immune attack by developing potent immunosuppressive mechanisms during cancer progression (Wang et al., 2017; Xu et al., 2019). Despite the numerous benefits of cancer vaccines, there are significant obstacles connected with cancer vaccination techniques. First, tolerance to the antigen develops, resulting in a reduced immunological response. Second, the heterogeneity of the cancer type introduces a variety of inherent and extrinsic factors, which hurt antitumor vaccination processes. Third, the immune invasion process was discovered to be a substantial impediment to vaccination effectiveness. This necessitates the development of viable alternate techniques for improving antitumor immunity (Antonarelli et al., 2021). Most vaccinations were proven to be insufficiently immunogenic when given alone. As a result, the next generation of adjuvants or more effective adjuvants are needed.

Oncolytic Virus Therapy

Cancer cells have been found to have a compromised antiviral defense; this makes them susceptible to Oncolytic virus (OV) infection. OVs are viruses that can be specially altered or selected to replicate in cancer cells and selectively destroy them. After an infection, Ovs work to destroy cancer cells, which release antigens and prompt the immune system to attack any remaining tumor cells. Interestingly, in the 1800s, it was noted that cancer patients, particularly those with leukemia who caught the flu, had a brief period of remission (Donnelly et al., 2013). OVs have two ways of functioning: they can selectively target and break down cancer cells while avoiding healthy tissue, or they can activate the immune response, enabling the body's natural defenses to eliminate tumors. Naturally occurring OVs, such as the non-pathogenic Reolysin reovirus present in the respiratory or digestive system, show great potential for effectively treating and eliminating cancer cells (Zou et al., 2019). T-Vec (Imlygic) is the only FDA-approved OV for treating various cancers. It contains granulocyte-macrophage colony-stimulating factor (GM-CSF) which stimulates immune cells, improving the inflammatory response. GM-CSF is used as an immunostimulant in cancer therapy (Zou et al., 2019). It is important to consider the specific biology of an organ or disease when identifying patients who may respond well to treatment. This is because tumor-derived GM-CSF can activate and expand immunosuppressive MDSC, which can decrease the activity of effector T-cells, potentially leading to treatment resistance (Thorn et al., 2016; Zou et al., 2019).

Limitations of Oncolytic Virus Therapy

Oncolytic viral treatment has limitations due to factors such as viral tropism, delivery platforms, viral dissemination, dosage techniques, antiviral immunity, and oncolysis by the OVs. Physical barriers provide a significant difficulty to viral transmission since viruses must pass through the endothelium layer to reach the target cells. In addition, abnormal lymphatic systems, excessive permeability of blood vessels in tumors, and the thick extracellular matrix (ECM) of solid tumors can lead to interstitial hypertension, which may hinder the penetration of viruses (Zheng et al., 2019). Another significant obstacle for OVs (oncolytic viruses) is the numerous individual barriers in the immunosuppressive TME (tumor microenvironment) of solid tumors. Physical restrictions, tumor heterogeneity, antiviral immunity, and immunosuppressive TME all pose challenges for OVs in selectively targeting tumor cells, penetrating tumors, and achieving effectiveness.

Currently, various methods are being studied to improve the efficiency of tumor targeting, the administration and dispersion of virions, as well as techniques for equipping them with therapeutic transgenes to increase efficacy without elevating toxicity and combining with other therapies.

Chimeric Antigen Receptor (CAR) T-cell Therapy

Figure 1 illustrates how chimeric antigen receptors (CARs) can modify the specificity and activity of T-lymphocytes and other immune cells. CARs are recombinant antigen receptors used in cancer immunotherapy to create tumor-targeted T-cells quickly. This approach circumvents the obstacles and delays of active immunization. Modified T-cells expressing CARs act as "living drugs" with both immediate and long-term effects due to their exceptional properties (Abbott & Ustoyev, 2019; Sadelain et al., 2013). T-cell-based therapies, including CAR T-cells, have been studied extensively since the early 2000s. Clinical responses were observed in lymphoma patients who received genetically modified T-cells. The introduction of CAR T-cell treatment in immunotherapy has been hailed as a breakthrough since 2013, thanks to clinical trials yielding impressive results (Sadelain et al., 2013).

The FDA approved tisagenlecleucel, also called CAR T-cell therapy, in 2017 as a treatment option for pre-B-cell ALL in people 25 years old and under. Abbott and Ustoyev's clinical trials formed the foundation for this innovative therapy, which has emerged as one of the most hopeful experimental treatments for malignant

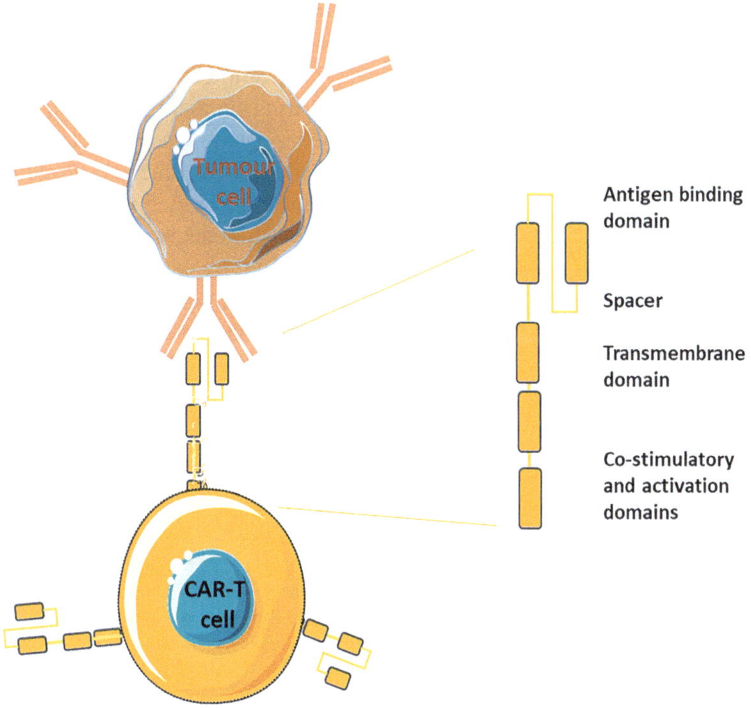

Fig. 1 Schematic diagram showing how a chimeric antigen receptor (CAR) T-cell interacts with a tumor cell

neoplasms. Many clinical trials are currently underway to investigate the potential of CAR T-cell therapy.

The roles of T-cell receptor (TCR), MHC, and other coreceptors were established in previous scientific publications, forming the basis for CAR T-cell therapy. TCRs are found in T-lymphocytes and consist of two polypeptide chains belonging to the immunoglobulin superfamily, but with a simpler structure (without an Fc segment). Antibodies attach to antigenic epitopes on natural protein molecules on the cell membrane. TCRs recognize antigen peptide fragments that are associated with the MHC molecule on the cell surface. The CD3 complex is linked to the polypeptide chains of the TCR dimer chains (Singh et al., 2016). Combining the antigen-binding variable domain of antibodies with the constant domain of TCR into one polypeptide can be advantageous in allowing TCR to recognize and react to antigens independently of MHC. This approach, known as first-generation CAR, is based on the structural similarities between TCR and immunoglobulin.

The efficacy of CAR T-cell therapy varies depending on the target. For example, CD19 T-cells were found to be highly effective in treating B-linear ALL, as well as B-cell lymphoma and CLL (Sadelain et al., 2013). However, first-generation CAR T-cells were found to be insufficient for some applications, leading to the development of second-generation CARs. These newer designs incorporate CD3-chain receptors along with the cytoplasmic domain of a costimulatory receptor, such as CD28, 4-1BB, DAP10, OX40, or ICOS. In studies on animals, a new version of CARs with two costimulatory domains and an activation domain in their cytoplasmic domain appear to be more effective in targeting tumors using T-lymphocytes. These third-generation CAR T-cells showed better performance in terms of growth and stability compared to cells that were transduced with the second-generation CAR vector, especially in patients with mild illness and low B cells in circulation (Sadelain et al., 2013; Singh et al., 2016). The fourth-generation of CAR T-cells is based on the second-generation design, which includes a cassette that induces the production of a transgenic cytokine (in this case, IL-12) in the absence of a cytokine. Another fourth-generation construct called 4SCAR has a secretory signal peptide, scFv (such as CD19), and transmembrane domains CD28, CD27, and CD3z. It also contains a 2A sequence and an inducible switch caspase 9 (iCasp9) to increase safety and reduce the toxic effects of T-cells in adaptive treatment (Tu et al., 2019) (Di Stasi et al., 2011; Tu et al., 2019).

One approach to enhancing the effectiveness of CAR-targeted T-cells is to genetically alter them to secrete proinflammatory or pro-proliferative cytokines. This method aims to enhance the tumor microenvironment and activate the body's natural immune response. Additionally, by expressing cytokines from the T-cells themselves, the potential for harmful systemic toxicity from cytokines is reduced (Sadelain et al., 2013; Singh et al., 2016). CD19 is a highly researched target for CAR-based therapy, mainly due to its presence in most B-cell leukemias and lymphomas but not in regular tissue except for the B-cell lineage. The FDA approved the first CAR T-cell therapy, Tisagenlecleucel (Kymriah, CTL019; Novartis), in 2017, representing a revolutionary approach to cancer management. Tisagenlecleucel is designed for patients under 25 with B-cell precursor acute lymphoblastic leukemia (ALL) who have not responded to standard therapy or have experienced recurrence at least twice. The treatment involves genetically modifying a patient's T-cells to produce CARs that target the cancer cells' CD19 surface protein (First-Ever CAR T-cell Therapy Approved in U.S., 2017).

Limitations of CAR-based Therapy

While CAR cellular therapy has proven to be highly effective in treating tumors, it often comes with dangerous side effects that must be overcome for successful use. These side effects can range from mild to severe, with the latter potentially posing a threat to life (Curran et al., 2012; Sadelain et al., 2013). Additionally, a side effect of CAR cellular treatment is "on-target/off-tumor" toxicity (OTOTT), which can only be prevented if the target antigen is strictly limited to the tumor. Unfortunately, many of the antigens that CAR cells target are also present in normal tissue, leading to OTOTT (Curran et al., 2012).

Combination Therapy

The efficacy of cancer treatment can be improved by using combination therapies that reverse immunosuppression. The development of cancer vaccines is an ongoing process that involves identifying various immunogenic antigens, generating potent vaccine vectors, and overcoming the immunosuppression caused by solid tumors. This progress is essential for the success of cancer treatment, and researchers worldwide are working tirelessly to develop effective cancer vaccines.

Epigenetic Modelling in Breast Cancer Therapy

Epigenetics refers to changes in gene expression without changing DNA sequence. This includes DNA methylation, histone posttranslational modifications, chromatin remodeling factor recruitment, and production of non-coding RNA (miR and lncR) (Szczepanek et al., 2023). Breast cancer growth and resistance can result in changes to DNA methylation, histone alterations, and chromatin remodeling. These epigenetic features are potential targets for therapy, as epigenetic therapeutics can overcome clinical resistance to standard treatments for breast cancer (Romagnolo et al., 2016). However, there has been limited success in advancing epigenetic therapies for breast cancer from preclinical to clinical phases. Nevertheless, the promise of novel epigenetic therapies remains high, especially with the rise of personalized medicine and improved genomic assessment.

Epidrugs

Various factors can lead to epigenetic alterations, including both external factors like stress and diet, and internal factors such as genes and ageing. These changes can impact the structure of chromatin and gene expression in the body. Different mechanisms like changes to histones, DNA methylation, dysregulation of non-coding RNA, and interactions with proteins or nucleic acids can influence the structure of chromatin. If these epigenetic processes become deregulated, they can impact different pathways such as EMT, Hippo signaling, the p53 pathway, and AMPK signaling. Ultimately, deregulation of these processes can lead to senescence or mutations, increasing the risk of cancer (Kim et al., 2023; Wang et al., 2020).

Figure 2 shows that aberrant epigenetic processes are influenced by enzymes that modify DNA methylation and histones, including DNA methyltransferases (DNMTs), histone methyltransferases (HMTs), histone demethylases (HDMs), and histone deacetylases (HDACs), according to Yang et al. (2021). To combat these abnormal modifications, small-molecule inhibitors called Epidrugs target the enzymes responsible for the modifications, reducing their activity.

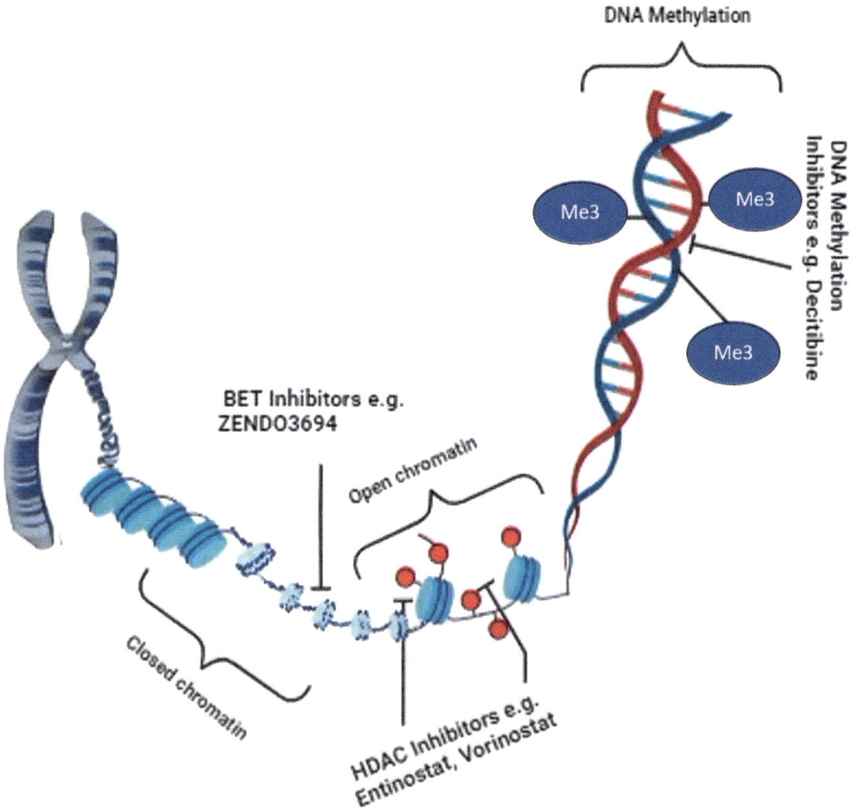

Fig. 2 Illustration of sites of action targeted by epigenetic therapies in breast cancer

DNA Methyltransferase Inhibitors (DNMTi) in Breast Cancer

According to Wang et al. (2020), DNMT is responsible for DNA methylation. This process does not modify the DNA sequence, but it can affect the structure of chromatin, the stability of DNA, and interactions between DNA and proteins. DNMT plays a role in regulating gene expression, controlling embryonic development, managing cellular function, and contributing to the development and progression of cancer (Yang et al., 2021). There are three families of DNMTs known as DNMT1, DNMT2, and DNMT3. Among these enzymes, DNMT1 is the most researched since it plays an essential role in DNA replication repair and methylation maintenance (Kim et al., 2023). Currently, DNMT1 inhibitors such as azacytidine and decitabine are being studied as epigenetic medications for cancer therapy. These are the only two DNMT inhibitors approved by the FDA for specific cancer treatments, including breast cancer (Kim et al., 2023; Wang et al., 2020).

Although first-generation DNMTis hold promise, studies have found that they can be harmful to the human body when used in high quantities (Su et al., 2018). To minimize toxicity, it is recommended to use low concentrations for long-term exposure. Therefore, there is a need to develop second-generation DNMTis that can address the issue of inadequate sensitivity. In cancer therapy, techniques such as DNMT suppression and gene reactivation have been utilized in the development of DNMTis (Kim et al., 2023). After being tested on breast cancer, it was found that DNMTis can effectively inhibit cell growth and induce cell cycle arrest (Su et al., 2018; Wang et al., 2020). These results suggest that DNMTis could be a promising treatment option for cancer (Su et al., 2018). Decitabine (5-aza-2′-deoxycytidine), an FDA-approved DNMTis, is a demethylating drug that permanently fuses DNA. This complex subsequently binds to DNMTs, making them ineffective in the process (Kim et al., 2023).

Treatment for breast cancer has shown promise with the use of DNMTis. Decitabine, in particular, has been effective in treating TNBC with great sensitivity. Studies have shown that Decitabine promotes autophagy in breast cancer cells, which can be seen through an increase in the autophagy marker LCB-II (Vernier et al., 2020). Meanwhile, Azacitidine has also been identified as a potential treatment for preclinical breast cancer by inhibiting breast cancer brain metastasis (Kim et al., 2023). Azacitidine has been observed to suppress the Wnt signaling pathway, cell migration, cell invasion, and tumorigenesis in brain-colonizing cells both in vitro and in vivo (Butler et al., 2020).

According to research done by Terranova-Barberio et al. (2017), using a combination of azacitidine and vorinostat treatment can lead to an increase in PD-L1 mRNA expression. Guadecitabine may serve as a suitable alternative to standard DNMTis like decitabine and azacytidine due to its usage in front-line therapy. Gilmer found that combining guadecitabine and HDACis can reprogram aggressive TNBC cells. Furthermore, guadecitabine can also enhance MHC class I and II expression in TNBC and promote the recruitment of CD8+ T-cells to the tumor microenvironment in vivo (Wong, 2021). Recent studies have shown that guadecitabine could potentially be used as an antitumor drug for patients with breast cancer (Wong, 2021). Additionally, the anti-diabetic medication liraglutide has demonstrated DNMTi properties in both in vitro and in vivo studies with mice tumor models, specifically in breast cancer (Butler et al., 2020). This medication affects cell viability, migration, and DNMT activity and has an anti-proliferative effect, which can inhibit the migration and motility of mesenchymal breast cancer cell lines (Kim et al., 2023). Further research has discovered that when liraglutide is combined with half-dose chemotherapeutic drugs, adverse effects such as toxicity and reproductive dysfunction can be greatly reduced (Chequin et al., 2021). As a result, liraglutide may now be considered a novel adjuvant to enhance breast cancer therapy (Kim et al., 2023; Vernier et al., 2020).

Histone Deacetylase Inhibitors (HDACis) in Breast Cancer

Histone deacetylase inhibitors (HDACis) are a special group of anticancer medicines that induce temporary modifications in gene expression without causing permanent changes in DNA sequence (Minucci & Pelicci, 2006; Terranova-Barberio et al., 2017). HDACis can be hydroxamic acids (hydroxamates), short-chain fatty acids, benzamides, cyclic tetrapeptides, and sirtuin inhibitors (Cappellacci et al., 2020). The response of cells to HDACis causes a complex physiological reaction that regulates histone and non-histone proteins through posttranslational acetylation, which plays a critical role in several cancer-related pathways (Marks, 2010). In addition to its impact on cancer signaling, HDACi also plays a crucial role in immune-modulatory activities, including the regulation of Treg, Foxp3 expression, and changes in the composition of tumor-infiltrating lymphocytes (TILs) (Terranova-Barberio et al., 2016). The epigenetic regulation of T-cell infiltration, differentiation, and PD-L1 expression is increasingly important (Terranova-Barberio et al., 2016; Woods et al., 2015). Furthermore, HDACs are necessary for the expression of key genes that are involved in carcinogenesis (Cappellacci et al., 2020).

Targeting HDACs with HDACis is a potential therapeutic method for cancer cell elimination. Combination treatment with HDAC is extensively used in cancer clinical studies (Terranova-Barberio et al., 2016; Woods et al., 2015). Vorinostat was approved by the FDA as the first HDACi. It acts by decreasing TNBC cell growth by increasing miRNA expression, which boosts tumor suppressor gene expression (Zou et al., 2019). Vorinostat combined with simvastatin (a cholesterol-lowering medicine) was found to trigger apoptosis in TNBC via interfering with Rab7 prenylation and suppressing autophagosome-lysosome fusion (Terranova-Barberio et al., 2016). A recent study discovered that by combining vorinostat with letrozole (an aromatase inhibitor), breast cancer cell growth, apoptosis, and osteoclast differentiation of peripheral blood mononuclear cells can be reduced (Patra et al., 2022). This combo may help lower the risk of osteoporosis in patients with breast cancer. Additionally, when vorinostat is combined with immune checkpoint blockers like PD-1 and CTLA-4, it can trigger tumor apoptosis and regression in TNBC (Zucchetti et al., 2019).

Panobinostat, an FDA-approved HDACi, may enhance H3 and H4 histone acetylation, the cell cycle, and death in breast cancer (Woods et al., 2015). One in vivo investigation suppressed proliferation while increasing histone acetylation in TNBC cells (Qin et al., 2019). As a result, panobinostat can resensitize suppressed estrogen receptor alpha in TNBC to tamoxifen (Wawruszak et al., 2021). An anti-HER2 therapy that combines panobinostat and trastuzumab has been employed (Kim et al., 2023). Researchers found that using Panobinostat and letrozole together was effective in suppressing aromatase expression in hormone-responsive breast cancer cells (Qin et al., 2019). This suggests that these combined treatments may be a promising new approach for treating hormone receptor-positive/aromatase-positive breast cancer (Kim et al., 2023; Laengle et al., 2020).

Additionally, recent studies have shown that the antiepileptic medication valproic acid (VPA) could be a viable option for cancer treatment (Laengle et al., 2020). Research has shown that a substance called VPA has powerful anticancer effects both in vitro and in vivo. When used alone or in combination with demethylating cytotoxic drugs, it has resulted in positive clinical trial outcomes. VPA has been found to inhibit the development of HER2+ breast cancer cells by increasing the expression of p21 WAF1 (Wawruszak et al., 2021). It also induces apoptosis and histone H3 acetylation by inhibiting hsp90 function (Wu et al., 2021). In one study, when VPA was combined with 5-aza-2′-deoxycytidine (a DNA methyltransferase inhibitor), it was able to reactivate transcription of the RA receptor 2 tumor suppressor gene in breast cancer (Wawruszak et al., 2021), leading to the death of breast cancer stem cells.

Epidrugs with Nanotechnology

The use of nanotechnology could offer a solution for delivering drugs to cancer cells with precision. Cancer nanotechnology has the potential to improve pharmacokinetics and target anticancer medications to tumors, which may reduce systemic toxicity (Kim et al., 2023). Nanoparticles are a type of nanotechnology that can target tumor cells and regulate the tumor microenvironment in breast cancer. These include membrane-camouflaged, exosome-disguised, albumin, and lactoferrin nanoparticles (Zhang et al., 2023; Kim et al., 2023). Epigenetics-based nano-delivery can promote cell death and interfere with proliferation and migration (Zhang et al., 2023). By combining nanomedicine with new-generation drugs, it may be possible to improve the effectiveness of treatment-resistant tumors. Overall, nanoscale applications in medicine offer new possibilities for enhancing drug delivery, stability, solubility, and reducing off-target effects.

Limitations and Prospects of Epigenetic Modelling in Breast Cancer Therapy

When using epigenetic medicines to treat cancer, there are four main concerns to consider: cytotoxicity, tolerance, selectivity, and potency. Research has shown that when drugs are used alone, about one-third of patients with early-stage ER+ breast cancer develop medication resistance in BC (Jones et al., 2016). To address this issue, potential approaches include using multiple medication therapy (MMT), multi-compound medication (MCM), and multi-target-directed ligand (MTDLs). These methods may increase efficacy, provide better therapeutic effects, reduce adverse effects, and lower the potential for drug resistance (Jones et al., 2016; Li et al., 2017).

The utilization of MMT presents an opportunity to augment chromatin's accessibility to DNA-damaging chemotherapy drugs, resulting in a higher degree of treatment efficacy when multiple medications are used. In cases where the resistance to drug therapy is caused by CpG island methylation, the MMT approach can be implemented by combining Zebulon and decitabine to achieve demethylation (Benedetti et al., 2015). Even at modest doses, MMT can boost therapeutic impact by reducing drug resistance and associated negative effects when compared to solitary therapy (Daher-Reyes et al., 2019). This will provide the option to choose from several pharmacological dosages for individualized therapy. MCM also makes use of combination treatment, with each aim serving as a "polyvalent pill" (Benedetti et al., 2015; Xu et al., 2022). The strategy of MTDLs endeavors to combat cancer by merging HDACis with other medicines to create a single molecule with multiple target sites (Daher-Reyes et al., 2019).

A different method called MMT is more successful in treating refractory metastatic TNBC. This approach addresses the limitations of using just one medication. Jones et al. (2016) found that a combination of HDACi, romidepsin, cisplatin, and nivolumab was effective (Maccallini et al. 2022). However, as Li et al. (2017) point out, using multiple drugs may not always lead to positive results. For instance, atezolizumab alone did not show a significant difference in overall response rate or progression-free survival. Combination therapy also had drawbacks, as reported by Jones et al. (2016) and Xu et al. (2022). Therefore, new techniques are needed to treat drugs in combination with various therapies to improve antitumor effects (Xu et al., 2022).

Gene Therapy

Research into the molecular foundations of breast cancer has led to the development of gene therapy as a promising treatment option for this illness. Gene therapy involves the introduction of genetic material into specific cells using a vector, followed by the correction, addition, or suppression of genes (McCrudden & McCarthy, 2014). To effectively treat cancer, it is crucial to focus on targeting cancer cells while avoiding healthy ones. Recent clinical trials have shown that this approach is less harmful than traditional medicines (Sheikh-Hosseini et al., 2020). As per the European Commission's 2003/63 directive, a gene therapy product involves administering a fragment of nucleic acid either in vivo or ex vivo for therapeutic, diagnostic, or preventive purposes (McCrudden & McCarthy, 2014).

The process of gene therapy involves introducing foreign genetic material, such as DNA and RNA, into the desired cells. This is followed by gene editing, gene expression, and gene silencing. The development of recombinant DNA technology between the 1960s and 1990s paved the way for the emergence of gene therapy. The goal of gene therapy is to create a working version of a faulty gene, increase the presence of genes that modify diseases, or reduce the activity of an impaired gene (Colella et al., 2018).

Gene Therapy Strategy for Breast Cancer Treatment

Originally, gene therapy was developed as a treatment method for genetic disorders caused by a single gene. However, recent research has revealed that it can also be effective in treating cancer, especially solid or hematological malignancies (Bottai et al., 2017). As genetic changes and gene expression play a crucial role in the development and progression of breast cancer (BC), gene therapy has emerged as a promising option (Pahle & Walther, 2016). Various gene therapy techniques are currently utilized to treat BC, such as gene correction, suicide gene therapy, gene suppression, transcriptional factor targeting using decoy oligodeoxynucleotides, miRNA targeting, Aptamer targeting of BC cells, and DNA or RNA vaccination (Sheikh-Hosseini et al., 2020; Pahle & Walther, 2016).

Gene Correction

A potential method for treating cancer involves exchanging the abnormal gene with the normal variant, which can inhibit the cancerous behavior of cells. While this method alone might not be very effective, research has indicated that when combined with chemo or radiation therapy, it has the potential to cure cancer (Bottai et al., 2017). Tumor suppressor genes like TP53 can mutate and lead to cancer (Dastjerd et al., 2022; Bottai et al., 2017). To prevent the development of breast cancer and facilitate apoptosis, the abnormal TP53 gene can be replaced with a functional one (Bottai et al., 2017; Dastjerd et al., 2022).

Gene Editing

Modern gene editing techniques have revolutionized gene therapy, offering new avenues for treating a range of conditions such as cancer and inheritable or infectious diseases. These cutting-edge methods rely on vectors to transport genetic material and utilize gene editing devices to directly target cells via in vivo or ex vivo procedures. This approach enables genes to be added, corrected, or deactivated, resulting in long-lasting effects (Mout et al., 2017). During the process of gene editing, nuclease enzymes play a critical role by binding to target DNA and creating double-stranded breaks (DSBs). Zinc finger nuclease (ZFN), transcription activator-like effector nuclease (TALEN), and clustered regularly interspaced short palindromic repeats (CRISPR)-associated nuclease Cas9 (CRISPR/Cas9) are the three primary nucleases utilized in this process (Dastjerd et al., 2022). However, incorporating two nucleases (ZFN and TALEN) into building technologies can be challenging, expensive, and time-consuming, which limits their clinical applications. In contrast, CRISPR/Cas9-based technology is better suited for ex vivo gene editing, and its therapeutic applications are rapidly expanding (Dastjerd et al., 2022; Mout et al., 2017).

Breast cancer can be targeted by CRISPR/Cas9 technology which addresses mutations in genes that regulate crucial cellular processes such as cell survival, motility, proliferation, and apoptosis. These mutations can cause disruptions in gene function resulting in uncontrolled cellular growth and tumor formation. Researchers have identified many of these genes as contributors to tumorigenesis, as seen in a recent article by Ahmed et al. (2021). This article delves into the essential genes involved in breast cancer formation and explores the potential of CRISPR/Cas9 technology as a gene editing strategy that could lead to the development of effective breast cancer treatments.

Based on Fig. 3, CRISPR/Cas9 technology has the potential to target multiple genes involved in different stages of cancer, such as initiation, promotion, progression, and metastasis. The BRCA1 and BRCA2 proteins play a crucial role in repairing DNA through the homologous recombination mechanism. However, mutations in these genes can cause cells to lose their DNA repair ability, increasing the risk of cancer through non-homologous end joining. This can lead to further DNA alterations and deletions (Jazieh et al., 2020). Recently, researchers successfully transfected BRCA1-targeting gRNAs into HAP1-Cas9 cell lines. They used targeted

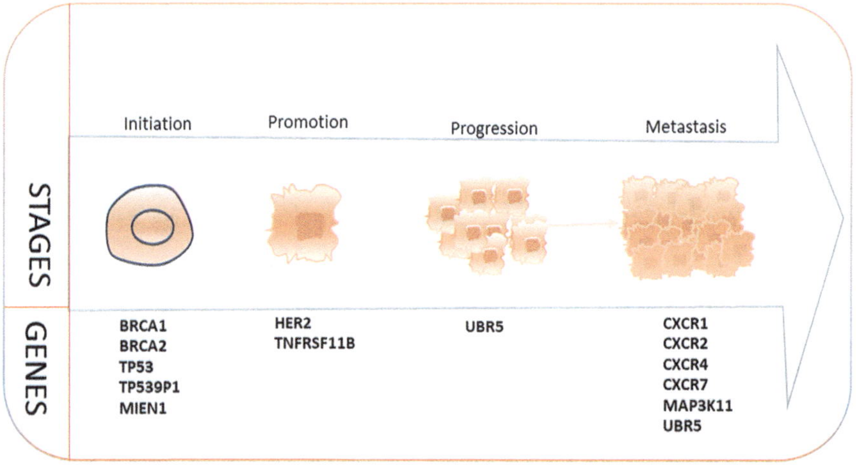

Fig. 3 The several phases involved in the carcinogenesis of breast cancer about some of the genes involved

deep sequencing to detect mutation frequencies and observed a significant decrease in relative indel frequencies over time (Kweon et al., 2020). The LOF mutations in BRCA1 variations can help evaluate cell viability and assess the function of BRCA1 (Jazieh et al., 2020; Kweon et al., 2020).

According to research by Feng et al. (2018), replication stress transfer responsible for precancerous lesions can lead to mis-segregation during the cell cycle. This is because the deletion of BRCA2 leads to the formation of 53GP1 nuclear bodies during the G1 phase. When the p53-dependent G1 is seized, this eventually leads to cell inviability, as confirmed by studies utilizing CRISPR/Cas9-mediated gene targeting of BRCA genes (Ahmed et al., 2021; Mout et al., 2017).

In the context of breast cancer, the HER2 gene codes for the HER2 protein, a membrane receptor tyrosine kinase that belongs to the ERBB family of proteins (HER1-4). Overexpression of HER2 protein due to HER2 amplification has been shown to play a significant role in the carcinogenesis of HER2-positive breast cancer subtype (Slamon et al., 1987). The use of CRISPR/Cas9 technology to target HER2 has been found to inhibit cell proliferation and carcinogenesis in breast cancer cells. However, this impact is limited to HER2+ cell lines, according to research conducted by Wang and Sun in 2017. Scientists are also exploring the potential of targeting other genes involved in cancer initiation, such as TP53PB1 and MKI67. Breast cancer cells are known to metastasize to various parts of the body, which is responsible for most cancer-related deaths (Redig & McAllister, 2013).

A new oncogene, MIEN1, has been discovered and is commonly found in various types of breast cancer, including HER-2 and luminal B subtypes. Researchers employed the CRISPR/Cas9 tool to target the MIEN1 gene in MDA-MB-231 breast cancer cells. By using a co-transfection technique that involved two sgRNA, they were able to ensure stability and knock out a portion of the gene. The researchers' findings indicate that co-transfection improves on-target efficiency, resulting in a significant reduction of MIEN1 protein expression in most cell lines (Van Treuren & Vishwanatha, 2018).

The CX3CR1 gene encodes the CX3 chemokine receptor 1 (CX3CR1) protein, which has been associated with the spread of cancerous cells, as well as cell survival and viability (D'Haese et al., 2010). In vitro experiments on MDA-MB-231 cell lines have shown that suppressing CX3CR1 transcription using CRISPR results in the absence of CX3CR1 protein expression (Shen et al., 2016). Other genes that contribute to metastasis, such as CXCR2, CXCR4, CXCR7, MAP 3K11, TNFRSF11B, and UBR5, are still being studied as potential targets for CRISPR-mediated technology.

Gene Suppression and Silencing

This method involves disrupting the process of gene transcription and translation to decrease the activity of oncogenes that contribute to the growth of cancer, its spread, and the formation of new blood vessels. To do this, specific gene transcripts are targeted using antisense oligodeoxynucleotides (AS-ODNs) to prevent their expression. This approach has the potential to slow down the progression of cancer or improve the effectiveness of chemotherapy or radiation therapy (Bottai et al., 2017). This method involves the use of siRNA, which is a type of RNA interference (RNAi). RNAi involves the suppression of specific genes in cancer cells, and it is used in gene silencing treatment (Belete, 2021). In breast cancer therapy, some of the targets for siRNA include cell cycle regulators, proto-oncogenes, signaling proteins, drug resistance proteins, and angiogenic factors (Bottai et al., 2017). SiRNA is crucial because most genes lack inhibitors, making it challenging to select a specific target due to a lack of ligand binding sites and amino acid sequence similarity with other proteins. RNA interference comes in various forms, including microRNA (miRNA), Small Interfering RNA (siRNA), and short hairpin RNA (shRNA) (Takeshita & Ochiya, 2006).

The use of RNAi-based cancer treatment, which targets tumor suppressor genes, oncogenes, cancer progression genes, and drug resistance genes, has shown promise in selectively silencing genes and causing fewer adverse effects than traditional chemotherapy (Hu et al., 2019). Research on animals has demonstrated the anticancer effects of siRNA targeting key cell cycle proteins such as PKN3, KSP, and PLK1 (Hossen et al., 2023). Currently, various liposomal siRNA dosage formulations, including those for pancreatic cancer (PKN3 siRNA), liver cancer (CEBPA siRNA), and neuroendocrine tumors (PLK1 siRNA), are in the early stages of clinical studies (Belete, 2021; Hossen et al., 2023).

Suicide Gene Therapy

In this strategy for transfecting cancer cells, suicide genes like Cytosine deaminase (CD), Herpes simplex virus thymidine kinase (HSV-TK), Cytochrome P450-2B1, and Nitroreductase are utilized. When these genes become active in a cancer cell, they produce enzymes which can convert non-toxic prodrugs into poisonous metabolites. Ultimately, this results in the elimination of both the cancer cells and nearby cells as a bystander effect (Izmirli & Sönmez, 2016). Through suicide gene therapy, cancer cells are specifically targeted and eliminated, while healthy cells remain unaffected. This process involves the use of non-human genes, often originating from viruses or bacteria (Thoidingjam et al., 2023). Additionally, this therapy has a bystander effect, damaging and killing neighboring tumor cells due to the spread of toxic metabolites. As tumor cells die, they can release necrotic materials and tumor antigens into the bloodstream, which can activate the immune system and lead to the elimination of distant tumor metastases (Amer, 2014).

The latest research on suicide genes has focused on optimizing their activity through mutant variations or fusion proteins. These improvements have resulted in more efficient conversion of dangerous metabolites and the ability to adjust substrate specificity, leading to the development of alternative prodrugs for cancer treatment (Mangipudi et al., 2009). Some gene therapy attempts have utilized bacterial or plant toxins' suicidal ability, like saporins. One recent example is the Clostridium perfringens enterotoxin (CPE), a pore-forming toxin that has effectively destroyed claudin-3 and -4 overexpressing epithelial tumor cells both in vitro and in vivo (Amer, 2014; P, 2013). These discoveries suggest that toxin gene therapy could potentially be used to eradicate tumors.

Various gene therapy products have been approved for cancer treatment, such as gendicine, oncorine, rexin-G, imlygic, delytact, and eight types of CAR T-cells, including kymriah, yescarta, tecartus, breyanzi, abecma, ARI-0001, carteyva, and carvykti (Arabi et al., 2022). Suicide gene therapy for breast cancer currently involves the use of the HSV-TK suicide gene system, Her2/neu proto-oncogene, and epidermal growth factor variant III (EGFRvIII) biomarkers (Izmirli & Sönmez, 2016). Although suicide gene therapy shows great potential in treating cancers, there are still challenges that need to be addressed. For instance, difficulties arise in activating prodrugs, introducing suicide genes into malignant cells without harming healthy cells, and overcoming the host immune response to the vector and suicide gene product (Izmirli & Sönmez, 2016). To make suicide gene therapy more effective for cancer patients, it is important to conduct focused research to address these challenges.

Targeting Transcription Factors by Decoy Oligodeoxynucleotides (ODN)

In order to suppress cancer-causing genes, a method using two-strand ODNs with transcription factor-specific sequences has been employed. These ODNs competitively inhibit transcription factors and gene transcription (Benizri et al., 2019). Gene silencing can be achieved through two promising techniques: Antisense DNA (ASO) and RNA interference (RNAi). ASO utilizes a DNA fragment that complements the target mRNA sequence, while RNAi targets the mRNA with small interfering RNAs (siRNAs). Antisense oligonucleotides can inhibit gene expression in both the cytoplasm and the nucleus (Khvorova & Watts, 2017). Exicure, an oligonucleotide currently in clinical trials, shows potential as an effective therapy option for cancer treatment, either on its own or in combination with pembrolizumab (Benizri et al., 2019). To target tumors, lipid nanoparticles (LNP) were loaded with siRNA, which targeted the Polo-Like Kinase 1 (PLK1) protein found in the triple-negative breast cancer cell line (MDA-MB-231). Intravenous injection of the LNPs resulted in blocked PLK1 protein production and reduced tumor development, which is an interesting finding (Okamoto et al., 2018).

Although the clinical application of oligonucleotides is still in its nascent stages, their potential for treating cancer patients is promising. In order to enhance their efficacy and safety, they can be combined with other cancer treatments to target one or more mRNAs or even bioconjugated with a small chemical or protein. While some bioconjugated oligonucleotides have been approved for clinical use, others are still undergoing research. However, the challenge of effectively delivering

ODNs to their intended targets remains, necessitating larger doses and increasing safety risks and adverse events (Benizri et al., 2019).

Targeting miRNA

Breast cancer development has been linked to microRNAs (miRNAs). Studies have shown that breast cancer patients have altered levels of several miRNAs in their plasma or expression of miRNAs in their breast tissue (Dastjerd et al., 2022). These molecules regulate gene expression at the post-transcriptional level and play a role in various cellular processes, such as proliferation, differentiation, response to DNA damage, apoptosis, and interaction with the cancer microenvironment (Ebrahimpour et al., 2021). Various miRNAs can contribute to cancer development, progression, metastasis, suppression, or response to therapy. Some miRNAs, known as oncomiRNAs or metastatic RNAs, promote tumor growth and can cause a metastatic phenotype by increasing metastasis or inhibiting tumor suppressor activity (Dastjerd et al., 2022). Some types of miRNAs can act as onco-suppressors by targeting miRNAs that encode for oncoproteins, as noted by El-Kenawy et al. (2019). While miR-21, miR-29, and miR-155 are oncogenic, miR-34 and let-7 are tumor suppressors, and miR-181a, miR-21, and miR-1 can promote therapy response, according to Ji et al. (2017). Both miRNA imitators and inhibitors have been shown to regress breast cancer. In one study, an antisense-oligonucleotide (miR-155 ASO) was developed and transferred to MDA-MB-157 breast cancer cells, which decreased their proliferation and promoted apoptosis (Xin et al., 2017).

Targeting BC Cells by Aptamers

Aptamers are short DNA or RNA strands that identify targets with high accuracy and sensitivity. They are becoming more popular as a unique type of nucleic acid probe (Varty et al., 2021). The oligonucleotides in question are synthesized in vitro through the SELEX process, which stands for the Systematic Evolution of Ligands by Exponential enrichment (Arabi et al., 2022; Varty et al., 2021). Although DNA and RNA aptamers share similarities, each has its own set of distinct benefits. DNA aptamers, for instance, are generally less expensive, more stable, and easier to produce. RNA aptamers, on the other hand, can improve binding selectivity and sensitivity by adopting specific structures. Aptamers are also capable of targeting breast cancer cells, penetrating them, and transferring genes without relying on viral vectors. Among the aptamers that have been developed, two DNA aptamers, HeA2-1 and HeA2-3, have been specifically designed to recognize the HER-2 protein in HER-2-positive breast cancer cell lines (Dastjerd et al., 2022). A noteworthy instance is S6, an RNA aptamer that seeks out the SKBR-3 cell line, a type of breast cancer with an overexpression of the Her2 gene (Wu et al., 2017). Research conducted on a mouse tumor model called PNDA-3 demonstrated that a DNA aptamer could significantly impede the growth of the tumor and stop it from spreading to other areas (Wu et al., 2017). This fascinating discovery suggests that PNDA-3 could be a promising option for targeted breast cancer treatment (Wu et al., 2017).

Aptamers can improve BC treatment with conjugates like siRNA, LNA, miRNAs, chemotherapy agents, NPs, PDT agents, and immunotherapy (Varty et al., 2021; Wu et al., 2017). Currently, many solutions are being explored, but a significant portion of them are still in the preclinical and early clinical trial phases.

Gene Therapy Ongoing Clinical Trials

Gene therapy options are now in clinical studies for the therapy of a variety of diseases, especially breast cancer. Table 1 highlights a few examples of clinical investigations on BC gene therapy.

Challenges and Limitations of Gene Therapy

The main causes for cancer gene therapy failure or limited success include not just technological, but also ethical, policy, and economic difficulties. Cancer gene therapy also carries risks of health problems connected with insertional mutagenesis, and the prospect of passing genetic mutations on to offspring is a point of contention

Table 1 Clinical studies involving BC gene therapy (data retrieved from www.clinicaltrials.gov)

Description	Condition	Trial phase	Identifier
Adenovirus-mediated human interleukin-12	Breast cancer	Phase 1	NCT00849459
Retroviral Transduction of the MDR1 gene Into Peripheral Blood Progenitor Cells (PBPCs)	Breast cancer	Phase 2	NCT00001493
CD34+ Derived Dendritic Cells HER-2/Neu	Breast cancer	Phase 1	NCT00197522
Ad5CMV-p53 gene and chemotherapy	Breast cancer	Phase 1	NCT00004038
Ad5CMV-p53 gene and chemo-drug: docetaxel, doxorubicin hydrochloride	Breast cancer	Phase 2	NCT00044993
AdV-tk and valacyclovir	Breast cancer	Phase 1	NCT01997190
Recombinant adenovirus-hIFN-beta	Breast cancer	Phase 1	NCT00066404

in the discussion over human cancer gene therapy. Gene treatments are beneficial in just a subgroup of cancer patients in some cases, making each gene therapy agent an orphan medication (Das et al., 2015).

Conclusions and Future Perspectives

Significant advancement has been achieved in the realm of cancer treatment development, notably in the discovery of BC drugs. Some notable advances include immunotherapy, gene therapy, and epigenetics modelling. In these therapeutic models, research has been conducted and is still ongoing, with promising results. The growing drive for personalized treatment creates chances for techniques such as gene therapy research, and hence more studies to investigate such strategies. Many preclinical and clinical trials are underway to identify and evaluate novel anticancer bioactivity compounds. However, most of these candidates fall short in terms of effectiveness, low toxicity, or lack of other negative effects. In recent years, combining more than one therapeutic drug has emerged as an essential aspect of cancer therapy. Combinations of anticancer drugs target important pathways synergistically or cumulatively, possibly decreasing resistance to therapies, growth of tumors, and potential for metastatic disease. A variety of combinatory strategies have been tested in breast cancer studies. Nonetheless, no new drugs have materially altered the current scenario.

Numerous studies in BC have shown that carefully selected pharmaceutical combinations give more therapeutic benefits than single-agent therapy, and drug combinations may assist in minimizing acquired drug resistance and increase breast cancer treatment efficacy. One of the key issues connected with cancer therapeutic strategies is off-target toxicity generated by other cancer drugs. New emerging technologies, such as nanotechnology, can assist in resolving these issues. The nanoparticle-mediated delivery strategy ensures that the targeted drug or therapeutic intervention reaches its intended target, in this case, a malignant cell/tumor, without causing unintended effects on other neighboring healthy cells. Immunotherapy has demonstrated encouraging results in reinvigorating the body's defense systems against cancer cells by harnessing the strength of the immune system. Immune checkpoint inhibitors and adoptive T-cell therapies have shown promise in overcoming medication resistance by focusing on particular molecular processes that drive cancer cells to reject conventional treatments.

By addressing the genetic determinants of medication resistance, gene therapy provides a personalized approach. This method has the potential to cure medication resistance and restore the efficacy of traditional therapies by delivering therapeutic genes or altering defective genes. Gene delivery system improvements and CRISPR-based technologies have cleared the road for more accurate and efficient treatments. The complicated regulatory mechanisms behind drug-resistant breast cancer can be revealed using epigenetic modelling. Understanding how epigenetic changes lead to drug resistance allows researchers to create innovative medicines that reverse these changes, restoring medication sensitivity. To restore normal cellular activity and sensitize resistant cancer cells to therapy, epigenetic medicines and treatments targeting chromatin remodeling enzymes are being investigated. Ultimately, immunotherapy, gene therapy, and epigenetic modelling offer potentially a new front in the fight against drug-resistant breast cancer. As our knowledge grows and technology progresses, the possibilities for more effective, targeted, and personalized therapy choices for patients with drug-resistant breast cancer become increasingly appealing.

References

Abbott, M., & Ustoyev, Y. (2019). Cancer and the immune system: The history and background of immunotherapy. *Seminars in Oncology Nursing, 35*(5), 150923.

Abdou, Y., Goudarzi, A., Yu, J. X., Upadhaya, S., Vincent, B., & Carey, L. A. (2022). Immunotherapy in triple-negative breast cancer: Beyond checkpoint inhibitors. *npj Breast Cancer, 8*(1), 121.

Ahmed, M., Daoud, G. H., Mohamed, A., & Harati, R. (2021). New insights into the therapeutic applications of CRISPR/Cas9 genome editing in breast cancer. *Genes (Basel), 12*(5), 723.

Amer, M. H. (2014). Gene therapy for cancer: Present status and future perspective. *Molecular and Cellular Therapies, 2*, 27.

Antonarelli, G., Corti, C., Tarantino, P., Ascione, L., Cortes, J., Romero, P., Mittendorf, E. A., Disis, M. L., & Curigliano, G. (2021). Therapeutic cancer vaccines revamping: Technology advancements and pitfalls. *Annals of Oncology, 32*, 1537–1551.

Arabi, F., Mansouri, V., & Ahmadbeigi, N. (2022). Gene therapy clinical trials, where do we go? An overview. *Biomedicine & Pharmacotherapy, 153*, 113324.

Ayers, M., Lunceford, J., Nebozhyn, M., Murphy, E., Loboda, A., Kaufman, D. R., Albright, A., Cheng, J. D., Kang, S. P., Shankaran, V., Piha-Paul, S. A., Yearley, J., Seiwert, T. Y., Ribas, A., & McClanahan, T. K. (2017). IFN-γ–related mRNA profile predicts clinical response to PD-1 blockade. *The Journal of Clinical Investigation, 127*, 2930–2940.

Balkwill, F. (2009). Tumour necrosis factor and cancer. *Nature Reviews Cancer, 9*(5), 361–371.

Belete, T. M. (2021). The current status of gene therapy for the treatment of cancer. *Biologics, 15*, 67–77.

Benedetti, R., Conte, M., Iside, C., & Altucci, L. (2015). Epigenetic-based therapy: From single- to multi-target approaches. *The International Journal of Biochemistry & Cell Biology, 69*, 121–131.

Benizri, S., Gissot, A., Martin, A., Vialet, B., Grinstaff, M. W., & Barthélémy, P. (2019). Bioconjugated oligonucleotides: Recent developments and therapeutic applications. *Bioconjugate Chemistry, 30*, 366–383.

Bottai, G., Truffi, M., Corsi, F., & Santarpia, L. (2017). Progress in nonviral gene therapy for breast cancer and what comes next? *Expert Opinion on Biological Therapy, 17*, 595–611.

Butler, C., Sprowls, S., Szalai, G., Arsiwala, T., Saralkar, P., Straight, B., Hatcher, S., Tyree, E., Yost, M., Kohler, W. J., Wolff, B., Putnam, E., Lockman, P., & Liu, T. (2020). Hypomethylating agent azacitidine is effective in treating brain metastasis triple-negative breast cancer through regulation of DNA methylation of keratin 18 gene. *Translational Oncology, 13*(6), 100775.

Cappellacci, L., Perinelli, D. R., Maggi, F., Grifantini, M., & Petrelli, R. (2020). Recent Progress in histone deacetylase inhibitors as anticancer agents. *Current Medicinal Chemistry, 27*(15), 2449–2493.

Chequin, A., Costa, L. E., de Campos, F. F., Moncada, A. D. B., de Lima, L. T. F., Sledz, L. R., Picheth, G. F., Adami, E. R., Acco, A., Gonçalves, M. B., Manica, G. C. M., Valdameri, G., de Noronha, L., Telles, J. E. Q., Jandrey, E. H. F., Costa, E. T., Costa, F. F., de Souza, E. M.,

Ramos, E. A. S., & Klassen, G. (2021). Antitumoral activity of liraglutide, a new DNMT inhibitor in breast cancer cells in vitro and in vivo. *Chemico-Biological Interactions, 349*, 109641.
Colella, P., Ronzitti, G., & Mingozzi, F. (2018). Emerging issues in AAV-mediated *in vivo* gene therapy. *Molecular Therapy - Methods & Clinical Development, 8*, 87–104.
Curran, K. J., Pegram, H. J., & Brentjens, R. J. (2012). Chimeric antigen receptors for T cell immunotherapy: Current understanding and future directions. *Journal of Gene Medicine, 14*(6), 405–415.
D'Haese, J. G., Demir, I. E., Friess, H., & Ceyhan, G. O. (2010). Fractalkine/CX3CR1: Why a single chemokine-receptor duo bears a major and unique therapeutic potential. *Expert Opinion on Therapeutic Targets, 14*(2), 207–219.
Daher-Reyes, G. S., Merchan, B. M., & Yee, K. W. L. (2019). Guadecitabine (SGI-110): An investigational drug for the treatment of myelodysplastic syndrome and acute myeloid leukemia. *Expert Opinion on Investigational Drugs, 28*, 835–849.
Das, S. K., Menezes, M. E., Bhatia, S., Wang, X. Y., Emdad, L., Sarkar, D., & Fisher, P. B. (2015). Gene therapies for cancer: Strategies, challenges and successes. *Journal of Cellular Physiology, 230*(2), 259–271.
Dastjerd, N. T., Valibeik, A., Rahimi Monfared, S., Goodarzi, G., Moradi Sarabi, M., Hajabdollahi, F., Maniati, M., Amri, J., & Samavarchi Tehrani, S. (2022). Gene therapy: A promising approach for breast cancer treatment. *Cell Biochemistry and Function, 40*, 28–48.
Debien, V., De Caluwé, A., Wang, X., Piccart-Gebhart, M., Tuohy, V. K., Romano, E., & Buisseret, L. (2023). Immunotherapy in breast cancer: An overview of current strategies and perspectives. *npj Breast Cancer, 9*, 7.
DeMaria, P. J., & Bilusic, M. (2019). Cancer Vaccines. *Hematology/Oncology Clinics of North America, 33*, 199–214.
Di Stasi, A., Tey, S.-K., Dotti, G., Fujita, Y., Kennedy-Nasser, A., Martinez, C., Straathof, K., Liu, E., Durett, A. G., Grilley, B., Liu, H., Cruz, C. R., Savoldo, B., Gee, A. P., Schindler, J., Krance, R. A., Heslop, H. E., Spencer, D. M., Rooney, C. M., & Brenner, M. K. (2011). Inducible apoptosis as a safety switch for adoptive cell therapy. *The New England Journal of Medicine, 365*(18), 1673–1683.
Donnelly, O., Harrington, K., Melcher, A., & Pandha, H. (2013). Live viruses to treat cancer. *Journal of the Royal Society of Medicine, 106*, 310–314.
Ebrahimpour, A., Sarfi, M., Rezatabar, S., & Tehrani, S. S. (2021). Novel insights into the interaction between long non-coding RNAs and microRNAs in glioma. *Molecular and Cellular Biochemistry, 476*, 2317–2335.
El-Kenawy, A., Benarba, B., Neves, A. F., De Araujo, T. G., Tan, B. L., & Gouri, A. (2019). Gene surgery: Potential applications for human diseases. *EXCLI Journal, 18*, 908–930.
Emens, L. A., Esteva, F. J., Beresford, M., Saura, C., De Laurentiis, M., Kim, S.-B., Im, S.-A., Wang, Y., Salgado, R., Mani, A., Shah, J., Lambertini, C., Liu, H., de Haas, S. L., Patre, M., & Loi, S. (2020). Trastuzumab emtansine plus atezolizumab versus trastuzumab emtansine plus placebo in previously treated, HER2-positive advanced breast cancer (KATE2): A phase 2, multicentre, randomised, double-blind trial. *The Lancet Oncology, 21*, 1283–1295.
Fares, J., Kanojia, D., Rashidi, A., Ulasov, I., & Lesniak, M. S. (2020). Landscape of combination therapy trials in breast cancer brain metastasis. *International Journal of Cancer, 147*, 1939–1952.
Feng, Y., Spezia, M., Huang, S., Yuan, C., Zeng, Z., Zhang, L., Ji, X., Liu, W., Huang, B., Luo, W., Liu, B., Lei, Y., Du, S., Vuppalapati, A., Luu, H. H., Haydon, R. C., He, T.-C., & Ren, G. (2018). Breast cancer development and progression: Risk factors, cancer stem cells, signaling pathways, genomics, and molecular pathogenesis. *Genes & Diseases, 5*, 77–106.
Filin, I. Y., Solovyeva, V. V., Kitaeva, K. V., Rutland, C. S., & Rizvanov, A. A. (2020). Current trends in cancer immunotherapy. *Biomedicine, 8*(12), 621.
First-Ever CAR T-cell Therapy Approved in U.S. (2017). *Cancer Discovery, 7*. OF1–OF1.

Fujiwara, Y., Sun, Y., Torphy, R. J., He, J., Yanaga, K., Edil, B. H., Schulick, R. D., & Zhu, Y. (2018). Pomalidomide inhibits PD-L1 induction to promote antitumor immunity. *Cancer Research, 78*, 6655–6665.

Guha, P., Heatherton, K. R., O'connell, K. P., Alexander, I. S., & Katz, S. C. (2022). Assessing the future of solid tumor immunotherapy. *Biomedicine, 10*(3), 655.

Hossen, M. N., Wang, L., Chinthalapally, H. R., Robertson, J. D., Fung, K.-M., Wilhelm, S., Bieniasz, M., Bhattacharya, R., & Mukherjee, P. (2023). Switching the intracellular pathway and enhancing the therapeutic efficacy of small interfering RNA by auroliposome. *Science Advances, 6*, eaba5379.

Hu, B., Weng, Y., Xia, X.-H., Liang, X., & Huang, Y. (2019). Clinical advances of siRNA therapeutics. *The Journal of Gene Medicine, 21*, e3097.

Izmirli, M., & Sönmez, D. (2016). The war against cancer: Suicide gene therapy. *Advances in Modern Oncology Research, 2*, 139.

Jazieh, K., Bell, R., Agarwal, N., & Abraham, J. (2020). Novel targeted therapies for metastatic breast cancer. *Annals of Translational Medicine, 8*, 907–907.

Ji, W., Sun, B., & Su, C. (2017). Targeting microRNAs in cancer gene therapy. *Genes (Basel), 8*(1), 21.

Jiang, X., & Liu, Q. (2023). mRNA vaccination in breast cancer: Current progress and future direction. *Journal of Cancer Research and Clinical Oncology*, 1–16.

Jones, P. A., Issa, J.-P. J., & Baylin, S. (2016). Targeting the cancer epigenome for therapy. *Nature Reviews. Genetics, 17*, 630–641.

Jou, J., Harrington, K. J., Zocca, M. B., Ehrnrooth, E., & Cohen, E. E. W. (2021). The changing landscape of therapeutic cancer vaccines-novel platforms and neoantigen identification. *Clinical Cancer Research, 27*(3), 689–703.

Kennedy, L. B., & Salama, A. K. S. (2020). A review of cancer immunotherapy toxicity. *CA: a Cancer Journal for Clinicians, 70*, 86–104.

Khvorova, A., & Watts, J. K. (2017). The chemical evolution of oligonucleotide therapies of clinical utility. *Nature Biotechnology, 35*, 238–248.

Kim, A., Mo, K., Kwon, H., Choe, S., Park, M., Kwak, W., & Yoon, H. (2023). Epigenetic regulation in breast cancer: Insights on epidrugs. *Epigenomes, 7*(1), 6.

Kweon, J., Jang, A.-H., Shin, H. R., See, J.-E., Lee, W., Lee, J. W., Chang, S., Kim, K., & Kim, Y. (2020). A CRISPR-based base-editing screen for the functional assessment of BRCA1 variants. *Oncogene, 39*, 30–35.

Laengle, J., Kabiljo, J., Hunter, L., Homola, J., Prodinger, S., Egger, G., & Bergmann, M. (2020). Histone deacetylase inhibitors valproic acid and vorinostat enhance trastuzumab-mediated antibody-dependent cell-mediated phagocytosis. *Journal for Immunotherapy of Cancer, 8*(1), e000195.

Lai, J., Beavis, P. A., Li, J., & Darcy, P. K. (2021). Augmenting adoptive T-cell immunotherapy by targeting the PD-1/PD-L1 Axis. *Cancer Research, 81*, 5803–5805.

Larkin, J., Chiarion-Sileni, V., Gonzalez, R., Grob, J. J., Cowey, C. L., Lao, C. D., Schadendorf, D., Dummer, R., Smylie, M., Rutkowski, P., Ferrucci, P. F., Hill, A., Wagstaff, J., Carlino, M. S., Haanen, J. B., Maio, M., Marquez-Rodas, I., McArthur, G. A., Ascierto, P. A., Long, G. V., Callahan, M. K., Postow, M. A., Grossmann, K., Sznol, M., Dreno, B., Bastholt, L., Yang, A., Rollin, L. M., Horak, C., Hodi, F. S., & Wolchok, J. D. (2015). Combined nivolumab and ipilimumab or monotherapy in untreated melanoma. *New England Journal of Medicine, 373*, 23–34.

Lee Ventola, C. (2017). Cancer immunotherapy, part 1: Current strategies and agents. *P&T®, 42*(6), 375–383.

Li, J., Goh, E. L. K., He, J., Li, Y., Fan, Z., Yu, Z., Yuan, P., & Liu, D. X. (2023). Emerging intrinsic therapeutic targets for metastatic breast cancer. *Biology (Basel), 12*(5), 697.

Li, J., Hao, D., Wang, L., Wang, H., Wang, Y., Zhao, Z., Li, P., Deng, C., & Di, L. J. (2017). Epigenetic targeting drugs potentiate chemotherapeutic effects in solid tumor therapy. *Scientific Reports, 7*(1), 4035.

Lisi, L., Lacal, P. M., Martire, M., Navarra, P., & Graziani, G. (2022). Clinical experience with CTLA-4 blockade for cancer immunotherapy: From the monospecific monoclonal antibody ipilimumab to probodies and bispecific molecules targeting the tumor microenvironment. *Pharmacological Research, 175*, 105997.

Lollini, P.-L., Cavallo, F., Nanni, P., & Forni, G. (2006). Vaccines for tumour prevention. *Nature Reviews. Cancer, 6*, 204–216.

Lopes, A., Vandermeulen, G., & Préat, V. (2019). Cancer DNA vaccines: Current preclinical and clinical developments and future perspectives. *Journal of Experimental & Clinical Cancer Research, 38*, 146.

Maccallini, C., Ammazzalorso, A., De Filippis, B., Fantacuzzi, M., Giampietro, L., & Amoroso, R. (2022). HDAC inhibitors for the therapy of triple negative breast cancer. *Pharmaceuticals (Basel), 15*(6), 667.

Mangipudi, S. S., Canine, B. F., Wang, Y., & Hatefi, A. (2009). Development of a genetically engineered biomimetic vector for targeted gene transfer to breast cancer cells. *Molecular Pharmaceutics, 6*, 1100–1109.

Marks, P. A. (2010). Histone deacetylase inhibitors: A chemical genetics approach to understanding cellular functions. *Biochimica et Biophysica Acta (BBA) - Gene Regulatory Mechanisms, 1799*, 717–725.

McCrudden, C. M., & McCarthy, H. O. (2014). Current status of gene therapy for breast cancer: Progress and challenges. *Application of Clinical Genetics, 7*, 209–220.

Minucci, S., & Pelicci, P. G. (2006). Histone deacetylase inhibitors and the promise of epigenetic (and more) treatments for cancer. *Nature Reviews. Cancer, 6*, 38–51.

Mohamed, A., Krajewski, K., Cakar, B., & Ma, C. X. (2013). Targeted therapy for breast cancer. *American Journal of Pathology, 8*(2), 120–134.

Morse, M. A., Gwin, W. R., & Mitchell, D. A. (2021). Vaccine therapies for cancer: Then and now. *Targeted Oncology, 16*, 121–152.

Mout, R., Ray, M., Lee, Y.-W., Scaletti, F., & Rotello, V. M. (2017). In vivo delivery of CRISPR/Cas9 for therapeutic gene editing: Progress and challenges. *Bioconjugate Chemistry, 28*, 880–884.

O'Malley, W. E., Achinstein, B., & Shear, M. J. (2009). Action of bacterial polysaccharide on Tumors. II. Damage of sarcoma 37 by serum of mice treated with Serratia Marcescens polysaccharide, and induced tolerance. *Nutrition Reviews, 46*(11), 389–391.

Okamoto, A., Asai, T., Hirai, Y., Shimizu, K., Koide, H., Minamino, T., & Oku, N. (2018). Systemic administration of siRNA with anti-HB-EGF antibody-modified lipid nanoparticles for the treatment of triple-negative breast cancer. *Molecular Pharmaceutics, 15*, 1495–1504.

Pahle, J., & Walther, W. (2016). Vectors and strategies for nonviral cancer gene therapy. *Expert Opinion on Biological Therapy, 16*, 443–461.

Patra, S., Praharaj, P. P., Klionsky, D. J., & Bhutia, S. K. (2022). Vorinostat in autophagic cell death: A critical insight into autophagy-mediated, –associated and -dependent cell death for cancer prevention. *Drug Discovery Today, 27*(1), 269–279.

Qin, G., Li, Y., Xu, X., Wang, X., Zhang, K., Tang, Y., Qiu, H., Shi, D., Zhang, C., Long, Q., Lee, K., Zhai, Q., Wang, S., Chen, M., & Deng, W. (2019). Panobinostat (LBH589) inhibits Wnt/β-catenin signaling pathway via upregulating APCL expression in breast cancer. *Cellular Signalling, 59*, 62–75.

Ramírez, A., Conejo-García, A., Griñán-Lisón, C., López-Cara, L. C., Jiménez, G., Campos, J. M., Marchal, J. A., & Boulaiz, H. (2018). Enhancement of tumor cell death by combining gef gene mediated therapy and new 1,4-benzoxazepin-2,6-dichloropurine derivatives in breast cancer cells. *Frontiers in Pharmacology, 9*, 798.

Redig, A. J., & McAllister, S. S. (2013). Breast cancer as a systemic disease: A view of metastasis. *Journal of Internal Medicine, 274*, 113–126.

Robert, C. (2020). A decade of immune-checkpoint inhibitors in cancer therapy. *Nature Communications, 11*, 3801.

Romagnolo, D. F., Daniels, K. D., Grunwald, J. T., Ramos, S. A., Propper, C. R., & Selmin, O. I. (2016). Epigenetics of breast cancer: Modifying role of environmental and bioactive food compounds. *Molecular Nutrition & Food Research, 60*(6), 1310–1329.

Sadelain, M., Brentjens, R., & Rivière, I. (2013). The basic principles of chimeric antigen receptor design. *Cancer Discovery, 3*, 388–398.

Salvioni, L., Zuppone, S., Andreata, F., Monieri, M., Mazzucchelli, S., Di Carlo, C., Morelli, L., Cordiglieri, C., Donnici, L., De Francesco, R., Corsi, F., Prosperi, D., Vago, R., & Colombo, M. (2020). Nanoparticle-mediated suicide gene therapy for triple negative breast cancer treatment. *Advances in Therapy (Weinh), 3*(8).

Savas, P., Salgado, R., Denkert, C., Sotiriou, C., Darcy, P. K., Smyth, M. J., & Loi, S. (2016). Clinical relevance of host immunity in breast cancer: From TILs to the clinic. *Nature Reviews. Clinical Oncology, 13*, 228–241.

Shanmugaraj, B., Priya, L. B., Mahalakshmi, B., Subbiah, S., Hu, R.-M., Velmurugan, B. K., & Baskaran, R. (2020). Bacterial and viral vectors as vaccine delivery vehicles for breast cancer therapy. *Life Sciences, 250*, 117550.

Sheikh-Hosseini, M., Larijani, B., Gholipoor Kakroodi, Z., Shokoohi, M., Moarefzadeh, M., Sayahpour, F. A., Goodarzi, P., & Arjmand, B. (2020). Gene therapy as an emerging therapeutic approach to breast cancer: New developments and challenges. *Human Gene Therapy, 32*, 1330–1345.

Shen, F., Zhang, Y., Jernigan, D. L., Feng, X., Yan, J., Garcia, F. U., Meucci, O., Salvino, J. M., & Fatatis, A. (2016). Novel small-molecule CX3CR1 antagonist impairs metastatic seeding and colonization of breast cancer cells. *Molecular Cancer Research, 14*, 518–527.

Singh, N., Frey, N. V., Grupp, S. A., & Maude, S. L. (2016). CAR T cell therapy in acute lymphoblastic Leukemia and potential for chronic lymphocytic Leukemia. *Current Treatment Options in Oncology, 17*, 28.

Slamon, D. J., Clark, G. M., Wong, S. G., Levin, W. J., Ullrich, A., & McGuire, W. L. (1987). Human breast cancer: Correlation of relapse and survival with amplification of the HER-2/neu oncogene. *Science, 1979*(235), 177–182.

Solinas, C., Aiello, M., Migliori, E., Willard-Gallo, K., & Emens, L. A. (2020). Breast cancer vaccines: Heeding the lessons of the past to guide a path forward. *Cancer Treatment Reviews, 84*, 101947.

Su, Y., Hopfinger, N. R., Nguyen, T. D., Pogash, T. J., Santucci-Pereira, J., & Russo, J. (2018). Epigenetic reprogramming of epithelial-mesenchymal transition in triple-negative breast cancer cells with DNA methyltransferase and histone deacetylase inhibitors. *Journal of Experimental & Clinical Cancer Research, 37*, 314.

Szczepanek, J., Skorupa, M., Jarkiewicz-Tretyn, J., Cybulski, C., & Tretyn, A. (2023). Harnessing epigenetics for breast cancer therapy: The role of DNA methylation, histone modifications, and MicroRNA. *International Journal of Molecular Sciences, 24*(8), 7235.

Takeshita, F., & Ochiya, T. (2006). Therapeutic potential of RNA interference against cancer. *Cancer Science, 97*, 689–696.

Terranova-Barberio, M., Thomas, S., & Munster, P. N. (2016). Epigenetic modifiers in immunotherapy: A focus on checkpoint inhibitors. *Immunotherapy, 8*, 705–719.

Terranova-Barberio, M., Thomas, S., Ali, N., Pawlowska, N., Park, J., Krings, G., Rosenblum, M. D., Budillon, A., & Munster, P. N. (2017). HDAC inhibition potentiates immunotherapy in triple-negative breast cancer. *Oncotarget, 8*(69), 114156–114172.

Thoidingjam, S., Sriramulu, S., Freytag, S., Brown, S. L., Kim, J. H., Chetty, I. J., Siddiqui, F., Movsas, B., & Nyati, S. (2023). Oncolytic virus-based suicide gene therapy for cancer treatment: A perspective of the clinical trials conducted at Henry ford health. *Translational Medicine Communications, 8*(1), 11.

Thorn, M., Guha, P., Cunetta, M., Espat, N. J., Miller, G., Junghans, R. P., & Katz, S. C. (2016). Tumor-associated GM-CSF overexpression induces immunoinhibitory molecules via STAT3 in myeloid-suppressor cells infiltrating liver metastases. *Cancer Gene Therapy, 23*, 188–198.

Tu, S., Zhou, X., Guo, Z., Huang, R., Yue, C., He, Y., Li, M., Chen, Y., Liu, Y. C., Chang, L. J., & Li, Y. (2019). CD19 and CD70 dual-target chimeric antigen receptor T-cell therapy for the treatment of relapsed and refractory primary central nervous system diffuse large B-cell lymphoma. *Frontiers in Oncology, 9*, 1350.

Van Treuren, T., & Vishwanatha, J. K. (2018). CRISPR deletion of MIEN1 in breast cancer cells. *PLoS One, 13*, e0204976.

Varty, K., O'Brien, C., & Ignaszak, A. (2021). Breast cancer aptamers: Current sensing targets, available aptamers, and their evaluation for clinical use in diagnostics. *Cancers (Basel), 13*(16), 3984.

Vernier, M., McGuirk, S., Dufour, C. R., Wan, L., Audet-Walsh, E., St-Pierre, J., & Giguère, V. (2020). Inhibition of DNMT1 and ERRα crosstalk suppresses breast cancer via derepression of IRF4. *Oncogene, 39*, 6406–6420.

Wang, H., & Sun, W. (2017). CRISPR-mediated targeting of HER2 inhibits cell proliferation through a dominant negative mutation. *Cancer Letters, 385*, 137–143.

Wang, M., Zhao, J., Zhang, L., Wei, F., Lian, Y., Wu, Y., Gong, Z., Zhang, S., Zhou, J., Cao, K., Li, X., Xiong, W., Li, G., Zeng, Z., & Guo, C. (2017). Role of tumor microenvironment in tumorigenesis. *Journal of Cancer, 8*(5), 761–773.

Wang, Q., Yu, G., Ming, X., Xia, W., Xu, X., Zhang, Y., Zhang, W., Li, Y., Huang, C., Xie, H., Zhu, B., & Xie, W. (2020). Imprecise DNMT1 activity coupled with neighbor-guided correction enables robust yet flexible epigenetic inheritance. *Nature Genetics, 52*, 828–839.

Wawruszak, A., Halasa, M., Okon, E., Kukula-Koch, W., & Stepulak, A. (2021). Valproic acid and breast cancer: State of the art in 2021. *Cancers, 13*(14), 3409.

Wong, K. K. (2021). DNMT1: A key drug target in triple-negative breast cancer. *Seminars in Cancer Biology, 72*, 198–213.

Woods, D. M., Sodré, A. L., Villagra, A., Sarnaik, A., Sotomayor, E. M., & Weber, J. (2015). HDAC inhibition upregulates PD-1 ligands in melanoma and augments immunotherapy with PD-1 blockade. *Cancer Immunology Research, 3*, 1375–1385.

Wu, C.-H., Tsai, Y.-C., Tsai, T.-H., Kuo, K.-L., Su, Y.-F., Chang, C.-H., & Lin, C.-L. (2021). Valproic acid reduces vasospasm through modulation of Akt phosphorylation and attenuates neuronal apoptosis in subarachnoid Hemorrhage rats. *International Journal of Molecular Sciences, 22*(11), 5975.

Wu, X., Shaikh, A., Yu, Y., Li, Y., Ni, S., Lu, A., & Zhang, G. (2017). Potential diagnostic and therapeutic applications of oligonucleotide aptamers in breast cancer. *International Journal of Molecular Sciences, 18*(9), 1851.

Xin, Y., Huang, M., Guo, W. W., Huang, Q., Zhang, L. Z., & Jiang, G. (2017). Nano-based delivery of RNAi in cancer therapy. *Molecular Cancer, 16*, 134.

Xu, X., Li, J., Zou, J., Feng, X., Zhang, C., Zheng, R., Duanmu, W., Saha-Mandal, A., Ming, Z., & Wang, E. (2019). Association of Germline Variants in natural killer cells with tumor immune microenvironment subtypes, tumor-infiltrating lymphocytes, immunotherapy response, clinical outcomes, and cancer risk. *JAMA Network Open, 2*, e199292.

Xu, Y., Li, P., Liu, Y., Xin, D., Lei, W., Liang, A., Han, W., & Qian, W. (2022). Epi-immunotherapy for cancers: Rationales of epi-drugs in combination with immunotherapy and advances in clinical trials. *Cancer Communications, 42*, 493–516.

Yang, T., Yang, Y., & Wang, Y. (2021). Predictive biomarkers and potential drug combinations of epi-drugs in cancer therapy. *Clinical Epigenetics, 13*, 113.

Zhang, J., Huang, L., Ge, G., & Hu, K. (2023). Emerging epigenetic-based nanotechnology for cancer therapy: Modulating the tumor microenvironment. *Advanced Science, 10*(7), e2206169.

Zheng, M., Huang, J., Tong, A., & Yang, H. (2019). *Oncolytic viruses for cancer therapy: Barriers and recent advances* (Vol. 15, pp. 234–247). Molecular Therapy Oncolytics.

Zou, Y., Luo, Y., Zhang, J., Xia, N., Tan, G., & Huang, C. (2019). Bibliometric analysis of oncolytic virus research, 2000 to 2018. *Medicine (United States), 98*(35), e16817.

Zucchetti, B., Shimada, A. K., Katz, A., & Curigliano, G. (2019). The role of histone deacetylase inhibitors in metastatic breast cancer. *The Breast, 43*, 130–134.

Innovative Drug Delivery Systems for Drug-Resistant Breast Cancer

Langanani Mbodi, Koena A. Kgomo, Godfrey Grech, and Zodwa Dlamini

Abstract Breast cancer is the most common and one of the deadliest cancers affecting women worldwide. The mainstay treatment for breast cancer is surgery and adjuvant chemotherapy or radiotherapy. The management of BC is commonly challenged by factors such as recurrence which is a poor prognostic factor and chemoresistance. These factors impact negatively on patients' survival due to their association with increased risk of mortality. The chapter will concentrate on the creation and use of cutting-edge drug delivery technologies to combat breast cancer treatment resistance. Drug resistance poses a significant challenge in breast cancer treatment, and innovative delivery systems offer potential solutions. The chapter explores various approaches, including nanocarriers, liposomes, polymeric micelles, and targeted nanoparticles, which enhance drug delivery and improve therapeutic

L. Mbodi (✉)
Department of Obstetrics and Gynecology, Gynecologic Oncology Unit, University of the Witwatersrand, Parktown, South Africa

Department of Obstetrics and Gynaecology, Charlotte Maxeke Johannesburg Academic Hospital, Johannesburg, South Africa
e-mail: langanani.mbodi@wits.ac.za

K. A. Kgomo
Department of Obstetrics and Gynecology, Gynecologic Oncology Unit, University of the Witwatersrand, Parktown, South Africa

Department of Obstetrics and Gynaecology, Chris Hani Baragwanath Academic Hospital, Johannesburg, South Africa
e-mail: koena.kgomo@wits.ac.za

G. Grech
Department of Pathology, Faculty of Medicine and Surgery, University of Malta, Msida, Malta
e-mail: godfrey.grech@um.edu.mt

Z. Dlamini
SAMRC Precision Oncology Research Unit (PORU), DSI/NRF SARChI Chair in Precision Oncology and Cancer Prevention (POCP), Pan African Cancer Research Institute (PACRI), University of Pretoria, Pretoria, South Africa
e-mail: zodwa.dlamini@up.ac.za

Z. Dlamini (ed.), *Overcoming Breast Cancer Therapy Resistance*,
https://doi.org/10.1007/978-3-031-52860-6_14

efficacy. These systems can overcome drug efflux mechanisms, penetrate tumor tissues, and precisely target cancer cells. By utilizing innovative drug delivery systems, researchers aim to overcome drug resistance, improve treatment outcomes, and provide new therapeutic opportunities for patients with breast cancer lesions that are drug resistant.

Keywords Breast cancer · Drug resistance · Overcoming drug resistance · Nanotechnology · Targeted drug delivery

Introduction

The most frequent malignancy among women worldwide is breast cancer (BC). After lung cancer, it is also considered the deadliest cancer. The mainstay treatment for BC is surgery and adjuvant chemotherapy or radiotherapy. However, recurrence is still common and is considered a poor prognostic factor. The development of drug delivery systems such as nanotechnology in the past 10 years has brought hope to the development of cancer therapy as it enhances biological processes, promotes better compatibility, and generates functionalized tissues (Alshareeda et al., 2023). The use of engineered nanodevices and nanostructures for the monitoring, maintenance, building, and control of human biological systems at the molecular level is known as nanomedicine. This process allows for different medical functions including the process of diagnosing, treating, and of preserving and improving human health (Riehemann et al., 2009).

Definition of Nanotechnology

Nanotechnology has several definitions derived from the size of particles, the effects, and the interaction with processes. The word "*nanos" implies "dwarf"* and is often used for the description of the length scale between 0.1 and 100 nanometers (1 nm = 10^{-9} m). Since 1 nm = 10^{-9} m, the term "nanos" (which means "dwarf") is frequently used to describe the length scale between 0.1 and 100 nanometers. A more detailed explanation of nanotechnology is that it is "the field concerned with materials and systems whose structures and components exhibit novel and significantly improved physical, chemical and biological properties, phenomena and processes due to their nanoscale size" (Riehemann et al., 2009). Nanotechnology can also be described as "the exploitation of matter on an atomic, molecular, and super molecular scale" (Hammed et al., 2016). The phrase "nanotechnology" is credited to Norio Taniguchi, who is supposed to have created it in 1971 even though the research in this filed can be traced back to a lecture by Nobel Laurate Richard Feynman in 1959 entitled "There's Plenty of Room at the Bottom: An Invitation to Enter a New Field of Physics" to the American Physical Society. It was a prediction of innovation termed "swallowable doctors," "small computers that can read and recognize faces," "micro devices for health," and "microscopes that can see DNA," etc. Nanotechnology can also be described as "the science of manipulating materials at very small scales, i.e., at the atomic and molecular levels" (United Nations, 2020).

With the use of nanotechnology, scientists may create and work with particles that are 1–100 nm long (the size of a big protein structure) (Musee et al., 2013). The simplest form of nanoparticle is the liposome which can penetrate through fenestrated tumor neovasculature (Haq et al., 2009). Modernized and modified nanomedicine may introduce different, better, and improved ways to treat breast cancer, cancer recurrence and reduce incidences of tumor resistance (Alshareeda et al., 2023).

Nanotechnology in Healthcare

Although the nanotechnology-based approach is a few decades old, Nanomedicine is still a novel field in healthcare. As early as 1965, Scientists introduced the first lipid-based vesicles, liposomes. However, the polymer system that is used for the controlled release of macromolecules was only introduced around 1976 and the long-circulating stealth nanoparticles in 1994. The quantum dots were formally described in 1998 whereas the nanosensor is a recent twenty-first century invention (Muhammad et al., 2018). All these nanotechnology-based inventions have been used in healthcare and in cancer and most of them are still further investigated. Figure 1 illustrates an example of nanotechnology (drug and nanoparticle delivery system) used in therapeutics to enhance the drug efficacy and probably reduce cancer cells' resistance to chemotherapeutic agents.

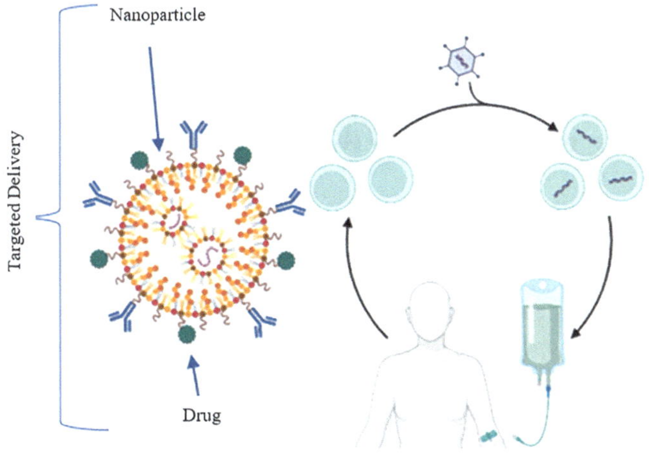

Fig. 1 Graphical representation of the therapy and drug delivery systems

Diagnostics

Nanodevices and nano-biosensors are used in monitoring the biomolecules even at very low concentrations and therefore they have found an application in the early diagnosis of diseases including cancer. Biosensors are not only able to diagnose cancers early but also assist in differentiating malignant versus benign lesions early. In diagnostic imaging, nanoparticles can selectively generate an image of the affected area as opposed to the global image generated by conventional radiological methods (Patel et al., 2015).

Therapeutics

The Nanoparticles (NPs) are also an ideal carrier to deliver chemotherapeutic agents specifically to the targeted diseased cells without affecting the healthy cells. As a result, there is minimum damage to the surrounding normal cells and hence less adverse effects related to normal cell damage as well as improving proficiency of chemotherapeutic drugs through intracellular molecules targeting of the gene-encoding DNA as an example as opposed to the cell itself (Klein & Wagner, 2014; Patel et al., 2015).

Although there are few NP medicines that are licensed to treat breast cancer, there is a growing transition toward more advanced therapies including combining specific gene therapies, and growth factors to NP to engineer local drug delivery through attachment. The above illustration demonstrates how targeted drug delivery will increase treatment effectiveness due to its benefits in terms of size, materials employed, production techniques, biocompatibility, and biodegradability for cancer therapies. Through the conjugation of different ligands to different NPs, the high multiple abilities encourage the combined targeted administration of medicine at the exact place to selectively eliminate tumor cells at lower doses and with less adverse effects on healthy, non-cancerous cells.

Mechanisms of Resistance in Breast Cancer

Drug resistance, which may be intrinsic or acquired and may arise against a single or multiple agents, limits the efficacy of any cancer treatment (Chu & Rubin, 2022). Patients with metastatic cancer who experience therapy failures are typically affected by a variety of drug resistance mechanisms (Bar-Zeev et al., 2017). The Goldie-Coldman hypothesis, which states that most cancer cells start with an innate response to chemotherapeutic agents but evolve spontaneous resistance at varying rates, has been used to describe the growth of cancer cells and has significant clinical implications (Chu & Rubin, 2022). The leading mechanism of drug resistance is an increased efflux of chemotherapeutic drugs from malignant cells with consequent subtherapeutic drug accumulation (Gote et al., 2021). The removal of medicines from cancer cells is carried out by ATP-binding cassette (ABC) superfamily transmembrane transporters (Bar-Zeev et al., 2017). There are 49 ABC efflux transporters that have been identified in humans, and only 15 were found to directly affect chemotherapeutic drugs. The most well-studied of these transporters are the breast cancer resistance protein (BCRP; gene ABCG2), multidrug resistance-associated protein 1 (MRP1; gene ABCC1), and the P-glycoprotein (P-gp/MDR1; gene ABCB1) (Bar-Zeev et al., 2017). Overexpression of some of these transporters in a variety of MDR cancer cells has resulted in extensive suppression of chemotherapeutic efficacy. Breast cancer resistance to chemotherapy is described as multifactorial and involves several mechanisms including, but not limited to: Cell membrane influences on drug absorption, transport, and efflux; Membrane glycoproteins action as efflux pumps; Enzyme system inactivation of chemotherapeutic drugs through their metabolism; The extent and affinity of hormone receptors alteration, Cancer-related genes, Cancer cells DNA repair, Cancer stemness, and Tumor microenvironment (Ji et al., 2019). The expression of a class of ATP-binding cassette transporters is involved in the multidrug resistance mechanism. These transporters use ATP to remove chemotherapy from cancer cells, reducing intracellular drug buildup (Cao et al., 2021).

In Breast Cancer gene (BRCA), PTEN/PI3K/AKT/mTOR, NF-kB, and JAK/STAT are implicated. Their survival, growth, and invasion are controlled through an intricate network signaling (Cao et al., 2021). PTEN/PI3K/AKT/mTOR controls survival, growth, proliferation, and motility in cancer cells. NF-kB, a pro-inflammatory transcription factor is a regulator of triple-negative breast cancer and in BRCA tumors, it is closely related to chemoresistance and metastasis (Cao et al., 2021; Nedeljković & Damjanović, 2019). JAK/ STAT pathway activation contributes to tumor growth and progression. The STATs (STAT3 and STAT5) aid in the growth and advancement of BRCA, and therapy that targets the JAK/STAT pathway has the potential to overcome resistance (Cao et al., 2021; Mckenna et al., 2018). MicroRNAs are the non-coding RNAs that regulate intracellular and intercellular signaling in chemoresistance BRCA tumors. Dysregulation of the miRNAs leads to chemotherapy resistance and development of metastasis (Cao et al., 2021).

Cancer stem cells are a group of tumorigenic cells that promote tumor growth, metastasis, and the emergence of chemotherapeutic drug resistance by overexpressing ABC transporters, which aid in the removal of chemotherapy agents from the cells (Cao et al., 2021; Das et al., 2019; Dittmer, 2018). As a result, a drug delivery strategy that prevents cellular efflux, improves drug retention despite gradient concentration, and is linked to ABC transporter expression markers, such as utilization of nanodiamond particles, may help combat chemotherapeutic drug resistance (Lainetti et al., 2020; Toh et al., 2014).

Nanotechnology in Breast Cancer

Nano-missiles bear arsenals to assist in eradicating cancer or cancer cells. This is a targeted delivery system of the drug that improves drug efficacy. In breast cancer, nanoparticles are used for cancer diagnosis and therapy due to their biodegradability, biocompatibility, size, material used, and fabrication technology properties. The combination of targeted medication delivery to the precise cancer cell site on the breasts with accuracy is made possible by the conjugation of various ligands to various nanoparticles. This selectively kills cancer cells (Alshareeda et al., 2023). The encapsulation process in BC enhances the biological half-life of the chemotherapeutic drug and hence improves response to drug and reduces resistance, reduces the dose of drug required for the effect and reduces side effects. NPs can also be dual functioning as both (imaging) and treating (drug) agents in cancer. Such is described as theragnostic used in image-guided therapy (Alshareeda et al., 2023; Kalash et al., 2016). Nanotechnology has already been acknowledged and applied in Africa for industrial growth and to improve outcomes in health care services, clean water, and affordable renewable energy. However, not yet been rolled out in breast cancer treatment (Musee et al., 2013).

Commonly Described Drug Delivery Approaches

Table 1 describes the application of Nanotechnology in Medicine mostly under investigation or being researched further.

Chemotherapeutic medications are delivered using nanocarrier-based drug delivery technologies that affect several malignant cell locations. Systems based on organic and inorganic particles are most prevalent. Micelles, liposomes, polymers, dendrimers, and nanogels are some of these delivery methods (Singh et al., 2017). The majority of the delivery systems authorized for nanomedicines are drug conjugates (protein, polymer, and/or antibody) and liposomal formulations. By enhancing the PK/PD of the free medication and leveraging passive targeting in both therapy and imaging or imaging-based therapy, they act to enhance outcomes and address resistance (Musee et al., 2013). The mechanism of this Nanotechnology is that it affects van der Waals forces of attraction, hydrogen bonds, electrical charge, ionic bonds, and covalent bonds in molecules, atoms, and quantum dots. It provides a catalytic impact by increasing the surface-area-to-volume ratio. A few instances of nanoscale chemistry are provided in the following sections to demonstrate how chemistry has helped Africa progress (Musee et al., 2013).

Due to its ease of structural manipulation at molecular level, nanotechnology offers several benefits over conventional drug design, including high and quick

Table 1 The broad application of Nanotechnology in Medicine that is currently being investigated

Organics	Application	Inorganics
Liposomes Protein-based organics Nucleic acids Extracellular vesicles Polymeric carrier	Enhanced delivery Lymph node tracer Early detection Bioimaging Targeted biopsy Enhanced radiation	Quantum dots Silica Nanopores Carbon based Metals and metal oxides

dissolving rates, higher medication bioavailability, improved stability of sensitive agents, and improved administration. Because nanoparticles can be created to recognize diseases at the cellular level, visualize afflicted organs through imaging studies, and transport therapeutic substances, this is achievable (Musee et al., 2013). The encapsulating of medications by nanoparticles allows for control over drug delivery, delivery site, dosage, and drug release characteristics (pharmacodynamics and pharmacokinetics), allowing for the penetration of cell barriers by nano-enabled drugs (Vijayakumar et al., 2013). Figure 2 illustrates some of the common nanotechnology-based drug delivery systems that are both registered for use, used in trials, and those under research for future use. The commonly used are the organics and receptor-based delivery systems.

Organic Drug Delivery Approaches

Figure 3 illustrates how the organic drug delivery system functions. It compares the outcome of the nanoparticle-coated chemotherapeutic drug to the use of conventional drugs without nanoparticle coating. The nanoparticle particle, among other things, increases the uptake of the drug, reduces efflux, and increases its

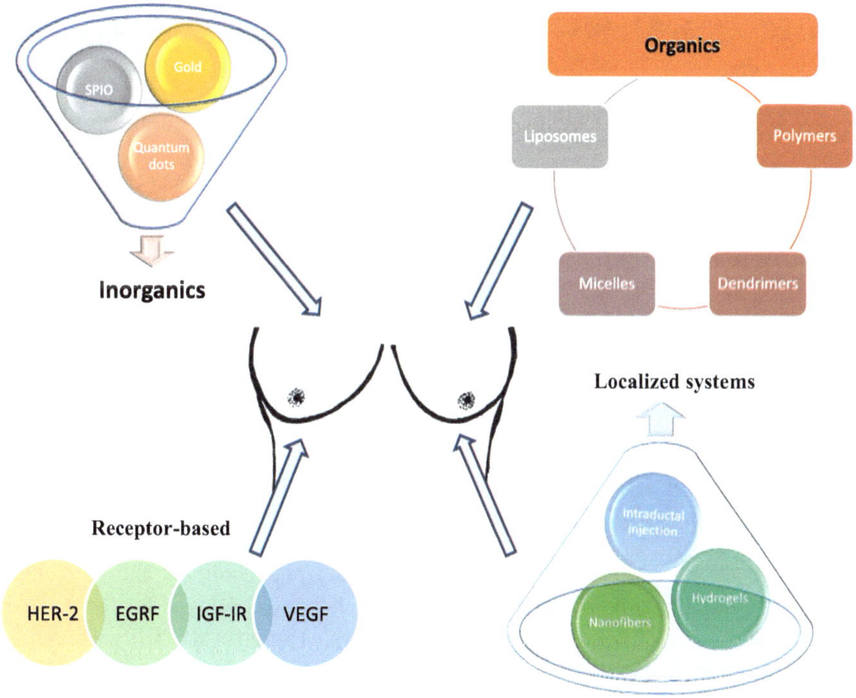

Fig. 2 The different nanotechnology-based drug delivery systems

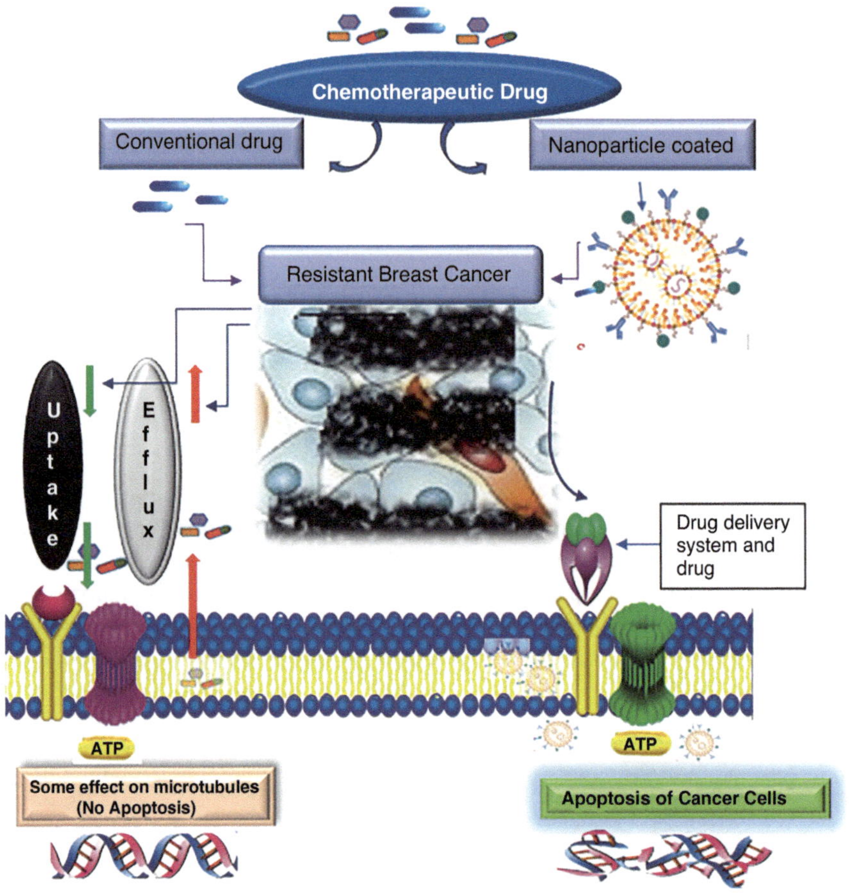

Fig. 3 Mechanisms of organic drug delivery systems

bioavailability with a resultant cell-specific increase in apoptosis and therefore destroys the cancer cells. This mechanism can bypass the resistance that is formed by most breast cancer cells. The drug delivery system presents the drug-nanoparticle mechanism directly to the malignant cells.

Micelles

Polymeric micelles (PMs) are made by combining phospholipids and surfactants with water-soluble colloidal particle polymers. They are employed for the delivery of chemotherapy medicines that are not water soluble (Singh et al., 2017). Therefore, they can accumulate in poorly vascularized tumors with good permeability and their enhanced retention (overcome efflux) ensures an increase in the drug's half-life. Through receptor-mediated endocytosis and an increase in the intracellular concentration of a particular drug, cytotoxicity is amplified. Anti-HER-2 monoclonal antibody (mAb) in combination with antibody-conjugated lysosomal P (LA-co-TMCC)-g-PEG-furan micelles is another method of enhancing cytotoxicity. These immunological micelles, which have antibodies attached to their surfaces, are used to treat HER-2-positive breast cancer. In the HER-2-negative breast cancer cells, the antibody–micelles complex formulation improves the efficacy of taxol chemotherapy as opposed to its use alone (Mohajer et al., 2007; Yuan et al., 2016). Micelles increase the response rate in patients with metastatic breast cancer to roughly 58% when compared to using only chemotherapy agents (Singh et al., 2017). Fig. 4 depicts the structure of the micelle.

Figure 4 illustrates a micelle that is formed by an aggregation of the hydrophilic head which contacts solvent and hydrophobic single tail in the center. Micelles generally act as emulsifiers where they permit a compound that would have been generally insoluble to be incorporated into the core through their interaction with the heads that render it favorable to interact.

Liposomes

Liposomes are spherical microparticles that have a single or multiple bilayer membrane structure that ranges in size from 50 to 200 nm. They were initially described in 1965. They contain lipophilic and hydrophobic stable pharmaceuticals that are non-toxic, biocompatible, biodegradable, and immune-neutral (Kalepu & Nekkanti, 2015; Singh et al., 2017). Chemotherapeutic agents are encapsulated in the liposome to improve drug efficacy, prolong circulation, protect against mononuclear phagocytes, and reduce toxicity through biodistribution (Kalepu & Nekkanti, 2015; Kang et al., 2009; Straubinger & Papahadjopoulos, 1983). Figure 5 shows a depiction of a liposome.

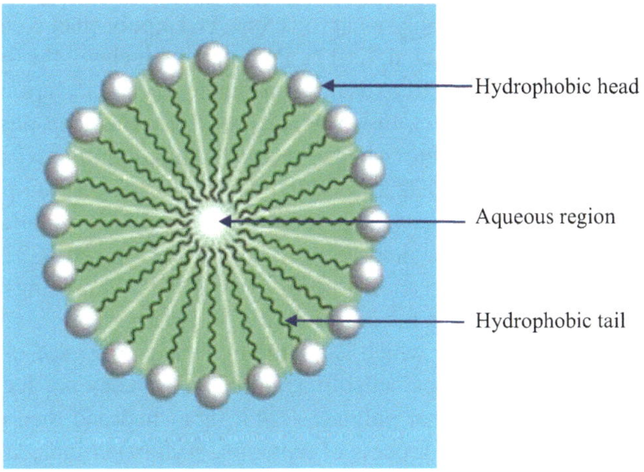

Fig. 4 A depiction of the of micelle

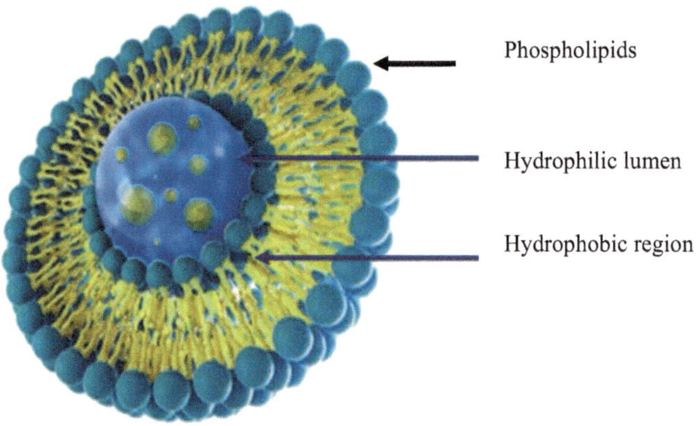

Fig. 5 Scheme depiction of a liposome drug delivery nanotechnology system

Figure 5 depicts a liposome which is a small, spherical, artificial, lipid bilayer that is used for drug delivery systems. Liposomes have both hydrophobic and hydrophilic properties which makes them a perfect vehicle for biological molecules encapsulation. For the delivery of drug molecules to the specific cell site, the liposome bilayer enables it to fuse with other bilayers such as the cell membrane. They are commonly made through disruption of biological membranes.

Polymers

Polymeric NPs are even smaller than liposomes in size (size 3–200 nm). They are divided into four categories: nonbiodegradable, biodegradable, synthetic and natural. Examples of natural polymers in use are cellulose, chitosan, alginate, and gelatin. Synthetic polymers include poly-ε-caprolactone (PCL), poly-(lactic-co-glycolide), and polylactide (PLA) (Singh et al., 2017). Polymers with chemotherapeutic drugs have been subjected to clinical trials as drug conjugates for use in various malignancies. Drugs including paclitaxel, doxorubicin, camptothecins, and platinates have enhanced stability, solubility, etc. when combined with polymeric NPs. The therapeutic index and efficacy of a nuclear PLGA NP are enhanced by a PEG-phospholipid copolymer envelope. The same was observed with the use of cisplatin. There is a synergistic impact and potential mode of action when targeting HER-2 receptors via extracellular (via TRZ binding) and intracellular (via PKI-166 binding) kinase (Lee & Nan, 2012). Figure 6 depicts the structure of a polymer.

Figure 6 depicts a polymer which is a large molecule composed of multiple or repeating subunits of molecules called macromolecules. They are formed from a linkage of linear molecules that polymerize into branched and then cross-linked macromolecules. Through the process of reptation, each macromolecule can move and entangle with other close chains. Its dynamicity and viscoelasticity make it a good molecular vehicle for drug delivery.

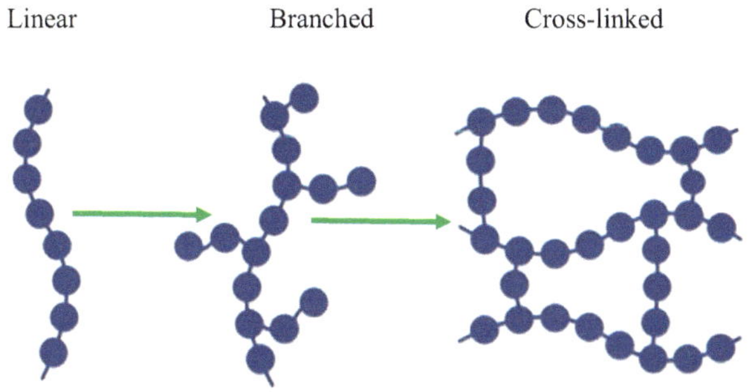

Fig. 6 Depiction of a polymer drug delivery nanotechnology system

Dendrimers

These are highly branched macromolecules that possess a low polydispersity index. This drug delivery system also improves biocompatibility and pharmacokinetics. They are reported as easy to predict and to control. Synthesized platforms include polyetherhydroxylamine (PEHAM), polyamidoamine (PAMAM), polyesteramine, polypropyleneimine, and polyglycerol. To increase effectiveness in the treatment of breast cancer, doxorubicin-G4-PAMAM complexes are additionally encapsulated into liposomes (Singh et al., 2017). Figure 7 depicts the structure of a typical dendrimer.

Figure 7 depicts the structure of a dendrimer as a highly ordered, spherical three-dimensional compound whose functional site allows it to mimic active site in biomaterials. They encapsulate hydrophobic compounds and as such can act as drug delivery systems.

Inorganic Drug Delivery Approaches

Gold Nanoparticles

Breast cancer cells' migration, invasion, angiogenesis, and metastasis were reported to be inhibited by gold nanoparticle-based drug delivery system for quercetin (Qu) [AuNPs-Qu-5]. Balakrishnan et al. targeted the Epidermal Growth Factor Receptor/Vascular Endothelial Growth Factor Receptor 2 (EGFR)/VEGFR-2) signaling pathway as well as studied significant inhibition of several proteins such as p-PI3K, Akt, Snail, Slug, vimentin, N-cadherin, and p-GSK3β using AuNPs-Qu-5 (Balakrishnan et al., 2016; Eissa et al., 2014; Singh et al., 2017). Another study by Eissa et al. investigated 120 patient samples for Estrogen Receptor (ER), Progesterone Receptor (PR), and Human Epidermal Growth Factor Receptor 2 (HER-2) with the use of histidine-rich glycoprotein RNA-AuNPs and found that there was 90% sensitivity and specificity. In triple-negative breast cancer MDA-MB-231, successful cancer

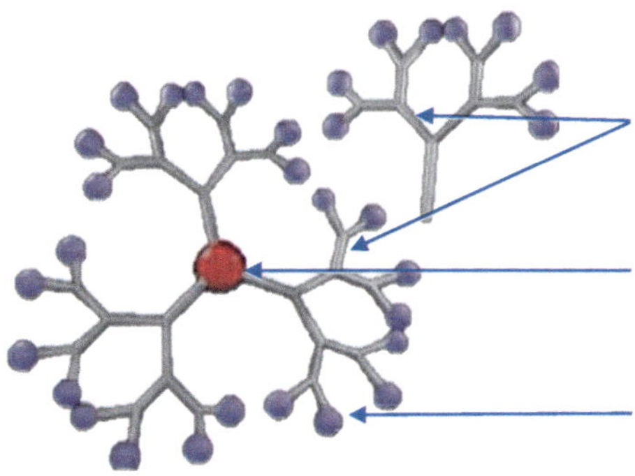

Fig. 7 Diagram of a typical Dendrimer

cell inhibition was achieved with the use of phytochemical compounds (for example, gallic acid) in combination with GNPs (Chen et al., 2016; Singh et al., 2017).

The Breast Cancer Receptor Cells and Receptor-Based Drug Delivery Approaches

Breast cancer cell growth is regulated by different receptors, and inhibition at the receptor as well as the use of drug delivery systems provides a new avenue for cancer therapy (Singh et al., 2017).

HER-2

HER-2 is overexpressed in breast cells. It is a member of the EGFR family that strongly correlates with tumorigenesis. Breast cancer treatment with anti-HER-2 therapy, nanocarriers (drugs), and antibody-directed therapy appears to be successful. An example of such is the effectiveness of the medication Trastuzumab (mAb), which demonstrated an overall response rate of 15–30% against HER-2-positive breast cancer when used alone as opposed to the combination with taxanes or vinorelbine, where the response rates were 50–80% (Singh et al., 2017). Using a targeted drug delivery system with these drugs may aid overcome resistance and improve overall survival as the mechanism not only block receptors in the use of trastuzumab-resistant tumors but also enhances biokinetics and increases its bioavailability (Montemurro & Aglietta, 2005; Valabrega et al., 2007).

EGFR

Poorly differentiated triple-negative and inflammatory breast cancer cells overexpress EGFR (Shimizu et al., 1981; Singh et al., 2017). HER-2 is overexpressed in breast cancer out of the known members of the EGFR family, which also includes

HER-1 (also known as ErbB1 and HER-1), HER-2 (also known as HER-2/neu and ErbB2), ErbB3 (HER3), and ErbB4 (HER4). There is an increase in gene copy number and protein overexpression in breast cancer that is ER negative, PR negative, and HER-2 negative (triple negative) (Burness et al., 2010; Guérin et al., 1989). Drugs such as cetuximab, lapatinib, and gefitinib are developed to target EGFR. However, the clinical outcomes of these drugs in triple-negative disease is still poor. Targeted drug delivery systems such as nanoparticles if developed for these cancers can offer better therapeutic outcomes and perhaps reduce resistance (Singh et al., 2017).

IGF-IR

The receptor tyrosine kinases (RTKs) regulate breast cancer growth and therefore its inhibition is seen as one of the targets for anticancer drugs. Normal breast cell proliferation and differentiation are also mediated by Insulin-like Growth Factor 1 Receptor (IGF-IR) signaling. Additionally, it promotes the mitogenesis and apoptosis of cancer cells (Singh et al., 2017). Breast cancer tumor growth is inhibited by the negative expression of IGF-IR, which is achieved via monoclonal antibodies, antisense IGF-IR, catechols, and transfection techniques. Thus, the use of nanoparticle drug delivery systems with IGF-IR inhibitors can be crucial in the treatment of breast cancer especially in resistant types (Prager et al., 1994; Sachdev et al., 2003).

VEGF

The upregulation of Vascular Endothelial Growth Factor (VEGF) by hormones, cytokines, and growth factors stimulates angiogenesis. VEGF is associated with breast cancer disease progression and development of metastasis. This is made possible by the expression of VEGF-2 (also known as flk/kdr), VEGFR-1 (also known as flt), and VEGF-C (homolog of the VEGF gene family) on receptors specific to vascular endothelial cells (Ferrara et al., 2003). Cancer metastasis and chemotherapy resistance also involve neovascularization and therefore, targeting endothelial growth factor cells by nanoparticles used in combination chemotherapeutic agents could be the future strategy for preventing and treating chemotherapy-resistant breast cancers (Singh et al., 2017).

Challenges of Nanotechnology Use

Nanotechnology and Nanomedicine are growing although not yet universally available and, in many fields, they are still undergoing clinical trials. There are barriers to rapid advancement in this field. Overcoming these barriers could revolutionize the treatment of several cancers including reversing resistance to chemotherapeutic drugs (Patel et al., 2015). Such barriers include lack of access especially in LMICs although there is much increase in research as well as advocacy for nanotechnology use and research in countries such as South Africa and Nigeria (Hammed et al., 2016; Masara et al., 2021; Musee et al., 2013). The limitations of nanotechnology in healthcare and the management of breast cancer may be attributed to a lack of understanding of the components and properties of nanoparticles, a lack of uniformity regarding toxicity, a lack of standardization in model systems and test assays, a lack of standard synthesis protocol, a lack of effective analytical tools, a lack of understanding of the impact on biological systems, a lack of in vivo monitoring systems, and a lack of standardized safety measures (Patel et al., 2015).

Conclusion

The pharmacokinetics and biodistribution of drugs are essential for the effect of drugs on the cell or disease site as they also affect resistance, recurrence, and resistance. Drug carrier systems control the pharmacokinetics and biodistribution of chemotherapeutic drugs. The use of nanoparticles in breast cancer affects the precise delivery of the chemotherapeutic drug to the target cancer cell site and is advantageous compared with conventional systems with regard to bioavailability, and biological half-life. This helps reduce drug resistance, reduce the dose of drug required for the effect, and reduce chemotherapeutic drug-related side effects. The nanoparticles can be integrated with other chemotherapeutic agents to improve outcomes and treat chemotherapeutic drug-resistant breast cancers.

References

Alshareeda, A. T., Nur Khatijah, M. Z., & Al-Sowayan, B. S. (2023). Nanotechnology: A revolutionary approach to prevent breast cancer recurrence. *Asian Journal of Surgery, 46*, 13–17.

Balakrishnan, S., Bhat, F. A., Raja Singh, P., Mukherjee, S., Elumalai, P., Das, S., Patra, C. R., & Arunakaran, J. (2016). Gold nanoparticle-conjugated quercetin inhibits epithelial-mesenchymal transition, angiogenesis, and invasiveness via Egfr/Vegfr-2-mediated pathway in breast cancer. *Cell Proliferation, 49*(6), 678–697.

Bar-Zeev, M., Livney, Y. D., & Assaraf, Y. G. (2017). Targeted nanomedicine for cancer therapeutics: Towards precision medicine overcoming drug resistance. *Drug Resistance Updates, 2017*(31), 15–30. https://doi.org/10.1016/j.drup.2017.05.002

Burness, M. L., Grushko, T. A., & Olopade, O. I. (2010). (2010). Epidermal growth factor receptor in triple-negative and basal-like breast cancer: Promising clinical target or only a marker? *Cancer Journal, 16*(1), 23–32.

Cao, J., Zhang, M., Wang, B., Zhang, L., Zhou, F., & Fang, M. (2021). Chemoresistance and metastasis in breast cancer molecular mechanisms and novel clinical strategies. *Frontiers in Oncology, 11*, 658552. https://doi.org/10.3389/fonc.2021.658552

Chen, Y. J., Lee, Y. C., Huang, C. H., & Chang, L. S. (2016). Gallic acid-capped gold nanoparticles inhibit EGF-induced MMP-9 expression through suppression of p300 stabilization and NFκB/

c-Jun activation in breast cancer MDA-MB-231 cells. *Toxicology and Applied Pharmacology, 2016*(310), 98–107.
Chu, C. S., & Rubin, S. C. (2022). Basic principles of chemotherapy and other systemic therapies. In *DiSaia and Creasman's clinical gynaecologic oncology* (pp. 443–463). Elsevier.
Das, S., Mukherjee, P., Chatterjee, R., Jamal, Z., & Chatterji, U. (2019). Enhancing chemosensitivity of breast cancer stem cells by downregulating SOX2 and ABCG2 using wedelolactone-encapsulated nanoparticles. *Molecular Cancer Therapeutics, 18*(3), 680–692. https://doi.org/10.1158/1535-7163.MCT-18-0409
Dittmer, J. (2018). Breast cancer stem cells: Features, key drivers and treatment options. *Seminars in Cancer Biology, 2018*(53), 59–74. https://doi.org/10.1016/j.semcancer.2018.07.007
Eissa, S., Azzazy, H. M., Matboli, M., Shawky, S. M., Said, H., & Anous, F. A. (2014). (2014). The prognostic value of histidine-rich glycoprotein RNA in breast tissue using unmodified gold nanoparticles assay. *Applied Biochemistry and Biotechnology, 174*(2), 751–761.
Ferrara, N., Gerber, H. P., & Lecouter, J. (2003). (2003). The biology of VEGF and its receptors. *Nature Medicine, 9*(6), 669–676.
Gote, V., Nookala, A. R., Bolla, P. K., & Pal, D. (2021). Drug resistance in metastatic breast cancer: Tumor targeted nanomedicine to the rescue. *International Journal of Molecular Sciences, 22*(9), 4673. https://doi.org/10.3390/ijms22094673
Guérin, M., Gabillot, M., Mathieu, M. C., Travagli, J. P., Spielmann, M., Andrieu, N., & Riou, G. (1989). Structure and expression of c-erbB-2 and Egf receptor genes in inflammatory and non-inflammatory breast cancer: Prognostic significance. *International Journal of Cancer, 43*(2), 201–208.
Hammed, O., Adekunle, Y. A., Ebiesuwa, S., & Mensah-Agyei, G. O. (2016). Nanomedicine: Overview, problem, solution and future. *International Journal of Computer Science and Software Engineering (IJCSSE), 5*(9), 218.
Haq, A. I., Zabkiewicz, C., Grange, P., & Arya, M. (2009). Impact of nanotechnology in breast cancer. *Expert Review of Anticancer Therapy, 9*(8), 1021–1024. https://doi.org/10.1586/era.09.72
Ji, X., Lu, Y., Tian, H., Meng, X., Wei, M., & Cho, W. C. (2019). Chemoresistance mechanisms of breast cancer and their countermeasures. *Biomedicine & Pharmacotherapy, 114*, 108800. https://doi.org/10.1016/j.biopha.2019.108800
Kalash, R. S., Lakshmanan, V., Cho, C., & Park, I. (2016). Theranostics. In *Biomaterials nanoarchitectonics* (pp. 197–215). Elsevier. https://doi.org/10.1016/B978-0-323-37127-8.00012-1
Kalepu, S., & Nekkanti, V. (2015). Insoluble drug delivery strategies: Review of recent advances and business prospects. *Acta Pharmaceutica Sinica B, 5*(5), 442–453.
Kang, D. I., Kang, H. K., Gwak, H. S., Han, H. K., & Lim, S. J. (2009). Liposome composition is important for retention of liposomal rhodamine in P-glycoprotein-overexpressing cancer cells. *Drug Delivery, 16*(5), 261–267.
Klein, P. M., & Wagner, E. (2014). Bioreducible polycations as shuttles for therapeutic nucleic acid and protein transfection. *Antioxidants & Redox Signaling, 21*, 804–817.
Lainetti, P. F., Leis-Filho, A. F., Laufer-Amorim, R., Battazza, A., & Fonseca-Alves, C. E. (2020). Mechanisms of resistance to chemotherapy in breast cancer and possible targets in drug delivery systems. *Pharmaceutics, 12*(12), 1193. https://doi.org/10.3390/pharmaceutics12121193
Lee, J. H., & Nan, A. (2012). Combination drug delivery approaches in metastatic breast cancer. *Journal of Drug Delivery, 2012*(2012), 915375.
Masara, B., Van Der Poll, J. A., & Maaza, M. (2021). A nanotechnology-foresight perspective of South Africa. *Journal of Nanoparticle Research, 23*, 92. https://doi.org/10.1007/s11051-021-05193-6
Mckenna, M., Mcgarrigle, S., & Pidgeon, G. P. (2018). The next generation of PI3K-AktmTOR pathway inhibitors in breast cancer cohorts. *Biochimica Et Biophysica Acta. Reviews on Cancer, 1870*(2), 185–197. https://doi.org/10.1016/j.bbcan.2018.08.001
Mohajer, G., Lee, E. S., & Bae, Y. H. (2007). Enhanced intercellular retention activity of novel pH-sensitive polymeric micelles in wild and multidrug resistant MCF-7 cells. *Pharmaceutical Research, 24*(9), 1618–1627.

Montemurro, F., & Aglietta, M. (2005). Incorporating trastuzumab into the neoadjuvant treatment of HER2-overexpressing breast cancer. *Clinical Breast Cancer, 6*(1), 77–80.
Muhammad, W., Haroon, M., Shah, M., Ullah, M. A., & Haleem, I. (2018). Potential application of nanotechnology in health care: An insight. *Nanoscale Reports, 1*(2), 1–8. https://doi.org/10.26524/NR1821
Musee, N., Sikhwivhilu, L., & Gulumian, M. (2013). Relevance of nanotechnology to Africa: Synthesis, applications, and safety. In A. Gurib-Fakim & J. Eloff (Eds.), *Chemistry for sustainable development in Africa*. Springer. https://doi.org/10.1007/978-3-642-29642-0_8
Nedeljković, M., & Damjanović, A. (2019). Mechanisms of chemotherapy resistance in triple-negative breast cancer-how we can rise to the challenge. *Cells-Basel, 8*(9), 957. https://doi.org/10.3390/cells8090957
Patel, S., Nanda, R., & Sahoo, S. (2015). Nanotechnology in healthcare: Applications and challenges. *Medicinal Chemistry, 5*, 528–533. https://doi.org/10.4172/2161-0444.1000312
Prager, D., Li, H. L., Asa, S., & Melmed, S. (1994). Dominant negative inhibition of tumorigenesis in vivo by human insulin-like growth factor I receptor mutant. *Proceedings of the National Academy of Sciences of the United States of America, 91*(6), 2181–2185.
Riehemann, K., Schneider, S. W., Luger, T. A., Godin, B., Ferrari, M., & Fuchs, H. (2009). Nanomedicine--challenge and perspectives. *Angewandte Chemie (International Ed. in English), 48*(5), 872–897. https://doi.org/10.1002/anie.200802585
Sachdev, D., Li, S. L., Hartell, J. S., Fujita-Yamaguchi, Y., Miller, J. S., & Yee, D. (2003). A chimeric humanized single-chain antibody against the type I insulin-like growth factor (IGF) receptor renders breast cancer cells refractory to the mitogenic effects of IGF-I. *Cancer Research, 63*(3), 627–635.
Shimizu, N., Behzadian, M. A., & Shimizu, Y. (1981). Genetics of cell surface receptors for bioactive polypeptides: Binding of epidermal growth factor is associated with the presence of human chromosome 7 in human-mouse cell hybrids. *Proceedings of the National Academy of Sciences of the United States of America, 77*(6), 3600–3604.
Singh, S. K., Singh, S., Lillard, J. W., Jr., & Singh, R. (2017). Drug delivery approaches for breast cancer. *International Journal of Nanomedicine, 2017*(12), 6205–6218. https://doi.org/10.2147/IJN.S140325
Straubinger, R. M., & Papahadjopoulos, D. (1983). Liposomes as carriers for intracellular delivery of nucleic acids. *Methods in Enzymology, 1983*(101), 512–527.
Toh, T.-B., Lee, D.-K., Hou, W., Abdullah, L. N., Nguyen, J., Ho, D., & Chow, E. K. H. (2014). Nanodiamond–mitoxantrone complexes enhance drug retention in chemoresistant breast cancer cells. *Molecular Pharmaceutics, 2014*(11), 2683–2691.
United Nations. (2020). *Economic Commission for Africa; United Nations. Economic Commission for Africa Towards an African nanotechnology future: Trends, impacts and opportunities*. UN. ECA. https://hdl.handle.net/10855/43636. Accessed 15 July 2023
Valabrega, G., Montemurro, F., & Aglietta, M. (2007). Trastuzumab: Mechanism of action, resistance and future perspectives in HER2-overexpressing breast cancer. *Annals of Oncology, 18*(6), 977–984.
Vijayakumar, R., Ravindra Kumar, A., Selvaraj, J., Rahul Gandhi, P., & Ranjithkumar, R. (2013). Application of nanotechnology in medicine: A view. In *Diagnostics and therapeutics, chapter: 4* (Vol. 7, Nanotechnology ed.). Studium Press LLC.
Yuan, Y., Cai, T., Xia, X., Zhang, R., Chiba, P., & Cai, Y. (2016). Nanoparticle delivery of anticancer drugs overcomes multidrug resistance in breast cancer. *Drug Delivery, 23*(9), 3350–3357.

Addressing Breast Cancer Disparities in Advancements for Conquering Drug Resistance

Rahaba Marima, Olalekan Fadebi, Benny Mosoane, Afra Basera, Linomtha Gabada, Lydia Mphahlele, Amahle Nyalambisa, Egnesious Sambo, Thabo Patrick Dumakude, Melissa B. Davis, and Zodwa Dlamini

Abstract Breast cancer is a global concern with high morbidity and mortality rates. While incidence rates remain high in developed countries compared to low-middle-income countries (LMICs), relatively high mortality rates are reported in LMICs. Notably, such disproportions also exist within the same country, with rural areas often carrying the brunt of this disease. BC is a multifactorial concept where a broad research gap exists on the influence of non-scientific and inherent factors collide, leading to BC drug resistance. This chapter discusses the significance of addressing these disparities. Disparities exist in terms of equality and equity, including access to healthcare, quality of care, and representation in clini-

R. Marima (✉) · Z. Dlamini
SAMRC Precision Oncology Research Unit (PORU), DSI/NRF SARChI Chair in Precision Oncology and Cancer Prevention (POCP), Pan African Cancer Research Institute (PACRI), University of Pretoria, Pretoria, South Africa
e-mail: rahaba.marima@up.ac.za; zodwa.dlamini@up.ac.za

O. Fadebi · A. Basera · L. Gabada · L. Mphahlele · A. Nyalambisa · E. Sambo · T. P. Dumakude
SAMRC Precision Oncology Research Unit (PORU), DSI/NRF SARChI Chair in Precision Oncology and Cancer Prevention, Pan African Cancer Research Institute (PACRI), University of Pretoria, Pretoria, South Africa

Department of Medical Oncology, Faculty of Health Sciences, Steve Biko Academic Hospital, University of Pretoria, Pretoria, South Africa
e-mail: u22493591@tuks.co.za; u22800370@tuks.co.za; u22609114@tuks.co.za; u23013801@tuks.co.za; u23013720@tuks.co.za; u15201407@tuks.co.za; u23026406@tuks.co.za

B. Mosoane
Department of Anatomical Pathology, National Health Laboratory Service (NHLS), University of Pretoria, Pretoria, South Africa
e-mail: Benny.Mosoane@nhls.ac.za

M. B. Davis
Institute of Translational Genomic Medicine and Department of Microbiology Biochemistry and Immunology, Morehouse School of Medicine, Atlanta, GA, USA
e-mail: mbdavis@msm.edu

Z. Dlamini (ed.), *Overcoming Breast Cancer Therapy Resistance*,
https://doi.org/10.1007/978-3-031-52860-6_15

cal trials. Socioeconomic and structural barriers also exist and can contribute to differential outcomes in BC patients. In addressing these disparities, this chapter highlights the need for community engagement, inclusive research efforts, and tailored interventions to overcome these disparities. Furthermore, by addressing these gaps, which pose as primary barriers, an integrated patient-centered approach is warranted and will be the most valuable tool in ensuring more equitable outcomes in the fight against drug-resistant BC.

Keywords Breast cancer · Disparities · Diagnosis · Treatment · Equality · Equity · Exposome · Social · Cultural

Introduction

Breast cancer (BC) is the leading cause of cancer-related mortalities in females and the most commonly diagnosed cancer in the world (Bray et al., 2018). In 2020, an estimated 2.3 million new BC cases (11.7%) were reported, according to the GLOBOCAN statistics (Sung et al., 2021). Clinically, hormonal, targeted, and several immunotherapy drugs are (Ender et al., 2019) used as BC treatment and may be disproportionally available. In clinical trials, many immunotherapeutic drugs have demonstrated efficacy in BC treatment (Ender et al., 2019). The impact of the quality of BC treatment is also associated with the inability to access healthcare which then promotes chemotherapeutic resistance due to poor compliance by affected patients. Access to healthcare, quality of care, and representation in clinical trials are disparities that impact BC research and treatment, resulting in BC drug resistance. Access to healthcare potentially is a means of increasing access for individuals who are not insured or are underinsured. In addition, cultural, structural, and religious factors also contribute to these disparities. The disparities in BC research and treatment outcomes challenge the values of researchers and their sense of equity for all individuals (Wheeler et al., 2013). Addressing and creating awareness of these disparities among patients, their families, societies, networks, healthcare professionals, policymakers, and all stakeholders alike may bridge the gap that exists between affordable healthcare, quality BC treatment, and outcomes for all patients (Ghafouri-Fard et al., 2021). The hope of reducing BC disparities as a means of conquering drug resistance can be achieved by understanding the occurrence in communities that are affected by involving the leaders and members of the community who are keen to advance their health as a community.

In underrepresented communities, inclusive research and engaging the community result in quality research outcomes. Community engagement is referred to as the advantageous actions or mutual values to promote shared respect, power, and authenticity between researchers and community members (Jones & Wells, 2007). The demonstration of respect for the community members has intrinsic importance. This approach allows for knowledge sharing between researchers and the community to locate, contact, and recruit distal community members to participate in public health-related workshops and trials. In addition, it contributes to participation in clinical trials, and it is crucial in promoting equity in trials. Thus, communities must normalize engaging thoroughly in research, programs, and proposed actions to fight BC disproportions. This approach has been implemented in several ways in BC research (Jones & Wells, 2007). However, it is not clear how inclusive BC research and community engagement suppress the societal values influencing disparities in access to screening, diagnosis, and treatment. This chapter will focus on the disparities in access to screening, diagnosis, and treatment; structural, cultural, and societal factors influencing disparities; and strategies for reducing disparities and promoting equity.

Intrinsic and Extrinsic Factors Contributing to BC Disparities

Intrinsic Factors

Genetic, Family History, and Ethnicity

Genetic predisposition has been consistently identified as one of the most famous risk factors of BC, accounting for approximately 10–30% of BC cases (Apostolou & Fostira, 2013). Recently, several genes that are linked to a high risk of BC have been identified, and they include *BRCA1* and *BRCA2* (Yoshida, 2021). These genes are tumor suppressors responsible for maintaining genomic stability. However, loss of heterozygosity followed by hereditary mutations in these genes increases chromosomal instability and poses a high risk to cancer progression, as well as playing vital roles in malignant transformation. In BC, Germline mutations in *BRCA1* and *BRCA2* genes are the main inherited factors (Mahdavi et al., 2019). Several hereditary factors promote incidences of BC, with approximately 40% of BC cases caused by inherited autosomal mutations in the *BRCA1* and *BRCA2* genes (Cobain et al., 2016). A study revealed that 50%–65% of carriers of *BRCA1* mutations and 45% of *BRCA2* mutations develop cancer by the age of 70 years (Godet & Gilkes, 2017). A cohort study reported that the risk of BC at the age of 80 years was 72% in carriers of *BRCA1* mutation and 69% in carriers of *BRCA2* mutations (Kuchenbaecker et al., 2017). Alterations in human interferon α-2b may also be implicated in the progression of BC coupled with other risk factors (Momenimovahed & Salehiniya, 2019).

Family history is a major risk factor for BC in several studies (Bravi et al., 2018; Momenimovahed & Salehiniya, 2019; Thakur et al., 2017). It has been suggested that 15–25% of women have a relative who has cancer. Women with a family history of BC who test negative for *BRCA* mutations are 11 times more likely to develop BC (Metcalfe et al., 2009). Early onset of BC is a risk factor in the progression of BC in carriers of *BRCA1* and *BRCA2* (Narod et al., 2014). It has been reported in a case-control study that the history of BC is associated with a double-fold increase in the risk of onset of contralateral BC (Narod et al., 2014). Accordingly, there should not be a difference in the clinical management of women with or without breast cancer and awareness of the significance of underlying mutations (Melvin et al., 2016). However, a family history of breast cancer may qualify an individual for chemoprevention in the developed parts of the world (Metcalfe et al., 2009).

Breast cancer estimated global incident rate of 1.67 million in the past 5 years was reported (Singh et al., 2017). A significant shift in global cancer distribution is speculated to shift toward low- and middle-income countries (LMICs), affecting all age groups due to population growth, adoption of Westernized lifestyles, and increased life expectancy (Singh et al., 2017). Contradictory reports on BC incidence rates are documented. However, consistent mortality rates across different parts of the world in non-white women have been reported. Thus, the incidence of BC varies widely across racial, ethnic, and geographical regions. Researchers reported that the incident rate of BC is equal for black and white women, but the difference is seen in women below the age of 45 years, where the incidence rate is higher in black than in white women, whereas it is higher in white than black women of ages between 60 and 84 years (Yedjou et al., 2019). There are several subtypes of breast cancer: estrogen receptor-positive (ER+) and human epidermal growth factor receptor 2 [HER2 (+/−)], and basal-like breast cancer, which is triple negative, the most aggressive, and a high-grade tumor subtype. The incidences of these aggressive subtypes are higher in women from LMICs (Haiman et al., 2011). Pregnancy and higher birth rates have been reported to increase the risk of basal-like breast cancer and, invariably, reduce the risk of estrogen receptor/progesterone receptor (ER+/PR+) breast cancer (Yedjou et al., 2019). Contrarily, pregnancy has also been shown to reduce the incidence of basal-like breast cancer (Haiman et al., 2011). Black women from LMICs have more parity at younger ages with a lower rate of breastfeeding, hence predisposing them to a triple-negative subtype of breast cancer (Yedjou et al., 2019). Notably, these reports are contradictory despite the evident BC disparities in underrepresented communities.

Cultural, Societal, Socioeconomic, and Religious Factors

Some religious and cultural communities may have beliefs or practices that prohibit obtaining medical care, particularly for women's health issues like BC. In some religious communities, a lack of knowledge and instruction regarding BC and early detection techniques may result in delayed diagnosis and worse results, with women often depending on a spiritual and higher power. Receiving prompt and thorough breast cancer treatment can be significantly hampered by low-income communities' limited access to health insurance. Socioeconomically disadvantaged groups with low health literacy may struggle to comprehend medical information, making it a challenge to make knowledgeable decisions about BC treatment. Language barriers can hinder communication with healthcare providers, leading to misunderstandings and inadequate information about BC prevention and treatment options.

These social, cultural, and economic issues have impacted the experiences of women about BC as well as the general knowledge and comprehension of the disease and how it is being managed (Mdondolo et al., 2003; Schlebusch & Van Oers, 1999; Thorne & Murray, 2000; Wright, 1997). Among rural women, for example, social beliefs and economics associated with women's bodies in sub-Saharan Africa

(SSA) are instrumental in noncompliance to treatment regimens or termination of treatment for BC (Adesunkanmi et al., 2006; Anyanwu et al., 2011; Clegg-Lamptey & Hodasi, 2007; Opoku et al., 2012). Cultural beliefs about the cause of breast diseases and associations of female breasts with emotional support, motherhood, and femininity influence the diagnosis and treatment of BC in SSA. Additionally, women's experiences of BC are not only influenced by social and cultural factors and social perceptions of the disease but also by the availability of resources for the management of the disease (Mdondolo et al., 2003; Omonzejele, 2008; Schlebusch & Van Oers, 1999; Thorne & Murray, 2000; Wright, 1997). In African communities that lean more on tradition, good health is perceived as a prudent relationship between the living and the dead and peaceful habitation, even among individuals. Hence, it is believed that the disease is a result of an absence of supernatural and ancestral forces and the malfunctioning of a body organ (Omonzejele, 2008). This affects the diagnosis, treatment, and management of the disease and how the disease is experienced overall. In SSA, the resolution to seek complementary therapy, such as healing and prayer camps, is a result of the belief of the society that BC is associated with supernatural forces. Several women in SSA first use complementary medicine in conjunction with other treatments and only report to the hospitals when the BC is at an advanced stage (Clegg-Lamptey et al., 2009; Mdondolo et al., 2003; Opoku et al., 2012; Schlebusch & Van Oers, 1999). This delay in clinical reporting may also be attributed to the socioeconomic and health literacy of these women. The guilt associated with the perception that BC is caused by supernatural forces results in the loss of control over the disease from several SSA women (Schlebusch & Van Oers, 1999). The belief that the living cannot contend with the dead makes women feel guilty that they have offended their ancestors, and hence, they are being punished with BC.

Although not all Africans believe in ancestral spirits, on some occasions, health and illness are believed to be from supernatural forces, such as God, Allah, or ancestral spirits. Therefore, it is considered a norm to blend traditional and Western/modern medicine for the treatment of diseases (Omonzejele, 2008). Some intellects gave the impression that seeking complementary treatment for BC designates a preference for traditional medicine over Western/modern medicine in SSA (Tesfamariam et al., 2013; Wright, 1997). Traditional medicine is thought to be affordable, easily accessible, reliable, and comprehensive as opposed to Western medicine and as it is believed to involve the body, spirit, and soul (Asobayire & Barley, 2015; Omonzejele, 2008) in many non-white populations. Traditional healers are believed to incorporate both scientific and metaphysical causes and treatment for diseases such as cancers, which makes women have more trust in them (Benedict, 2014; Omonzejele, 2008; Wright, 1997). For example, Mdonlolo et al. reported that South African Xhosa women lean more toward traditional medicine in the treatment of BC because of the reduced pain, does not involve cutting the skin, and can be acquired much faster than Western medicine (Mdondolo et al., 2003). Similarly, Wright reported that Black BC patients preferred traditional treatment as opposed to Western medicine because it is appropriate and less harmful (Wright, 1997). These women also felt that a cancer ward in Western medicine lacks privacy as it is open and accessible to the public (Wright, 1997). This is crucial in the SSA context, where there is stigmatization of breast cancer, and women tend to choose privacy.

The diagnosis and management of BC in SSA are affected by another sociocultural factor in African tradition, that belief in the "whole" and beautiful body of a woman. The discernment of attractiveness and the ideal body shape varies from one culture to another, demonstrating particular social and cultural values (Reischer & Koo, 2004). Africans believe a woman is considered beautiful if she has all her body parts intact, especially parts that are feminine, especially the breasts. On the contrary, mastectomy, seen as the "mutilation" of a woman's body, is the regular form of treatment for BC in SSA (Clegg-Lamptey et al., 2009; Wright, 1997). Thus, this treatment for BC opposes the popular perception of a beautiful body. For example, it is reported that South African women who underwent mastectomy opt for reconstructive surgery because mastectomy contravenes the cultural notions about the "whole and beautiful body." The belief is common to the extent that men go out of their way to hinder their wives from undergoing mastectomy procedures or seeking treatment for breast diseases if they cannot afford the cost of reconstruction surgeries (Cooper & Mullin, 2001). However, some women prefer prosthetics to breast construction surgeries after mastectomies (van der Wiel, 2013). This designates women's awareness of cultural expectations of their body's physique, and they are supposed to present their postmastectomy bodies to society; women are faced with double challenges relating to their health and the presentation of their bodies to society after breast cancer diagnosis. Therefore, it does not come as a surprise that women in SSA often dismiss their risks of breast cancer, a situation that opposes interventions focused on early diagnosis. Unlike in other cultures in developed countries, developing countries such as African countries cannot afford to primarily focus on the scientific treatment for BC but rather equally incorporate sociocultural factors for improved patient outcomes, Fig. 1.

Exposome and Racial Disparities in Breast Cancer

The responsiveness of cells to stress-causing external conditions depends on a diverse set of strict regulatory processes. The epigenetic landscape is the interface between many environmental variables and the complicated genetic landscape, which leads to gene expression changes that influence many areas of wellness and ailments (Zhubi et al., 2014). Changes in gene expression that are independent of the genome sequence are studied through epigenetics. Toxicants are some external factors proven to produce a phenotype or disease in a person or their offspring via epigenetic changes (Skinner et al., 2010; Yu et al., 2020). Numerous epigenetic processes, notably alterations to histones, DNA (e.g., methylation), and non-coding RNAs (ncRNAs), can alter gene expression when exposed to external factors (Karlsson & Baccarelli, 2016).

Disparities in the physiological functions of the epigenetic apparatus trigger a variety of ailments given that these processes ("epigenome") are significantly responsive to the external status (lack of nutrient consumption, physicochemical exposures, and psychological stress) relative to the genes, particularly during infancy owing to the epigenetic landscape's naturally changing nature (Kubota,

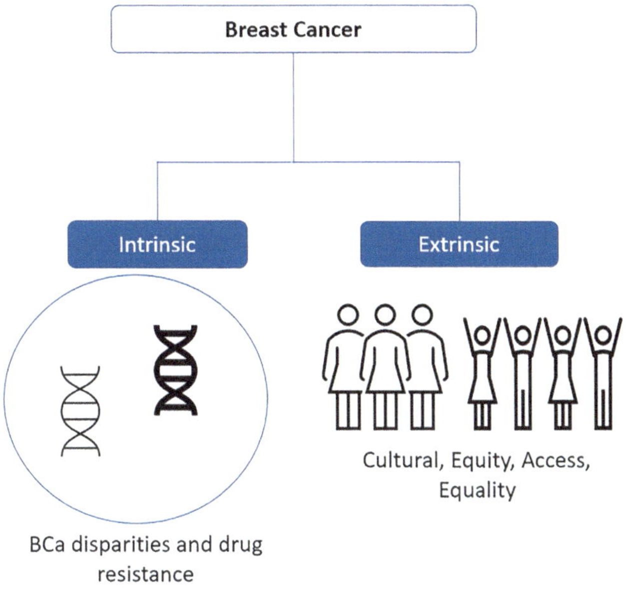

Fig. 1 BC disparities by managing the intrinsic and extrinsic factors. Equal efforts should be invested in both factor types and not exclusively on the tumor effects to overcoming drug resistance

2016). Contaminants such as dioxin, arsenic, cadmium, mercury, nickel, benzene, bisphenol A, and diethylstilbestrol are some components that may also alter the epigenetic modulation of the gene. These modifications can result in aberrant gene expression, leading to numerous cancers and other disorders (Fragou et al., 2011). In individuals, epigenetic contaminants alter the arrangement of chromatin and cause the hypermethylation of cell cycle regulatory genes, resulting in increased cell growth and cell transformation (Olmedo-Suárez et al., 2022). In BC, promoter hypermethylation has been observed in more than 70% of cases in the *GSTP1*, *BRCA1*, *CDH1*, and *p16 genes* (Esteller et al., 2001). Smoking and alcohol intake are some exposures linked to the hypomethylation within the *AHRR* (cg05575921) and *F2RL3* (cg03636183) genes (Gao et al., 2015) and CDC42BPB, respectively (Philibert et al., 2018). Furthermore, DNA methylation has been associated with exposure to DDT pesticides, increasing breast cancer susceptibility (Wu et al., 2020).

Environmental factors discussed above play a role in the racial disparities in BC. Racial differences in BC prevalence and outcomes are complicated and multidimensional, encompassing biological, and non-biological factors (Gonzales et al., 2018). Systematic disparities in housing, education, employment, criminal justice, and healthcare between racial and ethnic groups result in limited access to healthcare, transportation, and other resources. The disparities result in unfavorable health outcomes, not limited to residential areas but also the metropolitan areas (Collin et al., 2021). Due to system unfairness, structural racism, and socioeconomic statuses, people are exposed to distinct physical and social environments (Bailey et al., 2017; Ramirez & Trapido, 2020), which leads to behaviors including smoking, alcohol consumption, and lack of exercise (Nandi et al., 2014), which result in hypermethylation of DNA and BC (Gao et al., 2015; Philibert et al., 2018).

In the United States, African Americans' access to housing and employment is affected by racial discrimination (Williams et al., 2016) involving racially motivated policies and laws such as the Jim Crow law (Plascak et al., 2022). A phenomenon known as "redlining," where the state denied citizens mortgages based on race/ethnicity and lending bias—the denial of loans based on ethnicity culminated in the inability of African Americans to apply for housing loans (Hillier, 2003; Wisniewski, 1976; Zenou & Boccard, 2000). Loaning prejudice involves the same denial of housing loans, except it is individual specific rather than location based. In present times, redlining is a concern as it hinders financial strength and stability, which are paramount to wealth and health (Bailey et al., 2017).

The bias in mortgage results in residential separation, causing the individuals to occupy areas with air pollution and poverty (Williams & Wednesday, 2001). Air pollution and risk behaviors predispose individuals to BC (Goldberg et al., 2017; Taylor et al., 2007). Reports have revealed that residing in redlined areas is associated with a 60% increase in BC mortality, and non-Hispanic black females (80%) are the majority of occupants of these redlined areas, compared to 20% non-Hispanic white females (Collin et al., 2021).

In modern day, long-lasting place-based features and legislation (e.g., freeway and other built environment factors; zoning codes; school district zones; municipal tax rates, income, and expenditures), as well as the intergenerational transfer of socioeconomic variables, can inadvertently transform old systemic prejudice into negative health effects for individuals from marginalized ethnic and racial backgrounds who are alive currently who were not immediately affected by the since repelled laws. Historic system racism is correlated to better BC outcomes in affluent populations. Locations historically graded as "ideal" had decreased odds of late diagnosis, high tumor grade, triple-negative subtypes, and BC-specific death, but only among non-Hispanic white females (Plascak et al., 2022).

Racial inequalities in social and environmental subjection over a person's life may contribute to disparities in race in breast cancer by affecting transcription patterns and cellular physiology. Thus, gene–environment interactions controlled by epigenetic changes may play an important role in racial differences in BC occurrence and prognosis (Joshi et al., 2022).

Exposomic Factors

The history of hormone replacement therapy, alcohol consumption, reproductive history, and physical activity are some environmental factors related to BC risk (Huo et al., 2014; Yaghjyan et al., 2012). Environmental exposures, together with their related genetic factors, result in BC risks. The exposome is referred to as the overall measure of environmental influences such as drugs, dietary factors, behavioral factors, chemical pollutants, socioeconomic factors, and appropriate biological responses throughout the lifespan (Miller & Jones, 2013). Studies suggest that environmental chemicals are believed to partake in various biological roles in the development of BC, with some exposures occurring in the prime of life and others in the middle or late years of life. There are biological affirmation and epidemiological studies that a higher risk of BC could be a result of exposures to air pollution, dichlorodiphenyltrichloroethane (DDT), dioxin, and perfluorooctanesulfonamide (PFOSA) during the development of the breast, and for occupational exposures to chemicals and other mammary carcinogens like components of gasoline (Rodgers et al., 2018).

Most epidemiological studies exploring the environmental impact on BC risk have concentrated on a few sets of exposures and results based on previous knowledge and, therefore, are susceptible to omitting crucial relationships. Additionally, the focus of the study is to assess the risk of exposure to single chemicals. Discovering the underlying environmental risk factors may lower the burden of BC. Performing exposome-wide association studies (EWAS) is a promising approach to measuring molecular information of both endogenous and exogenous origins in biospecimens and recognizing links with BC (Rappaport, 2012; Wild et al., 2013). Computer-based approaches that use "omics" technologies are now sprouting as enormous ways of mapping the exposome to identify features related to BC higher risk.

Combining the omics and phenotypic measurements is beneficial in investigating the unique exposures. This will offer exceptional opportunities to discover new environmental risk factors for BC and shed more light on the molecular mechanisms of these relationships. The key innovative component approach on the identification of the differences between BC positive and BC negative participants can be achieved through the use and integration of omics BC risk factors, as well as the development of a new chemical library of pharmaceuticals, chemicals found in food and consumer products, and pollutants with biological activities similar to those of known breast carcinogens. The use of mass spectrometry (MS/MS) fragmentation profiles will enable critical structural information to acquire more confident identification of compounds. Another interesting method for creating a database of metabolomics compounds is to discover chemicals linked to BC by using recently available databases of short-term toxicity and exposure forecasts for thousands of chemicals. By presenting new information about human exposures to diet, lifestyle, and chemical factors linked to health outcomes and/or pathways related to BC, this omics approach will expand the list of environmental factors linked to BC and strengthen the scientific case for limiting exposure to such factors. This initiative will reveal endogenous mediators of the associations between exposures and breast cancer-related phenotypes, offering fresh insights into the underlying biological pathways. This will increase our knowledge of the relationship between genetics and the environment and how it affects women's health, which will ultimately aid in the creation of preventative measures and a decrease in the occurrence of BC. Exposomic factors may thus be unique to populations. Hence, creating and sharing exposome databases may aid in the identification of common or even distinctive exposure factors.

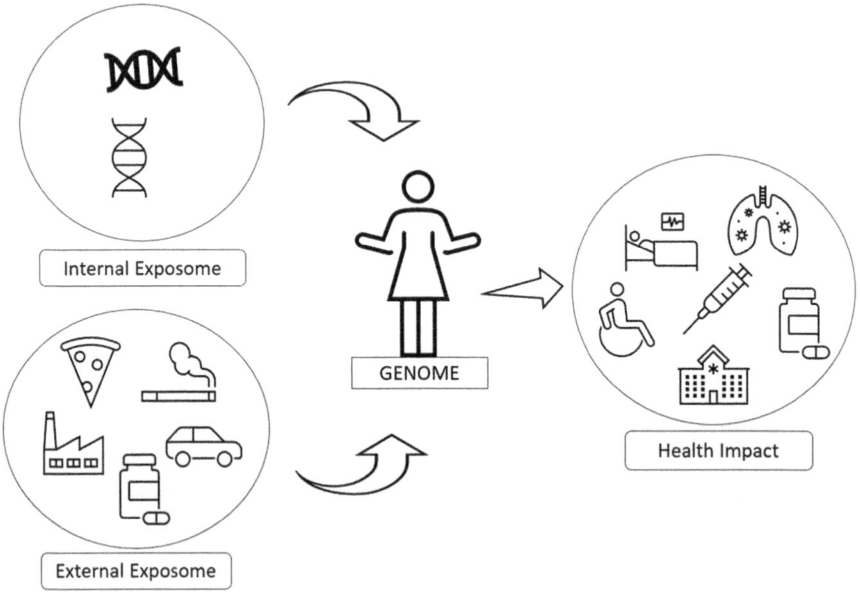

Fig. 2 Exposomic factors on BC disparities and drug resistance. The internal and the external exposomes influence the health outcomes of BC patients

Figure 2 illustrates exposomic factors that may contribute to BC and, thus, disparities.

Disparities in BC Medical Care and Management Between HICs and LMICs

BC Screening and Diagnosis

BC screening aids with early diagnosis and can significantly reduce mortality rates, especially observed in LMICs. Screening of the BC is done at multiple levels of self-examination, clinical breast examination (CBE) and imaging techniques, ultrasonography, mammography, magnetic resonance imaging (MRI), and digital breast tomosynthesis (DBT). The World Health Organization (WHO), American Cancer Society (ACS), United States Preventive Service Task Force (USPSTF), American College of Obstetricians and Gynecologists (ACOG), and National Comprehensive Cancer Network (NCCN) have published BC screening guidelines about age and other risk factors such as genetic mutations (Budh & Sapra, 2023). ACS recommends that regular screening should start at age 45, with annual screening from age 45 to 54 years and biannual screening after the age of 55 years (Ma et al., 2019). For the age group 40–49, USPSTF recommends that the screening be considered after evaluating and discussing the risks and benefits with the attending clinician. Biannual mammography in women aged between 50 and 69 years is recommended by the WHO, whereas ACOG recommends the same after the age of 55 years (Budh & Sapra, 2023).

CBE is not recommended by ACS, contrary to USPSTF, which advocates for CBE with mammography (Ma et al., 2019; Yaffe et al., 2018). NCCN recommends that women aged between 25–39 years have CBE every 1–3 years (Yaffe et al., 2018). American College of Physicians suggests that asymptomatic women at the age of 40 years should discuss with their attending clinicians the personal preferences, benefits, and potential harms of screening. The initiation of screening at an early age is considered for women with first-degree relatives with BC. Women who carry BRCA mutations should undergo annual breast MRI and mammography(Warner, 2018). Screening should stop after the age of 75 years or in women with 10 years of life expectancy or less (García-Albéniz et al., 2020).

Mammography remains the best screening tool, given that it can detect lesions before they are palpable and can demonstrate microcalcifications less than 10 μm (Albright et al., 2019). For standardized reporting, the Breast Imaging Reporting & Data System (BI-RADS) is used by radiologists to categorize breast lesions (Al Awfi & Al-Hubaishi, 2017; Xu et al., 2020). Each score carries a specific recommendation, Table 1.

Mammography sometimes leads to false-negative results, particularly in dense breasts. The application of digital mammography is recommended for a dense breast to diagnose BC (Institute of et al., 2005). MRI, although superior, is widely costly. Ultrasound is limited as a screening tool due to poor specificity and inability to detect microcalcifications. Ultrasound is operator dependent and limited due to the skills of the practitioner (Youk & Kim, 2010).

In LMICs, access to screening remains a major challenge even though early detection significantly improves BC prognosis. LMICs face barriers such as cost, geographical remoteness, and lack of awareness, whereas HICs have widespread mammography screening programs, regular checkups, and awareness campaigns. It is costly to implement such screening strategies, thereby impeding efficient screening of LMICs. Globally, BC awareness campaigns and initiatives help promote early detection, improve treatment outcomes, and decrease the burden of disease. However, there are significant differences in breast cancer awareness efforts between high-income countries (HICs) and LMICs. HICs have easy access to a wide range

Table 1 Breast imaging reporting and data system (BI-RADS)

BI-RADS score	Assessment	Recommendation
0	Incomplete assessment	Another mammogram may be needed
1	No abnormality	Routine screening continued
2	Benign breast condition	Routine screening continued
3	Probably benign finding	Mammogram repeated in the next 6 months
4	Cancer suspected	A biopsy may be needed
5	Highly suggestive of malignancy	Biopsy is needed

of media channels, including television, radio, and the Internet, which facilitates BC awareness campaigns. In contrast, limited access to media in some LMICs can impede awareness campaigns, necessitating innovative communication approaches, especially at the grassroots community level in LMICs.

Figure 3 is a global representation of the unequal distribution of cancer care and management medical devices.

BC Treatment

Optimal treatment outcomes for BC are dependent on a timely diagnosis followed by an organized, multidisciplinary approach to care. However, in LMICs, financial constraints, lack of resources, insufficient workforce, and inadequate infrastructure make it difficult to achieve effective care management. Surgical oncology aims to achieve local control of the tumor. Modified radical mastectomy (MRM) of Patey is the most preferred contemporary procedure as opposed to the previously practiced radical mastectomy of Halsted (Alkabban & Ferguson, 2023). The MRM procedure removes the whole breast procedure, a big part of the neighboring tissue, and axillary lymph nodes. This procedure spares the pectoralis muscles. A simple mastectomy procedure involves the removal of the breast tissue only, preferably when the tumor is small with sentinel lymph nodes (SLN). SNL refers to the regional nodes that directly drain from the primary tumor (Giammarile et al., 2022). Breast-conserving surgery removes the tumor with 1 cm margins of the normal breast tissue. Radiation therapy (RT) also contributes to local disease control, halving the risk of cancer recurrence in 10 years (Alkabban & Ferguson, 2023). RT is beneficial in larger tumors (>5 cm), skin or chest wall-invading tumors, positive lymph nodes, and widely metastatic tumors (Wang et al., 2018). RT can be delivered as an external radiation beam or brachytherapy.

Medical oncology entails hormonal therapy, chemotherapy, and targeted therapy. The administration of chemotherapy before surgery is referred to as neoadjuvant, and after surgery is called adjuvant (Montemurro et al., 2020). First-generation chemotherapy regimen includes cyclophosphamide, methotrexate, and 5-fluorouracil. Anthracyclins and texanes are the newer regimens used for BC. The duration of adjuvant and neoadjuvant chemotherapy can range from 3 to 6 months. As an adjuvant therapy, Tamoxifen (hormonal therapy) has been shown to halve the risk of BC recurrence for 10 years and reduce mortality by 30% in 15 years for patients with HR-positive tumors (Alkabban & Ferguson, 2023). Studies show that an extended duration of Tamoxifen or aromatase inhibitors like letrozole, up to 10 years, can reduce recurrence and mortality significantly (Bartlett et al., 2019; Goss et al., 2016; Vinayak & Davidson, 2019). Targeted therapy is indicated for tumors that express HER-2. Trastuzumab, a monoclonal antibody, reduces recurrence by 52% and death by 33% when combined with chemotherapy in HER-2-positive early BC (Dieci

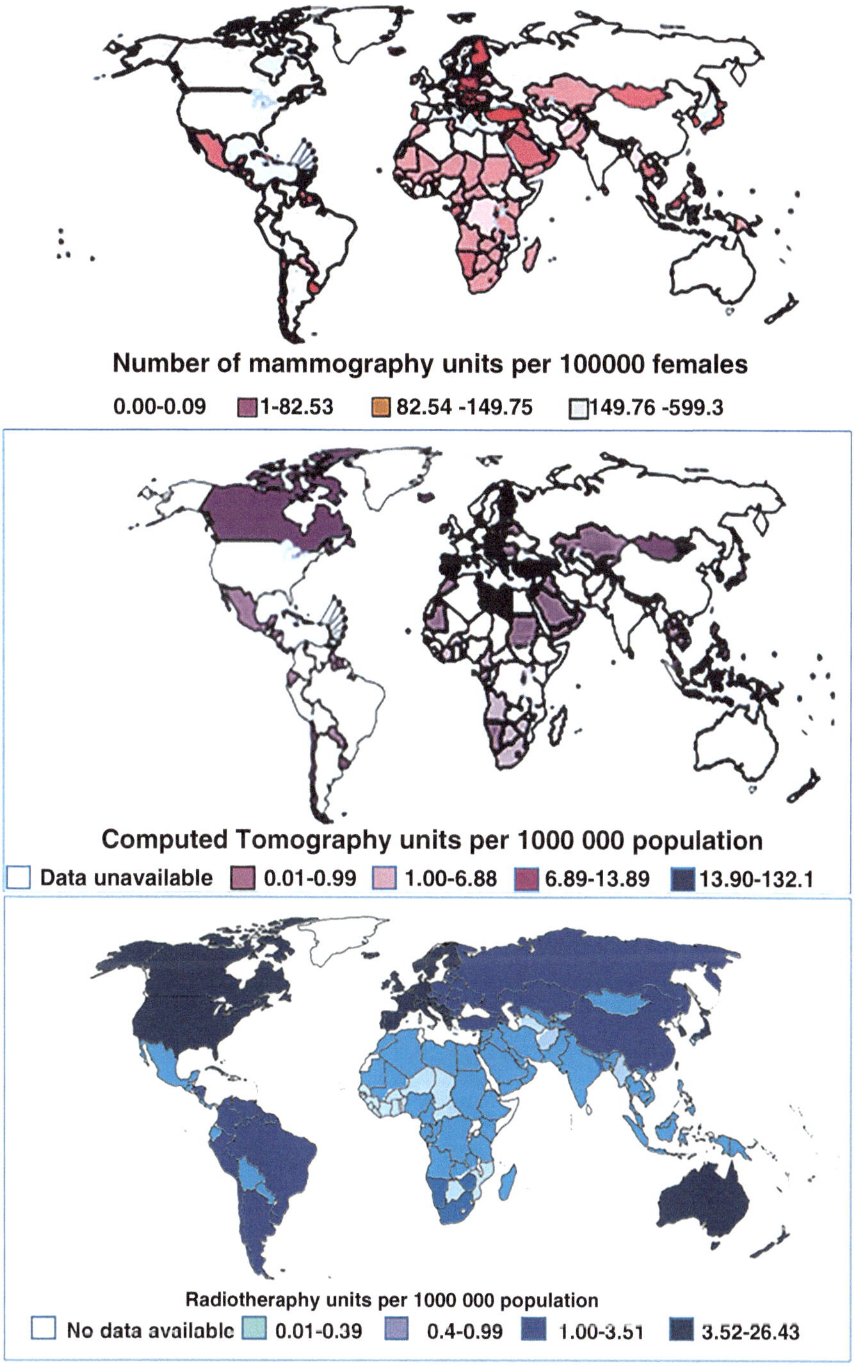

Fig. 3 Global BC care and management facilities (Globocan, 2020)

et al., 2019; Wu et al., 2018). Compared to European countries with >90% anticancer treatment availability, a WHO survey has reported that only 22–43% of African and Asian countries report on anticancer therapy availability, with no specifics.

Challenges and Limitations in BC Disparities and Drug Resistance

Early BC detection and diagnosis are key in BC management and averting therapy resistance. Unlike HICs, LMICs are still faced with several factors, such as limited resources and an effective healthcare infrastructure. Structural, cultural, and socioeconomic barriers are significant and yet are often overlooked factors that should be integrated into the BC management plan. This is especially true for African women and other women from LMICs, where women are generally not the primary decision-makers, even on matters concerning their health and well-being, but still have to submit to masculine authority. This is even worse for women living in rural areas. Furthermore, in other cultures, such as African cultures, decisions are made and affected by a structure, such as a family or a community, compared to isolated individual decisions. The underrepresentation of non-White women in BC clinical trials is another significant challenge. This is corroborated by the reluctance of these underrepresented women to even participate in genomic and clinical studies due to trust and ethical reasons that have been previously reported. As such, the lack of representation may be attributed to multiple factors. Religion is also a factor in BC and other disease management in other populations. In addition, education and awareness of BC in different socioeconomic classes cannot be facilitated with a one-size-fits-all approach but rather customized according to each class to yield positive results. While there may be various treatment modalities for BC, the road to accessing these treatments may be impeded by non-scientific barriers, which should be addressed to address BC disparities. Solutions to BC disparities and drug resistance in high-resource settings may not necessarily yield fruitful results in LMICs, with an influence of structural and socioeconomic barriers.

Redressing BC Disparities and Drug Resistance: A Multifaceted Approach

Despite improvements in cancer screening, diagnosis, and treatment, several populations continue to be afflicted by poor outcomes and higher mortality (Ver Hoeve et al., 2022). Delays in BC treatment of more than 3 months have been linked to more advanced stages and poorer survival (Ginsburg et al., 2020). Structural barriers such as poor coordination of services, lack of strong referral networks, and complex patient navigators exist in several healthcare systems, particularly in underserved populations and completing required cancer care. These structural barriers are prevalent within cancer care. The inability to access complex and, most times, confusing existing cancer care services creates disparities in BC care. Efforts to address these disparities, improve BC care services, and execute follow-ups to avert drug resistance.

The capacity to effectively diagnose and manage BC begins with capacity building, such as training in BC risk factors, CBE, and proper referral procedures, which may improve early detection and outcomes. It is important that care are trained to recognize early the signs and symptoms of BC for adequate referral through the health care system and also in the identification of complex, personal, multifactorial, and structural factors that can influence a woman's opportunities to seek and receive care (Ginsburg et al., 2018). Effective training of providers to recognize an early BC and refer patients for necessary diagnostic interventions in a fragmented healthcare system, which ordinarily would prevent patients from making their way through the whole care pathway, would avoid diagnostic delay. Once quality training is in place, accessible services to diagnose and early detection of screening programs to navigate the fragmented healthcare system would improve early detection and outcomes.

The geographical distribution of healthcare services impacts access to BC care. A major difficulty in improving diagnosis and achieving early detection of BC is associated with the unequal distribution of health services for BC care. There is a promising correlation between the availability of healthcare resources and the health status of the community (Ahmad Kiadaliri et al., 2011). Therefore, the distribution of healthcare is perceived to be one of the social factors that affect the outcome of healthcare management (Ahmad Kiadaliri et al., 2011). Centralization of care by reaching out to underrepresented communities could offer an opportunity to greatly increase the quality of care. Factors leading to BC disparities and drug resistance are interconnected. As such, addressing BC disparities should be done at multiple levels, considering the multiple factors involved will yield better results, especially in underserved communities, Fig. 4.

Conclusions and Perspectives

Addressing BC disparities warrants an all-around integrated approach, considering the lives worlds of BC patients, their families, and communities. A wide spectrum of scientific and non-scientific factors is involved and is an integral part of the solution to BC disparities and drug resistance. In some cultures, BC is still stigmatized, and this is a major barrier to early BC detection and drug resistance, especially in the African communities. Thus, all these factors should be integrated into BC awareness, education, and intervention efforts. With support from men and greater communities, structural and socioeconomic barriers can be conquered and pave the way for scientific factors such as early BC diagnosis, appropriate treatment, and conquering drug resistance.

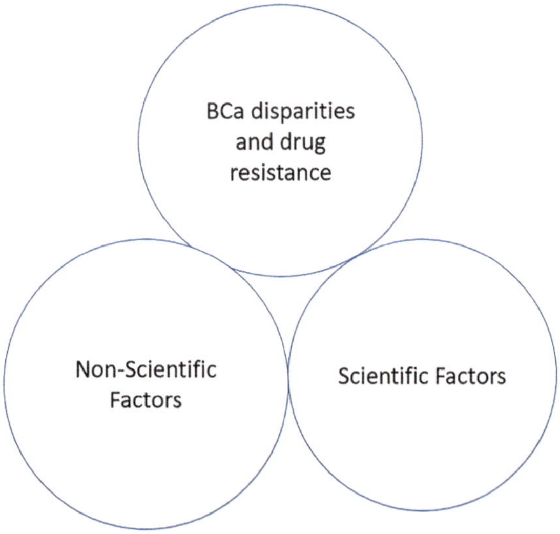

Fig. 4 Factors leading to BC disparities and drug resistance are interconnected. The administration of BC treatment should be an integrated approach

References

Adesunkanmi, A., Lawal, O., Adelusola, K., & Durosimi, M. (2006). The severity, outcome, and challenges of breast cancer in Nigeria. *The Breast, 15*, 399–409.

Ahmad Kiadaliri, A., Najafi, B., & Haghparast-Bidgoli, H. (2011). Geographic distribution of need and access to health care in rural population: An ecological study in Iran. *International Journal for Equity in Health, 10*, 39.

Al Awfi, M. M., & Al-Hubaishi, O. S. (2017). Characteristics and correlates of women eligible for targeted screening mammography in Oman. *Oman Medical Journal, 32*, 455–460.

Albright, F. S., Kohlmann, W., Neumayer, L., Buys, S. S., Matsen, C. B., Kaphingst, K. A., & Cannon-Albright, L. A. (2019). Population-based relative risks for specific family history constellations of breast cancer. *Cancer Causes & Control, 30*, 581–590.

Alkabban, F. M., & Ferguson, T. (2023). Breast cancer. In *StatPearls*. StatPearls Publishing.

Anyanwu, S. N., Egwuonwu, O. A., & Ihekwoaba, E. C. (2011). Acceptance and adherence to treatment among breast cancer patients in Eastern Nigeria. *The Breast, 20*, S51–S53.

Apostolou, P., & Fostira, F. (2013). Hereditary breast cancer: The era of new susceptibility genes. *BioMed Research International, 2013*, 747318.

Asobayire, A., & Barley, R. (2015). Women's cultural perceptions and attitudes towards breast cancer: Northern Ghana. *Health Promotion International, 30*, 647–657.

Bailey, Z. D., Krieger, N., Agénor, M., Graves, J., Linos, N., & Bassett, M. T. (2017). Structural racism and health inequities in the USA: Evidence and interventions. *The Lancet, 389*, 1453–1463.

Bartlett, J. M. S., Sgroi, D. C., Treuner, K., Zhang, Y., Ahmed, I., Piper, T., Salunga, R., Brachtel, E. F., Pirrie, S. J., Schnabel, C. A., & Rea, D. W. (2019). Breast Cancer Index and prediction of benefit from extended endocrine therapy in breast cancer patients treated in the Adjuvant Tamoxifen-To Offer More? (aTTom) trial. *Annals of Oncology, 30*, 1776–1783.

Benedict, A. O. (2014). The perception of illness in traditional Africa and the development of traditional medical practice. *International Journal of Nursing, 1*, 51–59.

Bravi, F., Decarli, A., & Russo, A. G. (2018). Risk factors for breast cancer in a cohort of mammographic screening program: A nested case–control study within the FR iCaM study. *Cancer Medicine, 7*, 2145–2152.

Bray, F., Ferlay, J., Soerjomataram, I., Siegel, R. L., Torre, L. A., & Jemal, A. (2018). Global cancer statistics 2018: Globocan estimates of incidence and mortality worldwide for 36 cancers in 185 countries. *CA: a Cancer Journal for Clinicians, 68*, 394–424.
Budh, D. P., & Sapra, A. (2023). Breast cancer screening. In *StatPearls*. StatPearls Publishing.
Clegg-Lamptey, J., Dakubo, J., & Attobra, Y. (2009). Psychosocial aspects of breast cancer treatment in Accra, Ghana. *East African Medical Journal, 86*, 54152.
Clegg-Lamptey, J., & Hodasi, W. (2007). A study of breast cancer in Korle Bu Teaching Hospital: Assessing the impact of health education. *Ghana Medical Journal, 41*, 55305.
Cobain, E. F., Milliron, K. J., & Merajver, S. D. (2016). Updates on breast cancer genetics: Clinical implications of detecting syndromes of inherited increased susceptibility to breast cancer. *Seminars in Oncology, 43*, 528–535.
Collin, L. J., Gaglioti, A. H., Beyer, K. M., Zhou, Y., Moore, M. A., Nash, R., Switchenko, J. M., Miller-Kleinhenz, J. M., Ward, K. C., & Mccullough, L. E. (2021). Neighborhood-level redlining and lending bias are associated with breast cancer mortality in a large and diverse metropolitan area. *Cancer Epidemiology, Biomarkers & Prevention, 30*, 53–60.
Cooper, S. E., & Mullin, V. C. (2001). Quality of life of cancer patients in underserved populations in South Africa. *Journal of Psychosocial Oncology, 19*, 39–56.
Dieci, M. V., Vernaci, G., & Guarneri, V. (2019). Escalation and de-escalation in HER2 positive early breast cancer. *Current Opinion in Oncology, 31*, 35–42.
Ender, F., Von Bubnoff, N., & Gieseler, F. (2019). Extracellular vesicles: Subcellular organelles with the potential to spread cancer resistance. *Anticancer Research, 39*, 3395–3404.
Esteller, M., Corn, P. G., Baylin, S. B., & Herman, J. G. (2001). A gene hypermethylation profile of human cancer. *Cancer Research, 61*, 3225–3229.
Fragou, D., Fragou, A., Kouidou, S., Njau, S., & Kovatsi, L. (2011). Epigenetic mechanisms in metal toxicity. *Toxicology Mechanisms and Methods, 21*, 343–352.
Gao, X., Jia, M., Zhang, Y., Breitling, L. P., & Brenner, H. (2015). DNA methylation changes of whole blood cells in response to active smoking exposure in adults: A systematic review of DNA methylation studies. *Clinical Epigenetics, 7*, 113.
García-Albéniz, X., Hernán, M. A., & Hsu, J. (2020). Continuation of annual screening mammography and breast cancer mortality in women older than 70 years. *Annals of Internal Medicine, 173*, 247.
Ghafouri-Fard, S., Abak, A., Tondro Anamag, F., Shoorei, H., Fattahi, F., Javadinia, S. A., Basiri, A., & Taheri, M. (2021). 5-Fluorouracil: A narrative review on the role of regulatory mechanisms in driving resistance to this chemotherapeutic agent. *Frontiers in Oncology, 11*, 1210.
Giammarile, F., Vidal-Sicart, S., Paez, D., Pellet, O., Enrique, E. L., Mikhail-Lette, M., Morozova, O., Maria Camila, N. M., Diana Ivonne, R. S., Delgado Bolton, R. C., Valdés Olmos, R. A., & Mariani, G. (2022). Sentinel lymph node methods in breast cancer. *Seminars in Nuclear Medicine, 52*, 551–560.
Ginsburg, O., Rositch, A. F., Conteh, L., Mutebi, M., Paskett, E. D., & Subramanian, S. (2018). Breast cancer disparities among women in low- and middle-income countries. *Current Breast Cancer Reports, 10*, 179–186.
Ginsburg, O., Yip, C.-H., Brooks, A., Cabanes, A., Caleffi, M., Dunstan Yataco, J. A., Gyawali, B., Mccormack, V., Mclaughlin De Anderson, M., Mehrotra, R., Mohar, A., Murillo, R., Pace, L. E., Paskett, E. D., Romanoff, A., Rositch, A. F., Scheel, J. R., Schneidman, M., Unger-Saldaña, K., Vanderpuye, V., Wu, T.-Y., Yuma, S., Dvaladze, A., Duggan, C., & Anderson, B. O. (2020). Breast cancer early detection: A phased approach to implementation. *Cancer, 126*, 2379–2393.
Globocan. (2020). Cancer Today [Online]. Available: https://gco.iarc.fr/today/online-analysis-map?v=2020&mode=population&mode_population=continents&population=900&population=900&key=asr&sex=2&cancer=20&type=1&statistic=5&prevalence=0&population_group=0&ages_group%5B%5D=0&ages_group%5B%5D=17&nb_items=10&group_cancer=1&include_nmsc=0&include_nmsc_other=0&projection=natural-earth&color_palette=default&map_scale=quantile&map_nb_colors=5&continent=0&show_ranking=0&rotate=%255B10%252C0%255D. Accessed 26 Oct 2023.

Godet, I., & Gilkes, D. M. (2017). BRCA1 and BRCA2 mutations and treatment strategies for breast cancer. *Integrative cancer science and therapeutics, 4*, 1000228.

Goldberg, M. S., Labreche, F., Weichenthal, S., Lavigne, E., Valois, M.-F., Hatzopoulou, M., Van Ryswyk, K., Shekarrizfard, M., Villeneuve, P. J., & Crouse, D. (2017). The association between the incidence of postmenopausal breast cancer and concentrations at street-level of nitrogen dioxide and ultrafine particles. *Environmental Research, 158*, 7–15.

Gonzales, M. C., Grayson, J., Lie, A., Yu, C. H., & Shiao, S. P. K. (2018). Gene-environment interactions and predictors of breast cancer in family-based multi-ethnic groups. *Oncotarget, 9*, 29019–29035.

Goss, P. E., Ingle, J. N., Pritchard, K. I., Robert, N. J., Muss, H., Gralow, J., Gelmon, K., Whelan, T., Strasser-Weippl, K., Rubin, S., Sturtz, K., Wolff, A. C., Winer, E., Hudis, C., Stopeck, A., Beck, J. T., Kaur, J. S., Whelan, K., Tu, D., & Parulekar, W. R. (2016). Extending aromatase-inhibitor adjuvant therapy to 10 years. *The New England Journal of Medicine, 375*, 209–219.

Haiman, C. A., Chen, G. K., Vachon, C. M., Canzian, F., Dunning, A., Millikan, R. C., Wang, X., Ademuyiwa, F., Ahmed, S., Ambrosone, C. B., Baglietto, L., Balleine, R., Bandera, E. V., Beckmann, M. W., Berg, C. D., Bernstein, L., Blomqvist, C., Blot, W. J., Brauch, H., Buring, J. E., Carey, L. A., Carpenter, J. E., Chang-Claude, J., Chanock, S. J., Chasman, D. I., Clarke, C. L., Cox, A., Cross, S. S., Deming, S. L., Diasio, R. B., Dimopoulos, A. M., Driver, W. R., Dünnebier, T., Durcan, L., Eccles, D., Edlund, C. K., Ekici, A. B., Fasching, P. A., Feigelson, H. S., Flesch-Janys, D., Fostira, F., Försti, A., Fountzilas, G., Gerty, S. M., Giles, G. G., Godwin, A. K., Goodfellow, P., Graham, N., Greco, D., Hamann, U., Hankinson, S. E., Hartmann, A., Hein, R., Heinz, J., Holbrook, A., Hoover, R. N., Hu, J. J., Hunter, D. J., Ingles, S. A., Irwanto, A., Ivanovich, J., John, E. M., Johnson, N., Jukkola-Vuorinen, A., Kaaks, R., Ko, Y. D., Kolonel, L. N., Konstantopoulou, I., Kosma, V. M., Kulkarni, S., Lambrechts, D., Lee, A. M., Marchand, L. L., Lesnick, T., Liu, J., Lindstrom, S., Mannermaa, A., Margolin, S., Martin, N. G., Miron, P., Montgomery, G. W., Nevanlinna, H., Nickels, S., Nyante, S., Olswold, C., Palmer, J., Pathak, H., Pectasides, D., Perou, C. M., Peto, J., Pharoah, P. D., Pooler, L. C., Press, M. F., Pylkäs, K., Rebbeck, T. R., Rodriguez-Gil, J. L., Rosenberg, L., Ross, E., Rüdiger, T., Silva Idos, S., et al. (2011). A common variant at the TERT-CLPTM1L locus is associated with estrogen receptor-negative breast cancer. *Nature Genetics, 43*, 1210–1214.

Hillier, A. E. (2003). Redlining and the homeowners' loan corporation. *Journal of Urban History, 29*, 394–420.

Huo, C. W., Chew, G. L., Britt, K. L., Ingman, W. V., Henderson, M. A., Hopper, J. L., & Thompson, E. W. (2014). Mammographic density—A review on the current understanding of its association with breast cancer. *Breast Cancer Research and Treatment, 144*, 479–502.

Institute Of, M., National Research Council Committee On New Approaches To Early, D. & Diagnosis Of Breast, C. (2005). The national academies collection: Reports funded by National Institutes of Health. In J. E. Joy, E. E. Penhoet, & D. B. Petitti (Eds.), *Saving women's lives: Strategies for improving breast cancer detection and diagnosis*. National Academies Press.

Jones, L., & Wells, K. (2007). Strategies for academic and clinician engagement in community-participatory partnered research. *JAMA, 297*, 407–410.

Joshi, S., Garlapati, C., & Aneja, R. (2022). Epigenetic determinants of racial disparity in breast cancer: Looking beyond genetic alterations. *Cancers (Basel), 14*, 1903.

Karlsson, O., & Baccarelli, A. A. (2016). Environmental health and long non-coding RNAs. *Current Environmental Health Reports, 3*, 178–187.

Kubota, T. (2016). Epigenetic alterations induced by environmental stress associated with metabolic and neurodevelopmental disorders. *Environmental Epigenetics, 2*, dvw017.

Kuchenbaecker, K. B., Hopper, J. L., Barnes, D. R., Phillips, K.-A., Mooij, T. M., Roos-Blom, M.-J., Jervis, S., Van Leeuwen, F. E., Milne, R. L., & Andrieu, N. (2017). Risks of breast, ovarian, and contralateral breast cancer for BRCA1 and BRCA2 mutation carriers. *JAMA, 317*, 2402–2416.

Ma, J., Jemal, A., Fedewa, S. A., Islami, F., Lichtenfeld, J. L., Wender, R. C., Cullen, K. J., & Brawley, O. W. (2019). The American Cancer Society 2035 challenge goal on cancer mortality reduction. *CA: a Cancer Journal for Clinicians, 69*, 351–362.

Mahdavi, M., Nassiri, M., Kooshyar, M. M., Vakili-Azghandi, M., Avan, A., Sandry, R., Pillai, S., Lam, A. K.-Y., & Gopalan, V. (2019). Hereditary breast cancer; Genetic penetrance and current status with BRCA. *Journal of Cellular Physiology, 234*, 5741–5750.
Mdondolo, N., De Villiers, L., & Ehlers, V. J. (2003). Cultural factors associated with the management of breast lumps amongst Xhosa women. *Health SA Gesondheid, 8*, 86–97.
Melvin, J. C., Wulaningsih, W., Hana, Z., Purushotham, A. D., Pinder, S. E., Fentiman, I., Gillett, C., Mera, A., Holmberg, L., & Van Hemelrijck, M. (2016). Family history of breast cancer and its association with disease severity and mortality. *Cancer Medicine, 5*, 942–949.
Metcalfe, K., Finch, A., Poll, A., Horsman, D., Kim-Sing, C., Scott, J., Royer, R., Sun, P., & Narod, S. (2009). Breast cancer risks in women with a family history of breast or ovarian cancer who have tested negative for a BRCA1 or BRCA2 mutation. *British Journal of Cancer, 100*, 421–425.
Miller, G. W., & Jones, D. P. (2013). The nature of nurture: Refining the definition of the exposome. *Toxicological Sciences, 137*, 1–2.
Momenimovahed, Z., & Salehiniya, H. (2019). Epidemiological characteristics of and risk factors for breast cancer in the world. *Breast Cancer: Targets and Therapy, 11*, 151–164.
Montemurro, F., Nuzzolese, I., & Ponzone, R. (2020). Neoadjuvant or adjuvant chemotherapy in early breast cancer? *Expert Opinion on Pharmacotherapy, 21*, 1071–1082.
Nandi, A., Glymour, M. M., & Subramanian, S. (2014). Association among socioeconomic status, health behaviors, and all-cause mortality in the United States. *Epidemiology, 25*, 170–177.
Narod, S., Tung, N., Lubinski, J., Huzarski, T., Robson, M., Lynch, H. T., Neuhausen, S., Ghadirian, P., Kim-Sing, C., & Sun, P. (2014). A prior diagnosis of breast cancer is a risk factor for breast cancer in BRCA1 and BRCA2 carriers. *Current Oncology, 21*, 64–68.
Olmedo-Suárez, M., Ramírez-Díaz, I., Pérez-González, A., Molina-Herrera, A., Coral-García, M., Lobato, S., Sarvari, P., Barreto, G., & Rubio, K. (2022). Epigenetic regulation in exposome-induced tumorigenesis: Emerging roles of ncRNAs. *Biomolecules, 12*, 513.
Omonzejele, P. F. (2008). African concepts of health, disease, and treatment: An ethical inquiry. *Explore, 4*, 120–126.
Opoku, S. Y., Benwell, M., & Yarney, J. (2012). Knowledge, attitudes, beliefs, behavior, and breast cancer screening practices in Ghana, West Africa. *Pan African Medical Journal, 11*, 89.
Philibert, R., Dogan, M., Noel, A., Miller, S., Krukow, B., Papworth, E., Cowley, J., Knudsen, A., Beach, S. R., & Black, D. (2018). Genome-wide and digital polymerase chain reaction epigenetic assessments of alcohol consumption. *American Journal of Medical Genetics Part B: Neuropsychiatric Genetics, 177*, 479–488.
Plascak, J. J., Beyer, K., Xu, X., Stroup, A. M., Jacob, G., & Llanos, A. A. M. (2022). Association between residence in historically redlined districts indicative of structural racism and racial and ethnic disparities in breast cancer outcomes. *JAMA Network Open, 5*, e2220908.
Ramirez, A. G., & Trapido, E. J. (2020). *Advancing the science of cancer in Latinos*. Springer.
Rappaport, S. M. (2012). Biomarkers intersect with the exposome. *Biomarkers, 17*, 483–489.
Reischer, E., & Koo, K. S. (2004). The body beautiful: Symbolism and agency in the social world. *Annual Review of Anthropology, 33*, 297–317.
Rodgers, K. M., Udesky, J. O., Rudel, R. A., & Brody, J. G. (2018). Environmental chemicals and breast cancer: An updated review of epidemiological literature informed by biological mechanisms. *Environmental Research, 160*, 152–182.
Schlebusch, L., & Van Oers, H. M. (1999). Psychological stress, adjustment and cross-cultural considerations in breast cancer patients. *South Africa Journal of Psychology, 29*, 30–35.
Singh, E., Joffe, M., Cubasch, H., Ruff, P., Norris, S. A., & Pisa, P. T. (2017). Breast cancer trends differ by ethnicity: A report from the south African National Cancer Registry (1994-2009). *European Journal of Public Health, 27*, 173–178.
Skinner, M. K., Manikkam, M., & Guerrero-Bosagna, C. (2010). Epigenetic transgenerational actions of environmental factors in disease etiology. *Trends in Endocrinology and Metabolism, 21*, 214–222.
Sung, H., Ferlay, J., Siegel, R. L., Laversanne, M., Soerjomataram, I., Jemal, A., & Bray, F. (2021). Global Cancer Statistics 2020: GLOBOCAN estimates of incidence and mortality worldwide for 36 cancers in 185 countries. *CA: a Cancer Journal for Clinicians, 71*, 209–249.

Taylor, T. R., Williams, C. D., Makambi, K. H., Mouton, C., Harrell, J. P., Cozier, Y., Palmer, J. R., Rosenberg, L., & Adams-Campbell, L. L. (2007). Racial discrimination and breast cancer incidence in US Black women: The black women's health study. *American Journal of Epidemiology, 166*, 46–54.

Tesfamariam, A., Gebremichael, A., & Mufunda, J. (2013). Breast cancer clinicopathological presentation, gravity and challenges in Eritrea, East Africa: Management practice in a resource-poor setting. *South African Medical Journal, 103*, 526–528.

Thakur, P., Seam, R. K., Gupta, M. K., Gupta, M., Sharma, M., & Fotedar, V. (2017). Breast cancer risk factor evaluation in a Western Himalayan state: A case–control study and comparison with the Western World. *South Asian Journal of Cancer, 6*, 106–109.

Thorne, S. E., & Murray, C. (2000). Social constructions of breast cancer. *Health Care for Women International, 21*, 141–159.

Van Der Wiel, R. (2013). "I am happy with one": Re-evaluating the relationship between gender, breast-cancer surgery, and survival. *Agenda, 27*, 55–64.

Ver Hoeve, E. S., Simon, M. A., Danner, S. M., Washington, A. J., Coples, S. D., Percac-Lima, S., Whited, E. C., Paskett, E. D., Naughton, M. J., Gray, D. M., Wenzel, J. A., Zabora, J. R., Hassoon, A., Tolbert, E. E., Calhoun, E., Barton, D. L., Friese, C. R., Titler, M. G., & Hamann, H. A. (2022). Implementing patient navigation programs: Considerations and lessons learned from the Alliance to Advance Patient-Centered Cancer Care. *Cancer, 128*, 2806–2816.

Vinayak, S., & Davidson, N. E. (2019). Extending adjuvant endocrine therapy in breast cancer: Who, what, why? *Oncology (Williston Park), 33*, 243–246.

Wang, X., Xu, L., Yin, Z., Wang, D., Wang, Q., Xu, K., Zhao, J., Zhao, L., Yuan, Z., & Wang, P. (2018). Locoregional recurrence-associated factors and risk-adapted postmastectomy radiotherapy for breast cancer staged in cT1-2N0-1 after neoadjuvant chemotherapy. *Cancer Management and Research, 10*, 4105–4112.

Warner, E. (2018). Screening BRCA1 and BRCA2 mutation carriers for breast cancer. *Cancers (Basel), 10*, 477.

Wheeler, S. B., Reeder-Hayes, K. E., & Carey, L. A. (2013). Disparities in breast cancer treatment and outcomes: Biological, social, and health system determinants and opportunities for research. *The Oncologist, 18*, 986–993.

Wild, C. P., Scalbert, A., & Herceg, Z. (2013). Measuring the exposome: A powerful basis for evaluating environmental exposures and cancer risk. *Environmental and Molecular Mutagenesis, 54*, 480–499.

Williams, D. R., Mohammed, S. A., & Shields, A. E. (2016). Understanding and effectively addressing breast cancer in African American women: Unpacking the social context. *Cancer, 122*, 2138–2149.

Williams, D., & Wednesday, R. (2001). Abstract# 32866 Racial residential segregation: A fundamental cause of racial disparities in health. In *The 129th annual meeting of APHA (October 24, 2001-9: 10 AM)*.

Wisniewski, R. E. (1976). Mortgage redlining (disinvestment): The parameters of federal, state, and municipal regulation. *U Det J Urb L, 54*, 367.

Wright, S. V. (1997). An investigation into the causes of absconding among black African breast cancer patients. *South African Medical Journal, 87*, 1540–1543.

Wu, H. C., Cohn, B. A., Cirillo, P. M., Santella, R. M., & Terry, M. B. (2020). DDT exposure during pregnancy and DNA methylation alterations in female offspring in the Child Health and Development Study. *Reproductive Toxicology, 92*, 138–147.

Wu, Y. T., Xu, Z., Zhang, K., Wu, J. S., Li, X., Arshad, B., Li, Y. C., Wang, Z. L., Li, H. Y., Wu, K. N., & Kong, L. Q. (2018). Efficacy and cardiac safety of the concurrent use of trastuzumab and anthracycline-based neoadjuvant chemotherapy for HER2-positive breast cancer: A systematic review and meta-analysis. *Therapeutics and Clinical Risk Management, 14*, 1789–1797.

Xu, P., Yang, M., Liu, Y., Li, Y. P., Zhang, H., & Shao, G. R. (2020). Breast non-mass-like lesions on contrast-enhanced ultrasonography: Feature analysis, breast image reporting, and data system classification assessment. *World Journal of Clinical Cases, 8*, 700–712.

Yaffe, M. J., Mittmann, N., Alagoz, O., Trentham-Dietz, A., Tosteson, A. N., & Stout, N. K. (2018). The effect of mammography screening regimen on incidence-based breast cancer mortality. *Journal of Medical Screening, 25*, 197–204.

Yaghjyan, L., Mahoney, M. C., Succop, P., Wones, R., Buckholz, J., & Pinney, S. M. (2012). Relationship between breast cancer risk factors and mammographic breast density in the Fernald Community Cohort. *British Journal of Cancer, 106*, 996–1003.

Yedjou, C. G., Sims, J. N., Miele, L., Noubissi, F., Lowe, L., Fonseca, D. D., Alo, R. A., Payton, M., & Tchounwou, P. B. (2019). Health and racial disparity in breast cancer. *Advances in Experimental Medicine and Biology, 1152*, 31–49.

Yoshida, R. (2021). Hereditary breast and ovarian cancer (HBOC): Review of its molecular characteristics, screening, treatment, and prognosis. *Breast Cancer, 28*, 1167–1180.

Youk, J. H., & Kim, E. K. (2010). Supplementary screening sonography in mammographically dense breast: Pros and cons. *Korean Journal of Radiology, 11*, 589–593.

Yu, J., Loh, X. J., Luo, Y., Ge, S., Fan, X., & Ruan, J. (2020). Insights into the epigenetic effects of nanomaterials on cells. *Biomaterials Science, 8*, 763–775.

Zenou, Y., & Boccard, N. (2000). Racial discrimination and redlining in cities. *Journal of Urban Economics, 48*, 260–285.

Zhubi, A., Cook, E. H., Guidotti, A., & Grayson, D. R. (2014). Epigenetic mechanisms in autism spectrum disorder. *International Review of Neurobiology, 115*, 203–244.

Advancing Beyond Breast Cancer Resistance: A Glimmer of Hope

Zodwa Dlamini, Rodney Hull, Richard Khanyile, Thulo Molefi, Zukile Mbita, and Alexandre Kokoua

Abstract This comprehensive exploration delves into the intricate landscape of breast cancer treatment resistance, offering insights into mechanisms and innovative strategies. Advances in precision medicine, artificial intelligence, immunotherapy, splicing alterations, gut microbiota, viral onco-resistance, panomics, druggable molecular aberrations, combination therapies, natural products, and nanotechnology are spotlighted as potential solutions. Additionally, the critical need to address disparities and cultural stigmas in breast cancer care is emphasized. The narrative calls for continued collaboration, research, and integration of diverse approaches to pave the way for a future where breast cancer is effectively managed and conquered.

Keywords Breast cancer · Treatment resistance · Precision medicine · Artificial intelligence · Immunotherapy · Splicing alterations · Gut microbiota · Viral onco-resistance · Panomics · Combination therapies

Z. Dlamini (✉) · R. Hull
SAMRC Precision Oncology Research Unit (PORU), DSI/NRF SARChI Chair in Precision Oncology and Cancer Prevention (POCP), Pan African Cancer Research Institute (PACRI), University of Pretoria, Pretoria, South Africa
e-mail: zodwa.dlamini@up.ac.za; rodney.hull@up.ac.za

R. Khanyile · T. Molefi
SAMRC Precision Oncology Research Unit (PORU), DSI/NRF SARChI Chair in Precision Oncology and Cancer Prevention (POCP), Pan African Cancer Research Institute (PACRI), University of Pretoria, Pretoria, South Africa

Department of Medical Oncology, Faculty of Health Sciences, Steve Biko Academic Hospital, University of Pretoria, Pretoria, South Africa
e-mail: richard.khanyile@up.ac.za; thulo.molefi@up.ac.za

Z. Mbita
Department of Biochemistry, Microbiology and Biotechnology, School of Molecular and Life Sciences, University of Limpopo, Polokwane, South Africa
e-mail: Zukile.Mbita@ul.ac.za

A. Kokoua
Laboratory of Anatomy, Experimental Surgery and Biomechanics (LANCEB), University of Félix Houphouët-Boigny, Abidjan, Côte d'Ivoire

Z. Dlamini (ed.), *Overcoming Breast Cancer Therapy Resistance*,
https://doi.org/10.1007/978-3-031-52860-6_16

Introduction

The journey through this comprehensive exploration of breast cancer treatment resistance has been both enlightening and challenging. We have traversed the intricate landscape of breast cancer, dissecting the mechanisms behind treatment resistance and delving into innovative strategies that hold the promise of changing the course of this disease (Fig. 1). As we conclude this journey, we are presented with a vision of hope—a future where breast cancer is no longer synonymous with despair, but rather a condition that can be effectively managed and even conquered.

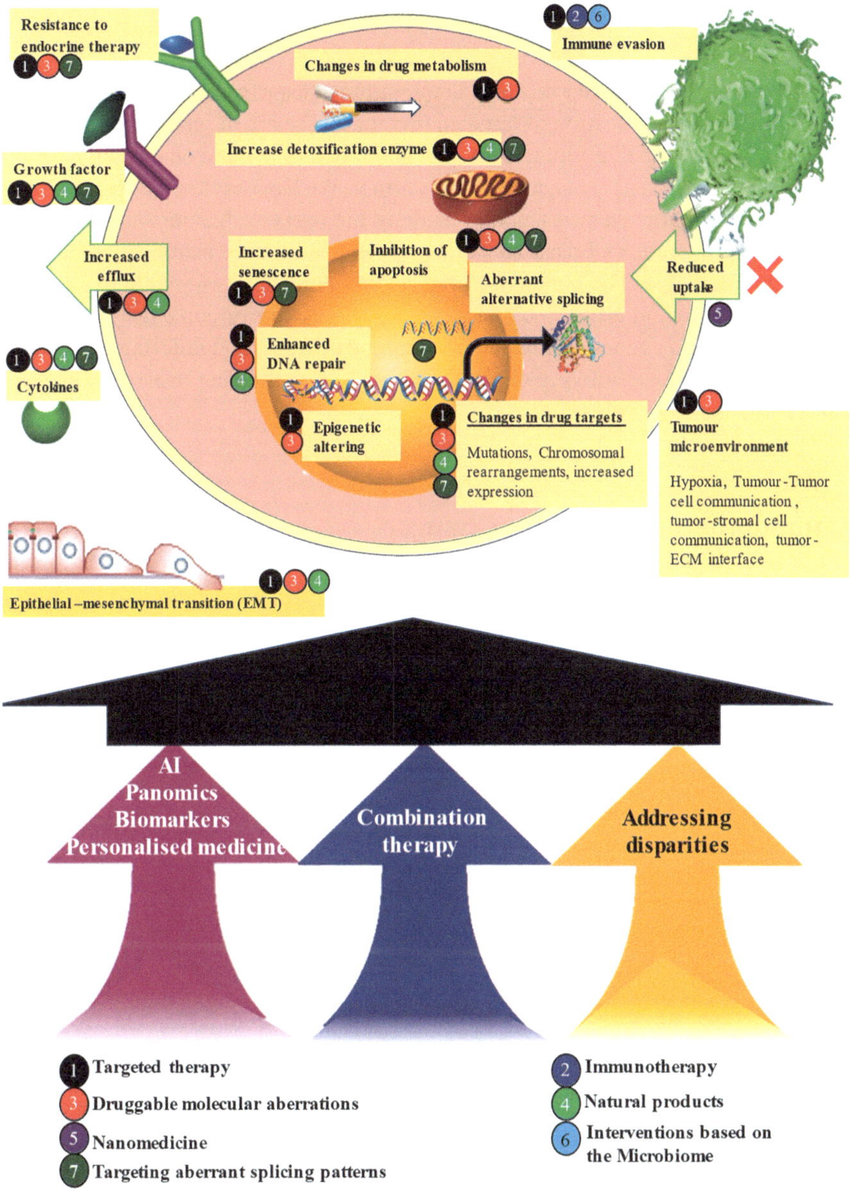

Fig. 1 Mechanisms to overcome treatment resistance in breast cancer. The three large arrows reflect the technologies and advancements that form the basis of new treatment options, the use of combination therapies as the first-line strategy to overcome resistance, and the need to overcome disparities in breast cancer treatment, diagnosis, and screening in different populations based on socioeconomic status, country of origin, ethnicity, and culture. The mechanisms of resistance are represented in the diagram of the cell with the various approaches to overcome each mechanism of resistance represented as numbers in the colored circles

The Evolution of Targeted Therapies

One of the most significant advancements in breast cancer treatment has been the development and application of targeted therapies. The era of one-size-fits-all treatments is gradually being replaced by precision medicine that considers the unique molecular characteristics of each patient's tumor. We have explored how the combination of stress-targeted drugs, comprehensive biomarker screening, and the molecular characterization of breast cancer subtypes has already begun to reshape the treatment landscape. The potential of precision medicine lies not only in its ability to improve treatment efficacy but also in its capacity to overcome drug resistance. By identifying key genes, unraveling signaling pathways, and tailoring therapies to the individual, we are moving closer to the goal of eradicating resistance in breast cancer treatment.

Immunotherapy: A Game Changer

Immunotherapy has ushered in a new era in oncology, particularly in the treatment of breast cancer. Mono- and combination therapies have shown promising clinical outcomes, offering renewed hope for patients with advanced disease. However, challenges such as immune-related adverse events, low response rates, and resistance continue to pose obstacles. To unlock the full potential of immunotherapy, research efforts must focus on better characterizing the breast cancer tumor microenvironment (TME) and identifying predictive markers for therapy response or resistance. Additionally, expanding clinical trials to include a more diverse patient population, including those from lower socioeconomic groups, is essential to ensure that the benefits of immunotherapy reach all patients.

Unraveling the Role of Splicing Alterations

Splicing alterations have emerged as a key player in breast cancer development and resistance to treatment. While targeting these alterations holds promise for therapeutic development, the complexity of mRNA splicing in normal cellular function presents challenges. Specific, non-toxic inhibitors of splicing factors and small molecule inhibitors are needed to harness the therapeutic potential of splicing alterations fully. Advancements in next-generation sequencing and the use of splice-switching oligonucleotides offer hope for more precise and effective treatments that minimize non-specific toxic effects. The journey to harnessing the power of splicing alterations may be complex, but it is a path worth pursuing for the potential it holds in overcoming resistance.

The Viral Onco-Resistance Challenge

Viruses have been identified as potential contributors to treatment resistance in breast cancer. Viral oncoproteins can manipulate cellular drug transporters, signaling pathways, and cell death responses, thus promoting resistance to chemotherapy. While current knowledge is based on in vitro studies, translating these findings into clinical practice requires further research. Innovative approaches, such as oncolytic virotherapy, which combines different oncolytic viruses to target distinct pathways, represent a promising avenue to combat viral onco-resistance. Continued investigation in real patient settings will be essential to validate these findings and unlock the potential of virotherapy in breast cancer treatment.

Natural Products: A New Frontier

Natural products have entered the arena as a potential solution to breast cancer treatment resistance. Compounds such as curcumin have shown their ability to sensitize drug-resistant breast cancer cells to chemotherapy, offering new possibilities for combination therapies. Biochemistry and molecular biology experts play a crucial role in customizing treatment plans that leverage natural products to enhance patient outcomes. Ongoing research and analysis in this field hold the promise of transforming breast cancer treatments, providing patients worldwide with more effective and personalized options.

The Role of Artificial Intelligence in Personalized Medicine

In tandem with precision medicine, artificial intelligence (AI) has emerged as a powerful tool in the fight against breast cancer resistance. AI-powered models and tools have demonstrated their ability to revolutionize early detection, drug discovery, and prediction of drug resistance. Through the integration of multi-omics data, clinical biomarkers, and bioinformatics, AI enables us to make more informed decisions regarding treatment options.

The potential benefits of AI in healthcare are vast. It not only enhances medical decision-making but also helps prevent treatment side effects, optimizes therapy for better patient outcomes, and reduces the cost of healthcare. However, the full integration of AI into clinical practice remains a work in progress, requiring increased funding, infrastructure, and a multidisciplinary approach to harness its transformative capacity fully.

The Promise of Panomics in Precision Medicine

Precision medicine, driven by molecular profiling technologies, has made significant strides in improving breast cancer diagnosis and prognosis. The integration of multi-omics tumor characterization, dynamic monitoring through liquid biopsies, and AI-guided annotation holds immense potential. Furthermore, enrolling patients in innovative clinical trials that test molecular profile-drug matches and drug-assignment algorithms can further advance precision cancer medicine. The future of precision medicine extends beyond genomics, encompassing education, engagement of end users, access to genotype-drug matching through innovative trial designs, and global data sharing to enhance our collective knowledge. Embracing a multi-omic approach and leveraging emerging technologies such as liquid biopsy and organoid studies will provide deeper insights into resistance mechanisms and potential novel combinations.

The Gut Microbiota Connection

The gut microbiota's influence on breast cancer development and response to treatment is a burgeoning area of research. Dysbiosis in the gut microbiota can lead to resistance to standard treatments, even in early-stage breast cancer. Addressing this issue involves restoring eubiosis through lifestyle interventions, probiotics, fecal transplantation, and bariatric surgery. Incorporating gut microbiota manipulation as an adjuvant therapy, especially for aggressive molecular subtypes and recurrent breast cancer, offers a promising avenue for improving treatment outcomes. As we move forward, further research into the intricate relationship between the gut microbiota and breast cancer will be crucial.

The Promise of Druggable Molecular Aberrations

The landscape of druggable tumor-specific molecular aberrations has expanded significantly, offering a survival benefit in several cancer types. Molecular pathology has become fundamental in guiding tumor diagnosis, prognosis, and therapeutic decisions. However, challenges remain in interpreting and translating comprehensive genomic data into clinical practice. The future of breast cancer treatment lies in a molecular-based personalized approach. Achieving this requires a deep understanding of molecular biology, multi-omic integration, and translational studies using innovative techniques. Research into clonal pressure and tumor heterogeneity can uncover resistance mechanisms, paving the way for novel combinations and optimized therapeutic strategies.

Combination Therapies: A Multifaceted Approach

Combination therapies have emerged as a cornerstone of breast cancer treatment, offering the potential to overcome resistance and improve patient outcomes. From immunotherapy to gene therapy and nanotechnology-driven drug delivery systems, combination approaches aim to target critical pathways in synergy. However, the challenge lies in optimizing drug-to-drug interactions, reducing toxicity, and maximizing therapeutic synergy. As we continue to explore novel combinations and refine existing regimens, the goal is to offer patients more effective and personalized treatment options that conquer resistance, recurrence, and relapse.

Nanotechnology and Drug Delivery

Nanotechnology-driven drug delivery systems offer precise control over drug pharmacokinetics and biodistribution. These systems have the potential to minimize resistance by ensuring targeted drug delivery to cancer cells, reducing drug doses, and minimizing side effects. As we continue to refine and expand the application of nanocarriers, we move closer to a future where resistance is a challenge of the past.

Addressing Disparities and Cultural Stigmas

Breast cancer disparities and cultural stigmas continue to impact healthcare access and outcomes. To address these issues comprehensively, we must integrate scientific and non-scientific factors into awareness, education, and intervention efforts. Collaboration with communities and addressing structural and socioeconomic barriers is essential to ensure equitable access to effective treatments.

Future Directions and Clinical Trials

As we look ahead, clinical trials will play a pivotal role in testing and refining emerging therapies. These trials will encompass a wide range of strategies, from precision medicine and immunotherapy to gene therapy and combination approaches. They will serve as the proving ground for innovations that can ultimately overcome resistance and transform breast cancer treatment. In conclusion, the path to overcoming breast cancer treatment resistance is complex and multifaceted. It requires a relentless commitment to research, innovation, and collaboration. As we move forward, we must harness the power of precision medicine, artificial intelligence, immunotherapy, splicing alterations, gut microbiota, viral onco-resistance, panomics, druggable molecular aberrations, combination therapies, natural products, nanotechnology, and cultural sensitivity. By embracing these diverse approaches and continuing to push the boundaries of breast cancer research, we can forge a future where resistance is conquered, and breast cancer becomes a disease with manageable outcomes. The journey is far from over, but together, we can pave the way for a brighter future in the battle against breast cancer treatment resistance.

Printed by Printforce, the Netherlands